The

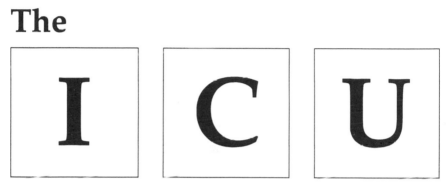

Book

PAUL L. MARINO, MD, PhD, FCCM

Clinical Associate Professor of Medicine and Surgery
University of Pennsylvania School of Medicine

Director, Critical Care Academic Program
Department of Surgery
Presbyterian Medical Center
Philadelphia, PA

Illustrations by Patricia R. Metzger
Photography by John Greim

The

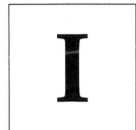 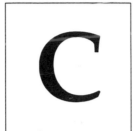 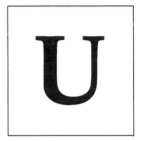

Book

 LEA & FEBIGER
Philadelphia
London

Lea & Febiger
200 Chester Field Parkway
Malvern, Pennsylvania 19355-9725
U.S.A.
(610) 251-2230

Library of Congress Cataloging-in-Publication Data

Marino, Paul L.
    The ICU book/Paul L. Marino.
      p. cm.
    ISBN 0-8121-1306-3
    1. Critical care medicine. I. Title.
    [DNLM; 1. Critical Care. 2. Intensive Care Units. WX 218
M3395i]
RC86.7.M369   1991
616'.028—dc20
DNLM/DLC
for Library of Congress   90-5622
                                                      CIP

PRINTED IN THE UNITED STATES OF AMERICA

Print number: 10 9

dedication

To the memory of Thomas Wade Lamb, MD, my mentor and my friend, who wore the heavy cloak of genius.

And to Daniel Joseph Marino, my two-year-old son, who has yet to feel the weight of his garments.

"Man is a mystery. It must be solved,
and if you spend all your life trying to solve it,
you must not say the time was wasted.
I have chosen to occupy myself with this mystery,
for I wish to be a man."

Fyodor Doestoevsky
August 16, 1839

preface

In recent years, the trend has been away from a unified approach to critical illness, as the specialty of critical care becomes a hyphenated attachment for other specialties to use as a territorial signpost. The landlord system has created a disorganized array of intensive care units (10 different varieties at last count), each acting with little communion. However, the daily concerns in each intensive care unit are remarkably similar because serious illness has no landlord. The purpose of THE ICU BOOK is to present this common ground in critical care and to focus on the fundamental principles of critical illness rather than the specific interests of each intensive care unit. As the title indicates, this is a "generic" text for all intensive care units, regardless of the name on the door.

The present text differs from others in the field in that it is neither panoramic in scope nor overly indulgent in any one area. Much of the information originates from a decade of practice in intensive care units, the last three years in both a Medical ICU and a Surgical ICU. Daily rounds with both surgical and medical housestaff have provided the foundation for the concept of generic critical care that is the theme of this book.

As indicated in the chapter headings, this text is problem-oriented rather than disease-oriented, and each problem is presented through the eyes of the ICU physician. Instead of a chapter on GI bleeding, there is a chapter on the principles of volume resuscitation and two others on resuscitation fluids. This mimics the actual role of the ICU physician in GI bleeding, which is to manage the hemorrhage. The other features of the problem such as locating the bleeding site, are the tasks of other specialists. This is how the ICU operates and this is the specialty of critical care. Highly specialized topics such as burns, head trauma, and obstetric emergencies are not covered in this text. These are distinct subspecialties with their own texts and their own experts, and devoting a few pages to each would merely complete an outline rather than instruct.

The emphasis on fundamentals in THE ICU BOOK is meant not only as a foundation for patient care but also to develop a strong base in clinical problem solving for any area of medicine. There is a tendency to rush past the basics in the stampede to finish formal training, and this leads to empiricism and irrational practice habits. Why a fever should or should not be treated, or whether a blood pressure cuff provides accurate readings, are questions that must be dissected carefully in the early stages of training, to develop the reasoning skills needed to be effective in clinical problem solving. The inquisitive stare must replace the knee-jerk approach to clinical problems if medicine is to advance. THE ICU BOOK helps to develop this stare.

Wisely or not, the use of a single author was guided by the desire to present a uniform view. Much of the information is accompanied by published works listed at the end of each chapter and anecdotal tales are held to a minimum. Within an endeavor such as this, several short-comings are inevitable, some omissions are likely and bias may occasionally replace sound judgment. The hope is that these deficiencies are few.

acknowledgments

Acknowledgments are few but deserving. First to Carroll Cann, Executive Editor at Lea & Febiger, whom I sought out to publish this work because he is without equal at his craft. Also to Kimberly LoDico, who edited the manuscript with an uncanny sense of the peculiar relationship that grows between the writer and the written. And to Thomas Colaiezzi, who expertly guided me through the production concerns and took the time to educate as well as to inform. And finally to Joe Marabito, whose kind advice many years ago culminates in this work. As for the staff at Lea & Febiger, they provided a view of what a publishing house should be like. They are professionals and it shows.

The artwork and photography in this book are all original works. The illustrations are from the pen of Patricia R. Metzger, who has a sense of perfection that marks only the gifted. This effort bears her personal mark, as I hoped it would. The photographs are from the camera of John M. Greim, whose abilities are far beyond the task he was given, but who is incapable of delivering anything less than his special skills.

Portions of the text were reviewed by Rhonda Albright, R.N., whose grammatical sense was a gift I sorely needed. Several problem chapters were refined thanks to the wisdom and encyclopedic knowledge of Dr. Kenneth Sutin. Finally, the chapters on nutrition were reviewed by Dr. Rolando Rolandelli, who provided an insight that was lacking.

Over the past 20 months, the housestaff in the Departments of Medicine and Surgery at The Graduate Hospital have worked extra hours in the intensive care units with little complaint and no reward, to allow me the time to write this book. They kept the fires burning, and kept my wheels greased when they started to creak. What is in my heart about these people can never be placed on paper, nor told in words. Without them this work would not have seen sunlight, and I hope only that the result justifies their sacrifices and their faith.

contents

SECTION XI
NUTRITION AND METABOLISM

SECTION XII
INFECTIOUS DISEASE

APPENDICES

REFERENCE TABLES

PHARMACOTHERAPY

RESUSCITATION

section 1
CRITICAL CARE PHYSIOLOGY

In science, you don't have to be polite, you only have to be right.
Max Perutz

1

CARDIAC PERFORMANCE

One of the hallmarks of serious illness is the direct link between cardiac performance and patient performance; that is, as the heart fails, the patient fails. Therefore, the forces that influence the stroke output of the heart also influence patient outcome. This chapter will review these forces and how they interact under normal conditions and in various stages of heart failure.[1-4] Most of the terms and concepts in this chapter are old friends from the physiology classroom, but now you can take them to the bedside.

MUSCLE MECHANICS

Because the heart is a muscle, the mechanical behavior of a muscle fiber can be used to describe the mechanical performance of the heart. The model used here is a single muscle fiber suspended from a rigid strut, as shown in Figure 1–1 (A–C).

1. If a weight (P) is attached to the free end of the muscle (M), the muscle will be stretched to a new resting length. The force that stretches the muscle prior to contraction is called the **Preload**.

2. The length that the muscle stretches when the preload is added is determined by the "elasticity" of the muscle. Elasticity is defined as the tendency of an object to return to its original shape when deformed. Therefore, the more elastic the muscle, the less it will be stretched by the preload. The traditional term for describing the elastic properties of muscle is **compliance**, which is the reciprocal of elastance.

3. If a clamp (C) is placed on the muscle, a second weight (A) can be attached to the preload weight without stretching the muscle further. If the muscle is stimulated with an electrical impulse and the clamp is removed, the muscle will begin to contract and lift both weights. The

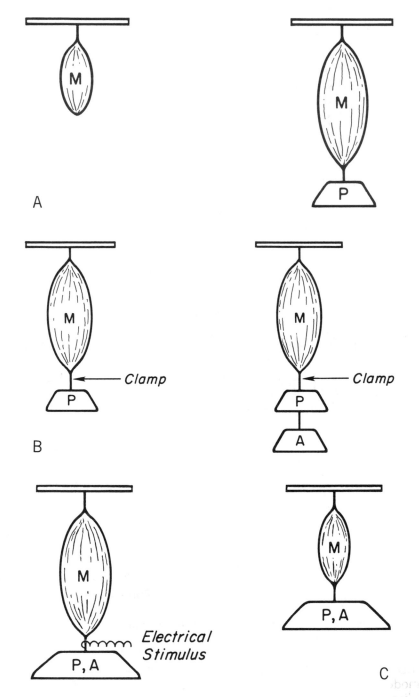

FIG. 1–1. (a) Muscle fiber (M) suspended from a rigid strut and stretched by preload weight (P). (b) Weight A added after muscle length is fixed with a clamp. Total weight to be moved by muscle contraction = weights P and A. (c)

TABLE 1–1. DETERMINANTS OF CARDIAC PERFORMANCE	
Preload	— The load that stretches the resting muscle to a new length
Afterload	— The load that must be moved during muscle contraction
Contractility	— The velocity of muscle shortening with a constant preload and afterload
Compliance	— The length the muscle is stretched by the preload

weight that must be moved by muscle contraction is called the **afterload**. Note that afterload includes the preload.

4. The ability of the muscle to lift both weights is an index of the strength of muscle contraction and the term used to describe this force is **contractility**.

DEFINITIONS

The mechanical behavior of the muscle is therefore determined by four distinct forces, each defined in Table 1–1. These forces act on the muscle either in the resting condition or during active muscle contraction. The resting muscle is influenced by the preload that is imposed and the elastic properties (compliance) of the tissue elements. The contracting muscle is influenced by the contractile behavior of the muscle (contractility) and the load that must be moved (afterload). The intact heart behaves in the same fashion, as shown next.

PRESSURE-VOLUME CURVES

The pressure-volume curves shown in Figure 1 2 describe the mechanical behavior of the left ventricle and the forces that influence this behavior.

The enclosed loop in the graph describes the events of one cardiac cycle.

THE CARDIAC CYCLE

1. The ventricle begins to fill at point A, when the mitral valve opens and blood rushes in from the left atrium. The volume in the ventricle increases progressively (along the horizontal axis) until the pressure in the chamber exceeds left atrial pressure and the mitral valve closes (point B). The volume in the ventricle at this point is the end-diastolic volume (EDV). This volume is analogous to the preload weight in the muscle model because it will stretch the (ventricular) muscle to a new resting (diastolic) length. In other words: **End-diastolic volume is equivalent to Preload.**

2. At point B, the ventricle begins to contract while both aortic and mitral valves are closed (isovolumic contraction). The chamber pressure

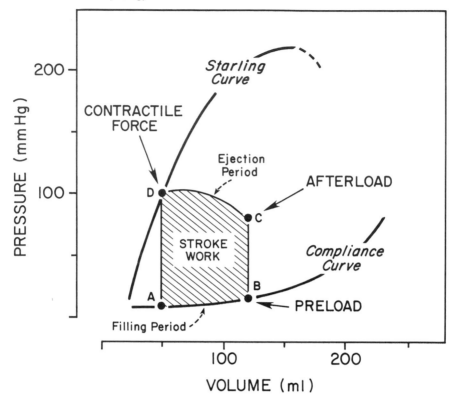

FIG. 1–2. Pressure-volume curves for the intact ventricle.

quickly rises until it exceeds the pressure in the aorta and forces the aortic valve open (point C). The pressure at this point is analogous to the afterload weight in the muscle model because it is imposed on the ventricle after the onset of contraction (systole), and is a force that must be overcome before the ventricle can eject the stroke volume. Therefore: **Aortic pressure is equivalent to Afterload.** (Afterload actually involves more than the aortic pressure, as will be discussed later.)

3. Once the aortic valve opens, the stroke volume is ejected into the aorta along the horizontal axis from point C to point D. When the pressure in the ventricle falls below the aortic pressure, the aortic valve will close at point D. The contractile force of the ventricle determines the volume of blood ejected along the horizontal axis at a given preload and afterload. In other words, the pressure at point D will be a function of contractility when point B (preload) and point C (afterload) are constant. Stated another way: **The systolic pressure is equivalent to contractility** when the load conditions are constant.

When the aortic valve closes at point D, the ventricular chamber pressure falls precipitously (isovolumic relaxation) until the mitral valve opens again at point A and the cycle begins again.

4. The area within the pressure-volume loop defines the work performed by the ventricle during one cardiac cycle (work is defined as the

force needed to move an object a defined distance). Any process that increases this area (i.e., an increase in preload, afterload, or contractility) will increase the "stroke work" of the heart. Stroke work is an important concept because work determines the energy expenditure (oxygen consumption) of the heart. This is developed further in Chapter 14.

THE STARLING CURVE

The output of the normal heart is influenced primarily by the volume of blood in the ventricles at the end of diastole. This was first described in a frog heart preparation by Otto Frank in 1885. Ernest Starling extended this observation to the mammalian heart in 1914 and received much of the credit for the discovery. The Starling curve (or Frank-Starling curve) is indicated in Figure 1–2 as the one relating end-diastolic volume to systolic pressure. Note the steep ascending portion of the curve.

> The steep slope of the Starling curve indicates the importance of preload (volume) for augmenting the output of the normal heart.

This is one of the fundamental truths in cardiovascular physiology, but is unexplained. The "sliding filament" hypothesis for muscle contraction has been suggested as a mechanism, but there is little to support this explanation at present.[2]

The Descending Limb

As the end-diastolic volume becomes excessive, the systolic pressure can begin to fall, creating a descending limb in the Starling curve. This phenomenon was originally ascribed to overstretch of the cardiac muscle fibers, which would pull the contractile filaments past each other and reduce the contact needed to maintain contractile force. However, the original description of the descent in the Starling curve may have been produced by an increase in afterload and not an increase in end-diastolic fiber length.[2] If afterload is held constant, the end-diastolic pressure must be in excess of 60 mmHg to decrease ventricular stroke output.[2] Because these pressures are rarely encountered in the clinical setting, the significance of the descending limb in the Starling curve is now in question.[5]

> There is no evidence for a descending limb in the Starling curve in clinical settings. This means that hypervolemia should not decrease cardiac output and diuresis should not augment cardiac output.

This is an important point to emphasize because of the present preoccupation with diuretic therapy for heart failure. This topic is presented in more detail in Chapter 14.

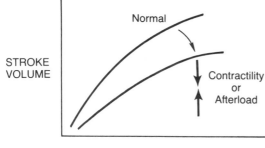

FIG. 1–3. Ventricular function curves.

THE VENTRICULAR FUNCTION CURVE

The clinical counterpart of the Starling curve is the Ventricular Function Curve shown in Figure 1–3. Note that stroke volume replaces systolic pressure and end-diastolic pressure (EDP) replaces end-diastolic volume (EDV). Both measurements can be obtained at the bedside using pulmonary artery catheters (see Chapter 9).

The slope of the ventricular function curve is determined by the contractile state of the myocardium **and** by the afterload.[1-3,6] As shown in Figure 1–3, a decrease in contractility or an increase in afterload will decrease the slope of the curve. The influence of afterload is important to remember because it means that **ventricular function curves are not reliable for evaluating the contractile state of the myocardium**, as is sometimes assumed.[6]

COMPLIANCE CURVES

The ability of the ventricle to fill during diastole can be determined by the relationship between pressure and volume at the end of diastole (EDP and EDV). This is illustrated in Figure 1–4. The slope of the diastolic pressure-volume curves is a measure of the compliance of the ventricle.[7]

$$\text{Ventricular Compliance} = \Delta\ EDV \div \Delta\ EDP$$

As shown in the figure, a decrease in compliance will shift the curve down and to the right, so that the EDP is higher at any given EDV. An increase in compliance would produce the opposite effect.

Preload is the stretch imposed on the resting muscle and should be equivalent to diastolic volume rather than diastolic pressure. However, EDV cannot be measured routinely at the bedside, and EDP is the usual clinical measure of preload (see Chapter 9). The problem with EDP as a measure of preload is that it is influenced by changes in compliance.[7] In the example shown in Figure 1–4, the EDP could be elevated while the EDV (preload) is actually reduced. In other words, the EDP will overestimate preload when ventricular compliance is reduced.

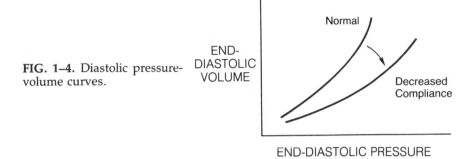

FIG. 1–4. Diastolic pressure-volume curves.

End-diastolic pressure is a reliable index of preload only when the compliance of the ventricle is normal or unchanged.

There are several processes in critically ill patients that can decrease the compliance of the ventricles (e.g., positive-pressure ventilation) and this limits the value of the EDP as an index of preload. This topic is discussed further in Chapter 14.

AFTERLOAD

Afterload was defined earlier as the force that impedes or opposes ventricular contraction. This force is equivalent to the tension developed across the wall of the ventricle during systole. The components of transmural wall tension are shown in Figure 1–5.

According to the LaPlace Law ($T = Pr$), the transmural wall tension is a function of the systolic pressure and the chamber radius. The systolic pressure is determined by the outflow impedance in the aorta, while the chamber size is a function of the EDV (i.e., preload). As shown in the original muscle model, **preload is part of the afterload**, or the total load that must be moved by the ventricle.

VASCULAR RESISTANCE

Impedance is a concept applied to pulsatile flow and has two components: (1) a compliance factor that opposes the rate of change in flow, and (2) a resistance factor that opposes the mean flowrate.[6] There is no routine clinical measure for arterial compliance, so the arterial resistance is used as the clinical measure of afterload. The arterial resistance is measured as the difference between inflow (mean arterial) pressure and outflow (venous) pressure, divided by the flowrate (i.e., the cardiac output). The pulmonary vascular resistance (PVR) and the systemic vascular resistance (SVR) are determined as follows:

$$PVR = PAP - LAP / CO$$

$$SVR = SAP - RAP / CO$$

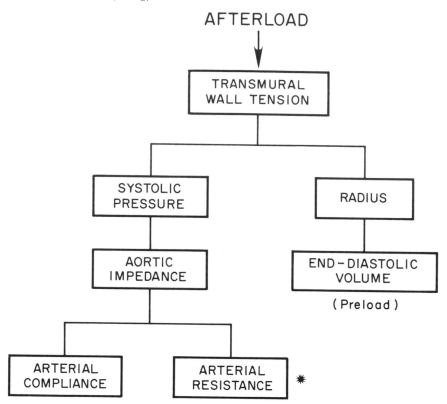

FIG. 1–5. The components of afterload.

where CO: cardiac output, PAP: mean pulmonary artery pressure, LAP: left atrial pressure, SAP: mean systemic arterial pressure, and RAP: right atrial pressure.

These equations are similar to the equation used to describe the resistance to the flow of electric current (Ohm's Law). The behavior of an electrical resistor may be far removed from the impedance to flow in a vascular circuit that is exposed to pulsatile flow and contains capacitive elements (the veins).

TRANSMURAL FORCES

The true afterload is a transmural force and, therefore, has a component that is not a part of the vascular system; the surrounding pleural pressure. A negative pleural pressure will add to the afterload because it increases transmural pressure at a given intracavitary pressure, while a positive pleural pressure will have the opposite effect.[8] This explains why systolic blood pressure (stroke volume) decreases during a negative-pressure (spontaneous) inspiration. The influence of intrapleural pressure on cardiac performance is discussed in more detail in Chapter 27.

In summary, there are several problems associated with vascular re-

FIG. 1–6. Effects of cardiac output on end-diastolic pressure EDP and systemic vascular resistance (SVR).

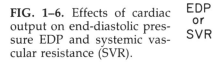
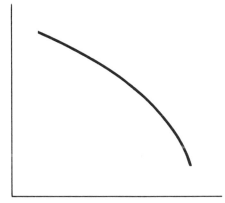

EDP
or
SVR

CARDIAC OUTPUT

sistance as an index of afterload, and the evidence from experimental studies indicates that vascular resistance is unreliable as a measure of ventricular afterload.[9] The vascular resistance measurement can be valuable when used as a determinant of blood pressure. That is, mean arterial pressure is the product of flow (cardiac output) and vascular resistance, so the vascular resistance measurement can help to sort out the specific hemodynamic problem in hypotension. The use of systemic vascular resistance in the diagnosis and management of clinical shock states is covered in more detail in Chapter 12.

THE HEMODYNAMICS OF HEART FAILURE

The circulatory adjustments that occur in heart failure can be described by making cardiac output the independent variable, while EDP and vascular resistance become the dependent variables. This is shown in Figure 1–6. As cardiac output is decreased, both EDP and SVR will increase.[6,10,11] This explains the clinical features of heart failure:

Increased EDP = Venous Congestion and Edema

Increased SVR = Vasoconstriction and Hypoperfusion

These hemodynamic changes are at least partly the result of activation of the renin-angiotensin-aldosterone (RAA) system.[12] The renin release in heart failure is the result of a reduction in renal perfusion pressure. The renin then forms angiotensin II, which is a potent vasoconstrictor that increases both arterial and venous resistance. Renin-mediated aldosterone release from the adrenals causes sodium retention, which leads to elevated venous pressures and edema formation.

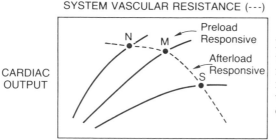

SYSTEM VASCULAR RESISTANCE (- - -)

CARDIAC OUTPUT

LEFT VENTRICULAR END-DIASTOLIC PRESSURE (—)

FIG. 1–7. Hemodynamic alterations in heart failure. N: normal cardiac function. M: mild heart failure; and S: severe heart failure. See text for explanation.

PROGRESSIVE HEART FAILURE

The hemodynamics of progressive heart failure can be described using the curves in Figure 1–7.[11] The solid curves define the relationship between preload and cardiac output (i.e., ventricular function curves) and the dashed curve defines the relationship between vascular resistance (afterload) and cardiac output. The point at which the curves intersect, therefore, defines the relationship between preload, afterload, and cardiac output at each stage of ventricular dysfunction.

1. Mild Heart Failure

When ventricular function begins to decrease, the slope of the ventricular function curve decreases, and the intersection point moves to the right along the vascular resistance curve. In early, mild heart failure, the slope of the preload curve is still steep, and the intercept point (point M) falls on the flat part of the afterload curve. In other words,

> In mild heart failure, the ventricle is preload responsive and afterload unresponsive.[11]

The ability to respond to preload in mild heart failure means that forward flow can be maintained but at a higher than normal filling pressure. This explains why the predominant symptom in mild heart failure is dyspnea.

2. Severe Heart Failure

As cardiac function decreases further, the ventricle becomes less responsive to preload (i.e., the slope of the ventricular function curve decreases) and the cardiac output begins to fall. The ventricular function curve now moves onto the steep portion of the afterload curve (Point S):

> In severe heart failure, the ventricle is preload unresponsive and afterload responsive.[11]

Both of these factors contribute to the decrease in forward flow seen in the later stages of heart failure. The afterload plays a particularly important role since the arterial vasoconstriction not only reduces cardiac output but also diminishes peripheral blood flow. The increasing importance of afterload in progressive stages of heart failure provides the basis for vasodilator therapy in heart failure. This is presented in more detail in Chapter 14.

BIBLIOGRAPHY

Berne RM, Levy MN. Cardiovascular physiology. 3rd ed. St. Louis: C.V. Mosby, 1981.
Little RC. Physiology of the heart and circulation. 3rd ed. Chicago: Year Book Medical Publishers, 1985.

REFERENCES

REVIEWS

1. Parmley WW, Talbot L. Heart as a pump. In: Berne RM ed. Handbook of physiology: The cardiovascular system. Bethesda: American Physiological Society, 1979; 429–460.
2. Braunwald E, Sonnenblick EH, Ross J Jr. Mechanisms of cardiac contraction and relaxation. In: Braunwald E. ed. Heart disease. A textbook of cardiovascular medicine. 3rd ed. Philadelphia: W.B. Saunders, 1988; 383–425.
3. Weber K, Janicki JS, Hunter WC, et al. The contractile behaviour of the heart and its functional coupling to the circulation. Prog Cardiovasc Dis 1982; 24:375–400.
4. Rothe CF. Physiology of venous return. Arch Intern Med 1986; 146:977–982.

SELECTED REFERENCES

5. Katz AM. The descending limb of the Starling curve and the failing heart. Circulation 1965; 32:871–875.
6. Nichols WW, Pepine CJ. Left ventricular afterload and aortic input impedance: Implications of pulsatile blood flow. Prog Cardiovasc Dis 1982; 24:293–306.
7. Harizi RC, Bianco JA, Alpert JS. Diastolic function of the heart in clinical cardiology. Arch Intern Med 1988; 148:99–109.
8. Robotham JL, Scharf SM. Effects of positive and negative pressure ventilation on cardiac performance. Clin Chest Med 1983; 4:161–178.
9. Lang RM, Borow KM, Neumann A, et al. Systemic vascular resistance: An unreliable index of left ventricular afterload. Circulation 1986; 74:1114–1123.
10. Zelis R, Flaim SF. Alterations in vasomotor tone in congestive heart failure. Prog Cardiovasc Dis 1982; 24:437–459.
11. Cohn JN, Franciosa JA. Vasodilator therapy of cardiac failure (first of two parts). N Engl J Med 1977; 297:27–31.
12. Dzau VJ, Colucci WS, Hollenberg NK, Williams GH. Relation of the renin-angiotensin-aldosterone system to clinical state in congestive heart failure. Circulation 1981; 63:645–651.

chapter

2

OXYGEN TRANSPORT

The first concern in any life-threatening illness is to maintain an adequate supply of oxygen to sustain oxidative metabolism. This chapter will introduce the components of the oxygen transport system and will present the mechanisms that govern the supply of oxygen to the tissues in health and in serious illness. The reference list at the end of the chapter contains several comprehensive reviews[1-6] for those who wish to pursue the subject further.

THE OXYGEN TRANSPORT VARIABLES

The components of the oxygen transport system are shown in Figure 2–1. The four factors that are most important are the oxygen content of whole blood, the oxygen delivery, the oxygen uptake, and the fractional extraction of oxygen from capillary blood. The following is a brief description of each component.

OXYGEN CONTENT

The oxygen in blood is either bound to hemoglobin or dissolved in plasma. The sum of both fractions is called the oxygen content. The content of oxygen in arterial blood (CaO_2) is calculated below using a hemoglobin (Hb) of 14 g/dL, arterial O_2 saturation (SaO_2) of 98%, and arterial PO_2 (PaO_2) of 100 mmHg.

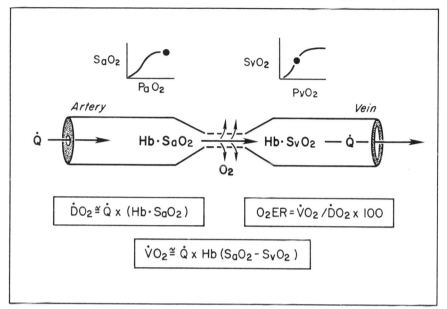

FIG. 2–1. The components of the oxygen transport circuit. See text for terms and abbreviations.

$$CaO_2 = (1.3 \times Hb \times SaO_2) + (0.003 \times PaO_2)$$

$$Normal \ CaO_2 = (1.3 \times 14 \times .98) + (0.003 \times 100)$$

$$= 18.1 \ ml/100 \ ml \ (or \ vol\%)$$

The first term in the equation $(1.3 \times Hb \times SaO_2)$ is the oxygen carried by hemoglobin. This term states that one gram of hemoglobin binds 1.3 ml oxygen when completely saturated ($SaO_2 = 100\%$). The second term $(0.003 \times PaO_2)$ defines the amount of oxygen dissolved in plasma, which is 0.003 ml/mmHg.

Note that the PaO_2 contributes little to the oxygen content. Despite its popularity, **the PaO_2 is not an important measure of arterial oxygenation.** The SaO_2 is the more important blood gas variable for assessing the oxygenation of arterial blood while the PaO_2 should be reserved for evaluating the efficiency of gas exchange in the lungs.

OXYGEN DELIVERY

The oxygen delivery ($\dot{D}O_2$) is the rate of oxygen transport in arterial blood. It is defined as the product of the cardiac output ($\dot{Q}$) and the arterial oxygen content (CaO_2). The normal $\dot{D}O_2$ is determined using a

| TABLE 2–1.   OXYGEN TRANSPORT VARIABLES ||
Parameter	Normal Range
Oxygen Delivery	520–720 ml/min·m²
Oxygen Uptake	110–160 ml/min·m²
Oxygen Extraction	22–32%
Serum Lactate	0–4 mEq/L
Mixed Venous P_{O_2}	33–53 mmHg
Mixed Venous S_{O_2}	68–77%
Note that O_2 delivery and O_2 uptake are indexed to body surface area	

Ca_{O_2} = 18 vol% and a cardiac "index" of 3 L/min·m² (cardiac output indexed to body surface area).

$$\dot{D}_{O_2} = \dot{Q} \times Ca_{O_2}$$

$$= \dot{Q} \times (1.3 \times Hb \times Sa_{O_2}) \times 10$$

$$\text{Normal } \dot{D}_{O_2} = 3 \times (1.3 \times 14 \times .98) \times 10$$

$$= 540 \text{ ml/min} \cdot m^2$$

(the factor 10 converts volumes percent to ml/s). If the normal range for the cardiac index is 2.5 to 3.5 L/min · m²,[1] then the normal range for $\dot{D}_{O_2}$ is 520 to 720 ml/min · m². Table 2–1 lists the normal ranges for all the oxygen transport variables included in this chapter.

OXYGEN UPTAKE

The oxygen uptake is the final step in the oxygen transport pathway and its represents the oxygen supply for tissue metabolism. The Fick equation defines the oxygen uptake ($\dot{V}_{O_2}$) as the product of cardiac output ($\dot{Q}$) and the arteriovenous difference in oxygen content ($Ca_{O_2} - Cv_{O_2}$). The oxygen uptake is calculated below using a venous oxygen saturation (Sv_{O_2}) of 73%.

$$\dot{V}_{O_2} = \dot{Q} \times (Ca_{O_2} - Cv_{O_2})$$

$$= \dot{Q} \times (13 \times Hb) \times (Sa_{O_2} - Sv_{O_2})$$

$$\text{Normal } \dot{V}_{O_2} = 3 \times (13 \times 14) \times (.97 - .73)$$

$$= 130 \text{ ml/min} \cdot m^2$$

Note the term (13 × Hb) is separated because it is a shared component of the oxygen content equations. Using a normal range for cardiac index of 2.5 to 3.5 L/min · m², the normal range for $\dot{V}O_2$ is 110 to 160 ml/min · m² (see Table 2–1).

Oxygen Uptake and Metabolic Rate

Most tissues are unable to store oxygen (except muscle, which can store oxygen by binding it to myoglobin) and the oxygen uptake from the capillaries is considered equivalent to the metabolic consumption of oxygen. This is a reasonable assumption unless there is a defect in the ability to extract oxygen from the capillaries. When oxygen uptake is impaired, the $\dot{V}O_2$ will underestimate the rate of metabolism. This situation may be common in critically ill patients and is well described in sepsis, burns, and multiple trauma. Therefore, the reliability of the $\dot{V}O_2$ as an index of metabolic rate must be determined for each individual patient. This is explained in more detail in Chapter 12.

OXYGEN EXTRACTION RATIO

The oxygen extraction ratio (O_2ER) is the fractional uptake of oxygen from the capillary bed, and is derived as the ratio of oxygen uptake to oxygen delivery.

$$O_2ER = \dot{V}O_2/\dot{D}O_2 \times 100$$

$$\text{Normal } O_2ER = 130/540 \times 100$$

$$= 24\%$$

The rate of O_2 delivery normally exceeds the rate of O_2 uptake by a wide margin, which means that only a small fraction of the available oxygen is extracted from capillary blood under normal conditions (22 to 32%). This allows the tissues to adjust to decreases in blood flow by increasing extraction, as presented next.

THE CONTROL OF OXYGEN UPTAKE

The uptake of oxygen from the microcirculation is a set point that is maintained by adjusting the extraction ratio to match changes in oxygen delivery. The ability to adjust O_2 extraction can be impaired in serious illness and this may be the one feature that identifies an illness as a life-threatening one.

THE NORMAL RESPONSE

The normal compensatory response to a decrease in blood flow is an increase in O_2 extraction sufficient enough to keep $\dot{V}O_2$ in the normal range.[3,4] This adjustment is illustrated in the example below:

$$\dot{V}O_2 = \dot{Q} \times Hb \times 13 \times (SaO_2 - SvO_2)$$

$$\dot{Q} = 3 \text{ L/min} \cdot m^2: \dot{V}O_2 = 3 \times 14 \times 13 \times (.97 - .73)$$

$$= 110 \text{ ml/min} \cdot m^2$$

$$\dot{Q} = 1 \text{ L/min} \cdot m^2: \dot{V}O_2 = 1 \times 14 \times 13 \times (.97 - .37)$$

$$= 109 \text{ ml/min} \cdot m^2$$

The drop in cardiac index is balanced by the increased ($SaO_2 - SvO_2$) difference and $\dot{V}O_2$ remains unchanged. Note the drop in SvO_2 from 73 to 37% from the increased extraction. The association between SvO_2 and O_2ER is the basis for SvO_2 monitoring (see end of chapter).

The ability to adjust extraction when blood flow decreases is a feature of all vascular beds except the coronary circulation and the diaphragm. These capillary beds extract the maximum amount of oxygen under normal conditions so that the oxygen levels in the tissues are vulnerable to even small changes in blood flow. The flow-dependency of the coronary circulation is a well described phenomenon and it stresses the need to maintain cardiac output in patients with coronary artery disease.

THE $\dot{D}O_2$ – $\dot{V}O_2$ CURVE

The relationship between O_2 delivery and O_2 uptake for normal subjects is shown in Figure 2–2. The flat portion of the curve is the region where the O_2 extraction varies in response to changes in blood flow. The $\dot{V}O_2$ is independent of blood flow in this region of the curve. The point at which the $\dot{V}O_2$ begins to decrease corresponds to **the point where the O_2 extraction is maximal** and cannot increase further. This point **is called the critical level of oxygen delivery**[7] and it represents the threshold $\dot{D}O_2$ needed for adequate tissue oxygenation. If the $\dot{D}O_2$ falls below this threshold level, the oxygen supply will fall to subnormal levels.

The critical level of $\dot{D}O_2$ has been measured in different clinical situations. A value of 300 ml/min $\cdot$ m^2 has been reported after cardiac bypass surgery and in patients with acute respiratory failure.[7,8] However, other studies have found no consistent threshold level for $\dot{D}O_2$ in critically ill patients.[9,10] The lack of a common threshold for patients with serious illness indicates the need to monitor $\dot{D}O_2$ and $\dot{V}O_2$ on an individual basis.

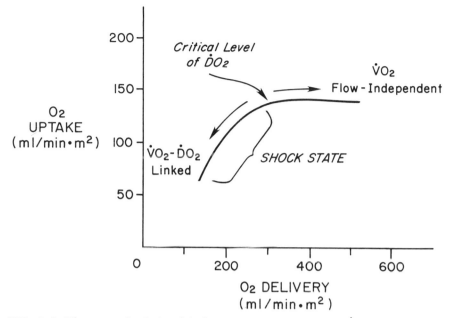

FIG. 2–2. The normal relationship between oxygen delivery ($\dot{D}_{O_2}$) and oxygen uptake ($\dot{V}_{O_2}$). See text for explanation.

FLOW DEPENDENT $\dot{V}_{O_2}$

The linear portion of the curve in Figure 2–2 is characterized by a direct link between oxygen delivery and oxygen uptake. The $\dot{V}_{O_2}$ is defined as being "flow-dependent" when this occurs.

> Oxygen uptake will become flow-dependent when oxygen extraction does not change in response to alterations in blood flow. This flow-dependence is common in serious illness.[5,6,9,10]

The linear relationship between $\dot{D}_{O_2}$ and $\dot{V}_{O_2}$ indicates a defect in oxygen extraction from the microcirculation. In critically ill patients, oxygen extraction can remain fixed, and the $\dot{V}_{O_2}$ becomes flow-dependent over a wide range of changes in $\dot{D}_{O_2}$. This is shown in Figure 15–2 for patients with septic shock. In this situation, it is imperative to maintain cardiac output to maintain oxygen supply to the tissues. The relationship between oxygen delivery and oxygen uptake is developed in the chapters in Section IV.

MIXED VENOUS OXYGEN

The relationship between cardiac output and oxygen extraction shown earlier predicts that venous oxygen levels will vary directly with changes in cardiac output. This is the rationale for the use of "mixed venous" (pulmonary artery) oxygen saturation to monitor changes in cardiac output.[12,13]

TABLE 2–2.   THE CAUSES OF LOW MIXED VENOUS OXYGEN
$$S\bar{v}O_2 \;=\; SaO_2 \;-\; (\dot{V}O_2/\dot{Q} \times Hb \times 13)$$ $$\boxed{1} \qquad\quad \boxed{2}\;\; \boxed{3} \qquad \boxed{4}$$ 1. Hypoxemia 2. Increased Metabolic Rate 3. Low Cardiac Output 4. Anemia

DETERMINANTS OF VENOUS OXYGEN

The determinants of venous oxygen are identified by rearranging the Fick equation.

$$\dot{V}O_2 \;=\; \dot{Q} \times Hb \times 13 \times (SaO_2 - S\bar{v}O_2)$$

$$S\bar{v}O_2 \;=\; SaO_2 - (\dot{V}O_2/\dot{Q} \times Hb \times 13)$$

The most prominent factor in the $S\bar{v}O_2$ equation is the ratio of oxygen uptake to cardiac output ($\dot{V}O_2/\dot{Q}$). If oxygen delivery is substituted for cardiac output, the ratio becomes the oxygen extraction ratio ($O_2ER = \dot{V}O_2/\dot{D}O_2$). This derives the inverse relationship between $S\bar{v}O_2$ and oxygen extraction. Table 2–2 lists the causes of low mixed venous oxygen using the components of the $S\bar{v}O_2$ equation.

OXIMETRY

The oxygen saturation in arterial blood is estimated from the arterial blood gas variables (PO_2, PCO_2, and pH), while the venous O_2 saturation must be measured directly. This is due to the shape of the oxyhemoglobin dissociation curve (see Figure 2–1). The arterial O_2 saturation falls on the flat part of the curve and can be estimated with little risk for error. However, the venous O_2 saturation falls on the steep portion of the curve (normal $S\bar{v}O_2$ is 68 to 77%) and can vary significantly with small errors in estimation. This is the reason that mixed venous oxygen saturation must be measured directly.

The method for measuring hemoglobin saturation with oxygen is called spectrophotometry and is based on the fact that different configurations of hemoglobin will reflect light of different wavelengths. This is applied to mixed venous blood in two ways.

1. An **in vitro method** that measures the transmission of light through a blood sample placed in a special cuvette. This is called transmission spectrophotometry and it is the traditional method for measuring $S\bar{v}O_2$.

2. An **in vivo method** that uses a pulmonary artery catheter to transmit light directly to blood flowing in the pulmonary artery.[13] The light reflected back to the catheter from the hemoglobin in the bloodstream

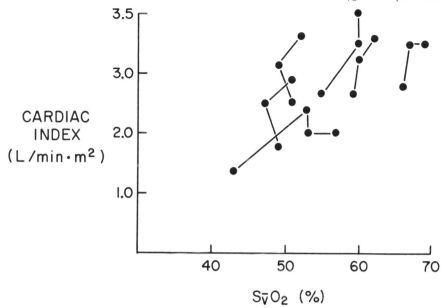

FIG. 2–3. The relationship between oxygen saturation in mixed venous (pulmonary artery) blood ($S\bar{v}O_2$) and cardiac index (CI) in patients with adult respiratory distress syndrome. See text for explanation.

is carried back along fiberoptic bundles to the proximal end of the catheter. The catheter is connected to a photodetector that measures the intensity of the reflected light beam. This method is called reflectance spectrophotometry and it provides a continuous on-line measurement of $S\bar{v}O_2$.

The benefit of the in vitro method is its reliability and the ability to detect all forms of hemoglobin (methemoglobin and carboxyhemoglobin). The value of the in vivo method is the ability to monitor $S\bar{v}O_2$ continuously at the bedside. We have been using the in vivo method for the past 3 years in postoperative cardiac surgery patients and it has proven reliable in most patients.

PITFALLS

There is a tendency to assume that all patients can respond to reduced blood flow by augmenting oxygen extraction. This creates the misconception that $S\bar{v}O_2$ monitors blood flow or cardiac output. Remember that seriously ill patients are often unable to mount this compensatory response to low blood flow. In these patients, venous oxygen levels will change little in response to changes in cardiac output.[10] The reliability of venous oxygen for monitoring changes in cardiac output in critically ill patients is shown in Figure 2–3. The patients in this study had respiratory failure from the adult respiratory distress syndrome and each line represents the measurements obtained on a single patient. As indicated, there was little correlation between the venous oxygen saturation and the cardiac index in this study group. This is typically seen in patients with clinical shock, but can also be seen in any patient who is seriously ill. Therefore, it is important to determine the relationship between cardiac output and mixed venous oxygen levels in each patient before using $S\bar{v}O_2$ or $P\bar{v}O_2$ to monitor changes in DO_2 or VO_2.

LACTIC ACID

The oxygen transport variables define the oxygen supply to the tissues but provide no information about the adequacy of this supply. That is, **a normal VO_2 is not necessarily an adequate VO_2** if the metabolic rate is excessive. When the metabolic rate exceeds the rate of oxygen supply, the tissues will switch to anaerobic metabolism and produce lactic acid. Therefore, the serum lactate concentration can be used to evaluate the balance between VO_2 and the metabolic demand for oxygen.

LACTATE KINETICS

Lactic acid is the end-product of anaerobic glycolysis but is also produced in aerobic conditions. The normal rate of lactic acid production is estimated at 1 mEq/kg per hour,[14] or 1800 mEq per day in the average 70 kg adult. Lactic acid readily crosses cell membranes and enters capillary blood. The lactate anion is cleared by the liver and used for gluconeogenesis (Cori cycle). The kidneys can clear lactate from the blood, but renal clearance is not prominent until the serum lactate levels reach 6 to 7 mEq/L.[14]

GUIDELINES

The serum lactate level can be measured in either the superior vena cava, pulmonary artery, or in peripheral arteries.[16] A lactate assay for whole blood is now available that can be performed in a matter of seconds and requires only a few microliters of blood.[14] A normal serum lactate is usually defined as 2 mEq/L or less,[14] but stressed patients in the ICU can have normal levels that reach to 4 mEq/L.[14,15] The rate of lactate clearance from the blood can help to distinguish normal from pathologic lactate production. The elimination half-life is 1 hour in normal conditions and exceeds 2 hours in pathologic processes.[16]

RELIABILITY

The major problem with serum lactate as a marker of tissue ischemia is the sensitivity and specificity of the measurement.

Sensitivity. The sensitivity of serum lactate levels is not known. However, the consensus is that the measurement is an insensitive marker for tissue ischemia. This seems reasonable, because tissues that are ischemic will have little venous effluent to contribute to the total venous pool and this will dilute the lactate emanating from the ischemic tissue. In fact, the greater the reduction in inflow to an organ (and the more the ischemia), the less the outflow will contribute to the total venous pool, and the greater the dilution of the lactate emanating from the organ. This limits the value of serum lactate as a marker of regional hypoperfusion.

Specificity. The major concern in specificity is the role of hepatic insufficiency in promoting elevated lactate levels. Liver failure alone does not seem to produce an increase in serum lactate levels.[18] However, when impaired lactate clearance is combined with increased lactate reduction (as can be seen in shock states), the liver may participate in the elevation of the serum lactate level. Hepatic clearance of lactate can be maintained until hepatic blood flow is reduced to 70% of control levels or hepatic venous P_{O_2} falls to below 24 mmHg.[19] This means that the liver may play little role in promoting lactate accumulation in low-flow states unless the venous P_{O_2} falls to low levels. The consensus at this time is that lactate accumulation in the blood reflects an increase in lactate production rather than reduced clearance.

Certain clinical disorders are associated with elevated serum lactate levels without widespread organ ischemia. These include thiamine deficiency, bacterial pneumonia, generalized seizures, respiratory alkalosis, and generalized trauma.[14-16] These disorders must be considered in any patient with an elevated serum lactate level.

SUMMARY

The serum lactate can be used to determine if the $\dot{V}_{O_2}$ is matched to the metabolic rate. An increase in serum lactate above 4 mEq/L that persists beyond a few hours is taken as evidence for tissue ischemia. However, a normal serum level probably does not rule out tissue ischemia. When inadequate tissue oxygenation is suspected but the serum lactate level is normal, serial determinations might help uncover the problem. See Chapter 12 for more information on the use of serum lactate in clinical shock syndromes.

BIBLIOGRAPHY

Snyder JV, Pinsky MR, eds. Oxygen transport in the critically ill. 2nd ed. Chicago: Year Book Medical Publishers, 1987.

Dantzger DR, ed. Cardiopulmonary critical care. Orlando: Grune & Stratton, 1986.

REFERENCES

REVIEWS

1. Shoemaker WC. Pathophysiology, monitoring, outcome prediction, and therapy of shock states. Crit Care Clin 1987; 3:307–358.

2. Shoemaker WC. Relationship of oxygen transport patterns to the pathophysiology and therapy of shock states. Intensive Care Med 1987; 13:230–243.
3. Fahey JT, Lister G. Oxygen transport in low cardiac output states. J Crit Care 1987; 2:288–305.
4. Schumacher PT, Cain SM. The concept of critical oxygen delivery. Intensive Care Med 1987; 13:223–229.
5. Rackow EC, Astiz M, Weil MH. Cellular oxygen metabolism during sepsis and shock. JAMA 1988; 259:1989–1993.
6. Dantzger D. Oxygen delivery and utilization in sepsis. Crit Care Clin 1989: 5:81–9.

CONTROL OF OXYGEN UPTAKE

7. Komatsu T, Shibutani K, Okamoto K, et al. Critical level of oxygen delivery after cardiopulmonary bypass. Crit Care Med 1987; 15:194–197.
8. Rashkin MC, Bosken C, Baughman RP. Oxygen delivery in critically ill patients. Relationship to blood lactate and survival. Chest 1985; 87:580–584.
9. Mohsenifar Z, Goldbach P, Tashkin DP, et al. Relationship between O_2 delivery and O_2 consumption in the adult respiratory distress syndrome. Chest 1983; 84:267–272.
10. Danek SJ, Lynch JP, Weg J, Dantzger DR. The dependence of oxygen uptake on oxygen delivery in the adult respiratory distress syndrome. Am Rev Respir Dis 1980; 122:387–395.
11. Astiz ME, Rackow EC, Kaufman B, et al. Relationship of oxygen delivery and mixed venous oxygenation to lactic acidosis in patients with sepsis and acute myocardial infarction. Crit Care Med 1988; 16:655–662.

MIXED VENOUS OXYGEN

12. Kandel G, Aberman A. Mixed venous oxygen saturation. Its role in the assessment of the critically ill. Arch Intern Med 1983; 143:1400–1402.
13. Birman H, Haq A, Hew E, Aberman A. Continuous monitoring of mixed venous oxygen saturation in hemodynamically unstable patients. Chest 1984; 86:753–756.

LACTIC ACID

14. Mizock BA. Lactic acidosis. Disease-A-Month 1989; 5:235–300.
15. Haljamae H. Lactate metabolism. Intensive Care World 1987; 4:118–121.
16. Weil MH, Michaels S, Rackow E. Comparison of blood lactate concentrations in central venous, pulmonary artery, and arterial blood. Crit Care Med 1987; 15:489–490.
17. Clark L Jr, Noyes LK, Grooms TA, Moore MS. Rapid micro-measurement of lactate in whole blood. Crit Care Med 1984; 12:461–464.
18. Kruse JA, Zaidi SAJ, Carlson RW. Significance of blood lactate levels in critically ill patients with liver disease. Am J Med 1987; 83:77–82.
19. Tashkin DP, Goldstein PJ, Simmons DH. Hepatic lactate uptake during decreased liver perfusion and hypoxemia. Am J Physiol 1972; 223:968–974.

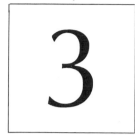

c h a p t e r

3

BEDSIDE ASSESSMENT OF GAS EXCHANGE

The first lecture I delivered as an instructor in medical school was greeted with a chorus of blank stares that spelled certain doom for an anticipated career in academics. I learned later that this reaction was the result of poor comprehension and not didactic boredom. The principles in this chapter are the same as those presented 15 years ago, but the focus is more on clinical applications. If you feel a blank stare coming on, several reviews at the end of the chapter might improve clarity.[1-5]

VENTILATION-PERFUSION BALANCE

The alveolar-capillary units in Figure 3–1 can be used to describe the different patterns of gas exchange. These patterns are defined using the ratio of alveolar ventilation ($\dot{V}$) to capillary perfusion ($\dot{Q}$), commonly called the $\dot{V}/\dot{Q}$ ratio. The patterns of gas exchange and associated $\dot{V}/\dot{Q}$ ratios are shown in Figure 3–1. Panel A shows a perfect match between ventilation and perfusion and a $\dot{V}/\dot{Q}$ ratio of unity. This ratio is the reference point for describing the abnormal patterns of gas exchange in the following sections.

DEAD SPACE VENTILATION

The ventilation that does not participate in gas exchange is called "dead space" ventilation. The $\dot{V}/\dot{Q}$ ratio in this case is greater than 1.0 (panel B). There are two types of dead-space ventilation.

1. **Anatomic dead space** is the gas in the large conducting airways

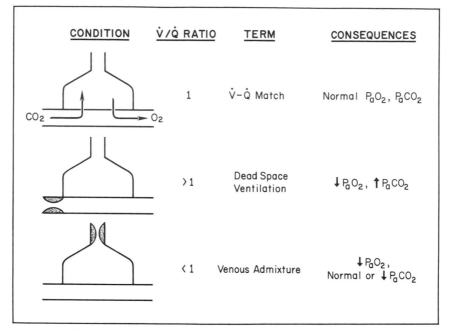

FIG. 3–1. The different types of ventilation-perfusion balance.

that does not come in contact with capillaries. About 50% of the anatomic dead space is in the pharynx.

2. **Physiologic dead space** is the alveolar gas that does not equilibrate fully with capillary blood. This represents excess ventilation relative to capillary perfusion.

The combined dead space (anatomic plus physiologic) represents 20 to 30% of the total minute ventilation in normal subjects (V_D/V_T is 0.2 to 0.3).[1,6] An increase in dead space produces both hypoxemia and hypercapnia. The CO_2 retention usually appears when V_D/V_T rises above 0.5.[6]

Etiologic Factors. Dead space ventilation is caused by overdistension of alveoli or low flow states. The former is seen in obstructive lung disease and PEEP ventilation. The latter is seen in heart failure (right or left), acute pulmonary embolism, and emphysema.

SHUNT FRACTION

The fraction of the cardiac output that does not fully equilibrate with alveolar gas is called the "shunt fraction" (Qs/Qt). The $\dot{V}/\dot{Q}$ ratio in this case is less than 1.0 (lower panel, Figure 3–1). There are two types of shunt:

1. **True shunt** indicates the absence of gas exchange between blood and alveolar gas ($\dot{V}/\dot{Q}$ equal to zero). This is equivalent to an anatomic shunt.

2. **Venous admixture** represents the capillary blood that does not fully

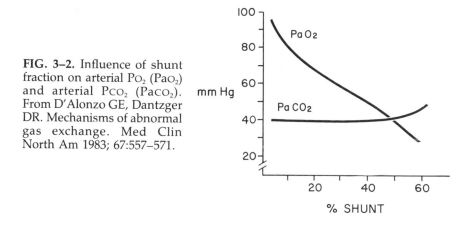

FIG. 3–2. Influence of shunt fraction on arterial P_{O_2} (Pa_{O_2}) and arterial P_{CO_2} (Pa_{CO_2}). From D'Alonzo GE, Dantzger DR. Mechanisms of abnormal gas exchange. Med Clin North Am 1983; 67:557–571.

equilibrate with alveolar gas. As venous admixture increases, it behaves more like true shunt.

The effect of shunt fraction on arterial blood gases is shown in Figure 3–2. The normal Qs/Qt is a little less than 10%, which means that over 90% of the cardiac output participates in gas exchange.[1,2] As shunt fraction increases, the Pa_{O_2} falls progressively but the arterial P_{CO_2} does not increase until Qs/Qt exceeds 50%.[2] The Pa_{CO_2} is often below normal in patients with intrapulmonary shunting and is the result of hyperventilation from the disease process or from associated hypoxemia.

The shunt fraction determines the ability of inspired oxygen to increase the arterial P_{O_2}. This is shown in Figure 3–3. As Qs/Qt increases, an increase in fractional concentration of inspired oxygen (FI_{O_2}) produces less of an increase in Pa_{O_2}. When Qs/Qt exceeds 50%, the Pa_{O_2} becomes unresponsive to changes in FI_{O_2}.[2] At this level, the intrapulmonary shunt behaves like a true (anatomic) shunt rather than venous admixture. When toxic levels of inspired oxygen are being used and the shunt fraction is over 50%, the FI_{O_2} can be reduced to lower levels without

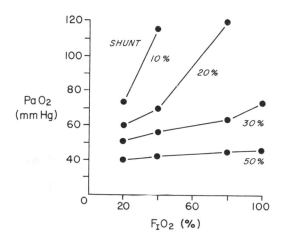

FIG. 3–3. Influence of shunt fraction on the relationship between the FI_{O_2} and Pa_{O_2}. From D'Alonzo GE, Dantzger DR. Med Clin North Am 1983; 67:557–571.

producing a significant drop in arterial P_{O_2}. This will help limit the risk for oxygen toxicity.

Etiologic Factors. The common causes of increased shunt fraction include pneumonia, pulmonary edema (cardiac and noncardiac), and pulmonary embolism. In pulmonary edema (particularly noncardiac) and pulmonary embolism, the gas exchange abnormality behaves more like true shunt and the Pa_{O_2} responds poorly to changes in FI_{O_2}. In pulmonary embolism, the shunt is the result of diversion of blood away from the embolized region and overperfusion of the remainder of the lung.[3]

GAS EXCHANGE CALCULATIONS

The following equations can be used to determine if a ventilation-perfusion abnormality exists and to quantitate the severity of the problem. These equations can be useful in the management of patients with respiratory failure.

DEAD SPACE (VD/VT)

The dead space calculation is based on the difference between exhaled P_{CO_2} and end-capillary (arterial) P_{CO_2}. In the normal lung, the capillary blood equilibrates fully with alveolar gas and the expired P_{CO_2} is roughly the same as the arterial P_{CO_2}. As dead space ventilation (VD/VT) increases, the expired P_{CO_2} (Pe_{CO_2}) will fall below the arterial P_{CO_2} (Pa_{CO_2}). The Bohr equation for calculating VD/VT is based on this principle.[6]

$$VD/VT = \frac{Pa_{CO_2} - Pe_{CO_2}}{Pa_{CO_2}}$$

Normal VD/VT = 0.3

The Pe_{CO_2} is determined by collecting expired gas in a large collection bag and using an infrared CO_2 analyser to measure the mean P_{CO_2} in the gas. This is easy to do and is usually done by the respiratory therapy department on request.

SHUNT FRACTION (Qs/Qt)

The shunt fraction (Qs/Qt) is determined using the O_2 content in arterial blood (Ca_{O_2}), mixed venous blood ($C\bar{v}_{O_2}$), and pulmonary capillary blood (Cc_{O_2}).

$$Qs/Qt = \frac{Cc_{O_2} - Ca_{O_2}}{Cc_{O_2} - C\bar{v}_{O_2}}$$

Normal Qs/Qt = 0.1

Because CcO_2 cannot be measured directly, pure oxygen breathing is recommended to produce complete saturation of hemoglobin in the pulmonary capillaries (i.e., ScO_2 = 100%). In this situation, Qs/Qt measures true shunt. When less than 100% oxygen is inhaled, Qs/Qt measures both true shunt and venous admixture.

THE A-a PO_2 GRADIENT

The difference in PO_2 between alveolar gas and arterial blood is called the "A-a gradient." This is derived using the alveolar gas equation shown below.

$$PAO_2 = PIO_2 - (PacO_2/RQ)$$

This equation states that the alveolar PO_2 (PAO_2) is proportional to the inspired oxygen (PIO_2) and inversely related to the alveolar (arterial) PcO_2. The PIO_2 is a function of the fractional concentration of inspired oxygen (FIO_2), the barometric pressure (P_B) and the partial pressure of water vapor (PH_2O) in the humidified gas ($PIO_2 = FIO_2 (P_B - PH_2O)$). The PH_2O is assumed to be 47 mm Hg at body temperature. The respiratory quotient (RQ) is the ratio of CO_2 and O_2 exchange across the interface between alveoli and capillaries ($RQ = \dot{V}CO_2/\dot{V}O_2$). In a normal subject breathing room air at sea level, the A-a PO_2 gradient is calculated as follows (FIO_2 = 0.21, P_B = 760 mm Hg, PAO_2 = 90 mm Hg, $PacO_2$ = 40 mm Hg, RQ = 0.8).

$$PAO_2 = FIO_2 (P_B - PH_2O) - (PacO_2/RQ)$$

$$= 0.21 (713) - (40/0.8)$$

$$= 100 \text{ mm Hg}$$

Normal A-a PO_2 = 10 to 20 mm Hg

The normal A-a PO_2 gradient varies with age and with the inspired oxygen. The influence of age is shown in the Appendix at the end of the book. The influence of FIO_2 is shown in Figure 3–4.[9]

The usual range for A-a PO_2 gradient in the normal adult at sea level is shown below for room air and pure oxygen breathing.[10,11]

FIO_2	Normal A-a PO_2
0.21	10 to 20 mm Hg
1.0	60 to 70 mm Hg

The A-a PO_2 gradient increases about 5 to 7 mmHg for every 10% increase in FIO_2. The influence of FIO_2 on the A-a PO_2 gradient is explained by the elimination of the hypoxic stimulus for vasoconstriction that would normally divert blood away from poorly ventilated areas. This allows

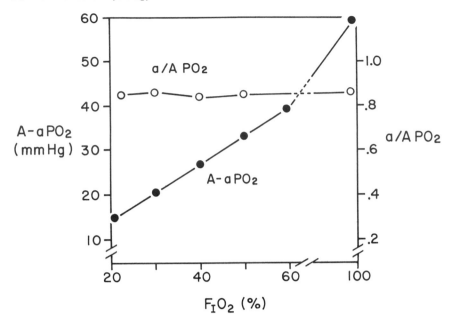

FIG. 3–4. Influence of FIO_2 on the A-a PO_2 gradient and the a/A PO_2 ratio in normal subjects. From Gilbert R, Kreighley JF. Am Rev Respir Dis 1974; 109:142–145.

blood to be returned to the poorly ventilated areas and this can increase shunt fraction.

Mechanical Ventilation. Positive-pressure ventilation will elevate the PIO_2 because P_B is above 760 mmHg. The mean airway pressure can be added to the barometric pressure to improve the accuracy of the calculation.[8] In the above example, a mean airway pressure of 30 cm H_2O would increase the A-a PO_2 gradient to 16 mm Hg, which represents a 60% increase. Although you should be aware of this correction factor, the clinical significance is questionable.

THE a/A PO_2 RATIO

The a/A PO_2 ratio is relatively unaffected by the FIO_2, as shown in Figure 3–4.[9] The equation below explains this.

$$\text{a/A } PO_2 = 1 - (\text{A-a } PO_2)/P_{AO_2}$$

The P_{aO_2} is in both numerator and denominator of the equation and this should eliminate the influence of FIO_2 on the P_{aO_2}. In other words, the a/A PO_2 ratio is a mathematical method for eliminating the influence of FIO_2 on gas exchange calculations. Normal values for the a/A PO_2 ratio are as follows.[9]

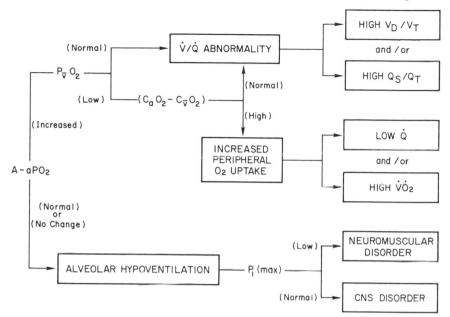

FIG. 3–5. Flow diagram for approaching hypoxemia. See text for explanation.

FIO$_2$	Normal a/A PO$_2$
0.21	0.74 to 0.77
1.0	0.80 to 0.82

THE PaO$_2$/FIO$_2$ RATIO

The ratio of arterial PO$_2$ to FIO$_2$ is a simple method that has been shown to correlate with changes in Qs/QT. The following correlations have been reported.[11]

PaO$_2$/FIO$_2$	Qs/Qt
<200	>20%
>200	<20%

APPROACH TO HYPOXEMIA

The approach to hypoxemia can be organized like the flow diagram in Figure 3–5. This approach requires a pulmonary artery catheter and is applicable only to patients in the ICU. The first step uses the A-a PO$_2$ gradient to determine the origin of the problem. A normal gradient indicates a process that does not involve the lungs (like neuromuscular weakness). An increased gradient signifies a ventilation-perfusion abnormality or a low mixed venous oxygen. The influence of mixed venous oxygen on the arterial PO$_2$ is explained in the next section.

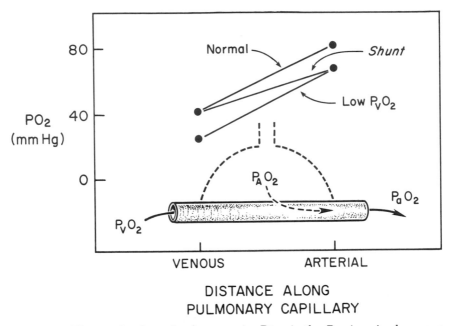

FIG. 3–6. The mechanisms for hypoxemia. $P\bar{v}O_2$ is the PO_2 in mixed venous (pulmonary artery) blood, PaO_2 is arterial PO_2. See text for explanation.

MIXED VENOUS OXYGEN

The oxygen in arterial blood represents the sum of the oxygen in mixed venous (pulmonary artery) blood and the oxygen added from alveolar gas. When lung function is normal, alveolar oxygen is the major determinant of arterial PO_2 (PaO_2). When gas exchange is impaired, alveolar oxygen contributes less and venous oxygen contributes more to the final PaO_2. This is illustrated in Figure 3–6. The horizontal axis in this figure represents the distance along the capillaries and the rate of rise in PO_2 represents the rate of oxygen exchange from alveoli to capillaries. When oxygen exchange decreases (denoted as shunt in the figure), the arterial PO_2 decreases. When the rate of rise is constant but the mixed venous PO_2 ($P\bar{v}O_2$) is lower, the end-point (arterial) PO_2 is the same in both situations. This shows why the lungs may not always be the culprit in cases of hypoxemia.[1,5]

The influence of mixed venous oxygen on the arterial PO_2 will depend on the shunt fraction. When shunt fraction is normal, the venous PO_2 has little influence on arterial PO_2. As shunt fraction increases, the venous PO_2 becomes progressively more important as a determinant of the arterial PO_2. The extreme example would be a 100% shunt, when the $P\bar{v}O_2$ would be the sole determinant of the PaO_2. Therefore, the mixed venous PO_2 will be important only in patients with an existing pulmonary problem.

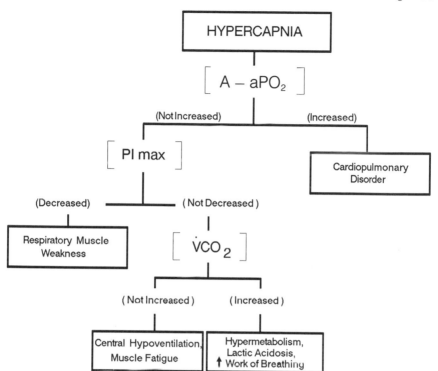

FIG. 3–7. Flow diagram for approaching hypercapnia. See text for explanation.

CARBON DIOXIDE RETENTION

The carbon dioxide in arterial blood is determined by the balance between metabolic production of CO_2 and elimination by the lungs.

$$Paco_2 = K \times (\dot{V}co_2/\dot{V}_E)$$

where $Paco_2$ is arterial Pco_2, $\dot{V}co_2$ is the rate of CO_2 production, $\dot{V}_E$ is expired minute volume, and K is a proportionality constant.[12] Alveolar ventilation can be derived by the relationship ($\dot{V}_E$ (1 - V_D/V_T) where V_D/V_T is anatomic dead space) and the equation can be rewritten as:

$$Paco_2 = K \times [\dot{V}co_2 /V_E (1 - V_D/V_T)]$$

where $\dot{V}_E$ is the expired minute ventilation. This identifies the main causes of CO_2 retention as 1) increased CO_2 production, 2) decreased minute ventilation, and 3) increased dead space ventilation.[13] These can be identified in the flow diagram in Figure 3–7. Each of these components is presented briefly in the following sections.

ENHANCED CO_2 PRODUCTION

The CO_2 production can be measured in intubated patients with the "metabolic cart" that is used for indirect calorimetry. This apparatus has an infrared CO_2 analyser that measures the CO_2 in each exhalation. The respiratory rate is then used to determine the CO_2 elimination rate.

Respiratory Quotient. The rate of CO_2 production is determined by the metabolic rate and the nutrient substrate (carbohydrate, fat, protein) being metabolized. The normal rate of CO_2 production ($\dot{V}CO_2$) in an average size adult is 200 ml/min, or about 80% of the oxygen consumption (normal $\dot{V}O_2$ is 250 ml/min). The ratio $\dot{V}CO_2/\dot{V}O_2$ is called the respiratory quotient (RQ) and this ratio is used to determine the pattern of fuel utilization in individual patients. The metabolism of carbohydrates, protein, and fat produces a specific RQ for each substrate. Carbohydrate produces the highest RQ (1.0), followed by protein (0.8) and lipids (0.7). The total body RQ is the averaged contribution from the metabolism of all three substrates. The RQ is normally 0.8 in the average adult with a diet consisting of 70% carbohydrate calories, and 30% fat calories. The RQ is presented in more detail in Chapter 39.

Etiologic Factors. The common causes of elevated $\dot{V}CO_2$ are sepsis, multiple trauma, burns, increased work of breathing, excess carbohydrates, the postoperative state, and the organic acidoses. Sepsis is probably the most common cause of increased $\dot{V}CO_2$. Increased work of breathing can lead to CO_2 retention during weaning from mechanical ventilation if the ability to eliminate CO_2 through the lungs is impaired. Excess carbohydrate calories can elevate the RQ to 1.0 or higher and promote CO_2 retention. However, the important determinant of arterial PCO_2 is the $\dot{V}CO_2$ and not the RQ. That is, the $\dot{V}CO_2$ can be elevated when the RQ is normal (if the $\dot{V}O_2$ is also elevated). Therefore, the RQ can be misleading if interpreted in isolation.

ALVEOLAR HYPOVENTILATION SYNDROMES

The hypoventilation syndromes produce a decrease in minute ventilation without altering intrinsic lung function (similar to breath holding). As indicated in Figure 3–7, the A-a PO_2 gradient is an important measurement for identifying alveolar hypoventilation syndromes. The A-a PO_2 gradient should be normal or unchanged if alveolar hypoventilation is present. Conversely, cardiopulmonary disorders should be accompanied by an increase in the A-a PO_2 gradient. The exception is severe CO_2 retention from lung disease, where the A-a PO_2 gradient may be close to normal. In this situation, the increase in airway resistance is so severe that almost no air is reaching the alveoli (similar to breath holding). The classification of alveolar hypoventilation syndromes is shown in Table 3–1. The list is restricted to the disorders that are likely to be encountered in the ICU patient population. If the A-a PO_2 gradient is normal or unchanged, then the respiratory muscle strength should be evaluated using the maximum inspiratory pressure described in the next section.

TABLE 3–1. CAUSES OF ALVEOLAR HYPOVENTILATION IN THE ICU	
Brainstem Depression	1. Opiates, lidocaine, etc.
Muscle Weakness	1. Shock or low-flow states
	2. Sepsis
	3. Phosphorus/magnesium depletion
	4. Hypoxia/hypercapnia
Neuropathic Disorders	1. Phrenic injury from cardiac surgery
	2. Neuropathy of critical illness (?)
	3. Myasthenia/Guillain Barre syndrome
Idiopathic Disorders	1. Obesity-hypoventilation
	2. Sleep apnea syndrome

Respiratory Muscle Weakness. There are several factors that can predispose to respiratory muscle weakness in the ICU patient population. The more common ones are sepsis, clinical shock, electrolyte abnormalities, and cardiac surgery. The mechanism in sepsis and shock may be low flow to the diaphragm.[14] Phrenic nerve injury can occur during cardiopulmonary bypass from local cooling of the surface of the heart (see Chapter 2).

Inspiratory muscle weakness can be identified by measuring the maximum inspiratory pressure (PImax) at the bedside.[15] This is done by having the patient exhale to residual volume and then inhale with a maximum effort against a closed valve. The normal ranges for the PImax depend on age and sex (see Table 30–2) and range from 80 to 130 cm H_2O for most adults.[15] Carbon dioxide retention appears when the PImax falls below 30 cm H_2O Remember that the PImax measures all muscles of inspiration, not just the diaphragm. This means that isolated diaphragm dysfunction (e.g., phrenic nerve injury) can be missed by the PImax because the accessory muscles can still maintain the PImax above the desirable level.

Idiopathic Syndromes. The idiopathic hypoventilation syndromes are classified according to body weight and time of day (or night). Daytime hypoventilation in an obese patient is called the obesity-hypoventilation syndrome (OHS) and the same problem in a lean patient is called primary alveolar hypoventilation (PAH). The sleep apnea syndrome is characterized by periodic breathing during sleep and does not necessarily include daytime hypoventilation.[13] OHS and sleep apnea improve with weight loss while OHS also responds to progesterone (see Chapter 26). Phrenic nerve pacing has met with limited success in PAH and otherwise this disorder is untreatable.

BIBLIOGRAPHY

Forster RE, DuBois AB, Briscoe WA, Fisher A, eds. The lung. 3rd ed. Chicago: Year Book Medical Publishers, 1986.
Tisi GM. Pulmonary physiology in clinical medicine. Baltimore: Williams & Wilkins, 1980.

REFERENCES

REVIEWS

1. Dantzger DR. Pulmonary gas exchange. In: Dantzger DR. ed. Cardiopulmonary critical care. Orlando: Grune & Stratton, 1986:25–46.
2. D'Alonzo GE, Dantzger DR. Mechanisms of abnormal gas exchange. Med Clin North Am 1983; 67:557–571.
3. Dantzger DR. Ventilation-perfusion inequality in lung disease. Chest 1987; 91:749–754.
4. Dantzger DR. The influence of cardiovascular function on gas exchange. Clin Chest Med 1983; 4:149–159.
5. Shapiro B. Arterial blood gas monitoring. Crit Care Clin 1988; 4:479–492.

VENTILATION-PERFUSION INEQUALITY

6. Buohuys A. Respiratory dead space. In: Fenn WO, Rahn H. eds. Handbook of physiology: Respiration. Bethesda: American Physiological Society, 1964:699–714.
7. Dean JM, Wetzel RC, Rogers MC. Arterial blood gas derived variables as estimates of intrapulmonary shunt in critically ill children. Crit Care Med 1985; 13:1029–1033.
8. Carroll GC. Misapplication of the alveolar gas equation. N Engl J Med 1985; 312:586.
9. Gilbert R, Kreighley JF. The arterial/alveolar oxygen tension ratio. An index of gas exchange applicable to varying inspired oxygen concentrations. Am Rev Respir Dis 1974; 109:142–145.
10. Harris EA, Kenyon AM, Nisbet HD, Seelye ER, Whitlock RML. The normal alveolar-arterial oxygen tension gradient in man. Clin Sci 1974; 46:89–104.
11. Covelli HD, Nessan VJ, Tuttle WK. Oxygen derived variables in acute respiratory failure. Crit Care Med 1983; 11:646–649.

ALVEOLAR HYPOVENTILATION SYNDROMES

12. Glauser FL, Fairman P, Bechard D. The causes and evaluation of chronic hypercapnia. Chest 1987; 91:755–759.
13. Praher MR, Irwin RS. Extrapulmonary causes of respiratory failure. J Intensive Care Med 1986; 1:197–217.
14. Rochester D, Arora NS. Respiratory muscle failure. Med Clin North Am 1983; 67:573–598.

section II
COMMON PROBLEMS AND PRACTICES

It is astonishing with how little reading a doctor can practise medicine, but it is not astonishing with how badly he may do it.

Sir William Osler

c h a p t e r

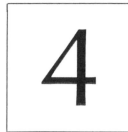

CENTRAL VENOUS ACCESS

The modern practice of critical care is not possible without cannulation of the large veins in the neck. This chapter will guide you through the common routes in the groin and neck, and will highlight some specific concerns related to the catheter insertion process. The information on the individual access routes is taken mostly from the reviews listed at the end of the chapter.[1-5]

THE ANTECUBITAL FOSSA

Long catheters can be placed into the basilic or cephalic vein in the arm and threaded into the thorax. The basilic vein is preferred because it follows a straighter path into the thorax. This method has a higher complication rate than the other routes used for central venous access.[7]

Advantages:
1. No risk for pneumothorax
2. Little risk for bleeding

Disadvantages:
1. High infection rate
2. High rate of thrombosis
3. Catheters difficult to thread, with a success rate as low as 60%[2]

ANATOMY

The surface anatomy of the veins in the antecubital fossa is shown in Figure 4–1. The **basilic vein** passes along the medial aspect of the fossa and is joined by the median basilic vein. It then ascends in the groove between the biceps and the pronator teres muscles on the medial aspect

39

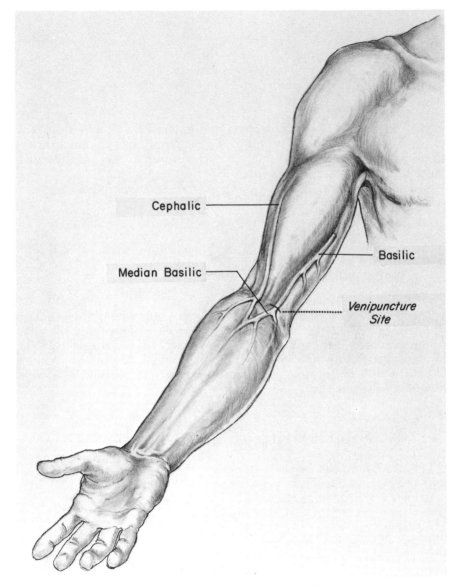

Cephalic

Basilic

Median Basilic

Venipuncture
Site

FIG. 4–1. The veins that run through the antecubital fossa.

of the arm, and courses deep in the upper arm to eventually form the axillary vein.

The **cephalic vein** passes along the lateral aspect of the antecubital fossa where it meets the median basilic vein. It ascends the arm in a groove along the lateral border of the biceps muscle and passes deep in the upper arm to join the axillary vein.

INSERTION TECHNIQUE

The basilic vein is preferred because the cephalic vein can have a variable course. The right arm is preferred for long catheters because of the shorter distance to the superior vena cava. *Never perform a cutdown unless absolutely necessary because of the high infection rate associated with cutdowns.*[2]

The patient need not be supine but the arm must be straight. The vein is distended with a tourniquet and entered by direct vision. The catheter is then advanced, using the distance from the venipuncture site to the junction between manubrium and sternum as the estimated distance to the superior vena cava.

A post-insertion chest x-ray is recommended because the advancing catheter tip can perforate the superior vena cava (this is rare).

BLIND INSERTION

If the basilic vein is not visible, measure the distance between the tip of the olecranon and the acromion and divide the distance into thirds. The basilic vein will be in the distal one-third segment, in the groove between the biceps and triceps. The vein is superficial to the brachial artery at this site and should be entered without inadvertent arterial puncture.

COMMENT

Avoid the antecubital fossa for central venous access because of the risk of infection and the need to replace the catheter every few days. The basilic vein, however, provides quick access for a peripheral venous line but is often overlooked. The vein is large and is easy to enter using the blind approach.

THE SUBCLAVIAN VEIN

The subclavian vein is the most common site for central venous cannulation. The vein can be entered from above or below the clavicle with equal success.

Advantages:
1. Ease of insertion
2. Patient comfort

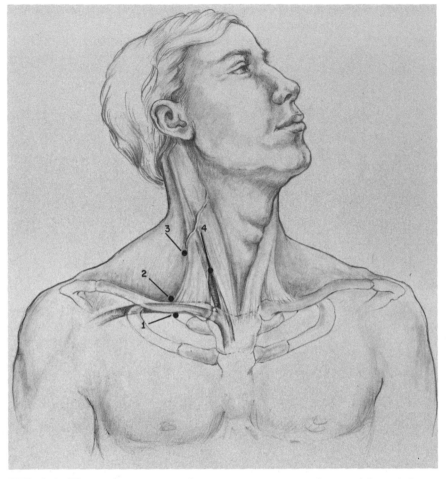

FIG. 4–2. The surface anatomy for percutaneous cannulation of the subclavian and jugular veins. Circular markers indicate skin insertion sites.

Disadvantages:
1. Pneumothorax (1 to 2% of attempted insertions)
2. Subclavian artery puncture (1% of attempted insertions)

ANATOMY

The surface anatomy for subclavian vein insertion is shown in Figure 4–2. The vein begins at the outer border of the first rib and runs underneath the clavicle until it meets the internal jugular vein behind the sternoclavicular joint. The vein lies just under the clavicle at the insertion site for the clavicular head of the sternocleidomastoid muscle. This is the site where the vein is entered. The vein lies on the anterior scalene muscle and the subclavian artery lies just underneath the muscle. The cupola of the lung is just deep to the artery.

TECHNIQUE

When inserting a catheter, the patient is placed supine with arms at the side and head faced away from the insertion side. A towel roll can be placed between the shoulder blades, although this should not be necessary routinely.

Infraclavicular Approach. Identify the insertion of the sternocleidomastoid muscle on the clavicle. After preparing the area and using appropriate local anesthesia, insert the needle under the clavicle at a point just lateral to the muscle insertion (point 1, Fig. 4–2). The needle is inserted with bevel upward and is advanced along a horizontal line drawn between the two shoulders. Keep the needle path just underneath the clavicle. When the vein is entered, turn the bevel of the needle to the 3-o'clock position so the guidewire will thread in the direction of the superior vena cava.

Supraclavicular Approach. Identify the clavicular insertion of the sternocleidomastoid muscle. The muscle and clavicle will form an angle where they meet (Fig. 4–2), and the needle is inserted to bisect this angle (point 2, Fig. 4–2). Keep the bevel of the needle facing upward and once the skin is penetrated, raise the needle and syringe 15 degrees upward in the coronal plane and begin to advance the needle. The vein should be entered at a distance of 1 to 2 cm from the skin surface.

COMMENT

The supraclavicular approach is the easiest access route because the vein is just under the skin at this point. The incidence of pneumothorax (2%) is the same with either method of insertion. If an initial attempt is unsuccessful, you must obtain a chest x-ray before crossing to the other side. In this situation, you can try an internal jugular vein approach on the same side without a chest film.

THE INTERNAL JUGULAR VEIN

The internal jugular (IJ) vein can be entered near the base of the neck just before it joins the subclavian vein under the sternoclavicular joint.
Advantage:
Minimal risk for pneumothorax. Preferred to the subclavian route for patients with hyperinflation, or for those receiving mechanical ventilation.
Disadvantage:
The major risk is carotid artery puncture. For this reason, the IJ approach is not recommended when the platelet count is less than 50,000/mm³, or the prothrombin time is 3 seconds above control.[2]

ANATOMY

The surface anatomy for the internal jugular vein approach is shown in Figure 4–2. The vein runs down the neck under the sternocleido-mastoid muscle. It follows an oblique course in relation to the overlying muscle, beginning at the medial edge of the muscle high in the neck, and ending at the lateral aspect of the muscle (the sternal insertion) at the base of the neck. With the head turned to the opposite side, the vein follows a straight line from the pinna of the ear to the sternocla-vicular joint. The vein lies in the carotid sheath, lateral to the vagus nerve and the carotid artery, in that order.

INSERTION TECHNIQUE

The vein can be entered from an anterior or posterior approach (Fig. 4–2). The right side is preferred because the vein runs a direct path to the right atrium. Transvenous pacemakers should always be placed on the right side when possible. The left-sided approach carries more risk for thoracic duct cannulation because the left thoracic duct is large and sits just underneath the left internal jugular vein.

To begin, position the patient in a supine or Trendelenburg position, arms at the side, and head turned away from the side to be cannulated. This position makes either of two approaches available.

The Anterior Approach. Identify the triangle created by the two heads of the sternocleidomastoid muscle (point 4, Fig. 4–2). Palpate the carotid artery at the apex of the triangle. Retract the artery medially and insert the needle at the apex of the triangle with the bevel facing up. Advance the needle in a 45 degree angle with the skin surface. If the vein is not encountered by a depth of 5 cm, withdraw the tip to the skin, aim a few degrees laterally, and repeat the approach.

When the vessel is entered, look for pulsations. If the blood is red and pulsating you have entered the carotid artery. In this situation, remove the needle and tamponade the area for 5 to 10 minutes. When the carotid artery has been punctured, no further attempts should be made on either side because puncture of both arteries can lead to serious consequences.

The Posterior Approach. This approach seems more awkward than the anterior approach, but there is less risk for carotid artery puncture. Identify the external jugular vein on the surface of the sternocleido-mastoid muscle (Fig. 4–2) and note the point where the vein crosses over the lateral edge of the muscle (point 3, Fig. 4–2). The insertion point is 1 cm superior to this point. Grasp the belly of the muscle and insert the needle with the bevel at a 3-o'clock position. Aim the needle at the suprasternal notch and advance the needle just under the belly of the muscle at an upward angulation of 15 degrees. You should enter the vessel 5 to 6 cm from the skin surface. Remember to stay just under the belly of the muscle because there is a tendency to plunge the needle too deep. The carotid sheath should be posterior and lateral to the trachea.

COMMENT

The disadvantages of the internal jugular approach far outweigh the single advantage (low risk of pneumothorax). Accidental puncture of the carotid artery occurs in 2 to 10% of insertions and can have serious consequences.[2] Patients frequently complain of the limited neck mobility associated with IJ lines. Inappropriate neck flexion often occurs in agitated patients and results in thrombosis of the line. In patients with tracheostomies, the catheter insertion site is near the tracheostomy site and can be exposed to infected secretions that drain from the tracheostomy.

THE EXTERNAL JUGULAR VEIN

The external jugular vein is easy to enter because it lies just under the skin surface (Fig. 4–2).
Advantages:
1. No risk for pneumothorax
2. Bleeding can be controlled
Disadvantages:
The major problem is difficulty advancing the catheter

ANATOMY

The external jugular vein runs obliquely across the surface of the sternocleidomastoid muscle and can be identified by inspecting the skin surface (Fig. 4–2). The vein passes under the muscle and joins the subclavian vein at an acute angle. The acute angle at this junction is the major impediment to advancing catheters from the external jugular vein into the chest.

INSERTION TECHNIQUE

Place the patient in the supine position and inspect the skin for the bulging vein. The Trendelenburg position may be needed to fill the vein enough to make it visible. However, up to 15% of patients will not have an identifiable vein even under optimal conditions.[1]
The external jugular vein has little support from surrounding structures and will move away from an advancing needle. The vein can be steadied by anchoring the vein between the thumb and forefinger when making the needle puncture. The needle should enter the vein with bevel pointed up and the needle pointed along the course of the vein. The catheter is advanced along the axis of the vein. If the catheter is not advancing easily, do not use unnecessary force because this can cause the catheter to perforate the vein at the junction of the subclavian vein.

COMMENT

The difficulty in threading catheters along the external jugular vein has limited the use of the approach. The usual indication is for patients with a severe coagulopathy. This approach also impairs neck mobility, and is not well tolerated by awake patients.

THE FEMORAL VEIN

The femoral vein is the easiest of the large veins to cannulate, with a success rate of 90% or greater.[1] Although the insertion site is in the groin area, the infection rate with femoral vein catheters left in place less than 3 days is no different than the infection rate seen with other central venous sites.[1]

Advantages:
1. Ease of insertion
2. No risk for pneumothorax

Disadvantages:
1. Limits flexion of the leg at the hip
2. Thrombosis (10%)
3. Femoral artery puncture (5% of attempts)

The femoral approach is particularly suitable for cardiopulmonary resuscitation because the physician inserting the catheter is away from the commotion around the thorax and there is no risk for pneumothorax.

ANATOMY

The surface anatomy for femoral vein cannulation is shown in Figure 4–3. The femoral vein is a direct continuation of the popliteal vein and it becomes the external iliac vein at the inguinal ligament. The vein lies within the femoral sheath and is medial to the femoral artery. At the inguinal ligament, the femoral sheath lies just a few centimeters below the skin surface.

INSERTION TECHNIQUE

Use a surgical prep for the groin area, including shaving the area. The catheter and needles should be longer than the usual length used for peripheral access. The following material should be adequate.

Seldinger Technique
1. 18-gauge needle, 6 to 7 cm in length
2. 0.035-inch guidewire
3. 16-gauge catheter, 16 to 20 cm in length

Catheter Through Needle Technique
1. 14-gauge needle, at least 5 cm in length
2. 16-gauge catheter, 16 to 20 cm in length

Palpate the femoral artery as it emerges from under the inguinal liga-

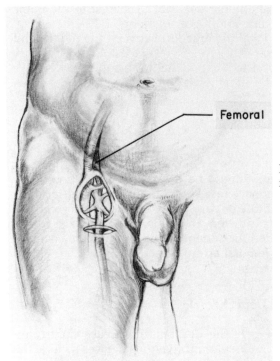

Femoral

FIG. 4–3. Anatomy of the femoral vein.

ment. The artery should be midway between a line from the anterior superior iliac spine to the symphysis pubis. The vein should be 1 to 2 cm medial to the palpated pulse. Enter the skin with the bevel of the needle pointed forward toward the shoulders, and advance the needle at a 45 degree angle to the skin surface. You should enter the vein about 2 to 4 cm from the skin surface. When a vessel has been entered, remove the syringe and watch for pulsations. Pulsating red blood indicates that the femoral artery has been entered. If the artery has been punctured, remove the needle and tamponade the groin for at least 10 minutes.

When the catheter or guidewire will not pass beyond the needle (and you are still in the vein), tilt the syringe to make the needle more parallel to the skin surface. This may move the bevel of the needle from the far side of the vessel wall into the lumen, and allow the catheter to be advanced.

Femoral vein catheters are usually 6 to 8 inches in length. Longer catheters are available that will reach the right atrium but these catheters increase the risk for damaging the vena cava, and often become thrombosed.[1]

BLIND INSERTION

If the femoral artery pulse is not palpable, the femoral vein can be located as follows:[8]

1. Visualize a line from the anterior superior iliac crest to the pubic tubercle and divide the line into three segments.
2. The femoral artery will lie at the junction between the medial and middle segments.
3. The femoral vein will be 1 to 2 cm medial to this junction.

This method for blind femoral vein catheterization has a reported success rate of 90 to 95%.[8]

COMMENT

Femoral vein catheterization should be the procedure of choice for venous access in cardiopulmonary resuscitation and for short-term access in patients who are comatose or paralyzed. The risk for thrombosis and infection is minimal if the catheters are left in place 3 days or less.[1,8] This route is not recommended for patients with a significant coagulopathy because of the risk of femoral artery puncture.[1]

PREPARING FOR CATHETERIZATION

The formal recommendations of the Centers for Disease Control regarding the proper insertion and care of intravenous devices include the following:[6]

A. Physician Preparation
1. Handwashing is mandatory, but soap and water are satisfactory.
2. Sterile gloves are required for all cannulations other than peripheral veins.
3. Caps, gowns, and masks are not mandatory, since their value is unproven.

B. Skin Preparation
1. A "defatting" substance like acetone is not necessary for preparing the insertion site.
2. Hair removal is not necessary. If hair is removed, a depilatory should be used instead of a razor to limit the risk of skin trauma and infection.
3. Iodine solution (1 to 2%) followed by 70% alcohol is effective, as is povidone-iodine solution.
4. Start the scrub at the proposed insertion site and work outward in a circular fashion.
5. The antiseptic should be left in contact with the skin for at least 30 seconds after the scrub.

C. Positioning the Patient
For spontaneously breathing patients, place in the supine position or the head-down (15 degrees below horizontal) position. This will distend the veins in the neck and will help to minimize the risk for venous air embolism. A semirecumbent position may be adequate for patients receiving positive-pressure ventilation or for those with acute heart failure.

INSERTING THE CATHETER

The original technique for inserting central venous catheters used a large-bore needle (usually 14 gauge) to enter the vessel, and then threaded the catheter through the needle. This "catheter-through-needle" method carried a high risk for damage to the vessel and associated structures and has largely been abandoned.

THE SELDINGER TECHNIQUE

The preferred method for insertion of central venous catheters is called the "catheter-over-guidewire" method or the Seldinger technique, after its founder.[9] This method is aimed at limiting the trauma to vessels and adjacent structures during the insertion. The sequence used in this method is illustrated in Figure 4–4. A small-bore needle (usually 20 gauge) is used to probe for the vein. When the vein is entered, the syringe is detached from the needle and a thin guidewire with a flexible tip (called a "J" wire) is passed through the needle. The needle is then removed over the guidewire and the guidewire is used to direct the catheter into the vessel. In Figure 4–4, the catheter system is an introducer catheter that is threaded over a dilator catheter. This catheter system is passed over the guidewire until it rests in the lumen of the vessel. The guidewire is then removed, leaving the infusion device in place.

The Seldinger technique has the following advantages. First, the small-bore probing catheter will limit damage to the vessel and surrounding structures. This may be particularly advantageous when an adjacent artery is accidentally punctured. Second, the insertion of the catheter over a guidewire will insure that the puncture hole in the vessel is no larger in diameter than the catheter, thereby minimizing the risk for bleeding from the puncture site in the vessel.

VENOUS AIR EMBOLISM

The most feared complication of catheter insertion is venous air embolism. This syndrome is produced by air that is entrained into the central veins through an open catheter system.[10] This occurs when the intrathoracic pressure is negative relative to atmospheric pressure (e.g., during a normal inspiration), and the catheter system is open to the room air. The air that enters the central veins will pass through the right side of the heart and obstruct the pulmonary circulation, producing acute right heart failure. This can be rapidly fatal, even when the pressure difference between the thorax and surrounding air is small.

A pressure gradient of 4 mmHg across a 14-gauge catheter can entrain 90 ml of air per second, and produce a fatal air embolus in one second.[3]

SELDINGER TECHNIQUE

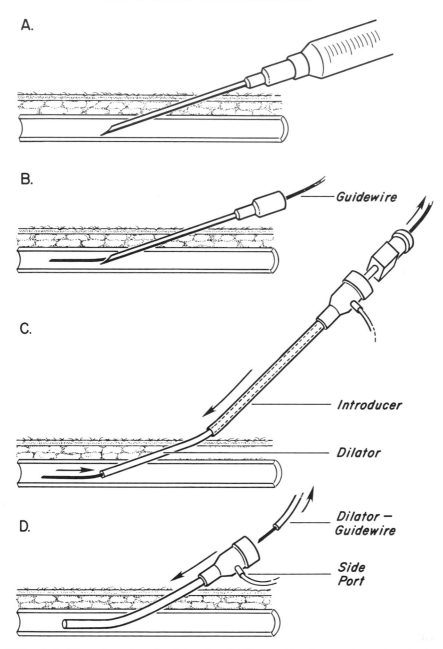

A.

B.

Guidewire

C.

Introducer

Dilator

D.

Dilator –
Guidewire

Side
Port

FIG. 4–4. The steps involved in the Seldinger "guidewire-through-needle" method of venous cannulation.

Preventive Measures. Prevention is the hallmark of venous air embolism because the mortality is at least 50% despite therapeutic maneuvers.[10] The pressure in the central veins is elevated during insertion by placing the patient in the Trendelenburg position with the head placed down (15 degrees below the horizontal plane). When changing connections in a central venous line, a temporary positive pressure can be created by having the patient hum audibly. This not only produces a positive intrathoracic pressure, it also allows you to hear when the pressure is positive.

Clinical Presentation. The usual presentation is acute onset of dyspnea that occurs during the procedure. Hypotension and cardiac arrest can develop rapidly. Air can escape across a patent foramen ovale and produce obstruction of the cerebral circulation, producing an acute stroke. A classic "mill wheel" murmur can be heard over the right heart, but this can be fleeting.

Therapy

Immediate therapy includes placing the patient with the left side down and aspirating blood and air directly from the venous line. If necessary, insert a needle into the right ventricle through the chest wall and aspirate as much air as possible. Unfortunately, there is little that is effective when the air embolism is severe and mortality has not been reduced by these therapeutic maneuvers.

POST-INSERTION CHEST FILMS

Chest films are recommended after all central venous catheter insertions. The goal is to locate the catheter tip and to search for evidence of pneumothorax, hemothorax, and cardiac tamponade.

TECHNIQUE

Portable (AP) films should be obtained in the upright position, during expiration. **Expiratory films** will magnify the pneumothorax because expiration decreases lung volume but does not decrease the volume of the pneumothorax. The pneumothorax will be more apparent because it is a larger fraction of the total volume of the involved hemithorax.

Upright films are not possible in some patients (e.g., coma). When supine films are obtained, remember that **pneumothoraces are usually not located at the lung apices in supine films** but are more commonly found in the subpulmonic recess or along the anteromedial mediastinum.[11] (See Chapter 29.)

Pneumothorax may not be evident immediately, but can appear 24 to 48 hours later.[12] The absence of pneumothorax on the immediate post-insertion film therefore does not exclude the disorder. The incidence of delayed pneumothorax is unknown. However, there is little evidence to justify serial chest films if the patient is asymptomatic.

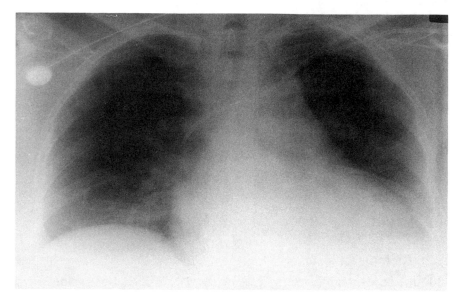

FIG. 4–5. Portable chest x-ray showing the tip of a left subclavian catheter against the far wall of the superior vena cava.

CATHETER TIP POSITION

The position of the catheter tip should raise some concern in the following situations.

1. **Tip abuts the caval wall**. Catheters threaded from the left-sided vessels can run directly into the far wall of the superior vena cava, as shown in Figure 4–5. A catheter tip left in this position can perforate the wall of the vena cava and produce hemothorax.[13] Therefore, the catheter should always be withdrawn a few centimeters when the tip is against the caval wall.

2. **Tip in the right atrium**. The superior vena cava meets the right atrium at the level of the third right costal cartilage. If the catheter tip is below this point it is probably in the right atrium or ventricle. These catheter tips can produce perforation of the free wall of the heart and pericardial tamponade.[3] For this reason, catheter tips should be positioned in the superior vena cava whenever possible.

BIBLIOGRAPHY

Peters JL ed. A manual of central venous catheterization and parenteral nutrition. Boston: Wright PSG, 1983.

Sprung CL, Grenvik A eds. Invasive procedures in critical care. Clinics in critical care medicine. New York: Churchill Livingstone, 1985.

Venus B, Mallory DL eds. Vascular cannulation. Problems in critical care. Philadelphia: J.B. Lippincott, 1988.

REFERENCES

REVIEWS

1. Seneff MG. Central venous catheterization: A comprehensive review, Part 1. Intensive Care Med 1987; 2:163–175.
2. Seneff MG. Central venous catheterization: A comprehensive review, Part 2. Intensive Care Med 1987; 2:218–232.
3. Sladen A. Complications of invasive hemodynamic monitoring in the intensive care unit. Curr Prob Surg 1988; (Feb)25:69–145.
4. Sitzmann JV. The technique of managing central venous lines. J Crit Illness 1986; 1:50–55.
5. Murphy LM, Lipman TO. Central venous catheter care in parenteral nutrition: A review. JPEN 1987; 11:190–201.

SELECTED TOPICS

6. Centers for Disease Control Working Group. Guidelines for prevention of intravascular infections. In: Guidelines for the prevention and control of nosocomial infections. VSDHHS-PHS, 1981.
7. Giuffreda DJ, Bryan-Brown CW, Lumb PD et al. Central vs. peripheral venous catheters in critically ill patients. Chest 1986; 90:806–809.
8. Getzen LC, Pollack EW. Short term femoral vein catheterization. Am J Surg 1979; 138:875–877.
9. Seldinger SI. Catheter replacement of the needle in percutaneous arteriography. Acta Radiol 1953; 39:368–372.
10. O'Quin RJ, Lakshminarayans S. Venous air embolism. Arch Intern Med 1982; 142:2173–2176.
11. Tocino IM, Miller MH, Fairfax WR. Distribution of pneumothorax in the supine and semirecumbent critically ill adult. Am J Radiol 1985; 144:901–905.
12. Slezak FA, Williams GB. Delayed pneumothorax: A complication of subclavian vein catheterization. JPEN 1984; 8:571–574.
13. Tocino IM, Watanabe A. Impending catheter perforation of superior vena cava: Radiographic recognition. Am J Radiol 1986; 146:487–490.

chapter

STRESS ULCERS

Stress ulcers are often viewed as a primary illness instead of a signal for mucosal ischemia. This misconception has created some confusion about the appropriate therapy for stress ulcers and specifically about the role of gastric acid suppression therapy. This chapter will introduce stress ulceration as a manifestation of mucosal ischemia and not a manifestation of gastric hyperacidity.

STRESS ULCER PRIMER

The term "stress ulcer" was introduced by Hans Selye in 1936 to describe the association between psychosomatic illness and peptic ulcer disease. However, stress ulcers are not deep craters like those seen in peptic ulcer disease, but are superficial erosions confined to the surface of the mucosa.[1-5] These erosions are often present within hours of admission to an intensive care unit.[7] Therefore, the goal of therapy is not so much to prevent their appearance but to limit the incidence of troublesome bleeding.

PATHOGENESIS

The gastric mucosa is covered by a protective layer of mucus that shields the mucosa from the corrosive effects of gastric acid. When blood flow to the mucosa is inadequate, this barrier dissolves and the underlying mucosa is eroded by the acid in the stomach lumen. The superficial erosions that result are called stress ulcers. According to this explanation, the fundamental problem in stress ulceration is inadequate blood flow to the stomach wall. Gastric hyperacidity is important only when the barrier is disrupted first by local ischemia.

CONSEQUENCES

Stress ulcers remain superficial in location and do not erode through the stomach wall to cause perforation. The major problem is blood loss,[1] which is occult in most cases and is detected only by testing for occult blood in gastric aspirates. Brisk bleeding is uncommon, but not rare.

Stress ulcer bleeding occurs in 20% of long term ICU inhabitants, but gross hemorrhage occurs in only 5% of patients.[1,7–9]

Most patients with occult blood loss will not progress to frank hemorrhage, and therefore monitoring occult blood in gastric secretions has no predictive value. Gross hemorrhage is self-limited in most cases, and is not slowed by either antacids or H2 blocking agents.[10] Massive hemorrhage is rare, but carries a mortality in excess of 80%.[1,7]

STRATEGIES FOR PROPHYLAXIS

Stress ulcers appear almost immediately after the onset of a serious illness, so that therapy is not aimed at preventing their appearance. Instead, therapy is aimed at preventing these lesions from bleeding. The following strategies have proven effective.

GASTRIC pH CONTROL

The traditional approach to stress ulcer prophylaxis is to inhibit acid production in the stomach with a histamine H2 receptor antagonist, or to neutralize the gastric pH with antacids. Both methods are effective and will reduce the incidence of bleeding from 20% to 5%.[7,8]

Antacids are more effective than H2 blockers if the end-point is occult blood loss, but both methods are equally effective if the goal is to prevent clinically significant bleeding.[7,8]

The clinical trials that compared antacids and H2 blockers, and used occult blood loss as an end-point, are now being questioned because the H2 blocker used in these trials (cimetidine) can produce a false-positive test for occult blood.[8] Furthermore, occult blood loss is not an appropriate end-point because it does not predict the appearance of significant hemorrhage. Therefore, antacids and H2 blockers are now considered equivalent in their ability to prevent significant stress ulcer bleeding.

LUMINAL NUTRIENTS

Infusion of enteral feedings or dextrose solutions into the stomach will protect against stress ulcer bleeding as effectively as antacids or H2 blockers.[11] The mechanism involved may be an antacid-like effect to neutralize gastric pH. The other possibility is a nutrient effect on the cells of the gastric mucosa; that is, the cells may use luminal nutrients as a source of energy to produce the protective surface lining.[12] Regardless of the mechanism, the protective effect of enteral feedings simultaneously solves the problems of nutrition and stress ulcer prophylaxis. See Chapter 40 for more information on enteral feeding and mucosal function.

CYTOPROTECTION

Cytoprotective agents will maintain the integrity of the mucosal barrier without altering gastric pH. This strategy seems to be the most logical approach because the problem in stress ulceration is disruption of the mucosal barrier and not gastric hyperacidity. The most popular cytoprotective agent at ths time is sucralfate, an aluminum salt of sucrose sulfate that is instilled directly into the stomach. The exact mechanism of action is unknown, but may involve prostaglandin-mediated improvements in mucosal blood flow.[13]

Sucralfate is comparable to antacids and H2 blockers for reducing the incidence of stress ulcer bleeding.[13-16]

There are a number of advantages to using sucralfate instead of H2 blockers or antacids. One advantage is cost; sucralfate can be half the cost of antacid therapy and 1/15th the cost of H2 blocker therapy.[17] The other advantage is the lack of toxicity. Sucralfate is virtually devoid of side effects. The only notable side effect is hypophosphatemia because the aluminum in the parent compound binds to phosphate in the gut.[18]

HEMODYNAMIC MANAGEMENT

The optimal strategy in preventing superficial erosions is to maintain splanchnic blood flow, yet this approach is rarely mentioned as an option in stress ulcer prophylaxis. The problem is monitoring splanchnic blood flow, which is not possible at the present time. Nevertheless, the appearance of stress ulcers should prompt a careful hemodynamic evaluation, including a pulmonary artery catheter if necessary. Remember that splanchnic flow is the first to become compromised in low-flow states, so there may be no other clues to the problem. The therapeutic approach to low-flow states includes **volume** to optimal filling pressures and **dobutamine** to promote cardiac output (see Chapters 12–14). Vasodilator therapy using **angiotensin converting enzyme inhibitors** may be valuable because the renin system is important in regulating splanchnic blood flow, at least in animal studies.[5] Until there are methods for monitoring splanchnic blood flow clinically, this approach will be difficult to implement.

GASTRIC ACID: FRIEND OR FOE?

The traditional approach to ulcer disease has centered on the control of gastric acidity, but this practice is now being questioned. There is now evidence to suggest that gastric acid is not the digestive aid it was once considered to be, but is an antibacterial defense mechanism.[19] The average adult produces 1 to 2 L of saliva each day, and as this saliva is swallowed, mouth organisms are introduced into the upper gastrointestinal tract. Most of the bacteria that is swallowed in saliva will survive less than 15 minutes in the stomach when the gastric pH is 3.0 or below.[19] However, when the gastric pH is 4.0 or above (which is the common end-point of acid suppression therapy), the bacteria will thrive and colonize the gastric contents. This bacterial colonization can lead to serious infections such as pneumonia and septicemia.

ASPIRATION PNEUMONIA

The most feared consequence of gastric colonization is the reflux of stomach contents into the upper airways. This retrograde movement of bacteria may be common in critically ill adults,[22] which means that acid suppression therapy carries a real risk for aspiration pneumonia. This is supported in preliminary studies.

> Nosocomial pneumonia is more common in ventilator patients receiving acid suppression therapy than in patients receiving cytoprotective therapy with sucralfate.[20-22]

This observation casts a shadow on the routine use of antacids or H2 blockers for stress ulcer prophylaxis, and supports the use of sucralfate. Further evaluation is needed before firm conclusions are possible.

TRANSLOCATION

Bacterial overgrowth in the stomach and small bowel can also lead to generalized septicemia if the pathogens gain access to the bloodstream through disrupted mucosa. The mucosal surface of the bowel normally serves as a barrier to pathogens in the gut lumen. When this barrier breaks down because of stress ulceration, bacteria and endotoxins can invade the mucosa and "translocate" from the bowel to the systemic circulation.[23] The consequence of this process is systemic sepsis and the "multiple organ failure syndrome." Translocation is now recognized as an important source of sepsis in the critically ill,[23] and the risk for this should discourage the practice of promoting bacterial overgrowth with H2-blockers and antacids.

SPECIFIC RECOMMENDATIONS

The following are some recommendations for stress ulcer prophylaxis in individual patients.

INDICATIONS

Several conditions are associated with stress ulcer bleeding. The following are some high-risk conditions and their proposed mechanisms.

Condition	Mechanism
1. Mechanical ventilation	Ischemia
2. COPD	Hyperacidity
3. Shock	Ischemia
4. Low cardiac output	Ischemia
5. Prolonged bowel rest	Barrier disruption
6. Steroids, Chemotherapy, Aspirin, Nonsteroidal anti-inflammatory agents.	Barrier disruption

The presence of any of the above is an indication for prophylaxis. However, any patient who is in the ICU for more than a few days is a candidate for prophylaxis.

GASTRIC EMPTYING

The ability of the stomach to empty can be used to select the therapy in individual patients, as outlined in Figure 5–1. Gastric emptying is evaluated by infusing a known volume (usually 50 to 100 ml) into the stomach, and measuring the volume that can be retrieved after 30 minutes. The volume should be infused over 30 minutes because bolus delivery and acute gastric distention can retard gastric motility. Small-bore feeding tubes do not often permit aspiration of gastric contents, and large-bore nasogastric tubes (18 to 22 French) are used for the test. If the volume retrieved is less than 50% of the infused volume, gastric emptying is considered adequate enough to begin oral or enteral feedings.

THERAPY

1. **Enteral Feeding** is the preferred method for prophylaxis if gastric emptying is adequate. Enteral feedings have a dual benefit because they provide nutrients to meet daily caloric needs and they provide effective prophylaxis for stress ulcer bleeding. If there is concern for regurgitation of stomach contents in the individual patient, methylene blue or food coloring can be added to the feeding solution, and the color of the upper airways secretions is monitored. This method is limited to patients who are intubated.

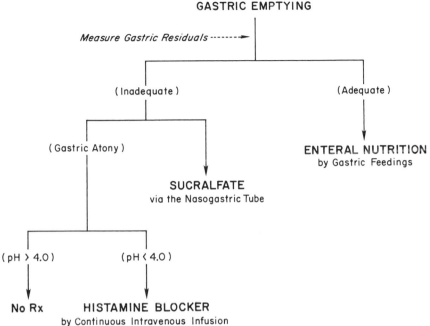

FIG. 5–1. Strategies for stress ulcer prophylaxis based on gastric motility.

2. **Sucralfate** is preferred if gastric emptying is inadequate for enteral tube feedings, but there is some movement of fluid out of the stomach into the small bowel.

Dose: A sucralfate suspension is made by diluting 1 g of the drug in 10 to 20 ml sterile water. The suspension is instilled into the stomach every 6 to 8 hours.

3. **Histamine (H2) Blockers** are given intravenously when gastric emptying is severely compromised. Continuous infusion is more effective than bolus administration of the drugs.[17,24] The recommended doses for two H2 blockers are shown below.

CIMETIDINE[17,24]

Start with a loading dose of 300 mg over 5 minutes. Follow with a continuous infusion at 37.5 mg/hr. Monitor gastric pH and increase infusion rate in increments of 25 mg/hr to keep gastric pH above 4.0. The maximum infusion rate is 100 mg/hr.

RANITIDINE[25]

Start with a loading dose of 0.5 mg/kg given over 30 minutes. Follow with a continuous infusion at 0.25 mg/kg/hr. **End-point:** pH > 4 in gastric aspirates obtained every 2 to 4 hours (see below).

4. **Antacids** are the least popular of the prophylaxis strategies, primarily because antacid titration is time-consuming and is no more ef-

fective than other regimens. The following antacid regimen has proven effective.[26]

Dose: Instill 30 ml of antacid and check gastric pH in 1 hour. If pH is below 4.0, give 60 ml and repeat sequence until pH is 4.0 or above. The antacid is given at 1 to 2 hr intervals and the pH is monitored at the time the antacid is instilled. Make sure to clamp the nasogastric tube between doses. If there is vomiting, apply nasogastric suction for 30 minutes each hour.

MONITORING PRACTICES

The gastric secretions can be monitored for pH and occult blood during prophylaxis, but this practice has its limitations.
Gastric pH
There are several problems with gastric pH monitoring:
1. There is no agreement on the optimal pH to maintain.
2. There is no correlation between the pH of gastric aspirates and the incidence of gross hemorrhage.[27]
3. There is poor correlation between the pH of gastric aspirates and the pH at the surface of the gastric mucosa.[28]
4. The use of pH monitoring does not reduce the incidence of significant bleeding.[8]
The last observation is particularly damaging to pH monitoring. To obviate pH monitoring and its problems, use sucralfate whenever possible.

Occult Blood Testing. One problem with occult blood testing has already been mentioned; that is, the presence of occult blood will not predict who will develop gross hemorrhage. The other shortcoming with this test is the large number of false-positive and false-negative reactions. Oral iron should not cause a false-positive reaction[29] and the important sources of error are listed below:[29-31]

False-Positive Reactions	False-Negative Reactions
1. Cimetidine	1. Antacids
2. pH = 2 to 4	2. pH < 2
3. Red Meat	3. Vitamin C
4. Horseradish	
5. Raw Turnips	
6. Apples/Oranges/Bananas	

The Hemoccult test (Smith, Kline & French) should be reserved only for stool, while the Gastroccult test (Smith, Kline & French) is meant only for gastric secretions. The latter test is specifically designed to eliminate false-negative tests resulting from low pH in gastric secretions.[31]

REFERENCES

REVIEWS

1. Zuckerman GR, Cort D, Shuman RB. Stress ulcer syndrome. Intensive Care Med 1988; 3:21–31.

2. Del Guercio LRM. Factors for stress ulceration: Sepsis, shock, hepatic failure. J Crit Illness 1989; 3(Suppl):S26–S30.
3. Shorrock CJ, Rees WDW. Overview of gastroduodenal mucosal protection. Am J Med 1988; 84(Suppl 2A):25–34.
4. Miller TA. Mechanisms of stress-related mucosal damage. Am J Med 1987; 83:(Suppl 6A):8–14.
5. Bailey RW, Bulkley GB, Hamilton SR, et al. The fundamental hemodynamic mechanism underlying gastric "stress ulceration" in cardiogenic shock. Ann Surg 1987; 205:597–612.

PROPHYLAXIS STRATEGIES

6. Peura DA, Johnson LF. Cimetidine for prevention and treatment of gastroduodenal mucosal lesions in patients in an intensive care unit. Ann Intern Med 1985; 103:173–177.
7. Zuckerman GR, Shuman R. Therapeutic goals and treatment options for prevention of stress ulcer syndrome. Am J Med. 1987; 83(Suppl 6A):29–35.
8. Shuman RB, Schuster DP, Zuckerman GR. Prophylactic therapy for stress ulcer bleeding: A reappraisal. Ann Intern Med 1987; 106:562–567.
9. Schuster DP, Rowley H, Feinstein S, et al. Prospective evaluation of the risk of upper gastrointestinal bleeding after admission to a medical intensive care unit. Am J Med 1984; 76:623–630.
10. Zuckerman G, Welch R, Douglas A, et al. Controlled trial of medical therapy for active upper gastrointestinal bleeding and prevention of rebleeding. Am J Med 1984; 76:361–366.
11. Pingleton SK, Hadzima S. Enteral alimentation and gastrointestinal bleeding in mechanically ventilated patients. Crit Care Med 1983; 11:13–15.
12. Pingleton SR. Gastric bleeding and/or (?) enteral feeding. Chest 1986, 90:2–3.
13. Szabo S, Hollander D. Pathways of gastrointestinal protection and repair: Mechanisms of action of sucralfate. Am J Med 1989; 86(Suppl A):23–31.
14. Borrero E, Bank S, Margolis I, et al. Comparison of antacid and sucralfate in the prevention of gastrointestinal bleeding in patients who are critically ill. Am J Med 1985; 79(Suppl 2C):62–64.
15. Tryba M. Risk of acute stress bleeding and nosocomial pneumonia in ventilated intensive care unit patients: Sucralfate versus antacids. Am J Med 1987; 83(Suppl 3B):117–124.
16. Driks MR, Craven DE, Celli BR, et al. Nosocomial pneumonia in intubated patients given sucralfate as compared with antacids or histamine type 2 blockers. N Engl J Med 1987; 317:1376–1382.
17. Kingsley AN. Prophylaxis for acute stress ulcers. Antacids or cimetidine. Am Surg 1985; 51:545–547.
18. Sherman RA, Hwang ER, Walker JA, Elsinger RP. Reduction in serum phosphorous due to sucralfate. Am J Gastroenterol 1983; 78:210–211.

GASTRIC ACID AND INFECTION

19. Howden CW, Hunt RH. Relationship between gastric secretion and infection. Gut 1987; 28:96–107.
20. Craven DE, Driks MR. Nosocomial pneumonia in the intubated patient. Sem Respir Med 1987; 2:20–33.
21. Craven DE, Kunches LM, Kilinsky V, et al. Risk factors for pneumonia and fatality in patients receiving continuous mechanical ventilation. Am Rev Respir Dis 1986; 133:792–796.

22. Pingleton SK, Hinthorn DR, Liu C. Enteral nutrition in patients receiving mechanical ventilation. Am J Med 1986; *80*:827–832.
23. Wilmore D, Smith RJ, O'Dweyer ST, et al. The gut: A central organ after surgical stress. Surgery 1988; *104*:917–923.

DOSE RECOMMENDATIONS

24. Ostro MJ, Russel JA, Soldin SJ, et al. Control of gastric pH with cimetidine: Boluses versus primed infusions. Gastroenterol 1985; *89*:532–537.
25. Rigaud D, Chastre J, Accary JP, et al. Intragastric pH during acute respiratory failure in patients with chronic obstructive pulmonary disease. Effect of ranitidine and enteral feeding. Chest 1986; *90*:58–63.
26. Glotzer D. Stress ulcer bleeding control in critically ill patients. J Crit Illness 1989; *3*(Suppl):S59–S64.

MONITORING

27. Fiddian-Green RG, McGough E, Pittinger G, Rothman E. Predictive value of intramural pH and other risk factors for massive bleeding from stress ulceration. Gastroenterol 1983; *85*:613–620.
28. Meiners D, Clift S, Kaminski D. Evaluation of various techniques to monitor intra-gastric pH. Arch Surg 1982; *117*:288–291.
29. McDonnell WM, Ryan JA, Seeger DM, Elta G. Effect of iron on the guaiac reaction. Gastroenterol 1989; *96*:74–78.
30. Layne E, Mellow MH, Lipman TO. Insensitivity of guiac slide tests for detection of blood in gastric juice. Ann Intern Med 1981; *94*:774–776.
31. Long PC, Wilentz KV, Sudlow G, et al. Modification of the hemoccult slide test for occult blood in gastric juice. Crit Care Med 1982; *10*:692–693.

6

NOSOCOMIAL DIARRHEA

Diarrhea can occur in 50% of the patients who stay in the ICU for more than a few days.[1] Although sometimes considered a nuisance more than an illness, diarrhea is now recognized as a potentially life-threatening disorder. This chapter will present the hospital-acquired diarrheas, particularly those caused by antibiotics and enteral tube feedings.

PATHOPHYSIOLOGY

There is surprisingly little agreement about the definition of diarrhea, despite its prevalence. The popular definitions include the following:[2]
1. Stool weight > 200 grams/day
2. Liquid stools
3. More than 3 or 4 stools/day
4. Any increase in number of stools/day

The major feature of nosocomial diarrhea is a liquid consistency.

CLASSIFICATION

There are four major types of diarrhea, each produced by different mechanisms.
1. **Osmotic Diarrhea.** Ingestion of poorly absorbed substances will draw water into the bowel lumen and produce liquid stools.
Common Causes:
1. Enteral feedings
2. Magnesium

The hallmark of osmotic diarrhea is the tendency to resolve when the inciting substance is removed.[1] The other feature of osmotic diarrhea is the **osmolar gap** in the stool, or the difference between measured and calculated osmolality of the stool. In osmotic diarrhea, the calculated osmolality is 100 mmole/L less than the measured value, while the difference is less than 100 mmole/L in the other types of diarrhea. The osmolality of a stool sample can be calculated as follows:[2]

$$Stool\ Osmolality = 2 \times (Na + K)$$

where Na is the sodium concentration and K is the potassium concentration in the stool.

2. **Secretory Diarrhea.** The small bowel normally secretes a large volume of electrolyte-rich fluid (9 L per day), but much of it is absorbed before reaching the colon. Any process that produces a net increase in secretion over absorption will produce a secretory diarrhea.

Common Causes:
1. Antibiotics
2. Drugs (e.g., theophylline)
3. Bile Acids
4. Laxatives (e.g., bisacodyl)

Secretory diarrhea does not resolve when osmotic fluids (e.g., enteral feedings) are withdrawn. In addition, there is no osmolar gap in the stool.

3. **Exudative Diarrhea.** This results from damage to the bowel mucosa, which allows protein and blood to spill into the bowel lumen.

Common causes:
1. Pseudomembranous enterocolitis
2. Intestinal Ischemia
3. Inflammatory Bowel Disease

Exudative diarrheas are characterized by the appearance of red blood cells and leukocytes in the stool. Gross blood is uncommon.

4. **Motility Diarrhea.** Either an increase or decrease in peristalsis can produce diarrhea. Hypermotility reduces absorption time, and hypomotility promotes stasis and bacterial overgrowth.

Common causes:
1. Diabetes Mellitus
2. Hyperthyroidism
3. Partial bowel obstruction

Motility diarrhea behaves much like the secretory diarrheas.

ANTIBIOTIC-ASSOCIATED DIARRHEA

Antibiotics may be the most common cause of diarrhea in the ICU by virtue of their widespread use in this patient population.

Any antibiotic is a potential offender, except oral vancomycin and possibly the aminoglycosides.[3,4]

Antibiotic-associated diarrhea can appear weeks after the antibiotic is stopped,[4] which means that virtually every case of nosocomial diarrhea in the ICU may be antibiotic related.

The diarrheal syndromes associated with antibiotic therapy can vary widely in severity,[5] according to the degree of inflammation produced in the bowel mucosa. The mildest syndrome is characterized by watery diarrhea with no inflammatory changes in the bowel, and is called "simple diarrhea." The advanced forms are associated with widespread inflammation of the large bowel and raised plaque-like lesions on the mucosal surface called pseudomembranes. The pseudomembranous form of colitis can be life-threatening, with a reported mortality of 10 to 20%.[5]

PATHOGENESIS

The consensus at the present time is that most cases of antibiotic-associated diarrhea are caused by *Clostridium difficile,* an enteric organism that proliferates when the normal bowel flora is altered by antibiotic therapy.[6–8] This organism is not invasive, but produces a cytotoxin that damages the mucosa of the large bowel.[6] *C. difficile* is readily transmitted from patient to patient by contact with contaminated objects (e.g., toilet facilities) or by the hands of hospital personnel.[6–8]

> *Clostridium difficile* has been isolated from the stool in as many as 40% of hospitalized patients, and is found on the hands of 50% of the hospital staff in contact with culture-positive patients.[6,7]

Over half of the patients who harbor the organism in their stool are asymptomatic.[6,7] Transmission via hospital staff can lead to widespread dissemination of the organism and epidemic outbreaks of diarrhea. This stresses the need for strict enteric isolation precautions to control the spread of this organism. The enteric isolation precautions recommended by the Centers for Disease Control are in the Appendix at the end of the book.

CLINICAL PRESENTATION

The diarrhea can appear during antibiotic therapy, but in almost half the cases it appears 2 to 10 weeks after antibiotic therapy is discontinued.[3,4] The diarrhea is usually watery and not grossly bloody.[4] Simple diarrhea is unaccompanied by other findings, while the inflammatory diarrheas are associated with fever and other signs of systemic illness. The manifestations of pseudomembranous colitis are listed in Table 6–1.

Toxic megacolon is a rare complication of pseudomembranous colitis,[9] but this condition can be fatal unless recognized early and treated aggressively. The cardinal signs of toxic megacolon are abdominal distention and ileus. Rebound tenderness is a variable finding. Abdominal films reveal dilated loops of colon and the mucosa and may show "thumbprinting".[9] When toxic megacolon is suspected, medical therapy

TABLE 6–1. CLINICAL MANIFESTATIONS OF
PSEUDOMEMBRANOUS COLITIS

Manifestation	Frequency
Watery Diarrhea	90–95%
Bloody Diarrhea	5–10%
Fever	80%
Leukocytosis	80%
Abdominal Pain	80–90%
Rebound Tenderness	10–20%

From Tedesco FJ. Pseudomembranous colitis: Pathogenesis and therapy. Med Clin North Am 1982; 66:655–664.

should be started immediately and emergency surgery should be considered.[9]

DIAGNOSIS

The diagnosis of *Clostridium difficile* enterocolitis requires an assay for the cytotoxin in the stool or an endoscopic examination of the large bowel mucosa.

Toxin Assay. The stool assay for *Clostridium difficile* cytotoxin may differ in different hospitals. The tissue culture assay is the most reliable method but is not available in many hospitals at the present time. The popular assay is a latex agglutination test, but this can be unreliable. The interpretation of the toxin assay must be determined by the experience at your hospital.

Using a tissue culture assay, a positive toxin assay secures the diagnosis, since false positive assays are rare.[3] The prevalence of positive toxin assays (tissue culture method) in different patient groups is shown in Table 6–2.

Asymptomatic carriers can have a negative toxin assay despite a positive culture.[3,7] One negative toxin assay should not exclude the diagnosis of *Clostridium difficile*, because the sensitivity of an assay can vary.[4] The value of repeat assays when the first is negative is not clear, but serial testing is recommended when there is a high suspicion for the disease.

TABLE 6–2. PREVALENCE OF *C. DIFFICILE* TOXIN BY TISSUE CULTURE ASSAY IN ANTIBIOTIC-ASSOCIATED DIARRHEA

Condition	% Positive Assays	Reference
1. Asymptomatic	2	3
2. Simple Diarrhea	20	5
3. Non-Specific Colitis	70	5
4. Pseudomembranous Colitis	>90	3

TABLE 6–3. TREATMENT FOR *CLOSTRIDIUM DIFFICILE* COLITIS		
Agent	**Dose**	**Comments**
Vancomycin (oral)	250–500 mg q 6 h	a. Agent of choice b. 20% relapse rate
Metronidazole (oral or IV)	500 mg q 6h	a. Effective when oral Rx not possible
Cholestyramine (oral)	4 gm q 8h	a. Effective as sole Rx in mild cases b. Binds antibiotics as well
Duration of Rx: 7 to 14 days		

Proctosigmoidoscopy. Endoscopic inspection of the large bowel mucosa is the procedure of choice for the diagnosis of inflammatory colitis. Proctosigmoidoscopy is easily performed at the bedside and is recommended for all cases of diarrhea when there is suspicion for *Clostridium difficile* colitis and the toxin assay is repeatedly negative. On occasion, inflammatory lesions are confined to the right side of the colon and will not be evident on proctosigmoidoscopy.[4]

TREATMENT

The first step in treating suspected antibiotic-associated colitis is to stop antibiotics if possible (except aminoglycosides) and place the patient on enteric isolation precautions (see Appendix). The drug therapy for *Clostridium difficile* colitis is shown in Table 6–3.

1. **Oral Vancomycin (250–500 mg PO every 6 hrs)** is presently the therapy of choice, although as many as 20% of patients will relapse after therapy is completed.[4] Symptoms usually subside within 2 to 3 days of starting therapy, but the therapy is continued for 7 to 14 days. Intravenous therapy is ineffective.

2. **Metronidazole (500 mg PO or IV every 6 hrs)** is an effective alternative to vancomycin,[4] and is indicated when oral therapy is not advised. Therapy is continued for 7 to 14 days in responsive cases.

3. **Cholestyramine (4 grams PO every 8 hrs)** is a resin that binds the cytotoxin and has been effective as sole therapy in mild cases of diarrhea.[4] This agent can also be added to vancomycin therapy but must be given between antibiotic doses because it binds antibiotics. **The use of resins is appealing because they will not suppress the normal bowel flora** and will not favor the persistence of *Clostridium difficile* in the stool.

The response to therapy is usually prompt and the clinical manifestations subside within 2 to 3 days.[4] Agents that reduce bowel motility (e.g., opiates) should be avoided because they increase the risk of toxic megacolon.[9] If the illness progresses during therapy, watch closely for toxic megacolon.

DIARRHEA FROM TUBE FEEDINGS

Diarrhea will develop in 30 to 60% of patients who are receiving enteral tube feedings.[1,12] The popularity of tube feedings is increasing and this will increase the prevalence of this diarrheal syndrome in the ICU.

PATHOGENESIS

Several factors may be responsible for promoting an osmotic diarrhea from enteral tube feedings. Some of these are listed below.[10-13]
1. Hyperosmolar or high lipid formulas
2. Bolus feedings or small bowel feedings
3. Atrophy of the small bowel mucosa
4. Hypoalbuminemia

The osmolality of feeding formulas has been given a prominent role in the diarrhea but the evidence is not convincing.[12] Many of the newer commercial feeding formulas are isotonic and should not pose a problem. Electrolyte and drug additives can be hyperosmolar and may promote diarrhea in some cases.[13]

Mucosal Atrophy. The mucosal surface of the small bowel shows degenerative changes when the bowel is placed at rest for more than a few days. This phenomenon is described in more detail in Chapter 40 and is shown in Figure 40–1. The loss of surface area for nutrient absorption results in malabsorption and an osmotic diarrhea. The atrophic changes appear during full intravenous nutrition and are believed to be the direct result of eliminating nutrients from the bowel lumen.[11,14] Atrophy of the small bowel mucosa is responsible for the refeeding diarrhea seen after prolonged periods of bowel rest.[14]

Hypoalbuminemia. A low serum albumin will reduce the serum colloid osmotic pressure and thereby promote the transudation of fluid out of the capillaries in the bowel wall (see Chapter 23). This has been used to explain the often noted association between hypoalbuminemia and diarrhea from tube feedings.[15] However, the results of other studies are conflicting.[12,16] Furthermore, other conditions that alter the Starling forces in favor of edema formation (e.g., portal hypertension) are not known to produce diarrhea.[17] At the present time, the role of hypoalbuminemia in promoting diarrhea from tube feedings is not clear. It is possible that hypoalbuminemia and diarrhea are merely markers of severe illness and are not causally linked. This area requires further study.

CLINICAL PRESENTATION

The onset of diarrhea usually occurs within 2 weeks after the commencement of tube feedings.[1] The stools are watery and devoid of blood. Fever should not be a feature of this diarrheal syndrome.

Necrotizing Enterocolitis is a rare but serious form of diarrhea that occurs during small bowel feeding in elderly patients with heart failure or peripheral vascular disease.[18] The clinical manifestations include fever, painful abdominal distention, and diarrhea that may be grossly bloody. The underlying problem is bowel ischemia and bacterial invasion of the bowel wall. The ischemia may be due to inability to increase mesenteric blood flow in response to the increase in mucosal activity associated with absorption of foodstuffs.

DIAGNOSIS

The hallmark of tube feeding diarrhea is its disappearance when the feedings are stopped. However, this may take a few days to become evident and this time delay could lead to serious consequences if the diarrhea is due to *Clostridium difficile* colitis. It is no surprise that C. *difficile* can appear during enteral tube feedings,[11] and this diagnosis should be eliminated in all patients who develop diarrhea during tube feedings and have received antibiotics within the past few weeks.

> The diagnosis of *Clostridium difficile* colitis must be entertained in all cases of diarrhea that appear during enteral feeding, even in the absence of fever.

The absence of fever is against the diagnosis of *Clostridium difficile* colitis, but 20% of patients with toxin-related diarrhea will not have a fever (see Table 6–1).

The osmolar gap of the stool might help to differentiate tube feeding (osmotic) diarrhea from toxin-related (secretory) diarrhea. However, the reliability of this test has not been evaluated in the ICU patient population.

TREATMENT

The goal of treating tube feeding diarrhea is to eliminate the responsible factor (e.g., hyperosmolar formulas), while avoiding total bowel rest to limit the tendency for mucosal atrophy and refeeding diarrhea.[10–14] The exception is necrotizing enterocolitis, where feedings must be stopped immediately. The following maneuvers may be effective:

1. **Reduce osmolality** by using isotonic feeding solutions and eliminating hyperosmolar additives. If the diarrhea occurs during isotonic feedings, it does not seem wise to dilute the feeding further because this will increase the water content in the bowel. In this situation, you can reduce the volume of the feeding by reducing the infusion rate (step C).

2. **Use intragastric feeding** if possible. The gastric secretions will reduce the osmolality of the solution entering the small bowel, and the gastric distention will slow the transit time. If there is a concern about regurgitation, add methylene blue or a suitable food coloring to the solution and observe the color of the tracheobronchial secretions.

3. **Reduce infusion rate** to reduce the total osmolar load on the bowel. The infusion rate can be cut in half or further if necessary. If this is

TABLE 6–4. MAGNESIUM CONTENT OF COMMONLY USED MEDICATIONS	
Preparation	Magnesium (mEq/5 ml)
Antacids	
1. Maalox Concentrate	10
2. Riopan	8
3. Mylanta	7
4. Gelusil	7
Laxatives	
1. Milk of Magnesia USP	13
2. Magnesium sulfate	8
From Oster JR, Epstein M. Management of magnesium depletion. Am J Nephrol 1988; 8:349–354.	

effective, the infusion rate is increased gradually over the next few days to the desired volume.[10]

4. **Avoid complete bowel rest** if possible, to maintain the absorptive surface of the bowel and limit the risk for refeeding diarrhea. Try to maintain enteral feedings at whatever volume is tolerated. The only situations where the feedings should be stopped completely are those where bowel ischemia or toxic megacolon are possible. Continue to deliver the nutritional requirements via the intravenous route until full enteral nutrition is resumed.

MISCELLANEOUS CONDITIONS

MEDICATIONS

The following agents may be responsible for diarrhea in selected patients. Only the agents that might be used in the ICU are included here.

Magnesium is a common constituent of antacid preparations, and can cause an osmotic diarrhea. The magnesium content of some commonly used medications is shown in Table 6–4. Laxatives are included for comparison.

The magnesium-containing antacids should be stopped in any patient with diarrhea, regardless of the etiology. Alternatives to antacids for the prophylaxis of stress ulcers are presented in the last chapter.

Cimetidine has been implicated as a cause of diarrhea in the ICU,[1] presumably as a result of bacterial overgrowth in the stomach and small bowel.[19] However, recent studies fail to show an association between diarrhea and histamine H2 blockers.[12] This issue requires further evaluation.

Theophylline can cause a secretory diarrhea by increasing the secretion of sodium and chloride in the distal small bowel.[20] The prevalence of diarrhea during theophylline therapy is not reported.

TABLE 6–5. CLINICAL FINDINGS IN 20 PATIENTS WITH BOWEL INFARCTION	
Clinical Finding	Number of Patients
Abdominal Pain	15
Abdominal Tenderness	15
Occult Blood in Stool	13
Metabolic Acidosis	9
Diarrhea	7
Bloody Diarrhea	5
Absent Bowel Sounds	7
Rigid Abdomen	3
Bowel Edema on X-Ray	1

From Cooke M, Sande MA. Diagnosis and outcome of bowel infarction on an acute medical service. Am J Med 1983; 75:984–991.

Quinidine can cause diarrhea in one-third of patients who take the drug orally.[21] The incidence of diarrhea during parenteral therapy is unknown.

ISCHEMIC INJURY

Ischemic damage to the bowel mucosa can cause an exudative diarrhea that may or may not be associated with gross blood in the stool. There is little published experience concerning the diarrhea from bowel infarction. The clinical presentation of bowel infarction in one study is shown in Table 6–5. Only 7 of 20 patients in this study had diarrhea, but the stools were visibly bloody in 5 of the 7 patients. Note that the characteristic features of bowel infarction (e.g., metabolic acidosis) were frequently absent, emphasizing the difficulty in making the clinical diagnosis of bowel infarction prior to laparotomy. Although this is a small study group, there are no other studies on the subject.

Diarrhea that appears within a few days of cardiac arrest or hypotension can signal the appearance of ischemic mucosal injury from reperfusion or the "no reflow" phenomenon (see Chapter 12). The diarrhea in this situation should contain blood, but there are no studies available on this aspect of postischemic syndromes.

BEDSIDE APPROACH TO DIARRHEA

The following bedside approach is recommended for all acute onset diarrhea except bloody diarrhea. The latter condition is a medical emergency that requires invasive hemodynamic monitoring and other measures not covered in the outline that follows. The flow diagram in Figure 6–1 shows the steps involved in this approach to diarrhea.

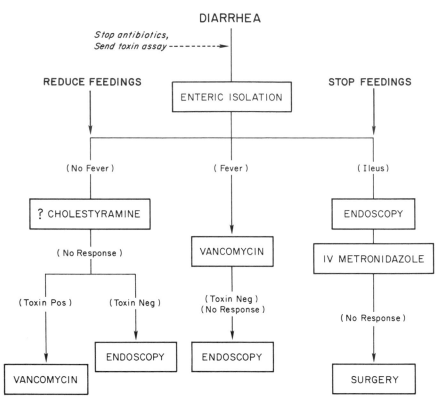

FIG. 6–1. Flow diagram for the bedside approach to nosocomial diarrhea. This approach does not apply to bloody diarrhea.

I. Universal measures
  A. Consider *Clostridium difficile* colitis.
    1. Send stool for *C. difficile* toxin.
    2. Institute enteric isolation precautions.

These measures are recommended in the initial approach to all diarrheas in the ICU because of the prevalence of *C. difficile* colitis in this patient population. If the toxin assay is not available, consider bedside endoscopy in high risk patients.

II. Specific Measures
    The presence of fever, ileus and other signs of sepsis will dictate the specific approach in each patient.
  A. Ileus and Abdominal Distention
    1. Stop all oral feedings.
    2. Consider emergent bedside endoscopy to look for ischemia, pseudomembranes or inflammation.
    3. Obtain abdominal films to look for partial obstruction, bowel wall edema, or other evidence of ischemia.
    4. Check hemodynamic status in select individuals, particularly

if there has been recent hypotension or cardiovascular instability.
5. Start intravenous metronidazole (500 mg every 6h) if there is
no evidence for ischemia or partial obstruction.

The major concerns with an ileus are ischemia, necrotizing enterocolitis,
pseudomembranous colitis, and toxic megacolon. The intravenous
metronidazole is started until a diagnosis is reached.
  B. Fever with or without other signs of sepsis.
    1. Start oral vancomycin (500 mg every 6h).
    2. Bedside endoscopy if the toxin assay is unavailable or negative.
      a. If mucosal inflammation is present, start therapy with van-
      comycin or metronidazole.
      b. If the mucosa appears normal, consider therapy with cho-
      lestyramine, and search for another cause of the problem.

Fever should not be a presenting feature of diarrhea from tube feedings,
and the leading diagnosis will be *Clostridium difficile* colitis. Most cases
of *C. difficile* will show some resolution of the fever and other symptoms
within 2 to 3 days of starting vancomycin. Diarrhea that persists beyond
this point suggests another underlying process.
  C. Diarrhea with no other findings.
    1. If tube feedings are present:
      a. Reduce lipid content if possible.
      b. Eliminate electrolyte and drug additives.
      c. Reduce daily volume by 50%.
    2. Discontinue any potentially offending drugs, including anti-
    biotics (if possible), theophylline, and magnesium-containing
    antacids.
    3. Consider trial of cholestyramine (4 g PO every 8h).
    4. If diarrhea does not subside:
      a. Start oral vancomycin.
      b. Obtain bedside endoscopy to search for mucosal inflam-
      mation.
      c. Repeat toxin assay if original assay was negative.

Diarrhea with no associated clinical findings could represent "simple"
antibiotic-associated diarrhea. Cholestyramine might help to bind any
toxin-mediated process. Diarrhea that persists after initial workup needs
repeat evaluation for *Clostridium difficile* colitis. Close observation is the
password in this situation.

REFERENCES

1. Kelly TWJ, Patrick MR, Hillman KM. Study of diarrhea in critically ill patients. Crit
   Care Med 1983; *11*:7–9.
2. Cooper BT. Diarrhoea as a symptom. Clin Gastroenterol 1985; *14*:599–613.

ANTIBIOTIC-ASSOCIATED DIARRHEA

3. Bartlett JG, Taylor NS, Chang T, et al. Clinical and laboratory observations in *Clostridium difficile* colitis. Am J Clin Nutr 1980; *33*:2521–2526.
4. Tedesco FJ. Pseudomembranous colitis: Pathogenesis and therapy. Med Clin North Am 1982; *66*:655–664.
5. Bartlett JG. New developments in infectious disease for the critical care physician. Crit Care Med 1983; *11*:563–573.
6. McFarland LV, Mulligan ME, Kwok RYY, Stamm WE. Nosocomial acquisition of *Clostridium difficile* infection. N Engl J Med 1988; *320*:204–210.
7. Kim KH, Fekety R, Batts DH, et al. Isolation of *Clostridium difficile* from the environment and contacts of patients with antibiotic-associated colitis. J Infect Dis 1981; *143*:42–50.
8. Fekety R, Kim KH, Brown D, et al. Epidemiology of antibiotic-associated colitis. Isolation of Clostridium difficile from the hospital environment. Am J Med 1981; *70*:906–908.
9. Van Ness MM, Cattau EL Jr. Fulminant colitis complicating antibiotic-associated pseudomembranous colitis: Case report and review of the clinical manifestations and treatment. Am J Gastroenterol 1987; *82*:375–377.

ENTERAL FEEDINGS

10. Cataldi-Betcher EL, Seltzer MS, Slocum BA, et al. Complications occurring during enteral nutrition support: A prospective study. J Parenter Ent Nutr 1983; *7*:546–552.
11. Koruda MJ, Geunter P, Rombeau JL. Enteral nutrition in the critically ill. Crit Care Clin 1987; *3*:133–154.
12. Gottschlich MM, Warden GD, Michel M, Havens P, et al. Diarrhea in tube-fed burn patients: Incidence, etiology, nutritional impact, and prevention. J Parenter Ent Nutr 1988; *12*:338–345.
13. Niemiec PW, Vanderveen TW, Morrison JI, et al. Gastrointestinal disorders caused by medication and electrolyte solution osmolality during enteral nutrition. J Parenter Ent Nutr 1983; *7*:387–389.
14. Randall HT. Enteral Nutrition: Tube feeding in acute and chronic illness. J Parenter Ent Nutr 1984; *8*:113–136.
15. Brinson RR, Kolts BE. Hypoalbuminemia as an indicator of diarrheal incidence in critically ill patients. Crit Care Med 1987; *15*:506–509.
16. Foreman ML, Dominquez BA, Lyman B, Cuddy PG, Pemberton MD. Enteral feeding with hypoalbuminaemia. J Parenter Ent Nutr 1989; *13*:13S.
17. Norman DA, Atkins JM, Seelig LL, et al. Water and electrolyte movement and mucosal morphology in the jejunum of patients with portal hypertension. Gastroenterol 1980; *79*:707–715.
18. Grant JP. Nutrition-related complications in critically ill patients. In: Lumb PL, Bryan-Brown CW eds. Complications in Critical Care Medicine. Chicago: Year Book Medical Publishers, 1988; 220–247.

MISCELLANEOUS

19. Ruddell WSJ, Losowsky MS. Severe diarrhea due to small intestinal colonisation during cimetidine treatment. Br Med J 1980; *281*:273.
20. Dobbins JW, Binder HJ. Pathophysiology of diarrhea: Alterations in fluid and electrolyte transport. Clin Gastroenterol 1981; *10*:605–625.
21. Huang SK, Marcus FI. Antiarrhythmic drug therapy of ventricular arrhythmias. Curr Probl Cardiol 1986; *11*:182–240.

c h a p t e r

THE THREAT OF
THROMBOEMBOLISM

Certain groups of patients are prone to thrombosis in the deep venous system of the legs. If the clots involve the large proximal veins in the thigh, they can embolize to the lungs. Fatal pulmonary embolism is the most feared consequence of leg thrombosis and occurs in up to 5% of patients at risk.[1-4] Several approaches are used to reduce the risk of thromboembolism in select patients, and these measures may save up to 8,000 lives each year.[4]

The approach that follows proceeds in three stages. The first stage identifies the patients at risk for thrombosis. The second stage selects the most appropriate preventive measures for each patient group. The final stage outlines an approach to suspected pulmonary embolism.

PATIENTS AT RISK

Table 7–1 lists the reported incidence of deep venous thrombosis (DVT) and fatal pulmonary embolism (PE) in different groups of patients in the absence of preventive measures.[1-5] Most of the patients at risk are in the postoperative period, with hip and knee surgery heading the list. Several factors promote thrombosis in the immediate postoperative period, including venous stasis, endothelial damage (from trauma or leg surgery), and a generalized hypercoagulable state (from thromboplastin release during surgery, and depressed levels of antithrombin III).

ORTHOPEDIC SURGERY

Reconstructive surgery of the hip and knee carries the highest risk for thromboembolism. Over 50% of these patients can develop DVT after

TABLE 7–1. RISK FACTORS IN THROMBOEMBOLISM[1,5]		
Patient Group	**DVT**	**Fatal PE***
Hip and Knee Surgery	40–70%	1–3%
General Surgery		
High Risk	30–60%	1–2%
Moderate Risk	10–40%	<1%
Low Risk	<3%	<.01%
Neurosurgery	25–50%	1–3%
Prostate Surgery	10–40%	
Medical Illness		
Acute MI	20–40%	<1%
Stroke	60%	
Other	10%	
*Indicates incidence without prophylaxis		

surgery, and 3% of patients will succumb to fatal pulmonary embolism. This group of patients is the most resistant to prophylaxis.

GENERAL SURGERY

The risk factors associated with DVT after elective procedures in the thorax and abdomen are classified as follows:[2]

High Risk: Recent history of DVT or PE; Extensive pelvic or abdominal surgery for malignancy.

Moderate Risk: Patient aged older than 40 years and procedure longer than 30 minutes.

Low Risk: Patient aged younger than 40 years with no other risk factors.

Over half of the patients in the high-risk group can develop postoperative DVT unless prophylactic measures are used (see Table 7–1). Patients with no risk factors have a minimal risk of thrombosis and routine prophylaxis is not necessary in these patients unless early ambulation is not possible.

OTHER SURGERY

Neurosurgery carries the same risk for postoperative DVT as does general surgery for high risk patients. Urologic procedures vary in risk from 10% (transurethral prostatectomy) to 40% (retropubic prostatectomy). Prophylaxis in these patient groups is guided by the risk of bleeding.

TABLE 7–2. STRATEGIES FOR PROPHYLAXIS[1,2]	
Patient Group	**Recommendations**
I. General Surgery	
A. High Risk	A. Low-dose heparin (q 8h) and pneumatic device or adjusted–dose heparin
B. Moderate Risk	B. Low–dose heparin (q 12h) or Dextran
C. Low Risk	C. TED stockings
II. Orthopedic	
A. Hip Surgery	A. Adjusted–dose heparin or adjusted–dose warfarin or Dextran and pneumatic device
B. Hip Fracture	B. Adjusted–dose warfarin or Dextran
C. Knee Surgery	C. Pneumatic calf compression
III. Neurosurgery and Prostate Surgery	Pneumatic calf compression
IV. Stroke and Acute MI	Low-dose heparin (q 12h)

MEDICAL CONDITIONS

There are only two medical conditions with a clearly defined risk for DVT and PE; these are stroke and acute myocardial infarction. **Obesity is not a proven risk factor for thromboembolism,** contrary to the popular belief.[5]

BLEEDING DISORDERS

The presence of an underlying coagulopathy does not eliminate the risk for DVT and PE.[6] However, the risk is small.

APPROACHES TO PROPHYLAXIS

Prophylaxis for thrombosis includes anticoagulants, leg compression devices, or filters placed in the inferior vena cava. The following is a brief outline of each method. Table 7–2 lists the recommended approaches for individual groups of patients.

LOW-DOSE HEPARIN

Dose: 5,000 IU subcutaneously every 8 to 12 hours. Start 2 hours prior to surgery, and continue until the patient is ambulatory.
Indications: All patients at risk, except those undergoing hip or knee surgery.
The principle behind low-dose heparin is the ability to inhibit thrombin formation with little or no risk of bleeding. The anticoagulant effect of heparin is produced in part by activation of antithrombin III, which

inhibits the conversion of prothrombin to thrombin. In the absence of active thrombosis, only small amounts of heparin are needed for this reaction. The dose is usually given every 12 hours but can be given every 8 hours in high-risk patients (Table 7–2). Coagulation does not need to be monitored during low-dose heparin therapy.

Low-dose heparin has been shown to reduce the incidence of postoperative DVT and fatal PE in large clinical trials,[1-4] but is without benefit following hip and knee surgery.

ULTRA LOW-DOSE HEPARIN

Dose: 1 IU/kg/hour as a continuous intravenous infusion.

Intravenous infusion of heparin has been recommended to reduce the discomfort and the hematomas associated with the subcutaneous route. This method is safe and effective,[7] but the clinical experience is limited at present.

ADJUSTED-DOSE HEPARIN

Dose: Start at 3,500 IU subQ every 8 hours, and adjust the dose to keep activated PTT at 1.5 times control.[8]

This regimen may be more effective than low-dose heparin for reducing the incidence of DVT after hip surgery.[8] However, postoperative DVT and PE continue to be a problem after hip surgery.

ADJUSTED-DOSE WARFARIN

Dose: Start at 10 mg PO each day, and adjust to keep the prothrombin time at 1.5 times control.

This regimen is equivalent to adjusted-dose heparin for prophylaxis,[2,9] but has a higher risk for bleeding. Despite this risk, oral anticoagulation is preferred by many for prophylaxis following hip and knee surgery.[2]

DEXTRAN

Dose: Dextran-40 at 500 ml per day, infused over 4 to 6 hours.

Dextrans are glucose polymers used as volume expanders (see Chapter 17). The major drawback to the dextrans has been their anticoagulant effects (e.g., reduced platelet adhesiveness). This property is used to advantage as a method of prophylaxis for postoperative DVT. Dextran-40 given in the above dose for 3 to 5 days after surgery has been effective in reducing postoperative DVT in moderate-risk abdominal surgery and elective hip surgery.[2] The major problem is the volume load in patients with left heart failure.

GRADED COMPRESSION (TED) STOCKINGS

TED (Thrombo Embolism Deterrent) stockings are designed to provide more compression distally (at the ankle) to propel blood towards the heart. These stockings are effective in routine prophylaxis for low-risk patients but are not recommended when there is a high risk for post-operative DVT.[2,10]

PNEUMATIC COMPRESSION DEVICES

Intermittent inflation of a pneumatic device wrapped around the lower leg is used to simulate the normal pumping action of the calf muscles (which can be lost during bed rest). These devices are effective in most high-risk patients,[2,3] but they do not prevent thigh thrombosis following hip surgery.[2] Pneumatic calf compression is devoid of side effects and is a popular method for neurosurgical or urologic patients who are at risk for bleeding.

SURGICAL PROPHYLAXIS

Surgical prophylaxis is aimed at preventing pulmonary embolism and does not itself prevent DVT in the legs. The popular method at present is to interrupt the inferior vena cava with a filter device. Indications for this approach include documented DVT above the knees or high-risk orthopedic surgery, plus any one of the following:[11]
1. Contraindication to anticoagulation
2. PE during full anticoagulation
3. Severe lung disease
4. Pulmonary hypertension

The most popular device at present is the Greenfield filter shown in Figure 7–1. This cone-shaped filter is mounted on a spring-loaded device and is inserted percutaneously via the internal jugular or femoral veins. Once situated below the renal veins, the filter is released and attaches to the vena cava by the hooks at the base. The long axis of the filter runs along the direction of blood flow and the elongated cone can trap clots without compromising the cross-sectional diameter of the vena cava.

The Greenfield filter is favored over other interruption devices because there is less tendency for caval obstruction and venous insufficiency in the legs. Once the filter is in place, the incidence of clinically evident pulmonary emboli is less than 3%.[11]

APPROACH TO SUSPECTED PULMONARY EMBOLISM

The prophylactic measures listed in Table 7–2 do not eliminate the risk for DVT and PE in high-risk patients, particularly orthopedic patients. Unfortunately, thrombosis in the thigh is often clinically silent

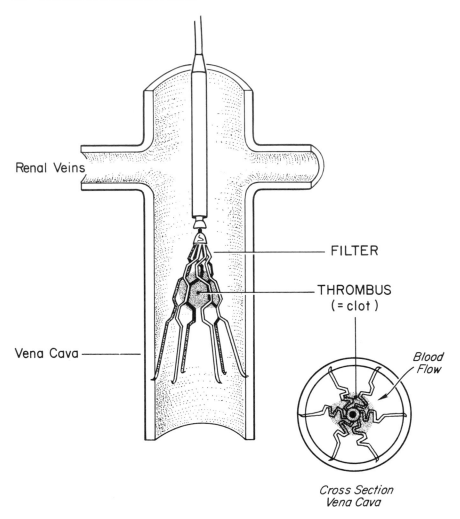

Renal Veins

FILTER

THROMBUS
(= clot)

Vena Cava

Blood
Flow

Cross Section
Vena Cava

FIG. 7–1. The Greenfield filter. Note how the cone traps the clot without compromising the cross sectional area of the vena cava.

and the problem is first suspected when a pulmonary embolus occurs. The following approach is, therefore, concerned with the patient who develops a clinical syndrome that is suggestive of acute pulmonary embolism.

CLINICAL PRESENTATION

The clinical features of pulmonary embolism are neither sensitive nor specific; i.e., there is no clinical finding that is always present (sensitivity) and no finding that is present in pulmonary emboli but not in other cardiopulmonary diseases (specificity). The sensitivity and specificity of

TABLE 7–3. CLINICAL FINDINGS IN PULMONARY EMBOLISM		
Finding	Sensitivity	Specificity
Dyspnea	0.74	0.38
Pleuritic Chest Pain	0.48	0.64
Hemoptysis	0.22	0.76
Tachypnea	0.48	0.80
Tachycardia	0.81	0.55
P_{O_2} below 80 mmHg	0.74	0.29
Infiltrate on Chest X-Ray	0.48	0.57

From Hoellerich VL, Wigton RS. Diagnosing pulmonary embolism using clinical findings. Arch Intern Med 1986; 146:1699–1704.

clinical findings in acute pulmonary embolism from one study are listed in Table 7–3.[12] Note that pleuritic chest pain is present in only half of the patients with documented emboli (sensitivity), while hypoxemia is absent in 25% of the patients. Because the clinical presentation will not confirm or exclude the presence of emboli, diagnostic tests are required in the evaluation. Figure 7–2 outlines an approach that can be used for any patient who is suspected of having pulmonary emboli.

THE SEARCH FOR LEG THROMBOSIS

The initial approach uses non-invasive tests to identify thrombosis in the thighs and does not attempt to document emboli in the lungs. The reason for this approach is simply that the emboli in the lungs are not the primary disease process but are manifestations of an underlying thrombosis in the legs.

> Most pulmonary emboli originate in the deep veins of the thigh, and thrombosis in these veins is evident by non-invasive testing in a majority of patients with acute pulmonary embolism.[13]

The routine therapy of uncomplicated pulmonary emboli is essentially the same as the therapy for leg thrombosis (i.e., anticoagulation) and the evaluation can stop if a thrombus is detected.

The evaluation of the legs will begin with two non-invasive tests that can be performed at the bedside. Contrast venography should be avoided whenever possible because of the cost and associated risks.

Impedance Plethysmography. Impedance plethysmography (IPG) is based on the principle that the electrical impedance of a tissue compartment is inversely related to the volume (of conducting electrolytes) of the compartment. Figure 7–3 illustrates the method used for detecting thrombosis in the deep veins of the thigh. Electrodes are wrapped around the upper calf and generate an imperceptible electric current through the lower leg. A blood pressure cuff placed around the thigh is inflated to impede venous outflow from the leg, causing a gradual increase in the volume of the calf (seen as an increase in the IPG tracing).

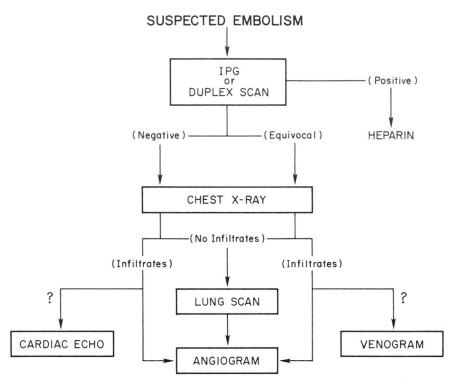

SUSPECTED EMBOLISM

FIG. 7–2. Flow diagram for the approach to a patient with suspected acute pulmonary embolism. See text for explanation.

When the cuff is suddenly deflated, the rate of venous outflow from the leg is equivalent to the rate of decline in the volume of the calf (seen as the slope of the terminal portion of the IPG tracing).

When the proximal thigh veins are filled with thrombi, two changes are evident in the IPG tracing (Fig. 7–3). First, the blood volume in the lower leg will be elevated and inflation of the cuff will produce less of an increment in the volume of the calf. As a result, the height of the IPG tracing will diminish. Second, the proximal vein thrombosis will reduce the rate of venous outflow and, therefore, the terminal slope of the IPG tracing will decrease.

> Impedance plethysmography is a reliable method for detecting thrombi in the deep veins of the thigh, but can miss thrombi in the veins below the knee.[15]

IPG has a sensitivity and specificity of about 90% for thigh thrombosis.[15] Only thrombi that completely obstruct the veins are detected and partially obstructing thrombi may be missed. The sensitivity for calf thrombosis is less than 70%.[15]

One of the problems with the IPG technique is the false-positive tests that are produced by increased venous pressure in the lower legs (e.g., heart failure and positive-pressure ventilation). These conditions are common in the ICU, and diminish the reliability of the test. A bilaterally

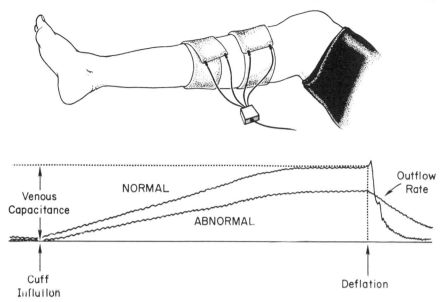

FIG. 7–3. Electrical impedance plethysmography for detecting proximal deep venous thrombosis.

abnormal IPG test result is of no value and only unilateral abnormalities are given diagnostic consideration.

Doppler Ultrasound. This is a promising technique that uses the reflection of an ultrasonic beam to evaluate blood flow. When the beam is directed at the femoral vein, moving blood cells will reflect the beam and change its frequency (the Doppler shift), whereas stationary blood cells in a thrombus will not alter the frequency in the reflected beam. The use of the Doppler ultrasound method in the evaluation of thromboembolism is in its infancy, but so far appears to be reliable when used properly.[16] However, reliability will be a function of the person performing the test, and the test must be validated at each center.

Contrast Venography. Venograms are reserved for patients who have equivocal findings on the IPG or Doppler ultrasound exams and who also have an abnormal chest x-ray. When the chest film is normal, a lung scan is preferred to venograms (see next section).

THE FINAL SEARCH FOR EMBOLI

The initial evaluation of the legs should curtail the need for lung scans and pulmonary angiograms. However, as many as 30% of patients with pulmonary emboli will show no evidence of leg thrombosis.[13] In other words, **normal tests for leg thrombosis do not rule out the possibility of an acute pulmonary embolus.** As shown in Figure 7–3, further tests to document the presence of emboli will be necessary when leg thrombosis is not evident.

Radionuclide Lung Scans. Lung scans should be reserved for situations where there is no evidence for leg thrombosis, and the chest x-ray shows clear lung fields or a small localized infiltrate only. **A normal lung scan can be used to rule out an embolus but an abnormal scan cannot always be used to rule in an embolus.** The practice of assigning a "probability" to an abnormal lung scan has become popular without any proof that this practice is valid. In other words, pulmonary angiograms have not been used to validate "low-probability" and "high-probability" scans. One study that compared scans and angiograms on all patients showed a poor correlation (i.e., low-probability scans could be associated with positive angiograms, and vice-versa).[14] The value of assigning a probability to abnormal lung scans is presently being studied.

Right Heart Ultrasound. Emboli may become fragmented as they pass through the right side of the heart, and these fragments can be visualized by an ultrasound examination of the right heart chambers.[17] Cardiac ultrasound has not shown a high yield in patients with acute PE,[17] but this test might prove valuable when the lung scan is not diagnostic and an angiogram is necessary (particularly if there is a risk associated with angiography).

Pulmonary Angiography. Contrast angiography should only be necessary when all other available tests are unrevealing or when immediate demonstration of emboli is desirable (e.g., when the patient is unstable). The goal of the approach just presented is to reduce the need for angiograms, along with their cost and associated risks.

REFERENCES

REVIEWS

1. Consensus conference. Prevention of venous thrombosis and pulmonary embolism. JAMA 1986; 256:744–749.
2. Hull RD, Raskob GE, Hirsh J. Prophylaxis of venous thromboembolism; An overview. Chest 1986; 89 (Suppl):374S–382S.
3. Goldhaber SZ. Prevention of venous thromboembolism. In: Goldhaber SZ ed. Pulmonary embolism and deep venous thrombosis. Philadelphia: W.B. Saunders, 1985.
4. Russel JC. Prophylaxis of postoperative deep venous thrombosis and pulmonary embolism. Surg Gynecol and Obstet 1983: 157:89–104.

RISK FACTORS

5. Cade JF. High risk of the critically ill for venous thromboembolism. Crit Care Med 1982; 10:448–450.
6. Phillips B, Woodring J. Anticoagulation does not exclude pulmonary emboli. Lung 1987; 165:37–43.

PROPHYLAXIS

7. Negus D, Friedgood A, Cox SJ, et al. Ultra low-dose intravenous heparin in the prevention of postoperative deep-vein thrombosis. Lancet 1980; *1*:874–890.
8. Leyvrax PF, Richard J, Bachman F, et al. Adjusted versus fixed-dose subcutaneous heparin in the prevention of deep vein thrombosis after total hip replacement. N Engl J Med 1983; *309*:954–958.
9. Hull R, Delmore T, Carter C, et al. Adjusted subcutaneous heparin versus warfarin sodium in the long-term treatment of venous thrombosis. N Engl J Med 1982; *306*:189–194.
10. Oster G, Tuden RL, Colditz GA. A cost effective analysis of prophylaxis against deep-vein thrombosis in major orthopedic surgery. JAMA 1987; *257*:203–208.
11. Kempczinski RF. Surgical prophylaxis of pulmonary embolism. Chest 1986; *89*:384S–388S.

DIAGNOSTIC APPROACHES

12. Hoellerich VL, Wigton RS. Diagnosing pulmonary embolism using clinical findings. Arch Intern Med 1986; *146*:1699–1704.
13. Hull RD, Hirsh J, Carter CJ, et al. Pulmonary angiography, ventilation lung scanning, and venography for clinically suspected pulmonary embolism with abnormal perfusion scans. Ann Intern Med 1983; *98*:891–899.
14. Hull RD, Hirsh J, Carter CJ, et al. Diagnostic value of ventilation-perfusion scanning in patients with suspected pulmonary embolism. Chest 1985; *88*:819–828.
15. Hull RD, Hirsh J, Carter CJ, et al. Diagnostic efficacy of impedance plethysmography for clinically suspected deep-vein thrombosis. Ann Intern Med 1985; *102*:21–28.
16. Sumner DS, Lamwith A.: Reliability of Doppler ultrasound in the diagnosis of acute venous thrombosis both above and below the knee. Am J Surg 1979; *138*:205–210.
17. Starkley IR, De Bono DP. Echocardiographic identification of right-sided cardiac intracavitary thromboembolus in massive pulmonary embolism. Circulation 1982; *66*:1322–1325.

section III
INVASIVE HEMODYNAMIC MONITORING

The trouble is not in science, but in the uses men make of it.
Wilder Penfield

c h a p t e r

ARTERIAL PRESSURE RECORDING

One of the disturbing revelations about modern medicine is how little physicians know about the blood pressure measurement, yet how often the measurement is used to make crucial decisions. For example, the diastolic pressure obtained with an arm cuff is used to decide about a lifetime of antihypertensive therapy, yet there is confusion about which phase of the Korotkoff sounds should be used as the diastolic pressure. The 1984 report from The National Committee on High Blood Pressure recommended phase IV (the muffling of the sound) as the diastolic pressure, while the 1988 report from the same Committee recommended phase V (disappearance of the sound) as the correct diastolic pressure.[1,2]

This chapter will concentrate mostly on the interpretation of arterial pressures obtained from direct intra-arterial recordings. The final section covers the technique for inserting catheters into the radial and femoral arteries.

PITFALLS OF THE CUFF METHOD

Few measurements are as popular and as unreliable as the blood pressure obtained with an inflatable arm cuff. The following is a capsule summary of the reported experience with the cuff method in different clinical situations.

COMMON SOURCES OF ERROR

The technique itself can introduce errors. For example, the process of inflating and deflating the cuff can produce an increase in blood volume and blood pressure in the ipsilateral arm that can last for several minutes.[3] This could explain why inconsistent readings are reported in healthy normotensive subjects.[4] In elderly hypertensive subjects, the diastolic pressure from a cuff can exceed the actual pressure by at least 10 mmHg in up to 70% of the subjects.[5] Cuff diastolic pressures can also be falsely elevated in obese subjects when the inflatable bladder on the cuff does not completely encircle the arm.[6] The same principle applies to thin patients, where cuff pressures can underestimate the actual pressure because the bladder overlaps on the arm.

LOW–FLOW STATES

Indirect cuff measurements are particularly prone to error in patients with a compromised hemodynamic status.

> The cuff method can underestimate the actual systolic pressure by an average of 34 mmHg in hypotensive patients and 64 mmHg in patients with heart failure.[7]

The inaccuracy of the cuff method in low–flow states is no surprise because the Korotkoff sounds are produced by blood flow. As flow diminishes, the sounds become less audible and the faint early sounds indicating systolic pressure can be missed. This will falsely lower the recorded pressure and can lead to inappropriate therapy with vasoactive drugs. This risk for error in low-flow states is the major reason that the indirect cuff method has largely been abandoned in critically ill patients.

DIRECT ARTERIAL RECORDINGS

The standard practice in seriously ill patients is to measure the arterial pressure directly via catheters placed in the radial or femoral artery. Unfortunately, the direct method is not without shortcomings, as will be demonstrated in the sections that follow.

THE ARTERIAL PRESSURE WAVEFORM

The arterial pressure waveform changes as the pressure wave moves from the proximal aorta towards the periphery. This is shown in Figure 8–1. The waveforms in this figure were obtained from the locations indicated by the straight lines.

> As the arterial pressure wave moves distally from the aorta, the systolic pressure gradually increases and the diastolic pressure gradually decreases.[8] The mean pressure remains relatively constant.

The systolic pressure can increase as much as 15 to 20 mmHg as the pressure wave travels distally.[9] The major change occurs from the proximal aorta to its major branches. In adults, there is no further change in the waveform from the brachial to the radial arteries.[10] However, in

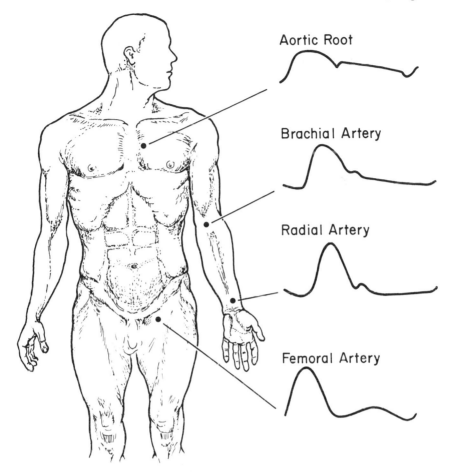

FIG. 8–1. The arterial pressure waveform recorded from different parts of the arterial tree.

infants, the systolic pressure in the pedal arteries can be 25 mmHg higher than in the radial artery.[11]

Wave Reflections. The change in the contour of the arterial pressure waveform is due to pressure waves that reflect back from narrowed peripheral vessels.[8] The arterial pressure waveform is produced by the combination of "incident" waves that travel from the proximal aorta toward the periphery, and "reflected" waves that bounce back from the peripheral vessels. Incident waves are a function of left ventricular stroke volume, and the compliance (distensibility) of the arterial tree. Reflected waves originate at bifurcation points and at points of arterial narrowing and are a function of the peripheral vascular resistance.

When the velocity of pressure propagation is high (when arterial compliance is low), the reflected waves return early and fuse with the systolic part of the pressure wave.[8] This produces an increase in the systolic pressure and a decrease in the diastolic pressure. An example of systolic amplification is shown in Panel B of Figure 8–2 (note the sharp peak in the waveform in Panel B compared to the waveform in Panel A). This augmentation from reflected waves is the mechanism for systolic hypertension in the elderly.[8] The increase in pressure causes an increase in left ventricular afterload, which can impair cardiac output. The effectiveness of peripheral vasodilator therapy in heart failure is explained in part by the ability of vasodilators to diminish the amplitude of reflected waves.[12]

Interpretation. Amplification of the systolic pressure is common in the ICU patient population because of the prevalence of elderly patients in this population. The magnitude of change will vary, depending on the patient and the site of the recording. The amplification should be greater in the radial arteries than in the femoral arteries and should be most apparent in the dorsalis pedis arteries.[11] Remember that the change in contour of the pressure waveform is not an artifact, and the recorded pressures from the artery are the actual pressures at that point in the arterial circuit.

The systolic and diastolic pressures in peripheral arteries may not be an accurate reflection of the pressures in the aorta. However, the mean pressure remains unchanged as the pressure wave moves peripherally,[8] and this pressure can be used as an index of central aortic pressure. The mean pressure in the aorta is valuable for determining the resistance to left ventricular emptying during systole (the afterload). The aortic diastolic pressure is the main driving force for coronary blood flow and would be valuable to monitor in selected patients with coronary artery disease. However, this is not possible because the peripheral diastolic pressure may underestimate the pressure in the aorta.

RECORDING ARTIFACTS

The systems used to measure the arterial pressure can produce artifacts that distort the pressure waveform. Failure to recognize these artifacts can lead to errors in management.

RESONANT SYSTEMS

The recording circuit consists of an arterial catheter connected to a pressure transducer through a fluid–filled tubing system. The fluid in the circuit creates a resonant system that can oscillate spontaneously and distort the arterial pressure waveform.[13,14]

The performance of a resonant system is defined by the "resonant frequency" and the "damping factor" of the system. The resonant frequency is the inherent frequency of oscillations produced in the system when it is disturbed. When the frequency of an incoming signal approaches the resonant frequency of the system, the resident oscillations will add to the incoming signal and amplify it. This type of system is called an "underdamped" system. The damping factor is a measure of the tendency for the system to attenuate the incoming signal. A resonant system with a high damping factor is called an "overdamped" system.

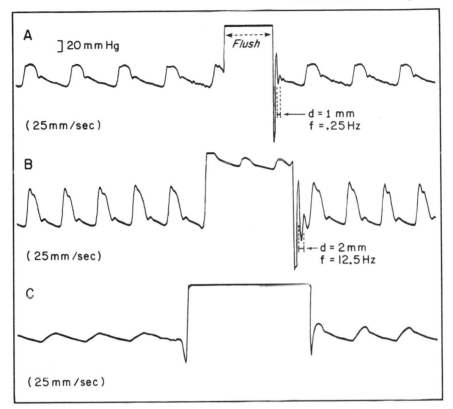

FIG. 8–2. The flush test to determine distortion of the arterial pressure waveform. (A) Normal test. (B) Underdamped system. (C) Overdamped system.

WAVEFORM DISTORTION

Three waveforms obtained from different recording systems are shown in Figure 8–2. The waveform in Panel A with the rounded peak and the dicrotic notch is the normal waveform expected from a recording system with no distortion. The waveform in Panel B with the sharp systolic peak is from an underdamped recording system. The recording systems used in clinical practice are naturally underdamped and these systems can amplify the systolic pressure by as much as 25 mmHg or more.[14] Limiting the length of the connector tubing between the catheter and transducer will limit the tendency for systolic amplification.

The waveform in Panel C of Figure 8–2 shows an attenuated systolic peak with a gradual upslope and downslope and a narrow pulse pressure. This waveform is from an "overdamped" system. Overdamping reduces the gain of the system and is sometimes the result of air bubbles trapped in the connector tubing or in the dome of the pressure transducer. Flushing the hydraulic system to evacuate air bubbles might help to improve an overdamped signal.

Unfortunately, it is not always possible to identify underdamped and overdamped systems using the arterial pressure waveform.[11] The test described in the next section can help in this regard.

THE FLUSH TEST

Applying a brief flush to the catheter-tubing system can be used to determine if the recording system is distorting the pressure waveform. Most commercially available transducer systems are equipped with a one-way valve that can be used to deliver a flush from a pressurized source. Figure 8–2 shows the results of a flush test in three different situations. In each case, the pressure increases abruptly when the flush is applied. However, the response at the end of the flush differs in each panel. In panel A, the flush is followed by a few oscillating waveforms. The frequency of these oscillations is the resonant frequency (f) of the recording system, which is calculated as the reciprocal of the time period between the oscillations. When using standard strip-chart recording paper divided into 1 mm segments, f can be determined by measuring the distance between oscillations and dividing this into the paper speed:[11]

$$f(Hz) = \frac{Paper\ Speed\ (mm/sec)}{Distance\ between\ oscillations\ (mm)}$$

In the test in panel A, the distance (d) between oscillations is 1.0 mm and the paper speed is 25 mm/sec, and therefore, f = 25 Hz (25 mm/sec ÷ 1.0 mm).

Signal distortion is minimal when the resonant frequency of the recording system is 5 times greater than the major frequency in the arterial pressure waveform.[1] Since the major frequency in the arterial pulse is approximately 5 Hz,[1] the resonant frequency of the recording system in panel A (25 Hz) is 5 times greater than the frequency in the incoming waveform, and the system will not distort the incoming waveform.

The flush test for the recording system in panel B reveals a resonant frequency of 12.5 Hz (f = 25 mm/sec ÷ 2 mm). This is too close to the frequency of arterial pressure waveforms, and therefore this system will distort the incoming signal and produce systolic amplification. A recording system with a resonant frequency of 8 Hz can cause a 27% increase in the systolic pressure recorded from the brachial artery.[10]

The flush test shown in the bottom panel of Figure 8–2 does not produce any oscillations. This indicates that the system is overdamped and will underestimate the actual arterial pressure.

When an overdamped system is discovered, the system should be flushed thoroughly (including all stopcocks in the system) to release any trapped air bubbles. If this does not correct the problem, the arterial catheter should be repositioned or changed.

THE MEAN BLOOD PRESSURE

The mean blood pressure is the driving pressure for peripheral blood flow and this pressure is preferred to the systolic and diastolic pressures for monitoring patients who are hemodynamically unstable. Furthermore, the mean pressure does not change as the pressure waveform moves distally along the arterial tree, nor is it altered by distortion from the recording systems.[13]

The mean pressure is measured electronically by first integrating the area under the arterial pressure waveform and then dividing by the duration of the cardiac cycle. Most electronic recording devices display the mean pressure continuously. Mean pressure is also estimated as the diastolic pressure plus one-third of the pulse pressure. However, this estimate is often unreliable and is never preferred to the electronically derived pressure.

ARTERIAL CANNULATION

The popular sites for arterial cannulation in adults are the radial and the femoral arteries. The brachial artery is rarely used because it is the sole blood supply to the forearm and hand. The dorsalis pedis artery is unpopular in adults because of the distortion produced in the pulse waveform at this site.[11]

THE RADIAL ARTERY

The radial artery is preferred because it is superficial, accessible, compressible, and the skin site is easy to keep clean. In addition, the hand receives generous collateral flow through the ulnar artery and the palmar arch, so that occlusion of the radial artery will not cause ischemic damage of the hand and digits. The major drawback of the radial artery is its small size, which limits the success of cannulation.

ANATOMY

The surface anatomy of the blood supply to the hand is shown in Figure 8–3. The radial and ulnar arteries are branches of the brachial artery and they supply blood to the hand through the superficial palmar arch. The radial artery runs down the anterior radial aspect of the forearm and is easily palpated at the wrist in a longitudinal groove just medial to the distal radius.

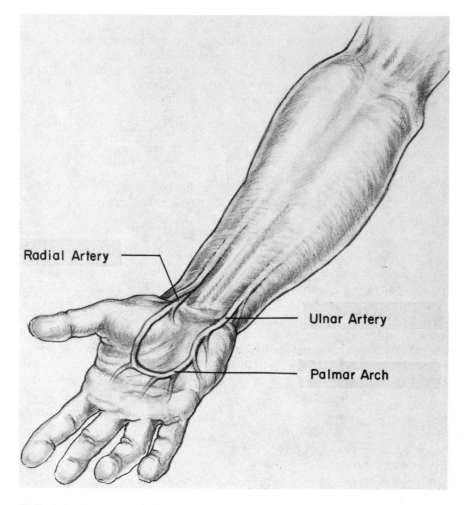

FIG. 8–3. Anatomy of the arterial supply to the hand.

THE ALLEN'S TEST

The Allen's test evaluates collateral flow to the hand when the radial artery is occluded. This test is designed to determine the safety of radial artery cannulation. The test is performed as follows:[15]

1. Occlude the radial and ulnar arteries with the thumb and forefinger of each hand.
2. Elevate the arm above the head, and have the patient open and close the hand until the fingers turn white.

3. Release the ulnar artery, and determine the time it takes for the normal color to return to the fingers.

Normal response time = 7 seconds

Inadequate collateral flow = 14 seconds or longer.

This test is universally recommended without proof of its value. In fact, a prospective study of 1,699 patients with radial artery catheters reported no cases of ischemic damage to the hands when the Allen's test showed poor collateral flow prior to radial artery cannulation.[16] The evidence at present fails to prove that the Allen's test is of any value prior to cannulation of the radial artery.

INSERTION TECHNIQUE

The wrist should be hyperextended to bring the artery closer to the surface. The wrist can be dorsiflexed over gauze roll, or the operator's free hand can be used to extend the wrist. Prepare the skin in the usual fashion (see Chapter 4) and wear gloves.

A 20-gauge, catheter-over-needle device is commonly used. The catheter should be short (2 inches) to minimize endothelial damage and waveform distortion. Hold the needle as you would hold a pencil, and remove the cap on the transparent hub of the needle so blood will flow into the hub when the artery is punctured. Palpate the artery just proximal to the head of the radius and insert the catheter-needle device through the skin at a 30 degree angle to the skin surface.

The through-and-through technique is used to place the catheter in the artery. When the needle tip first punctures the artery, blood will flow into the transparent hub of the needle. However, the catheter tip will not be in the lumen of the vessel at this point because it is back from the needle tip. To place the catheter tip in the vessel, the needle is passed completely through the artery and then withdrawn until blood returns again through the needle. At this point, the catheter tip should be in the lumen of the artery and the catheter can be advanced over the needle.

Repeated attempts to cannulate the artery can lead to thrombosis and permanent occlusion of the vessel. The present recommendation is that the site be abandoned after two unsuccessful attempts.[17]

COMPLICATIONS

Arterial occlusion has been reported in 25% of cannulations[16] and the occlusion is permanent in 3% of cases.[18] However, ischemic necrosis of the digits is extremely rare.[16-18] Doppler examination of pulses distal to the cannulation site is not predictive,[17] and routine Doppler evaluation is not necessary.

Catheter-related septicemia is reported in 1 to 2% of insertions, and infection rate **is no different with radial artery and femoral artery catheters.**[19]

THE FEMORAL ARTERY

The femoral artery is less popular than the radial artery because of its location. However, the femoral artery is easier to cannulate than the radial artery,[20] and the pressure in the femoral artery is a closer approximation to aortic pressure than the radial artery pressure.[8]

ANATOMY

The surface anatomy for the femoral artery and vein is illustrated in Chapter 4, Figure 4–3. The femoral artery is the continuation of the external iliac artery as it runs beneath the inguinal ligament. The artery passes midpoint between a line drawn from the anterior superior iliac crest to the symphysis pubis. The femoral vein lies medial to the artery in the femoral sheath.

INSERTION TECHNIQUE

Use a surgical prep for the groin area and remove the surrounding hair (a depilatory is preferred to a razor). The catheter should be long enough to stay in the vessel but not long enough to distort the arterial pressure waveform. A Seldinger technique is recommended to minimize trauma (see Chapter 4). The following material should be adequate:

1. 21-gauge needle, 6 to 7 cm in length
2. 0.021 inch guidewire
3. 18-gauge catheter, 16 to 20 cm in length

Draw an imaginary line from the anterior superior iliac crest to the symphysis pubis. The femoral artery should be midway along this line, and can be palpated as it passes from under the inguinal ligament. The artery should be punctured after the needle is advanced 2 to 4 cm from the skin surface. The femoral vein lies medial to the artery, and can be accidentally punctured. A venous puncture is identified by the lack of pulsations in blood returning from the needle.

COMPLICATIONS

The complication rate (7 to 10%) is the same for the femoral and radial arteries.[17] Although digital ischemia can occur in 3% of cannulations, there is little permanent damage.[17,20] Patients with peripheral vascular disease do not have a higher complication rate.[17] Infection rates are low

(1 to 3%) and equivalent to other arterial and central venous access sites.[19,20]

REFERENCES

NATIONAL REPORTS

1. The 1984 report of the joint national committee on detection, evaluation, and treatment of high blood pressure. Arch Intern Med 1984; *144*:1045–1057.
2. The 1988 report of the joint national committee on detection, evaluation, and treatment of high blood pressure. Arch Intern Med 1988; *148*:1023–1038.

PITFALLS OF THE CUFF METHOD

3. Bruner JMR, Krewis LJ, Kunsman JM, Sherman AP. Comparison of direct and indirect methods of measuring arterial blood pressure. Med Instr 1981; *15*:11–21.
4. Bruner JMR, Krewis LJ, Kunsman JM, Sherman AP. Comparison of direct and indirect methods of measuring arterial blood pressure, Part III. Med Instr 1981; *15*:182–188.
5. Hla KM, Vokaty KA, Feussner JR. Overestimation of diastolic blood pressure in the elderly. J Am Geriatr Soc 1985; *33*:659–663.
6. Linfors EW, Feussner JR, Blessing CL, et al. Spurious hypertension in the obese patient. Effect of sphygmomanometer cuff size on prevalence of hypertension. Arch Intern Med 1984; *144*.1482–1485.
7. Cohn JN. Blood pressure measurement in shock. Mechanism of inaccuracy in auscultatory and palpatory methods. JAMA 1981; *199*:972–976.

THE ARTERIAL PRESSURE WAVEFORM

8. O'Rourke MF, Yaginuma T. Wave reflections and the arterial pulse. Arch Intern Med 1984; *144*:366–371.
9. Rushmer RF. Cardiovascular dynamics. Philadelphia: W.B. Saunders, 1976; 179–182.
10. Kroeker EJ, Wood EH. Comparison of simultaneously recorded central and peripheral arterial pressure pulse during test, exercise and tilted position in man. Circ Res 1955; *3*:623–628.
11. Park MK, Robotham JL, German VF. Systolic pressure amplification in pedal arteries in children. Crit Care Med 1983; *11*:286–289.
12. Laskey WK, Kussmaul WG. Arterial wave reflection in heart failure. Circulation 1987; *75*:711–722.

RECORDING SYSTEMS

13. Gardner RM. Direct blood pressure measurement—dynamic response requirements. Anesthesiology 1981; *54*:227–236.
14. Rothe CF, Kim KC. Measuring systolic arterial blood pressure. Crit Care Med 1980; *8*:683–689.

ARTERIAL CANNULATION

15. Harman EM. Arterial cannulation. Prob Crit Care 1988; 2:286–295.
16. Slogoff S, Keats AS, Arlund C. On the safety of radial artery cannulation. Anesthesiology 1983; 59:42–47.
17. Russell JA, Joel M, Hudson RJ, et al. Prospective evaluation of radial and femoral artery catheterization sites in critically ill adults. Crit Care Med 1983; 11:936–939.
18. Weiss BM, Gattiker, RI. Complications during and following radial artery cannulation: A prospective study. Intensive Care Med 1986; 12:424–428.
19. Thomas F, Burke JP, Parker J, et al. The risk of infection related to arterial vs. femoral sites for arterial cannulation. Crit Care Med 1983; 11:807–812.
20. Gurman GM, Kriemerman S. Cannulation of big arteries in critically ill patients. Crit Care Med 1985; 13:217–230.

chapter

9

THE WORLD OF THE PULMONARY ARTERY CATHETER

Man cannot make principles; he can only discover them.
Thomas Paine

The pulmonary artery flotation catheter changed the face of cardio-vascular assessment at the bedside and gave an identity to the practice of critical care. It is more than an important development in critical care, it *is* critical care. This catheter is like a politician because it seems to perform well but you are never sure that you trust what it is telling you.

This chapter is an introduction to the pulmonary artery (PA) catheter and what it can measure. You must have an intimate knowledge of this catheter if you are to function in any ICU. The hemodynamic concepts in Chapters 1 and 2 should be reviewed if necessary before starting this chapter. Several excellent reviews of this subject are listed at the end of the chapter.[1-4]

THE FLOTATION CATHETER

The pulmonary artery (PA) catheter owes its origins to the motion of a sailboat. The principle is to use an inflatable balloon as a sail to carry the catheter along with a flowing stream of blood in the superior vena cava. The catheter is carried along through the right side of the heart and into the pulmonary arteries without need for fluoroscopic guidance. This "flotation" principle allows for a right heart catheterization at the bedside.

THE CATHETER

The features of most PA catheters include the following:

Length:	110 cm
Material:	Polyvinylchloride
Size:	7 French (double lumen)
	7.5 French (triple lumen)
Balloon:	1.5 ml capacity
Thermistor:	Mounted 4 cm from the distal tip
Ports:	One at the tip and another 30 cm from the tip. A third port is available on some catheters and is placed near the proximal port.
Accessories:	Fiberoptics for measuring O_2 saturation in pulmonary artery (mixed venous) blood. Pacing leads are also available.

Accessories are present only on specially designed catheters and are not available on standard thermodilution catheters.

ADVANCING THE CATHETER

The PA catheter is passed through a large bore (8.5 French) introducer catheter situated in the subclavian or internal jugular veins (see Chapter 13 for information on the introducer catheters). When the catheter tip emerges from the introducer catheter and is exposed to flowing blood, the balloon is inflated with 1.5 ml of air and the catheter is advanced slowly with balloon inflated. The pressure waveforms recorded from the advancing tip of the catheter are monitored to identify the position of the catheter tip. The waveforms encountered along the catheter route are illustrated in Figure 9–1. The description below proceeds in series as the catheter is advanced from the superior vena cava to the pulmonary arteries. The normal pressures in the thorax are shown in Table 9–1.

1. The pressure in the superior vena cava has a venous pattern (see next chapter) and is called the "central venous pressure" (CVP). The CVP is equivalent to the right atrial pressure.

2. When the catheter tip crosses the tricuspid valve and enters the right ventricle, a systolic pressure appears. The diastolic pressure remains the same.

3. When the catheter is carried across the pulmonic valve and into the pulmonary artery, the diastolic pressure suddenly rises and a dicrotic notch appears on the waveform. This is the pulmonary artery pressure waveform.

4. As the catheter tip is advanced along the pulmonary artery, the systolic component of the waveform will (or should) eventually disappear. This final pressure is called the "pulmonary capillary wedge pressure" (PCWP).

5. Once the PCWP is obtained, the balloon is immediately deflated and the pulmonary artery waveform should reappear. The balloon is kept fully deflated while the catheter is in place and is inflated only for brief periods of time to measure the wedge pressure.

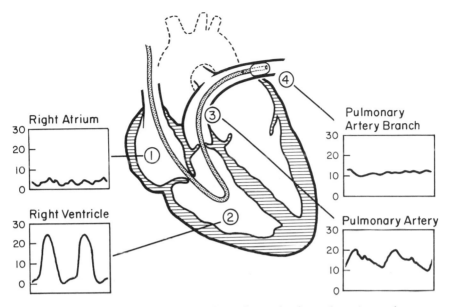

FIG. 9–1. The pressure waveforms along the path of an advancing pulmonary artery catheter. See text for explanation.

THE HEMODYNAMIC PROFILE

Once in place, the PA catheter is capable of generating a large number of measurements that can be organized into a "hemodynamic profile" like the one shown in Table 9–2. This profile has nine hemodynamic parameters and it provides a rather comprehensive evaluation of the cardiovascular system at the bedside. This profile shows the scope of measurements available when the PA catheter is used properly.

BEDSIDE MEASUREMENTS

The following measurements can be obtained directly from the catheter and do not require any calculations.

1. **Central venous pressure (CVP)**—The pressure recorded from the

TABLE 9–1. VASCULAR PRESSURES IN THE THORAX	
Pressure	Normal Values (mm Hg)
Right atrium	0–4
Right ventricle	15–30/0–4
Pulmonary artery	15–30/6–12
Pulmonary artery mean	10–18
Pulmonary wedge	6–12

TABLE 9–2. DERIVED HEMODYNAMIC PARAMETERS		
Parameter	Normal Value	Units
CI	2–4	l/min/m^2
SVI	36–48	ml/beat/m^2
LVSWI	44–56	gm·m/m^2
RVSWI	7–10	gm·m/m^2
SVRI	1200–2500	dyne·sec/cm^5/m^2
PVRI	80–240	dyne·sec/cm^5/m^2
$\dot{D}O_2$	500–600	ml/min/m^2
$\dot{V}O_2$	110–160	ml/min/m^2
O_2ER	22–32	

$(m^2 = $ indexed to body surface area$)$

proximal port of the catheter situated in the right atrium. Right atrial pressure should be equivalent to right ventricular end diastolic pressure (RVEDP) unless there is obstruction between the atrium and ventricles.

$$CVP = RVEDP$$

2. **Pulmonary capillary wedge pressure**—This is the pressure at the distal end when the balloon is lodged in the distal radicles of the pulmonary artery. This pressure is considered equivalent to the left atrial pressure or the left ventricular end-diastolic pressure (LVEDP).

$$PCWP = LVEDP$$

The wedge pressure is covered in detail in the next chapter.

3. **Cardiac output**—The thermistor at the distal end of the catheter will measure cardiac output by monitoring the change in temperature of the blood flowing in the pulmonary arteries after bolus injection of a solution that is colder than blood. This is called the "thermodilution" method and it is the subject of Chapter 11.

4. **Mixed venous oxygen saturation ($S\bar{v}O_2$)**—The oxygen saturation in the pulmonary artery can be measured either in vivo using a special PA catheter or in vitro using a blood sample obtained from the distal port of the catheter. The $S\bar{v}O_2$ is used as an index of the oxygen extracted from the peripheral microcirculation, as presented in Chapter 2.

INTERPRETING PRESSURES

The most important aspect of the PA catheter to learn is the limitations of the measurements that are obtained. The following statements highlight some of the limitations of these measurements.

1. The pressures can fluctuate during respiratory variations in intra-

thoracic pressure. They should be measured at the end of expiration, when pleural pressure is close to atmospheric pressure (see Chapter 10).

2. A pressure change should be 4 mm Hg or greater before it is considered clinically significant.[5]

3. The PCWP should never exceed the pulmonary artery diastolic pressure. When this occurs, the balloon is overinflated[6] and should be deflated immediately to prevent rupture of the artery. Excessive alveolar pressures can also result in a PCWP that exceeds the PAD, as discussed in Chapter 10.

4. The PAD can be falsely elevated when the heart rate exceeds 120 beats/min[7] because there is insufficient time for the pressure to return to baseline.

5. Neither the CVP or the PCWP are reliable measures of blood volume but changes in these pressures can correlate with changes in blood volume.[8] The poor correlation is explained by the relationship between ventricular filling pressures and ventricular compliance (see Chapter 1).

DERIVED PARAMETERS

The scope of the PA catheter is extended considerably by performing some simple calculations on the bedside measurements to derive a set of hemodynamic parameters like the ones in Table 9–2.[9] Note that the normal range for each parameter is included in the table along with the formulas and units that apply to each. All the variables are "indexed" or adjusted to body surface area (BSA).

1. **Cardiac Index (CI)**—This is the average cardiac output (thermodilution) divided by BSA.

$$CI = CO/BSA \quad l/min/m^2$$

Note that the units are reported in square meters. Whenever you see the m^2 in the units, the measurement is divided by BSA and will be lower than the actual cardiac output.

2. **Stroke Volume Index (SVI)**—The volume ejected during each systole.

$$SVI = CI/HR \times 1000 \quad ml/beat/m^2$$

3. **Left Ventricular Stroke Work Index (LVSWI)**—This represents the work performed by the ventricle to eject the stroke volume into the aorta. Work is determined by force (MAP − PCWP) and the mass (SVI) that is moved.

$$LVSWI = (MAP - PCWP) \times SVI \, (\times 0.0136) \quad gm \cdot m/m^2$$

The factor 0.0136 corrects pressure and volume to units of work.

4. **Right Ventricular Stroke Work Index (RVSWI)**—This is deter-

mined by the systolic pressure of the right ventricle (PAP − CVP) and the stroke volume.

$$RVSWI = (PAP - CVP) \times SVI \, (\times \, 0.0136) \quad gm \cdot m/m^2$$

5. **Systemic Vascular Resistance Index (SVRI)**—This is the vascular resistance across both arterial and venous circuits.

$$SVRI = (MAP - CVP) / CI \times 80 \quad dyne \cdot sec/cm^5 \cdot m^2$$

(The factor of 80 converts pressure and volume to dynes·sec/cm^5)

6. **Pulmonary Vascular Resistance Index (PVRI)**—This is the resistance across the entire lung, from pulmonary artery to left atrium. It is determined by the pressure difference across the lung (PAP − PCWP) and flow (CI).

$$PVRI = (PAP - PCWP) / CI \times 80$$

Remember that PCWP is equivalent to left atrial pressure, so (PAP − PCWP) represents the pressure drop across the whole lung, not just the pulmonary arteries.

7. **Oxygen Delivery Rate ($\dot{D}o_2$)**—The amount of oxygen delivered to the capillaries per minute, calculated as the cardiac index and the oxygen content of arterial blood (Cao_2).

$$\dot{D}o_2 = CI \times Cao_2 \quad ml/min/m^2$$

8. **Oxygen Uptake ($\dot{V}o_2$)**—The amount of oxygen taken up from the capillaries per minute. Calculated as the product of cardiac index and oxygen content difference across the capillaries ($Cao_2 - Cvo_2$).

$$\dot{V}o_2 = CI \times (Cao_2 - Cvo_2) \quad ml/min/m^2$$

Although the $\dot{V}o_2$ is often called the "oxygen consumption," it is not necessarily a measure of the metabolic consumption of oxygen.

9. **Oxygen Extraction Ratio (O_2ER)**—The fractional uptake of oxygen from the capillaries, or the balance between oxygen delivery and oxygen uptake.

$$O_2ER = \dot{V}o_2 / \dot{D}o_2$$

COMPUTER-GENERATED PROFILE

The hemodynamic profile just described is time-consuming and tedious to generate unless a microcomputer is used to generate the profile.

The computer is particularly adept at performing calculations and can save hours of time while also eliminating the risk for human error in performing the calculations. We have developed a computer program that not only generates hemodynamic profiles but also helps to interpret the data that is generated.[10]

The Appendix at the end of the book contains a computer program that will generate a hemodynamic profile containing the nine parameters listed in Table 9–2. This program is written in BASIC and can be used on IBM or compatible microcomputers.

USING PROFILES

The hemodynamic profile can be subdivided into several "modules" that are aimed at evaluating specific aspects of cardiovascular function. The following are some examples of how the profile can be tailored to a specific task.

VENTRICULAR DYSFUNCTION

The function of each ventricle can be evaluated using the ventricular filling pressures (preload), the systemic and pulmonary vascular resistances (afterload), and the stroke volume.

	Right Ventricle	Left Ventricle
Preload	CVP	PCWP
Stroke Output	SVI	SVI
Afterload	PVRI	SVRI

Stroke volume is used instead of cardiac output to eliminate the influence of heart rate. For example, a change in heart rate will produce a change in cardiac output, and this may be interpreted erroneously as a change in underlying ventricular function.

Stroke work can be monitored in patients with acute ischemia or infarction who have reduced cardiac output. The goal here is to increase cardiac output but reduce stroke work (see Chapter 14).

HYPOTENSION

Two variables determine mean arterial blood pressure (MAP):

$$MAP = CI \times SVRI$$

$$= (flow) \times (resistance)$$

The pattern of changes in these variables can help to identify and treat specific forms of clinical shock. The use of these two variables in shock is presented in detail in Chapter 12.

PERIPHERAL OXYGEN BALANCE

The changes in O_2 delivery ($\dot{D}O_2$) and O_2 uptake ($\dot{V}O_2$) can be valuable in the diagnosis and management of clinical shock.

	$\dot{D}O_2$	$\dot{V}O_2$	O_2ER
Hemorrhagic Shock	Low	Low	High
Septic Shock	High	High	Low

The $\dot{V}O_2$ is particularly valuable in shock because the hallmark of shock states is an inadequate $\dot{V}O_2$ for the needs of oxidative metabolism. The value of $\dot{V}O_2$ in clinical shock states is presented in Chapter 12.

The ability to tailor hemodynamic profiles to specific problems will increase the utility of the profiles, and will create more logical approaches to problems in individual patients.

COMPLICATIONS

Pulmonary artery catheterization is not without side effects, but few are life-threatening.[3,4,12] Many of these complications are non-specific and are seen with all types of intravascular catheters. However, a few complications are specific to the PA catheters.

Ventricular arrhythmias can occur in over 50% of insertions when the catheters are passed through the right side of the heart.[12] However, these arrhythmias are almost always benign and disappear when the catheter is withdrawn.[11,13] Prophylactic therapy with antiarrhythmic agents is not necessary.[13] Right bundle branch block develops in about 3% of insertions, but usually disappears within 24 hours.

Pulmonary artery rupture is rare, with 10 cases reported in the first 10 years of catheter use.[14] The usual presentation is acute hemoptysis, and the condition is often fatal. Occasional cases have been managed without surgery, but thoracotomy is usually required.

CRITICISMS

The PA catheter has become part of routine patient care in the ICU and has become so popular that its widespread use has been branded as a "cult."[15] Despite its popularity, there is little or no evidence to prove that this catheter has improved clinical outcome. One study has shown no difference in survival when PA catheters were used in patients with acute myocardial infarction.[16] However, nothing may help in this situation if there is no therapy that is effective.

The lack of improved survival with PA catheters is not surprising because these catheters are meant to be a monitoring device and not a therapy.

For example, you might insert a PA catheter in a patient who is hypotensive and discover cardiogenic shock. In this situation, the catheter has been valuable in helping to make the diagnosis but it will not improve survival because there is no effective therapy for cardiogenic shock.

Remember that the PA catheter is only a device for monitoring cardio-vascular function and is not a therapy or a panacea for hemodynamic problems.[17]

BIBLIOGRAPHY

Gore JM, Alpert JS, Benotti JR, Kotilainen PW, Haffajee CI eds. Handbook of Hemodynamic Monitoring. 1st ed. Boston: Little Brown & Co., 1985.

Sprung CL. The pulmonary artery catheter: Methodology and clinical application. Baltimore: University Park Press, 1983.

Grossman W ed. Cardiac catheterization and angiography. 3rd ed. Philadelphia: Lea & Febiger, 1985.

REFERENCES

REVIEWS

1. Weidemann HP, Matthay MA, Matthay RA. Cardiovascular-pulmonary monitoring in the intensive care unit (part I). Chest 1984; 85:537–549.
2. Matthay MA, Chatterjee K. Bedside catheterization of the pulmonary artery: Risks compared with benefits. Ann Intern Med 1988; 109:826–834.
3. Sladen A. Complications of invasive hemodynamic monitoring in the intensive care unit. Curr Probl Surg 1988; 25:1–130.
4. Putterman C. The Swan-Ganz catheter: A decade of hemodynamic monitoring. J Crit Care 1989; 4:127–146.

PRESSURE MEASUREMENTS

5. Niemens EJ, Woods SL. Normal fluctuations in the pulmonary artery wedge pressure in acutely ill patients. Heart Lung 1982; 11:393–398.
6. Wilson RF, Beckman B, Tyburski JG, et al. Pulmonary artery diastolic and wedge pressure relationships in critically ill and injured patients. Arch Surg 1988; 123:933–936.
7. Bouchard RJ, Gault JH, Ross J Jr. Evaluation of pulmonary arterial end-diastolic pressure as an estimate of left ventricular end-diastolic pressure in patients with normal and abnormal left ventricular performance. Circulation 1971; 44:1072–1079.
8. Shippy CR, Appel PL, Shoemaker WC. Reliability of clinical monitoring to assess blood volume in critically ill patients. Crit Care Med 1984; 12:107–112.

THE HEMODYNAMIC PROFILE

9. Fromm RE, Guimond JG, Darby J, Snyder JV. The craft of cardiopulmonary profile analysis. In: Snyder JV, Pinsky MR eds. Oxygen transport in the critically ill. 2nd ed. Chicago: Year Book Medical Publishers, 1987:249–269.
10. Marino PL, Krasner J. An interactive computer program for analysing hemodynamic problems in the ICU. Crit Care Med 1984; 12:601–602.

COMPLICATIONS

11. Gill JB, Cairns JA. Prospective study of pulmonary artery balloon flotation catheter insertion. J Intensive Care Med 1988; 3:121–128.
12. Patel C, Laboy V, Venus B, et al. Acute complications of pulmonary artery catheter insertion in critically ill patients. Crit Care Med 1986; 14:195–197.
13. Iberti TJ, Benjamin E, Gruppi L, et al. Ventricular arrhythmias during pulmonary artery catheterization in the intensive care unit. Am J Med 1985; 78:451–454.
14. Paulson DM, Scott SM, Sethi GK. Pulmonary hemorrhage associated with balloon flotation catheter. J Thorac Cardiovasc Surg 1988; 80:453–458.

CRITICISMS

15. Robin ED. The cult of the Swan-Ganz catheter. Ann Intern Med 1985; 103:445–449.
16. Gore JH, Goldberg RJ, Spodnick DH, Alpert JS, Dalen JE. A community-wide assessment of the use of pulmonary artery catheters in patients with acute myocardial infarction. Chest 1987; 92:721–727.
17. Sibbald WJ, Sprung CL. The pulmonary artery catheter. The debate continues. (editorial) Chest 1988; 94:899–901.

chapter

10

THE WEDGE PRESSURE

An exact science is dominated by the idea of approximation
Bertrand Russell

The pulmonary capillary wedge pressure (PCWP) is a tradition in critical care, and the "wedge pressure" has become a household term in clinical practice. Like all traditions, this measurement is often used but not often scrutinized. This chapter will emphasize the limitations of the wedge pressure and will point out some of the misconceptions that surround this measurement.

SALIENT FEATURES

There is a tendency to view the wedge pressure as a multipurpose measurement, but this is not the case. The following statements summarize the major features of this pressure. The wedge pressure . . .
1. is a measure of the pressure in the left atrium.
2. is NOT a measure of left ventricular preload.
3. can reflect the pressure in the surrounding alveoli.
4. is NOT a measure of the capillary hydrostatic pressure.
5. is NOT a transmural pressure.
Each of these statements will be explored in the sections that follow. For more information on the subject, see the reviews listed at the end of the chapter.[1-4]

WEDGE PRESSURE AND PRELOAD

The wedge pressure method is designed to measure the pressure in the left atrium. The information is used to assess intravascular volume and to evaluate the function of the left ventricle.

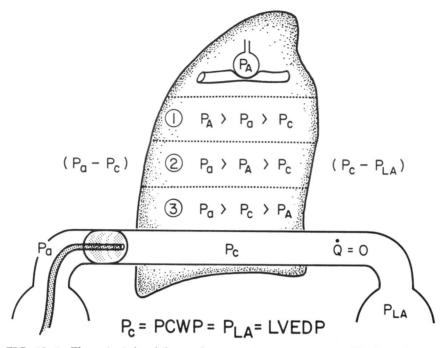

$$P_C = PCWP = P_{LA} = LVEDP$$

FIG. 10–1. The principle of the wedge pressure measurement. The lung is partitioned into three zones based on the relationship between the alveolar pressure (P_A), the mean pulmonary artery pressure (Pa), and the pulmonary capillary pressure (Pc). The wedge pressure (PCWP) is an accurate measure of left atrial pressure (LAP) only when Pc exceeds P_A (zone III). See text for further explanation.

THE PRINCIPLE

The principle of the wedge pressure measurement is illustrated in Figure 10–1. The balloon at the distal end of a pulmonary artery catheter is inflated to obstruct flow. This creates a static column of blood between the catheter tip and the left atrium and allows the pressures at both ends of the blood column to equilibrate. The pressure at the catheter tip is then equal to the pressure in the left atrium. This principle is expressed in the hydraulic equation below (where Pc is pulmonary capillary pressure, P_{LA} is left atrial pressure, Q is pulmonary blood flow, and Rv is pulmonary venous resistance).

$$Pc - P_{LA} = \dot{Q} \times Rv$$

$$\text{If } Q = 0: \qquad Pc - P_{LA} = 0$$

$$Pc = P_{LA} \, (= PCWP)$$

The pressure at the catheter tip during balloon occlusion is called the pulmonary capillary "wedge" pressure or PCWP. This pressure is considered equal to the left ventricular end-diastolic pressure (LVEDP) when there is no obstruction between the left atrium and left ventricle.

LVEDP AS PRELOAD

Chapter 1 defined preload as a force that stretched a muscle at rest and identified the end-diastolic volume (EDV) as the preload for the intact ventricle. Unfortunately, EDV is difficult to measure at the bedside (see Chapter 14) and the EDP has become the clinical measure of preload. The compliance (distensibility) of the left ventricle determines the accuracy of the EDP as a measure of preload. This is illustrated in the compliance curves in Chapter 1 (Figure 1–4) and in Figure 14–4 in Chapter 14. The problem can be summarized as follows:

> The end-diastolic (wedge) pressure is a reliable index of preload only when ventricular compliance is normal or unchanging.

The assumption that ventricular compliance is normal or unchanging is problematic in the adult ICU patient population. Although the prevalence of diastolic abnormalities has not been studied in critically ill patients, there are several conditions in these patients that can alter ventricular compliance. The most common of these may be positive-pressure mechanical ventilation, particularly when the inflation pressures are high (see Chapter 27). Other factors that can alter ventricular compliance are myocardial ischemia, ventricular hypertrophy, myocardial edema, pericardial tamponade, and select drugs like calcium channel blockers.[5] When ventricular compliance is low or decreasing, an elevated wedge pressure will not differentiate between systolic and diastolic heart failure. This is presented in more detail in Chapter 14.

WEDGE AND HYDROSTATIC PRESSURES

The wedge pressure is used as a measure of the capillary hydrostatic pressure to determine the tendency for individual patients to develop hydrostatic pulmonary edema. The problem here is that the PCWP is measured in the absence of blood flow and is not meant to simulate flow conditions in the capillaries. The specific relationship between the wedge pressure and the capillary hydrostatic pressure is illustrated in Figure 10–2. When the balloon at the end of the catheter is deflated and blood flow resumes, the pressure in the capillaries (Pc) will rise above the wedge pressure. The magnitude of difference (Pc − PCWP) is determined by the rate of flow (Q) and the resistance to flow in the pul-

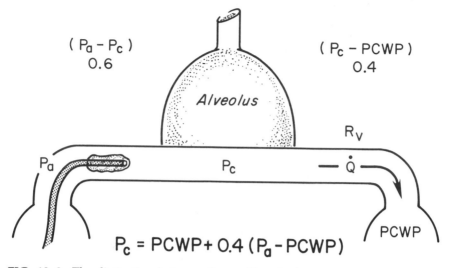

FIG. 10–2. The distinction between the capillary hydrostatic pressure (Pc) and the wedge pressure (PCWP).

monary veins (Rv). This is shown in the equation below (note that the PCWP has replaced P_{LA} in the equation shown earlier).

$$Pc - PCWP = \dot{Q} \times Rv$$

$$\text{If } Rv = 0: \quad Pc - PCWP = 0$$

$$Pc = PCWP$$

The conclusion from this equation is stated for emphasis.

> The wedge pressure is equal to the hydrostatic pressure only when the resistance in the pulmonary veins is negligible.

However, the veins in the lungs contribute a considerable fraction of the total resistance in the pulmonary circulation because the resistance in the pulmonary arteries is relatively low. The pulmonary circulation operates as a low pressure circuit (to accommodate the thin right ventricle) and the pulmonary arteries are not rigid conduits like the arteries in the systemic circulation. As a result of the low resistance in the pulmonary arteries, the pulmonary veins contribute a greater fraction to the total resistance across the lungs.

In animal studies, the pulmonary veins account for at least 40% of the total resistance in the pulmonary circulation.[6] The contribution in humans is not known but is assumed to be similar. Using a pulmonary venous resistance that is 40% of the total pulmonary vascular resistance, the pressure drop across the pulmonary veins (Pc − P_{LA}) will be 40% of the total pressure drop between the pulmonary artery and the left atrium (Pa − P_{LA}). This can be expressed as follows[4] assuming that PCWP is equivalent to P_{LA}:

$$Pc - PCWP = 0.4 \, (Pa - P_{LA})$$

$$Pc = PCWP + 0.4 \, (Pa - PCWP)$$

The difference between Pc and PCWP will be negligible in healthy subjects because the pulmonary artery pressure is low, as shown in the example below. However, there can be a considerable difference between the two pressures when pulmonary hypertension is present or when pulmonary venous resistance is elevated. This is shown below using the "adult respiratory distress syndrome" (ARDS) as an example of a clinical disorder associated with both pulmonary artery and pulmonary venous hypertension (see Chapter 23). A wedge pressure of 10 mmHg is used for both situations below.

$$PCWP = 10 \text{ mmHg}$$

Normal: $$PC = 10 + 0.4 \times (15 - 10)$$

$$= 12 \text{ mmHg}$$

ARDS: $$PC = 10 + 0.6 \times (30 - 10)$$

$$= 22 \text{ mmHg}$$

When the mean pulmonary artery pressure is doubled and venous resistance is increased by 50%, the hydrostatic pressure is more than double the wedge pressure (22 versus 10 mmHg). In this situation, therapy would be influenced by the method used to estimate hydrostatic pressure. If the adjusted pressure of 22 mmHg were used, therapy would include measures aimed at reducing the tendency for pulmonary edema. If the measured wedge pressure of 10 mmHg was used, no therapy is indicated. This illustrates how the measured wedge pressure can be misleading.

Unfortunately, the venous resistance in the lung cannot be measured directly and the adjustment equation shown here is not reliable for the individual patient. Nevertheless, this equation will provide a more accurate estimate of hydrostatic pressure than the wedge pressure, and it should be used whenever possible until a better estimate of Pc is discovered.

OCCLUSION PRESSURE PROFILE

The decline in pulmonary artery pressure at the outset of balloon occlusion is characterized by an initial rapid fall and a final slow descent. The inflection point between these two components has been suggested as the hydrostatic pressure in the pulmonary capillaries,[8] but this notion has been questioned because it does not conform to mathematical predictions.[9] In addition, a clear separation of a rapid and slow decay at the bedside is not always possible (personal observation). At present, this area awaits further investigation.

THORACIC PRESSURE ARTIFACTS

The influence of thoracic pressure on the wedge pressure is based on the distinction between intraluminal pressure (inside the vessel lumen) and transmural pressure (across the vessel wall). The intraluminal pressure is the conventional measure of vascular pressure, but the transmural pressure is the one that influences stretch (preload) and edema formation.

Alveolar pressure can be transmitted to pulmonary vessels and can change intraluminal pressure without altering transmural pressure. The equilibration of the pressure across the vessel wall depends on several factors (e.g., wall thickness and compliance) and this tendency will differ in individual patients. The following recommendation is meant to reduce errors in wedge pressure measurements from indeterminate contributions from thoracic pressure.

> In the thorax, the vascular pressure recorded from the lumen of the vessel will correspond to the transmural pressure only at the end of expiration, when the pressure in surrounding alveoli is equal to atmospheric (zero reference) pressure.

Remember that the vascular pressures recorded in the ICU are intraluminal pressures measured relative to atmospheric pressure (zero) and do not accurately reflect transmural pressure unless the extraluminal pressure is also atmospheric. This is particularly important when there are respiratory variations on the wedge pressure tracing, as shown next.

RESPIRATORY VARIATIONS

The influence of thoracic pressure variations on the wedge pressure is shown in Figure 10–3. The respiratory fluctuations in the wedge pressure are caused by thoracic pressure fluctuations that have been transmitted into the capillaries. The actual (transmural) pressure in these tracings may be constant throughout the respiratory cycle. The wedge pressure is read at the end of expiration and this corresponds to the lowest point on the tracing during mechanical ventilation and the highest point during spontaneous breathing. The electronic pressure monitors in most ICUs are designed to measure pressure in time intervals of four seconds (equivalent to one sweep across the oscilloscope monitor). These monitors display three different pressures: systolic, diastolic, and mean pressure. The systolic display is the highest pressure in each 4-second interval, the diastolic display is the lowest pressure, and the mean pressure is the average pressure over the 4-second time period. The wedge

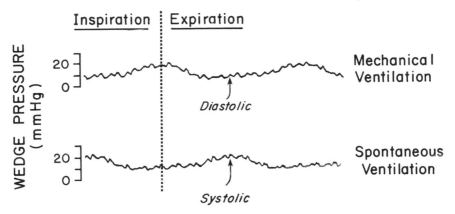

FIG. 10–3. Respiratory variations in the wedge pressure tracing during spontaneous ventilation and positive-pressure ventilation. The true (transmural) pressure is at the end of expiration, which corresponds to the systolic recording during spontaneous breathing, and the diastolic recording during mechanical ventilation.

pressure at end expiration can therefore be monitored by selecting the systolic display for spontaneous breathing and the diastolic display for mechanical ventilation. Note that the mean pressure is not monitored in the presence of respiratory variations.

POSITIVE END-EXPIRATORY PRESSURE

The alveolar pressure will not return to atmospheric pressure at the end of expiration in the presence of "positive end-expiratory pressure" (PEEP). As a result, the wedge pressure at end-expiration may overestimate the actual wedge pressure.[10] The PEEP can either be applied externally or can be intrinsic to the patient (auto-PEEP). Auto-PEEP is often an occult process caused by inadequate emptying of alveolar gas, and it may be common in patients with obstructive airways disease who are receiving mechanical ventilation. The important point to remember about auto-PEEP is its ability to go undetected in patients receiving mechanical ventilation unless you perform a maneuver (see Chapter 29).

> When there is a sudden or unexplained increase in wedge pressure in an agitated patient who is breathing rapidly, consider auto-PEEP as a cause of the problem.

Auto-PEEP is described in more detail at the end of Chapter 29.

The influence of PEEP on the wedge pressure is variable, and depends on the compliance of the lungs. If the wedge is first obtained during the application of PEEP, you can reduce the PEEP gradually to zero without separating the patient from the ventilator. Removing patients from ventilators during PEEP is a matter of debate. Some consider this a dangerous practice that can produce worsening gas exchange,[11] while others report only transient hypoxemia.[12] The risk from ventilator disconnect can be reduced or eliminated by maintaining positive pressure ventilation when PEEP is temporarily discontinued.

When PEEP is causing an increase in the wedge pressure, there are three possible interpretations:

1. The PEEP is not changing transmural capillary pressure.
2. The PEEP is compressing the capillaries, so the PCWP actually represents alveolar pressure and not left atrial pressure.
3. The PEEP surrounding the heart is decreasing the distensibility of the left ventricle, which will increase the PCWP at the same end-diastolic volume.

Unfortunately, it is not possible to identify which of these is operative in any single patient. The last two conditions could indicate hypovolemia (relative or absolute) and it is reasonable to infuse volume if possible when this situation arises.

THE LUNG ZONES

The accuracy of the wedge pressure requires a continuous fluid column between the catheter tip and the left atrium. If the pressure in surrounding alveoli exceeds capillary pressure and compresses the capillaries, the pressure at the tip of the PA catheter will reflect the alveolar pressure instead of the left atrial pressure. This concept has been used to divide the lung into three regions based on the relationship between alveolar pressure and the pressures in the pulmonary circulation.[1,4] This is illustrated in Figure 10–1.

The three lung zones are arranged in sequence from the apex of the lung to the base. Note that the most dependent zone (zone 3) is the only region where the capillary pressure exceeds the alveolar pressure. This is the region where the vascular pressures are the highest (because of gravity flow) and the alveolar pressures are the lowest.

> The tip of the pulmonary artery catheter should rest below the level of the left atrium (zone 3) to reduce or eliminate transmission of alveolar pressure to the capillaries.

This does not necessarily hold if the patient is hypovolemic or if high levels of PEEP are being used.[1]

There is no technique for directing catheters to zone 3 at the bedside without fluoroscopic guidance. Fortunately, most catheters are carried into dependent lung zones simply because the blood flow in these regions is highest. However, an average of one catheter for every three inserted will end up in lung regions above the left atrium.[1]

CLINICAL ACCURACY

There are numerous sources of error in the wedge pressure measurement. Technical problems have been reported in 30% of the measurements[13] and errors in interpretation are reported in 20% of the readings.[14] Inaccuracies in the measurement can also be the result of the pathologic process. The sections that follow will outline the practical issues of accuracy and reliability.

VERIFYING THE MEASUREMENT

Catheter Tip Position. The catheters are usually inserted while patients are supine and the tip of the catheter is often carried along with blood flow into the posterior lung regions. This should place the catheter tip below the level of the left atrium and satisfy zone 3 conditions. Unfortunately, portable chest x-rays will not localize the catheter tips in the anteroposterior plane, and lateral supine films have been suggested for this task.[1] The value of lateral films is being questioned because of reports showing no pressure change in dorsal versus ventral aspects of the lung (above and below the left atrium).[15] Bedside lateral films are tedious and expensive and not universally accepted. The following conditions may indicate nonzone 3 conditions without an x-ray:[1]

1. When there are marked respiratory variations in the pressure tracing.
2. When the wedge pressure increases by 50% or more of the amount of PEEP applied.

Wedged Blood Oxygenation. Aspiration of blood from the catheter tip during balloon inflation has been recommended to verify catheter position.[16] A specimen with an oxygen saturation of 95% or above is considered "arterialized" blood originating in the capillaries. In one study, 50% of the wedge pressures did not satisfy the oxygen saturation criteria,[13] indicating the possible impact of this practice on reducing errors in the wedge measurement. However, patients with pulmonary disease may not show the predicted increase in oxygen saturation because of local hypoxemia and not because of incorrect catheter tip placement.[15] It seems that a positive test might help but a negative test has little predictive value, particularly in patients with respiratory failure. We use continuous monitoring of mixed venous oxygen saturation routinely in our Surgical ICU and this provides a simple way to check each wedge pressure measurement with no added morbidity or cost.

Atrial Waveforms. The shape of the wedge pressure waveform can be used to verify the pressure as an atrial pressure.[13] The shape of an atrial waveform is illustrated in Figure 10–4 using an EKG to identify events on the tracing. The components of the waveform are defined as follows:[2]

1. The A wave—Produced by atrial contraction and is seen in association with the P wave on the EKG. These waves disappear in atrial fibrillation, atrial flutter and acute pulmonary embolus.
2. The X descent—Reflects atrial relaxation. A prominent descent is seen in pericardial tamponade.
3. The C wave—Marks the onset of ventricular systole when the mitral valve begins to close.
4. The V wave—Occurs during ventricular systole and is caused by the mitral valve bulging into the left atrium.
5. The Y descent—Caused by rapid atrial emptying when the mitral

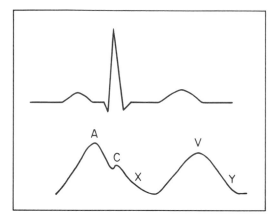

FIG. 10–4. Schematic representation of an atrial pressure waveform shown in relation to an electrocardiogram. See text for explanation.

valve opens at the onset of diastole. Attenuated or absent in pericardial tamponade.

The one abnormality in the atrial pressure waveform that receives the most attention is the giant V wave of mitral insufficiency. These waves are produced by regurgitant flow along the pulmonary veins that can reach the pulmonic valve.[2] Prominent V waves can produce a mean wedge pressure that is higher than the pulmonary artery diastolic pressure.[10] The mean wedge pressure in this situation will overestimate left ventricular filling pressure, and the diastolic mode is recommended for more accurate readings.

Prominent V waves are not pathognomonic of mitral insufficiency. Other conditions associated with this abnormality are left atrial enlargement (cardiomyopathy) and high flows in the pulmonary circulation (ventricular septal defect).

VARIABILITY

The inherent variability in the wedge pressure tracing is 4 mmHg in most patients but can reach up to 7 mmHg.[17] This means that a change in the wedge pressure must exceed 4 mmHg to be considered significant.

PCWP AND LVEDP

The PCWP is an accurate measure of LVEDP in most clinical situations.[1] However, the correlation between the two pressures can vary in the following conditions.

1. Aortic insufficiency—The LVEDP can be higher than the PCWP because the mitral valve closes prematurely while retrograde flow continues to fill the ventricle.

2. Noncompliant ventricle—Atrial contraction against a stiff ventricle produces a rapid rise in end-diastolic pressure that closes the mitral valve prematurely. The result is a PCWP that is lower than the LVEDP.[1]

3. Respiratory Failure—The PCWP can exceed the LVEDP in patients

with pulmonary disease.[15] The presumed mechanism is constriction of small veins in lung regions that are hypoxic. Accuracy cannot be predicted in any one patient. However, the risk for error may be reduced by placing the catheter in lung regions that are not involved in the pathologic process.

REFERENCES

REVIEWS

1. Marini JJ. Pulmonary artery occlusion pressure: Clinical physiology, measurement and interpretation. Am Rev Respir Dis 1983; 128:319–325.
2. Sharkey SW. Beyond the wedge: Clinical physiology and the Swan-Ganz catheter. Am J Med 1987; 83:111–122.
3. Raper R, Sibbald WJ. Misled by the wedge? The Swan-Ganz catheter and left ventricular preload. Chest 1986; 89:427–434.
4. Weidemann HP, Matthay MA, Matthay RA. Cardiovascular-pulmonary monitoring in the intensive care unit (part 1). Chest 1984; 85:537–549.

BASIC FEATURES

5. Harizi RC, Bianco JA, Alpert JS. Diastolic function of the heart in clinical cardiology. Arch Intern Med 1988; 148:99–109.
6. Michel RP, Hakim TS, Chang HK. Pulmonary arterial and venous pressures measured with small catheters. J Appl Physiol 1984; 57:309–314.
7. Allen SJ, Drake RE, Williams JP, et al. Recent advances in pulmonary edema. Crit Care Med 1987; 15:963–970.
8. Cope DK, Allison RC, Parmentier JL, et al. Measurement of effective pulmonary capillary pressure using the pressure profile after pulmonary artery occlusion. Crit Care Med 1986; 14:16–22.
9. Seigel LC, Pearl RG. Measurement of the longitudinal distribution of pulmonary vascular resistance from pulmonary artery occlusion pressure profiles. Anesthesiology 1988; 68:305–307.

THORACIC PRESSURE ARTIFACTS

10. Schmitt EA, Brantigan CO. Common artifacts of pulmonary artery and pulmonary artery wedge pressures: Recognition and management. J Clin Monit 1986; 2:44–52.
11. Weismann IM, Rinaldo JE, Rogers RM. Positive end-expiratory pressure in adult respiratory distress syndrome. N Engl J Med 1982; 307:1381–1384.
12. deCampo T, Civetta JM. The effect of short term discontinuation of high-level PEEP in patients with acute respiratory failure. Crit Care Med 1979; 7:47–49.

CLINICAL ACCURACY

13. Morris AH, Chapman RH, Gardner RM. Frequency of technical problems encountered in the measurement of the pulmonary artery wedge pressure. Crit Care Med 1984; 12:164–170.

14. Wilson RF, Beckman B, Tyburski JG, et al. Pulmonary artery diastolic and wedge pressure relationships in critically ill patients. Arch Surg 1988; *123*:933–936.
15. Henriquez AH, Schrijen FV, Redondo J, et al. Local variations of pulmonary arterial wedge pressure and wedge angiograms in patients with chronic lung disease. Chest 1988; *94*:491–495.
16. Morris AH, Chapman RH. Wedge pressure confirmation by aspiration of pulmonary capillary blood. Crit Care Med 1985; *13*:756–759.
17. Nemens EJ, Woods SL. Normal fluctuations in pulmonary artery and pulmonary capillary wedge pressures in acutely ill patients. Heart Lung 1982; *11*:393–398.
18. Johnston WE, Prough DS, Royster RL. Pulmonary artery wedge pressure may fail to reflect left ventricular end-diastolic pressure in dogs with oleic acid-induced pulmonary edema. Crit Care Med 1985; *13*:487–491.

c h a p t e r

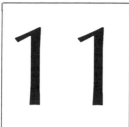

THERMODILUTION CARDIAC OUTPUT

The addition of a thermistor to the pulmonary artery flotation catheter increased the recording capabilities of the catheter from two measurements to ten measurements. The measurement that permitted this burst in capabilities was the cardiac output and the technique involved is called "thermodilution."

THE INDICATOR-DILUTION PRINCIPLE

The indicator-dilution principle predicts that when an indicator substance is added to a stream of flowing blood, the flowrate will be inversely proportional to the mean concentration of the indicator at a downstream site. The original indicator dilution method used a dye called indocyanine green as the indicator substance. The newer thermodilution method uses a cold solution as the indicator (a thermal indicator).

THE THERMODILUTION METHOD

The thermodilution method is illustrated in Figure 11–1.

A dextrose or saline solution that is cooler than blood is injected as a bolus through the proximal port of the pulmonary artery catheter and the solution mixes with the blood in the right heart chambers. This mixing lowers the temperature of the blood, and the cooled blood is carried into the pulmonary artery and flows past a thermistor on the distal end of the pulmonary artery catheter. The thermistor records the temperature change and sends this information to an electronic instru-

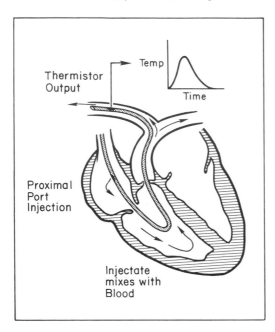

FIG. 11–1. Illustration of the thermodilution method. See text for explanation.

ment called a "cardiac output computer." This instrument monitors the temperature difference between the blood and the injectate solution and displays a temperature-time curve like the one depicted in Figure 11–1. The area under the curve is inversely related to the flowrate in the pulmonary artery. In the absence of intracardiac right-to-left shunts, the flowrate in the pulmonary artery is taken as the cardiac output.

THERMODILUTION CURVES

Some examples of thermodilution curves obtained at the bedside are shown in Figure 11–2. The curve in the upper panel represents a low cardiac output. Note the gradual rise and gradual descent of the curve and the relatively large area under the curve when compared to the curve in the middle panel. The latter curve depicts a high cardiac output and has an abbreviated peak and rapid washout. The cardiac output is inversely proportional to the area under these curves and the electronic cardiac output computers perform this integration and display the calculated output on the face of the instrument panel. There is a tendency to rely on this digital readout without question and this can be misleading, as demonstrated later.

TECHNICAL CONSIDERATIONS

The following features of the thermodilution technique deserve mention.

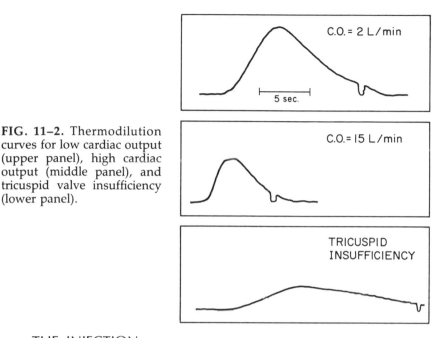

FIG. 11–2. Thermodilution curves for low cardiac output (upper panel), high cardiac output (middle panel), and tricuspid valve insufficiency (lower panel).

THE INJECTION

Solution: Either 0.9% saline or a 5% dextrose-water solution will produce equivalent measurements.[1]

Volume: Use 5 to 10 ml per injection in adults. Smaller volumes can yield unreliable measurements in adults,[1-4] and will falsely elevate the cardiac output. The 5 ml bolus produces satisfactory results with room temperature solutions,[4] and avoids the excess volume from multiple injections of the 10 ml bolus.

Injection Time: The injection should be completed within 4 seconds.[1] Prolonged injection times will produce falsely low measurements.

Injectate Temperature: Room temperature injectates produce reliable recordings and there is no evidence that iced solutions add to the accuracy.[5-8] In fact, iced solutions can cause a bradycardia that adds to inaccuracies and can have serious consequences.[10] At the present time, **there is no evidence to justify a preference for iced solutions over room temperature injectates in adults.**

NUMBER OF MEASUREMENTS

Serial measurements should be obtained at each recording period and the average value is taken as the cardiac output.[1-4] Two measurements are sufficient if they differ by 10% or less. The first measurement is often unreliable, and some recommend discarding the results of the first injection.[1] **Serial measurements that differ by more than 10 to 15% are considered unreliable.**[10]

TABLE 11–1. POTENTIAL SOURCES OF ERROR	
Condition	Direction of Change
Tricuspid Insufficiency	Decrease
Right to Left Shunt	Increase
Left to Right Shunt	Increase
?Low Cardiac Output	Decrease
Catheter Thrombus	Decrease

TIMING OF INJECTION

The cardiac output can vary significantly during the respiratory cycle, particularly during mechanical ventilation. This is because of the influence of positive-pressure lung inflation on cardiac output (see Chapter 27). Random thermodilution measurements obtained in different phases of the respiratory cycle can produce unacceptable variations (over 10 to 15%) while injections that are timed to the end of expiration can reduce the variability to 5%.[6] This has led to the recommendation that injections always be timed to the same part of the respiratory cycle, preferably end-expiration. However, it is difficult, if not impossible, to time injections so that the thermodilution curve is recorded at precisely the same time in the respiratory cycle. In fact, the injection times can be greater than a respiratory cycle in patients with rapid breathing.

A more reasonable goal is to time the onset of the injection to the same part of the respiratory cycle. If an average respiratory cycle is 4 seconds (respiratory rate of 15 breaths per minute) and the time required for the injectate to reach the thermistor 1 to 4 seconds, then starting the injection at the onset of inspiration should produce a thermodilution curve close to the end of expiration.

ACCURACY AND RELIABILITY

The accuracy of the thermodilution method is comparable to the direct Fick method (the gold standard for measuring cardiac output) in several groups of patients.[3,5,7,8] In fact, thermodilution may be more reliable than dye dilution in patients with low cardiac output.[8] The sources of error for the thermodilution technique are listed in Table 11–1.

TRICUSPID REGURGITATION

Tricuspid regurgitation may be one of the most common sources of error in the intensive care unit because of the high right-sided pressures produced by mechanical ventilators. A thermodilution curve produced by tricuspid insufficiency is shown in the lower panel of Figure 11–2. Note that the curve has a low peak and a prolonged washout. The low peak is produced by cold solution washing back into the vena cava (so that less cooling occurs in the pulmonary artery) and the delayed wash-out is produced by the delayed appearance of the injectate that moved retrograde into the vena cava (called recirculation). These features produce a curve that tends to underestimate the cardiac output.[9]

INTRACARDIAC SHUNTS

Right-to-left shunts produce falsely high readings because part of the cold injectate crosses the shunt and the cooling in the pulmonary artery is reduced. This produces a thermodilution curve with an abbreviated peak, like the thermodilution curve for tricuspid insufficiency.

Intracardiac left-to-right shunts also produce falsely elevated readings. In this situation, the blood volume in the right side of the heart is increased and the injectate is diluted, producing a curve with a reduced height.

LOW-OUTPUT STATES

Low cardiac outputs can delay the time for the injectate to reach the thermistor in the pulmonary artery and this will produce a thermodilution curve like the curve for tricuspid insufficiency in Figure 11–2. Despite the theoretical limitations of thermodilution in low-output states, **there is no convincing evidence that thermodilution is inaccurate in patients with low cardiac output.**[8,9] To ensure accuracy in low-output states, the thermodilution curves should be recorded and inspected routinely.

SUMMARY

The thermodilution method is reliable if performed properly. The only way to ensure accuracy is to record and inspect each thermodilution curve as it is generated and to pay particular attention to maintaining constant recording conditions for serial readings.

REFERENCES

1. Kadota LT. Theory and application of thermodilution cardiac output measurement: A review. Heart & Lung 1985; 14:605–614.
2. Fogler G. Measurement of cardiac output in anaesthetized animals by a thermodilution method. Q J Exp Physiol 1954; 39:153–164.
3. Elkayam U, Berkely R, Azen S, et al. Cardiac output by thermodilution technique. Effect of injectate volume and temperature on accuracy and reproducibility in the critically ill patient. Chest 1983; 84:418–422.
4. Pearl RG, Rosenthal MH, Nielson L, et al. Effect of injectate volume and temperature on thermodilution cardiac output determination. Anesthesiology 1986; 64:798–801.

5. Nelson LD, Anderson HB. Patient selection for iced versus room temperature injectate for thermodilution cardiac output determinations. Crit Care Med 1985; 13:182–184.
6. Stevens JH, Raffin TA, Mihm FG, et al. Thermodilution cardiac output measurement. Effects of the respiratory cycle on its reproducibility. JAMA 1985; 253:2240–2242.
7. Stetz CW, Miller RG, Kelly GE, et al. Reliability of the thermodilution method in the determination of cardiac output in clinical practice. Am Rev Respir Dis 1987; 126:1001–1004.
8. Hillis LD, Firth BG, Winniford MD. Analysis of factors affecting the variability of Fick versus indicator dilution measurements of cardiac output. Am J Cardiol 1985; 56:764–768.
9. Nadeau S, Noble WH. Limitations of cardiac output measurement by thermodilution. Can J Anaesth 1986; 33:780–784.
10. Nishikawa T, Namiki A. Mechanism for slowing of heart rate and associated changes in pulmonary circulation elicited by cold injectate during thermodilution cardiac output determinations in dogs. Anesthesiology 1988; 68:221–225.

section IV
CLINICAL SHOCK SYNDROMES

The patient in shock has the appearance of being seriously ill.
Norman E. Freeman, MD
1940

chapter

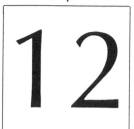

A STRUCTURED APPROACH TO CLINICAL SHOCK

This chapter will introduce you to a simple approach to shock that uses only six variables (most obtained with a pulmonary artery catheter) and proceeds in two stages. This approach does not define shock as hypotension or hypoperfusion but rather defines it as a state of inadequate tissue oxygenation. The final goals of the approach are to match the oxygen supply to the tissues with the metabolic rate. Restoration of pressure and flow are involved in the approach but are not the final goals. The principles used in this approach are housed in Chapters 1, 2 and 9 and are also reviewed in references 1–4 at the end of the chapter.

The approach to clinical shock in this book has one central theme: get as close to the tissue level as you can to assess the state of oxygenation. Shock is buried in the tissues and you will not find it by listening for sounds in the chest or by taking a blood pressure in the arm. The "black box" approach is certain failure with a machine as complex as the human body.

OVERVIEW

The variables used in this scheme are classified as Pressure/Flow Variables or Oxygen Transport Variables.

Pressure/Flow Variables
1. Pulmonary Wedge Pressure (PCWP)
2. Cardiac Output (CO)
3. Systemic Vascular Resistance (SVR)

Oxygen Transport Variables
4. O_2 Delivery ($\dot{D}O_2$)
5. O_2 Uptake ($\dot{V}O_2$)
6. Serum Lactate

1. The initial stage uses the Pressure/Flow Variables to identify and correct the major hemodynamic abnormality. The variables are arranged in patterns that are used to design strategies for diagnosis and management. The final goal of this stage is to restore pressure and flow (if possible) and to identify the underlying illness.

2. The second stage evaluates the effects of the initial therapy on tissue oxygenation. The goal here is to ensure that oxygen uptake ($\dot{V}O_2$) is matched to the metabolic rate. The serum lactate is used to determine the balance between $\dot{V}O_2$ and metabolic rate while the oxygen delivery ($\dot{D}O_2$) is used to manipulate the $\dot{V}O_2$ as needed.

STAGE I: HEMODYNAMIC PATTERNS

Each of the Pressure/Flow Variables is responsible for one of the major shock syndromes.

Variable	Syndrome	Etiology
PCWP	Hypovolemic	Hemorrhage
CO	Cardiogenic	Acute MI
SVR	Vasogenic	Sepsis

The relationships between variables in each of these syndromes will be organized into "patterns" that are used to generate an approach that is tailored to the specific patient. The normal interactions between these variables are presented in Chapter 1.[4]

The hemodynamic patterns in the three basic shock syndromes are shown in Figure 12–1. Each pattern is built as follows:

HYPOVOLEMIC SHOCK

The primary problem here is a decrease in ventricular filling (low PCWP) which leads to a drop in cardiac output (CO) and the low output produces vasoconstriction and an increase in systemic vascular resistance. The pattern will then look like this:

Low PCWP / Low CO / High SVR

CARDIOGENIC SHOCK

In this situation, there is a primary decrease in cardiac output, and this leads to venous congestion (high PCWP) and peripheral vasoconstriction (high SVR). The pattern of changes is then:

High PCWP / Low CO / High SVR

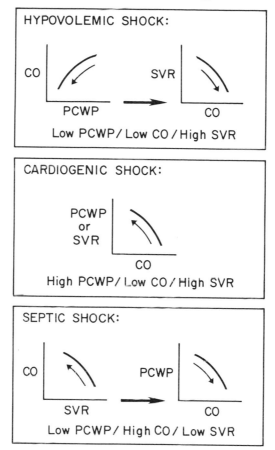

FIG. 12–1. The circulatory patterns in the three basic shock syndromes. In each panel, the primary hemodynamic problem is on the abscissa of the graph to the left. The final pattern is shown at the bottom of each panel. See text for explanation.

VASOGENIC SHOCK

The problem here is loss of vascular tone in the arteries (low SVR) and, to a variable degree, in the veins (low PCWP). The cardiac output is often elevated but can vary. One pattern in this type of shock is:

Low PCWP / High CO / Low SVR

The PCWP may be normal if venous tone is not altered or if the ventricle is stiff. These changes are discussed further in Chapter 15.

The common causes of the vasogenic shock pattern are:
1. Sepsis/Multiorgan Failure
2. Postoperative State
3. Pancreatitis
4. Trauma

TABLE 12–1. USING HEMODYNAMIC PATTERNS	
Information	Example
1. Create the pattern	Low PCWP/Low CO/Normal SVR
2. Identify the problem	Low vascular volume and vasodilatation
3. Select appropriate Rx	Volume until PCWP = 12 mmHg Dopamine (alpha-beta) if needed
4. Underlying disorder?	Adrenal insufficiency Sepsis Anaphylaxis

5. Adrenal Crisis
6. Anaphylaxis

COMBINED PROBLEMS

The three basic patterns outlined above can be combined in several ways to produce more complex problems. For example, when the pattern looks like this:

Normal PCWP / Low CO / High SVR

it can be separated into two basic patterns:

Cardiogenic shock: High PCWP / Low CO / High SVR

plus

Hypovolemic shock: Low PCWP / Low CO / High SVR

There are a total of twenty-seven possible patterns (three variables, each with three categories) and it is possible to interpret any one of these using the three basic patterns.

INTERPRETING HEMODYNAMIC PATTERNS

The information that can be generated from a hemodynamic pattern is illustrated in Table 12–1. First, the major hemodynamic problem(s) can be identified. In the example that is shown, the pattern is similar to hypovolemic shock except the SVR is normal instead of high. Therefore, the problem is "low volume plus low vascular tone." Therapy would then include volume and a drug that increases vascular tone (like dopamine). Finally, each pattern will suggest a list of underlying illnesses that might be responsible for the hemodynamic alterations. In Table 12–1, the disorders are ones that would present with volume loss and vasodilatation.

This shows the information that can be generated from one of these patterns. All you need to do is learn the three basic patterns and how they are generated.

HEMODYNAMIC MANAGEMENT

The following scheme shows how hemodynamic therapy can be matched to the hemodynamic patterns. The drugs presented in this section are covered in detail in Chapter 20. The drug effects are described using conventional terms; alpha: vasoconstriction, beta: vasodilatation and cardiac stimulation.

Condition   **Therapy**

1. Low or Normal PCWP........................... Volume infusion
   Fluids are always preferred to vasoactive drugs. The goal is to raise the PCWP to 18 to 20 mmHg or to a level that equals the colloid osmotic pressure (COP) of plasma. The COP measurement is discussed in the first part of Chapter 23.
2. Low CO
   a. High SVR... Dobutamine
   b. Normal SVR.......................................Dopamine
   A pure beta agonist like dobutamine is the therapy of choice for low cardiac output without hypotension. Dobutamine is less valuable in cardiogenic shock because it often does not elevate blood pressure; that is, the increase in cardiac output is offset by a decrease in SVR. In severe hypotension, a beta agent with some alpha vasoconstriction is more likely to increase the blood pressure because the alpha influence prevents the SVR from decreasing in response to the increase in cardiac output.
3. Low SVR
   a. Low or Normal CO........................... Alpha-Beta Agent
   b. High CO... Alpha agent (*)
   *NOTE
   Vasoconstrictors must be avoided whenever possible simply because these agents produce a pressure but at the expense of flow. The small vessel constriction from these agents can go unnoticed because the SVR is an insensitive measure of small vessel resistance.
   When some degree of vasoconstriction is needed, a combined alpha-beta agent is preferred to a pure alpha agent to decrease the tendency for profound vasoconstriction. **Dopamine** is often preferred as a combined agent because it also stimulates special dopamine receptors in the kidneys and **may help to preserve renal blood flow.**

Note that the number of hemodynamic drugs is limited. There should be no need for more agents than are listed below.

Desired Drug Effect   **Agents**

Beta, Cardiac Stimulation...........................Dobutamine
Alpha-Beta, Low BP ....Dopamine
Alpha-Beta, Second-Line ....Norepinephrine

Alpha Constriction. . . . . .High-Dose Dopamine or
Norepinephrine

The wide dose range for dopamine makes this a versatile drug. Because it works partly by displacing norepinephrine stores, it can lose effectiveness after a few days. Norepinephrine (Levophed) can substitute if necessary. If alpha constriction is needed for pressure control, the prognosis is likely to be poor and selection of agents is a minor issue. Remember to use fluids whenever possible instead of drugs. These adrenergic drugs stimulate metabolism and increase energy needs at a time when energy supply is dangerously compromised.

POSTRESUSCITATION INJURY

The period following the resuscitation of blood pressure can be associated with continued ischemia and progressive organ damage. Three syndromes of postresuscitation injury are presented briefly in this section to show you the value of monitoring tissue oxygenation and to justify the second stage of the approach.

NO-REFLOW

The no-reflow phenomenon is characterized by persistent hypoperfusion in the period following resuscitation from an ischemic insult.[5,6] The mechanism is believed to be calcium influx into vascular smooth muscle during the ischemic period which results in intense vasoconstriction that persists for hours after the resuscitation period. The splanchnic and cerebral circulations seem particularly vulnerable to this process and the consequences are serious. Splanchnic ischemia can damage the mucosal barrier in the bowel wall and allow intestinal organisms to "translocate" across the bowel wall and into the systemic circulation.[7] Persistent cerebral ischemia can produce permanent neurologic deficits and this may explain the prevalence of cerebral impairment following resuscitation from cardiac arrest.[6] The ultimate expression of the no-reflow phenomenon may be the "multiorgan failure syndrome"[8] which is just what the name implies and is often fatal.

REPERFUSION INJURY

Reperfusion injury differs from the no-reflow phenomenon because blood flow is restored after the ischemic insult. The problem here is that toxic substances have accumulated during the period of ischemia and these toxins are washed out in the reflow period and are swept along with the blood flow to distant organs.[9] The culprits are believed to be oxygen metabolites that are highly reactive and readily damage cell membranes. These oxygen radicals (a radical is a molecular species with an unpaired electron in its outer shell) have the ability to produce more

THE OXYGEN DEBT

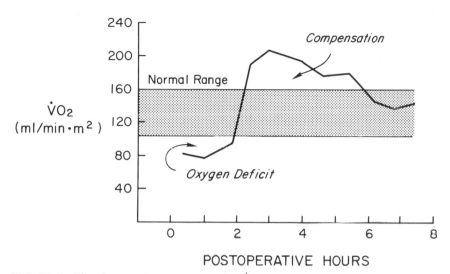

FIG. 12–2. The changes in oxygen uptake ($\dot{V}O_2$) during postoperative repayment of oxygen debt. See text for explanation.

radicals when they react with cell membrane lipids (peroxidation). This produces a "chain reaction" type of response that is well suited to the reperfusion period because one locus of toxin generation could rapidly grow to affect all distant organs The evidence for this mechanism is circumstantial and trials of antioxidant therapy for reperfusion injury have had mixed results.[11]

OXYGEN DEBT

The oxygen debt is an oxygen deficit that accumulates during a period of ischemia and must be compensated or "repaid" in the postischemic period. This concept is illustrated in Figure 12–2 for a patient in the immediate postoperative period following prolonged surgery for a ruptured viscus. The important feature to note is the shape of the $\dot{V}O_2$ changes in the immediate postoperative period. The $\dot{V}O_2$ is low at the end of the surgical procedure and then reaches supranormal levels (overshoot) in the first few hours after surgery. The contour looks similar to the phenomenon of reactive hyperemia that occurs after a brief period of occlusive ischemia. In the case of the $\dot{V}O_2$, the early period of subnormal values represents ongoing ischemia (not metabolic slowdown from anesthesia) and this is where the oxygen deficit builds. The period of supranormal $\dot{V}O_2$ levels is the compensatory period needed to "repay the debt" incurred during the ischemic period. Patients who are unable to mount this response carry a risk for persistent ischemia and organ damage.

The oxygen debt is a good example of the value of monitoring tissue oxygen balance following a period of ischemia. In the case of the oxygen debt, failure to observe a compensatory overshoot in the postischemic period indicates ongoing ischemia and the $\dot{V}O_2$ can be manipulated so that it reaches supranormal levels if necessary.[11] This may help to prevent organ damage and the poor outcome that often results.

STAGE II: TISSUE OXYGENATION

Since resuscitation of the blood pressure in stage I may not correct peripheral ischemia, a second stage is added to assess the state of tissue oxygenation.

OXYGEN UPTAKE ($\dot{V}O_2$)

Shock can be defined as a state where the $\dot{V}O_2$ is inadequate for the needs of aerobic metabolism.

The $\dot{V}O_2$ is the single best hemodynamic measurement for determining if the shock state is present.[2,3]

As discussed in Chapter 2, the $\dot{V}O_2$ is a measure of the oxygen taken up from the microcirculation and is not a measure of metabolic oxygen consumption. A lower than normal $\dot{V}O_2$ indicates an inadequate oxygen uptake into tissues unless the metabolic rate is decreased. Patients with a low $\dot{V}O_2$ have a higher morbidity and mortality than those with a normal or supranormal $\dot{V}O_2$.[2-4] However, the presence of a normal or high $\dot{V}O_2$ does not insure that the oxygen supply to tissue is adequate for the metabolic rate. Tissue ischemia will develop if the metabolic rate exceeds the oxygen uptake, regardless of the absolute level of the $\dot{V}O_2$. Therefore, in hypermetabolic states (e.g., sepsis), a normal $\dot{V}O_2$ may still be inadequate to meet the demands of the increased metabolic rate. When this occurs, lactic acid will begin to accumulate, and will eventually spill into the blood stream. Therefore, the serum lactate level can be used as a marker of anaerobic metabolism when the $\dot{V}O_2$ is in the normal range.

SERUM LACTATE

Serum lactate levels can be used to assess the balance between oxygen supply to tissues ($\dot{V}O_2$) and the metabolic oxygen consumption.[3] Lactate is usually measured in the arterial blood. The normal range is below 2 mM/L in healthy subjects and below 4 mM/L in stressed subjects.[9] The liver clears lactate from the bloodstream, but severe liver disease itself is not associated with lactate accumulation in the blood.[10]

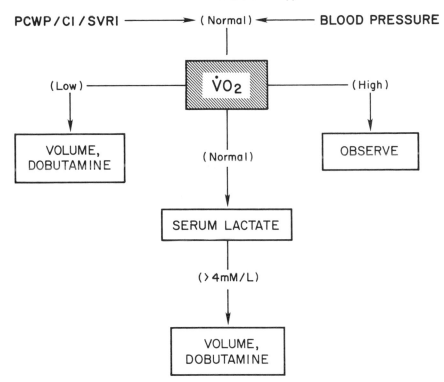

FIG. 12–3. The strategy in Stage II using the oxygen uptake ($\dot{V}O_2$) and arterial lactate level.

THE $\dot{V}O_2$ AND LACTATE AS END-POINTS

The approach used in stage II to assess tissue oxygenation is outlined in Figure 12–3. After the traditional hemodynamic parameters (PCWP/CO/SVR) are corrected, the $\dot{V}O_2$ should be determined.

Condition	Therapy
1. Low $\dot{V}O_2$	
a. PCWP < 18 mmHg	Volume Infusion
b. PCWP > 18 mmHg	Dobutamine/Dopamine

If the $\dot{V}O_2$ is low (less than 110 ml/min·M²), increase the cardiac output with volume or dobutamine. Volume is the obvious therapy in hemorrhagic shock, but may also benefit patients with septic shock and cardiogenic shock as long as the PCWP is not high enough to produce pulmonary edema. Volume is always preferred to hemodynamic drugs for improving peripheral blood flow. If volume can no longer be given, dobutamine should be given to increase cardiac output.

2. $\dot{V}O_2$ Normal or High	
a. Lactate High	Volume/Dobutamine
b. Lactate Normal	Observe

When the $\dot{V}O_2$ is not low, the arterial lactate level is used to determine the approach. If the arterial lactate is above 4 mM/L, increase the cardiac output (if possible) with volume or dobutamine, as was done for the low $\dot{V}O_2$. If the arterial lactate is not elevated, consider the management successful for the time being.

SUMMARY

The approach used here is different from the traditional approach to shock because it does not focus entirely on the blood pressure or the blood flow. Instead, these variables are used as goals of the initial management. The approach then moves to the tissue level to assess the adequacy of oxygenation. The hope is that the second stage will help to minimize the risk for post-resuscitation ischemia and its lethal consequences.

BIBLIOGRAPHY

Barrett J, Nyhus LM. Treatment of shock. 2nd ed. Philadelphia: Lea & Febiger, 1986.
Sibbald WJ, Sprung, CL eds. Perspectives on sepsis and septic shock. Society of Critical Care Medicine, 1986.
Snyder JV, Perisky MR eds. Oxygen Transport in the Critically Ill. Chicago, Year Book Medical Publishers, 1987.

REFERENCES

REVIEWS

1. Shoemaker WC. Circulatory mechanisms of shock and their mediators. Crit Care Med 1987; 15:787–794.
2. Shoemaker WC. Relationship of oxygen transport patterns to the pathophysiology and therapy of shock states. Intensive Care Med 1987; 13:230–243.
3. Rackow EC, Astiz ME, Weil MH. Cellular oxygen metabolism during sepsis and shock. JAMA 1988; 259:1989–1993.
4. Weber K, Janicki JS, Hunter WC, et al. The contractile behavior of the heart and its functional coupling to the circulation. Prog Cardiovasc Dis 1982; 24:375–400.

SELECTED REFERENCES

5. McNamara JJ, Suehiro GT, Suehiro A, et al. Resuscitation from hemorrhagic shock. J Trauma 1983; 23:552–558.
6. White BC, Winegar CD, Wilson RF, et al. Possible role of calcium blockers in cerebral resuscitation: A review of the literature and synthesis for future studies. Crit Care Med 1983; 11:202–207.
7. Sori AJ, Rush BF, Lysz, TW, et al. The gut as a source of sepsis after hemorrhagic shock. Am J Surg 1988; 155:187–191.

8. Cerra FB. The systemic septic response: Multiple systems organ failure. Crit Care Clin 1985; 2:591–607.
9. Haljamde H. Lactate metabolism. Intensive Care World 1987; 4:118–120.
10. Kruse JA, Zaidi SAJ, Carlson RW. Significance of blood lactate levels in critically ill patients with liver disease. Am J Med 1987; 83:77–82.
11. Waxman K, Nolan LS, Shoemaker WC. Sequential perioperative lactate determination. Physiological and clinical implications. Crit Care Med 1982; 10:96–99.

chapter

13

HEMORRHAGE AND HYPOVOLEMIA

The dominant concern in the bleeding patient is the intolerance of the human body to the loss of blood volume. The human can survive the loss of 80% of the liver and adrenals, 75% of the kidneys and red cell mass, and loss of more than one lung. However, acute loss of 35% of the blood volume can be fatal. The dangers of hemorrhage are related to a cardiovascular system that operates with a small volume and a steep Starling curve (volume-sensitive ventricle). The purpose may be to limit cardiac work and conserve energy. The consequence is illustrated in the numbers that follow.

BODY FLUIDS AND BLOOD LOSS

The distribution of body fluids for an adult male of 70 kg (154 lb) is shown below. Total body water (TBW) is taken as 60% of the lean body weight.[1]

Compartment	Volume (L)	% TBW
Intracellular	23.0	55
Interstitial Fluid	8.4	20
Bone	6.3	15
Plasma	3.2	7.5
Body Cavities	1.1	2.5
Total	42.0 L	100%

The plasma volume of 3.2 L corresponds to a blood volume of 5.7 L if the hematocrit is 45%. The blood volume therefore represents 13% of the total volume of body fluids. Assuming an acute loss of 35% of the blood volume can be fatal, the survival of the human is determined by

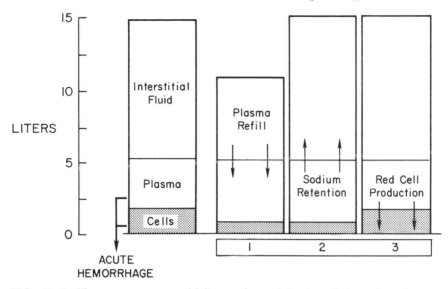

FIG. 13–1. The response to mild hemorrhage. Numbers below the columns correspond to the three phases explained in the text.

4% of the fluid in the body. Furthermore, your job is to prevent the bleeding patient from losing this 4% aliquot.

THE RESPONSE TO BLOOD LOSS

In the healthy adult, a 15% loss of blood volume does not require intervention with intravenous fluids.[2] This degree of blood loss is appropriate as a model for studying the natural response of the body to hemorrhage. The original studies of hemorrhage were performed on medical student volunteers (surprise!) and the response that was uncovered is divided into three phases.[2] These are depicted in the diagram in Figure 13–1, and each phase is summarized below.

Phase 1. Within an hour after blood loss begins, interstitial fluid begins to move into the capillaries. This shift or "transcapillary refill" continues for 36 to 40 hours and can reach a volume of 1 L.[3] The egress of fluid from the interstitial space leaves an interstitial fluid deficit.

Phase 2. The loss of blood volume activates the renin system and this leads to sodium conservation by the kidneys. Because sodium distributes primarily in the interstitial space (80% of sodium is extravascular), the retained sodium replenishes the fluid deficit in the interstitial space.

Phase 3. Within a few hours after the onset of hemorrhage, the marrow begins to produce erythrocytes, but the replacement of lost erythrocytes is a slow process. Only 15 to 50 ml of cell volume is produced daily, and complete replacement of lost cells can take up to 2 months.[2]

The early transcapillary refill leaves a fluid deficit in the interstitial space and not in the vascular space. This interstitial fluid deficit is the goal of early fluid therapy.

TABLE 13–1. CLASSIFICATION OF HEMORRHAGE*		
Class	**Clinical Signs**	**% Volume Loss**
I.	Tachycardia	15
II.	Orthostatic Hypotension	20–25
III.	Supine Hypotension Oliguria	30–40
IV.	Obtundation Cardiovascular Collapse	over 40

*From Committee on Trauma, American College of Surgeons. Early care of the injured patient. 3rd ed. Philadelphia: W.B. Saunders, 1982.

The goal of fluid therapy for mild hemorrhage is to fill the interstitial space, not the vascular space. This is the rationale for using saline (sodium chloride) fluids for the resuscitation of mild hemorrhage.

Saline fluids are designed to fill the interstitial space because sodium distributes evenly throughout the extracellular space and 80% of this space is extravascular. Infusing a fluid that remains in the vascular space (like albumin or blood) will not replace the interstitial fluid deficit and will prevent the activation of renin, thereby interfering with the sodium retention that the body uses to replace interstitial volume deficits.

The discussion above is an introduction to the topic of crystalloid (electrolyte) fluids versus colloid fluids for the resuscitation of acute hypovolemia. In the above example, crystalloid fluids should suffice. When the hemorrhage is more severe and rapid expansion of the vascular space is desirable, colloid fluids might be the fluids of choice. The debate concerning colloid and crystalloid fluids is presented in Chapter 17.

CLINICAL PRESENTATION

The clinical presentation can vary depending on acuity and extent of volume loss as well as the ability of the patient to mount a compensatory response to hypovolemia. The following areas deserve mention.

CLASSIFICATION OF VOLUME LOSS

The American College of Surgeons identifies four categories of hemorrhage based on the fractional loss of blood volume and the expected clinical findings.[4] These categories are shown in Table 13–1.

Class I. Loss of 15% or less of the total blood volume. This degree of blood loss can be silent clinically or can produce a resting tachycardia that appears first in the upright position. This "orthostatic tachycardia" is defined as a rise in heart rate of at least 20 beats/min when moving from the supine to upright position.

Class II. Loss of 20 to 25% of the blood volume. The major clinical finding at this stage is an orthostatic drop in systolic blood pressure of at least 15 mmHg. Supine blood pressure is often unchanged but can be diminished slightly. Urine flow is preserved at this stage.

Class III. Loss of 30 to 40% of the blood volume. At this stage there is hypotension in the supine position as well as oliguria (less than 400 ml/24h).

Class IV. Loss of more than 40% of blood volume. This is a potentially life-threatening condition that can lead to profound hypotension and cardiovascular collapse.

The demonstration of orthostasis requires a "body tilt" with the patient either standing or with the legs over the side of the bed. Sitting in bed with feet not in a dependent position is not satisfactory.

The severity of the blood pressure changes in hypovolemia will vary according to the acuity of the volume loss and the strength of the compensatory response. The early compensatory response of tachycardia and vasoconstriction can be blunted by several conditions including advanced age, diabetes, renal failure, and beta blocker or vasodilator therapy. In these conditions, the clinical presentation is marked by early hypotension and less severe (or absent) tachycardia.

CENTRAL VENOUS PRESSURES

The filling pressures of the right and left heart (CVP and PCWP) are often used to evaluate the vascular volume and to guide therapy. However, these measurements can be unreliable for assessing the state of the blood volume in critically ill adults.[5] Two problems can surface in hypovolemia. First, the central venous pressures are normally low and have little margin for change when hypovolemia develops. Secondly, these measurements are influenced by the compliance of the veins and ventricles and the compliance of both may decrease in hypovolemic states as a result of sympathetic activation.

Two practices can increase the sensitivity of the filling pressures. The first is to interpret changes in pressure over time rather than interpreting single measurements.[5] The second is to measure the pressures in both the supine and upright positions (if possible). A decrease in the CVP of 4 to 5 mmHg in the upright position can indicate hypovolemia.[6] This maneuver is valuable when the central filling pressures are in the normal range but hypovolemia is suspected.

THE HEMATOCRIT

Acute blood loss will not influence the hematocrit immediately because whole blood is being lost and the proportion of red cells to plasma volume should remain unchanged. The hematocrit will change acutely only when fluid replacement therapy begins. The influence of replacement therapy on the hematocrit is shown in Figure 13–2. Each column in the figure is partitioned to indicate the relative contributions of plasma

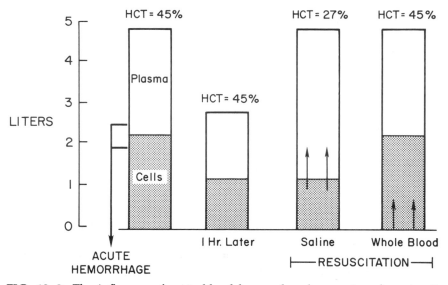

FIG. 13–2. The influence of acute blood loss and replacement on hematocrit (Hct). See text for explanation.

and red blood cells. The columns on the left show that an acute drop in blood volume of 2 L does not change the hematocrit. The columns on the right show that the replacement determines whether the hematocrit will change or not. Saline infusion will increase the plasma volume selectively and cause a decrease in hematocrit, while the infusion of whole blood expands both plasma and red cell volume equivalently and will not change hematocrit. This figure illustrates the role of the replacement therapy in determining the acute changes in hematocrit in the setting of acute hemorrhage.

> In acute hemorrhage, the hematocrit is a reflection of the replacement therapy and not the presence or extent of blood loss.

An acute drop in hematocrit indicates infusion of plasma expanders and does not signal active bleeding. In fact, the decrease in hematocrit can indicate adequate plasma expansion and be a sign of appropriate volume therapy.

PRINCIPLES OF FLUID THERAPY

The mortality in acute hemorrhage is highest in the first few hours,[7] therefore, the initial fluid infusion must be as effective as possible. The principles in this section will help you select the appropriate cannulation site, catheter, and fluid for each clinical situation.

THE CANNULATION SITE

Cannulation of the large central veins is almost universal when volume infusion is indicated for hypovolemia. The reason for this practice in all patients may be partly due to the misconception that the large central veins will permit faster infusion rates.

The maximum infusion rate for intravenous fluids is determined by the size of the catheter and not by the size of the vein that is cannulated.

The catheter diameter is always narrower than the diameter of the vein and the dimensions of the catheter will dictate the resistance to flow. This means that cannulating the large central veins does not ensure more rapid flowrates. In fact, as you will see in the next section, the long catheters used for central venous cannulation will impede flow much more than the short catheters used to cannulate peripheral veins.

CATHETER DIMENSIONS

The influence of catheter size on the infusion rate is described by the Hagen-Poisseulle equation.[8]

$$Q = \Delta P \frac{\pi r^4}{8\mu L}$$

This equation states that infusion rate ($\dot{Q}$) is directly related to the pressure gradient along the tube (P) and the fourth power of the catheter radius (r) and is inversely related to the length (L) of the catheter and the viscosity (μ) of the fluid. This means that flow will be lower in catheters that are long and narrow. Therefore, the flow of an intravenous fluid will be lower in catheters that are long and narrow and this explains why central venous catheters are associated with lower flowrates than short peripheral catheters.

The relationship between catheter size and flowrate is illustrated in Table 13–2. This table is from a study that used tap water as the fluid and kept the infusion pressure constant by suspending the fluid above the catheters at a constant height.[9] Note the flowrates for the 16-gauge catheter when the length is 2 inches and 12 inches. The infusion rate is almost four times higher in the short (2 inch) peripheral catheter than in the long (twelve inch) central venous catheter. The length of a central venous "multilumen" catheter is 17 ¾ inches, while the standard length of a peripheral venous catheter is only 2 inches. This illustrates the magnitude of change in flowrate that can be associated with a change from peripheral to central venous cannulation.

TABLE 13–2. INFLUENCE OF CATHETER SIZE ON INFUSION RATE		
Infusion Device	Length (inches)	Flowrate* (ml/mm)
9-French Introducer	5½	247
IV Extension Tubing	12	220
Peripheral		
14-Gauge Catheter	2	195
16-Gauge Catheter	2	150
Central		
16-Gauge Catheter	5½	91
16-Gauge Catheter	12	54

*gravity flow of tap water.
From Mateer JR, et al. Rapid fluid resuscitation with central venous catheters. Ann Emerg Med 1983; 12:149–152.

INTRODUCER CATHETERS

The adverse effects of catheter length in central venous cannulation can be overcome by using large bore "introducer sheath" catheters like the one shown in Figure 13–3. These catheters are available in sizes of 8.5 French (2.7 mm internal diameter) and 9.0 French (3 mm internal diameter). The 9-French catheter is nearly as wide as the standard tubing used for blood transfusions (3.0 versus 3.2 mm internal diameter for introducer and blood tubing, respectively). These catheters are used normally as conduits for multilumen catheters or pulmonary artery catheters but they can be used as "stand alone" catheters when rapid volume infusion is necessary. Most introducers have a side port that serves as an extra infusion line but the tubing in this line is narrow and limits

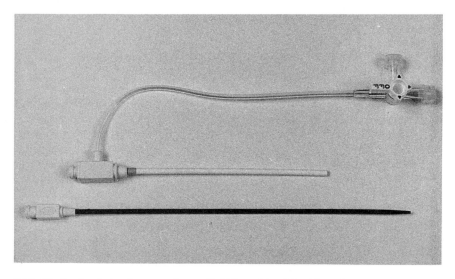

FIG. 13–3. An introducer catheter (8.5 French) with side infusion port.

TABLE 13-3. INFLUENCE OF FLUID TYPE ON INFUSION RATE	
Fluid	Flowrate (ml/min)*
Tap Water	100
5% Albumin	100
Whole Blood	65
Packed Cells	20

*gravity flow through a 16-gauge, 2-inch catheter.
From Dula DJ, et al. Flowrate variance of commonly used IV infusion techniques. J Trauma 1981; 21:480–482.

maximum infusion rates. This side port should be avoided when rapid infusion is desirable.

The infusion rate through a 9-French introducer catheter is shown in Table 13-2. Comparing the flow in the introducer with that in the 16-gauge catheter of similar length (5 ½ inches) reveals that the flow is almost three times faster in the introducer sheath. The IV tubing in Table 13-2 has a slower infusion rate than the introducer catheters but this is probably because of the longer length of the tubing. Although IV tubing is wider, the introducers can accommodate flowrates of up to 300 ml/min,[10] and at this rate the IV tubing would limit the maximum infusion rate.

FLUID VISCOSITY

The flow of fluids is characterized by the parallel movement of concentric layers of fluid sliding past each other. Viscosity is best described as the resistance to flow caused by friction between these concentric layers of fluid.[8] The common expression is the *relative viscosity*, defined as the flowrate of a fluid relative to water. The relative viscosity of plasma is 1.8, while whole blood has a relative viscosity of 3 to 4.[8]

The influence of viscosity on the flowrate of fluids is defined by the Hagen-Poisseulle equation presented earlier. The effect of viscosity on the infusion rate of blood and asanguinous fluids is shown in Table 13-3.[11] The catheter in this case was a 16-gauge catheter 2 inches in length (the dimensions of peripheral venous catheters) and the fluids were infused under the influence of gravity. Note that the infusion rate for water and 5% albumin is the same. This should dispel any myths about colloid solutions being sluggish compared to crystalloid fluids. Also, note the sluggish flow of the concentrated red cell preparation (packed cells). Infusion of the asanguinous fluids was five times faster than the packed red cell infusion, indicating that asanguinous fluids will be more effective than blood when rapid volume replacement is needed. The sluggish flow associated with red blood cell concentrates is improved by warming the blood and by diluting the cells with an equal volume of 0.9% saline. (Chapter 18 has more information on blood transfusion techniques.)

AUTOTRANSFUSION MANEUVERS

The autotransfusion maneuvers are designed to shift blood from the legs and increase venous return, thereby promoting the cardiac output. These maneuvers are used as temporary measures during patient transport or at the start of the resuscitation period. Unfortunately, the autotransfusion techniques provide little benefit and may even be harmful. The methods for autotransfusion involve either gravity maneuvers or pneumatic garments.

GRAVITY MANEUVERS

There are two maneuvers that use the force of gravity to promote venous return.[12-15]

1. **Legs Raised.** The legs are raised passively until they make an angle of 10 to 45° with the horizontal plane. This creates an illusion of "pouring" blood from the legs into the central veins.

2. **Head-Down Body Tilt.** The body is tilted with the head moving down from the horizontal plane until it rests 10 to 15° below the plane. This is the Trendelenburg position, introduced in the latter 19th century to facilitate suprapubic cystostomy, and adopted in World War I as an "antishock" position.

Clinical Efficacy. Neither of the gravity maneuvers has been shown to increase the volume of blood in the central veins[12,13] or to consistently improve cardiac output in either hypovolemic or normovolemic subjects.[14] The influence of the Trendelenburg position on carotid blood flow has been studied in animals only, but in these studies it caused a decrease in carotid flow.[15]

Misconceptions. The lack of efficacy of the gravity maneuvers is not surprising in light of the physical characteristics of the venous system. The assumption that raising the legs will create a pressure gradient from leg veins to central veins is not sound. The veins are a capacitance system and capacitance systems are designed to absorb pressure rather than to transmit pressure. In other words, pressure applied to one end of a vein will be absorbed or lost because the vein can bulge or act like a reservoir. This behavior makes it difficult to create a pressure gradient along the venous system unless the system is filled to capacity (the opposite of hypovolemia). The leg raising maneuver would be more likely to work if the veins were rigid tubes like the arteries.

The head down position in the Trendelenburg position is aimed at improving carotid blood flow but this neglects the influence of venous pressure in the cranium on cerebral flow. Cerebral blood flow is determined by the pressure gradient between the carotid arteries and the intracerebral veins. Placing the head in a dependent position will increase pressure in the intracranial venous sinuses and if the venous pressure increases more than the arterial pressure, carotid flow will diminish. This also means that the Trendelenburg position can increase intracranial pressure and this must be kept in mind in patients with head trauma or any other condition where increased intracranial pressure can be harmful.

Recommendation. Based on the available studies, passive leg raising cannot be recommended as effective and the Trendelenburg position cannot be recommended as effective or safe.

PNEUMATIC GARMENTS

Pneumatic garments are designed to encase the lower extremities and apply a "counterpressure" that partially compresses the small venules in the leg while sparing the arteries.[16] The goal is to increase the pressure in the small leg veins and promote venous return. These garments are used primarily for trauma victims in the field and are applied during transport. They are sometimes called medical antishock trousers or MAST garments.

Clinical Efficacy. The clinical experience with MAST garments is discouraging. The major observation that dominates all others is the lack of improved survival with the garment.[17] Other disturbing findings relate to the mechanism for the increase in pressure from the garment. In summary, the cardiac output is often decreased by the garment and the increase in mean arterial pressure is the result of an increase in systemic vascular resistance.[17] The latter is presumably because of arterial constriction from the garment. The benefits of the garment are to stabilize the lower torso for fractures and to tamponade bleeding sites. The increase in pressure can also improve coronary and cerebral blood flow.[16]

Recommendation. At the present time, there is no evidence to support the routine use of pneumatic garments as a life-saving measure.

RESUSCITATION STRATEGIES

The goal of all resuscitation efforts is to maintain oxygen uptake ($\dot{V}O_2$) into the tissues to support metabolism. The $\dot{V}O_2$ is described in Chapter 2. It is a function of the cardiac output ($\dot{Q}$), the serum hemoglobin concentration (Hb), and the difference in oxyhemoglobin saturation between arterial and venous blood ($SaO_2 - S\bar{v}O_2$).

$$\dot{V}O_2 = \dot{Q} \times Hb \times 13 \times (SaO_2 - S\bar{v}O_2)$$
$$\quad\quad * \quad\quad *$$

The asterisks indicate the components of the equation that are reduced as a result of blood loss. The immediate concern in acute hemorrhage is hypovolemia and low cardiac output. The secondary concern is anemia. The strategies below are separated according to these two concerns.

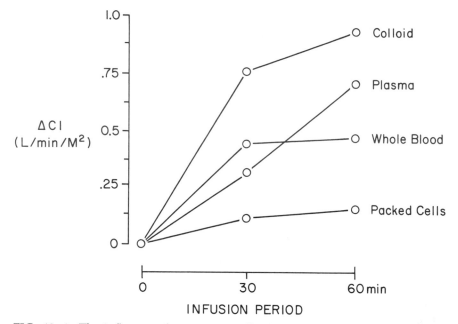

FIG. 13–4. The influence of resuscitation fluids on the cardiac index (CI). The colloid fluid is dextran-40. From Shoemaker WC. Intensive Care Med 1987; 13:230–243.

SUPPORTING THE CARDIAC OUTPUT

The selection of the initial resuscitation fluid in hemorrhagic shock is based on the ability of the fluid to increase the cardiac output. The ability of blood products and colloid fluids to promote cardiac output is shown in Figure 13–4. This figure is taken from a clinical study of adults with sepsis.[18] Each fluid was infused over a 1-hour period in a volume of 500 ml and the cardiac output was measured (thermodilution) at 30 and 60 minutes after the onset of infusion. Infusion of the colloid solution (dextran-40) caused the greatest increase in cardiac output while the red blood cell concentrate failed to augment cardiac output. The pattern of fluid response indicates that the ability of a fluid to augment cardiac output is inversely related to the density of cells in the fluid. The acellular fluids (colloid and plasma) were most effective for augmenting blood flow while the red cell concentrate was the least effective. Because the density of cells in the fluid is directly related to viscosity, the ability of the fluids to augment cardiac output in Figure 13–4 is another way of stating the Hagen-Poisseulle equation.

Colloid versus Blood. Colloid solutions are superior to blood products for improving cardiac output, as indicated in Figure 13–4. In fact, infusion of red cell concentrates can be associated with a decrease in cardiac output.[19] The viscosity of blood can increase at low flowrates,[8] so the influence of red cell infusions on the viscosity of circulating blood can be magnified in patients with a low cardiac output. All the information

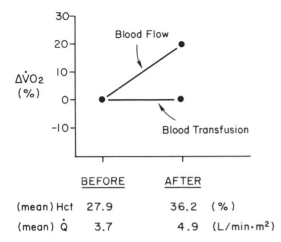

FIG. 13–5. The effects of cardiac index (CI) and hematocrit (HCT) on oxygen uptake ($\dot{V}_{O_2}$) in hemorrhagic shock. From McCormick M, et al. J Surg Res 1988; 44:499–505.

	BEFORE	AFTER	
(mean) Hct	27.9	36.2	(%)
(mean) $\dot{Q}$	3.7	4.9	(L/min·m²)

at present points to colloid solutions as the replacement fluid of choice for the immediate support of cardiac output in acute hemorrhage. This is a fortunate circumstance because whole blood is no longer stored routinely and cross-matched blood is not immediately available for trauma victims.

Colloid versus Crystalloid. The graph in Figure 13–4 does not include a crystalloid fluid but the results of several other studies indicate that colloids are able to increase cardiac output with one-third the volume required by crystalloid fluids.[20] Therefore colloids are the logical favorite for quick volume expansion. Crystalloids can achieve the same effect with a greater volume, and these fluids are preferred by many if the hemorrhage is not life-threatening. The debate over these two fluids will be hammered out in Chapter 17.

HEMOGLOBIN REPLACEMENT

Once cardiac output is supported, the concern shifts to replacing the hemoglobin that has been lost. The traditional approach to blood transfusion is aimed at maintaining a serum hemoglobin of 10 mg/dL or higher.[21] However, this practice seems steeped more in dogma than in scientific fact.[23] A more reasonable approach to blood transfusion might be to gauge the need for blood by monitoring the oxygen uptake ($\dot{V}_{O_2}$) as an index of the state of tissue oxygenation in individual patients. A normal $\dot{V}_{O_2}$ could be used as evidence for adequate tissue oxygenation (unless the patient is hypermetabolic).

The ability of blood transfusions to improve tissue oxygenation is shown in Figure 13–5. This graph is drawn from a clinical study of the influence of blood transfusions and cardiac output augmentation on the oxygen uptake during resuscitation from hemorrhagic shock.[22] Note that the $\dot{V}_{O_2}$ increased after the cardiac output was raised, but the $\dot{V}_{O_2}$ was not increased by raising the hematocrit with blood transfusion. The lack of an increase in $\dot{V}_{O_2}$ despite an increase in hemoglobin can be explained in two ways. First, the $\dot{V}_{O_2}$ may be on the flat portion of the curve

Normal Blood Volume

Males:	BV = 70 ml/kg	or	3.2 L/M²
Females:	BV = 60 ml/kg	or	2.9 L/M²

Fractional Blood Loss

	Loss (%)	Replace (%)
No Clinical Signs	<20	20
Orthostasis	20	20
Supine Hypotension	20–35	30
Organ Failure	>35	50

Volume Deficit

Volume Deficit = % Loss × Normal Blood Volume

Resuscitation Rules

Whole Blood	= 1.0 × Volume Deficit
Colloid	= 1.0 × Volume Deficit
Crystalloid	= 3.0 × Volume Deficit

FIG. 13–6. Estimating volume requirements for patients with acute hypovolemia.

relating oxygen delivery to oxygen consumption (see Chapter 2, Figure 2–2). Second, the blood transfusion may have decreased the cardiac output and counterbalanced the increase in serum hemoglobin.

The following aspect of blood transfusion therapy needs to be emphasized.

Blood transfusion to correct anemia does not ensure that tissue oxygenation is also improved. Therefore, the hemoglobin can be misleading as a guide for blood transfusion therapy.

A recent Consensus Conference on blood transfusion practices[23] concluded that more rational criteria for transfusions are needed. It seems that the oxygen uptake provides a much more rational guide for transfusion in individual patients than the serum hemoglobin.

ESTIMATING VOLUME REQUIREMENTS

The following approach can be used for a quick appraisal of the volume needs of each patient with acute hypovolemia. This is a useful exercise because there is a tendency to underestimate volume needs in these patients. The stepwise approach that follows is outlined in Figure 13–6.

1. **Estimate normal blood volume** for adults using 70 ml/kg for males and 60 ml/kg for females.[24] Use lean body weight for the estimate. For obese patients, use actual body weight and subtract 10%.

2. **Estimate the percent volume loss** using the classification system in Table 13–2. Remember that some patients (e.g., diabetics) will show

an exaggerated response to hypovolemia and will cause you to overestimate volume losses.

3. **Calculate the volume deficit** by multiplying the estimated normal blood volume and the percent loss. This is a quantitative estimate of the volume needs in each patient.

4. **Apply rules** to the replacement of blood and crystalloid fluids:
   a. If the fractional volume loss is 20% or less, blood replacement is not necessary unless there is a specific reason such as angina.
   b. If crystalloids are used, multiply the volume deficit by 3 to estimate the replacement volume.

The adjustment for crystalloid replacement is based on the observation that only 20 to 30% of infused crystalloid will remain in the vascular space.[20,24]

ENDPOINTS

The following variables can be used to gauge the success of the resuscitation effort.

THE CVP AND PCWP

The ventricular filling pressures are not always reliable for assessing blood volume in critically ill patients.[5] However, the following pressures are suggested as reasonable endpoints of the initial fluid resuscitation.

Immediate goals: CVP = 15 mmHg[25]

PCWP = 10 to 12 mmHg[26]

In patients with a history of hypertension or left heart failure, the PCWP can be increased to 18 to 20 mmHg or until the plasma colloid osmotic pressure is reached (see Chapter 14).

THE $\dot{V}O_2$ AND SERUM LACTATE

The use of the $\dot{V}O_2$ as an endpoint of therapy was introduced in the prior section on hemoglobin replacement. Remember that correction of the hypovolemia does not ensure that the peripheral ischemia has resolved, as discussed in Chapter 12. Therefore, it is necessary to monitor tissue oxygenation with the $\dot{V}O_2$ as well as the serum lactate in selected patients.

The $\dot{V}O_2$ should be low during hemorrhagic shock, and 40% reductions have been reported in animal models.[27] Fluid therapy should aim to restore the $\dot{V}O_2$ to the normal range and occasionally to a supranormal range if necessary. Remember that a normal $\dot{V}O_2$ is not proof of adequate tissue oxygenation because of the hypermetabolism that often accompanies shock states. When the $\dot{V}O_2$ is in the normal range, it is wise to monitor the serum lactate levels to detect tissue ischemia as early as possible.

Base deficit has been used as an indirect measure of serum lactate and has been suggested as a guide for volume therapy in trauma victims.[28] A base deficit that does not decrease or normalize during volume infusion is a signal for ongoing tissue ischemia and the need for continued aggressive management. The base deficit is readily obtained with the arterial blood gases using a nomogram (the Sigaard-Andersen nomogram), and many of the newer blood gas analyzers will automatically calculate base deficit. Normal range is $+2$ to -2. The value of this measure requires further study, but the topic is included here because the measurement is so easy to obtain.

REFERENCES

PHYSIOLOGY

1. Edelman IS, Leibman J. Anatomy of body water and electrolytes. Am J Med 1959; 27:256–263.
2. Moore FD. The effects of hemorrhage on body composition. N Engl J Med 1965; 273:567–577.
3. Haljamar H. Interstitial Fluid Response. In: Shires GT, ed. Shock and related problems. Clinical surgery international. Vol. 9. New York: Churchill Livingstone, 1984.

CLINICAL PRESENTATION

4. American College of Surgeons, Committee on Trauma. Early care of the injured patient. 3rd ed. Philadelphia: W.B. Saunders, 1982:24–26.
5. Shippy CR, Appel PL, Shoemaker WC. Reliability of clinical monitoring to assess blood volume in the critically ill patients. Crit Care Med 1984; 12:107–112.
6. Amoroso P, Greenwood RN. Posture and central venous pressure measurement in circulatory volume depletion. Lancet 1989; 1:258–260.
7. Bellamy RF. The causes of death in conventional land warfare: Implications for combat casualty care research. Military Med 1984; 149:55–62.

PRINCIPLES OF FLUID INFUSION

8. Chien S, Usami S, Skalak R. Blood flow in small tubes. In: Renkin EM, Michel CC eds. Handbook of physiology. Section 2: The cardiovascular system. Vol. IV. The microcirculation. Bethesda: American Physiological Society, 1984.
9. Mateer JR, Thompson BM, Aprahamian C, Darin JC. Rapid fluid resuscitation with central venous catheters. Ann Emerg Med 12:149–152, 1983.
10. Dailey RH. Large volume fluid resuscitation. West J Med 1985; 142:386–387.
11. Dula DJ, Muller A, Donovan JW. Flow rate of commonly used IV techniques. J Trauma 1981; 21:480–482.

AUTOTRANSFUSION

12. Bivins HG, Knopp R, dos Santos PAL. Blood volume distribution in the Trendelenburg position. Ann Emerg Med 1985; *14*:641–643.
13. Gaffney FA, Bastian BC, Thal ER, et al. Passive leg raising does not produce a significant autotransfusion effect. J Trauma 1982; *22*:190–193.
14. Sibbald WJ, Paterson NA, Holiday RL, et al. The Trendelenburg position: Hemodynamic effects in hypotensive and normotensive patients. Crit Care Med 1979; *7*:218–224.
15. Guneroth WG, Abel FL, Mullins GL. The effect of Trendelenburg's position on blood pressure and carotid flow. Surg Gynecol Obstet 1964; *117*:345–348.
16. McSwain NE, Jr. Pneumatic anti-shock garment: State of the art 1988. Ann Emerg Med 1988; *17*:506–525.
17. Pepe PE, Bass RR, Mattox KL. Clinical trials of the pneumatic antishock garment in the urban prehospital setting. Ann Emerg Med 1986; *15*:1407–1410.

STRATEGIES

18. Shoemaker WC. Relationship of oxygen transport patterns to the pathophysiology and therapy of shock states. Intensive Care Med 1987; *213*:230–243.
19. Shah DM, Gottlieb ME, Rahm RL, et al. Failure of red blood cell transfusion to increase oxygen transport and mixed venous PO_2 in injured patients. J Trauma 1982; *22*:741–746.
20. Rackow EC, Falk JL, Fein IA, et al. Fluid resuscitation in circulatory shock: A comparison of the cardiorespiratory effects of albumin, hetastarch and saline solutions in patients with hypovolemic and septic shock. Crit Care Med 1983; *11*:839–850.
21. Messmer KF. Acceptable hematocrit levels in surgical patients. World J Surg 1987; *11*:41–46.
22. McCormick M, Feustel PJ, Newell JC, et al. Effect of cardiac index and hematocrit changes on oxygen consumption in resuscitated patients. J Surg Res 1988; *44*:499–505.
23. Consensus Conference on Perioperative Blood Transfusions. JAMA 1988; *260*:2700–2703.
24. Arturson G, Thoren L. Fluid therapy in shock. World J Surg 1983; *7*:573–580.
25. Shoemaker WC, Fleming AW. Resuscitation of the trauma patient: Restoration of hemodynamic functions using clinical algorithms. Ann Emerg Med 1986; *12*:1437–1444.
26. Packman MI, Rackow EC. Optimum left heart filling pressure during fluid resuscitation of patients with hypovolemic and septic shock. Crit Care Med 1983; *11*:165–169.
27. Weil MH, Afifi AA. Experimental and clinical studies on lactate and pyruvate as indicators of the severity of acute circulatory failure (Shock). Circulation 1970; *51*:989–1001.
28. Davis JW, Shackford SR, Mackersie RC, Hoyt DB. Base deficit as a guide to volume resuscitation. J Trauma 1988; *28*:1464–1467.

c h a p t e r

14

ACUTE HEART FAILURE

The principles of cardiac performance in Chapter 1 can be used to design specific strategies for a bedside approach to heart failure. The approach in this chapter starts by identifying the side of the heart that is involved (right or left) then the phase of the cardiac cycle that is abnormal (systole or diastole). The strategies are designed according to the mechanical problem rather than the specific illness, although the two are closely related. Figure 14–1 shows some common causes of low cardiac output states in adults. This can serve as a reference guide for the initial bedside evaluation.

DIAGNOSTIC CONSIDERATIONS

The diagnosis begins with recognition of the early signs of heart failure, then proceeds to identify the side of the heart and phase of the cardiac cycle involved.[1,2]

EARLY RECOGNITION

The early signs of heart failure are shown in Figure 14–2. This record was obtained from a patient immediately following cardiac bypass surgery. The sequence of hemodynamic changes is as follows.

1. The earliest sign of ventricular dysfunction is an increase in pulmonary capillary wedge pressure (PCWP). The stroke output is maintained at this stage because the ventricle is still preload-responsive, that is, the Starling curve is still steep.

2. The next stage is marked by a decrease in stroke volume and an increase in heart rate. The tachycardia offsets the reduction in stroke

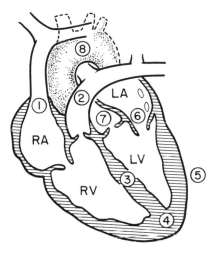

① Supraventricular Arrhythmias
② Pulmonary Embolus
③ Complete Heart Block
④ Ischemia / Infarction
   Ventricular Arrhythmias
⑤ Tamponade
⑥ Acute Mitral Insufficiency
⑦ Acute Aortic Insufficiency
⑧ Aortic Dissection

FIG. 14–1. Common causes of acute heart failure.

FIG. 14–2. Hemodynamic changes during progressive heart failure.

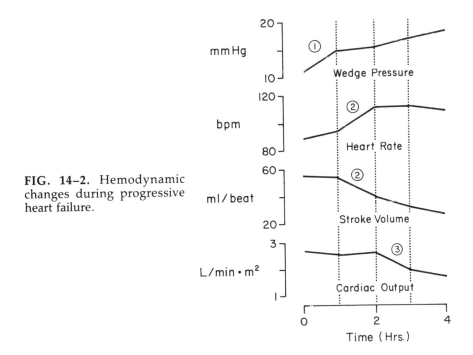

volume and the cardiac output is unchanged. This pattern of response illustrates the value of monitoring stroke volume as a marker of early heart failure instead of cardiac output. Remember that the cardiac output should always be interpreted in relation to the heart rate to detect early changes in stroke volume.

3. In the final phase, the tachycardia no longer compensates for the decreasing stroke volume and cardiac output begins to fall. This marks the transition from early compensated heart failure to cardiac decompensation. From here on, the peripheral vascular resistance increases progressively and the vasoconstriction eventually compromises peripheral blood flow and reduces cardiac output further.

In summary, the early stages of heart failure are characterized by a high filling pressure, low stroke volume, tachycardia, and a normal cardiac output. **The cardiac output is not reduced in the early stages of heart failure** because the ventricle is still responsive to preload. When the ventricle is no longer preload-responsive, cardiac output begins to fall and the decompensated stages of heart failure begin.

RIGHT VERSUS LEFT HEART FAILURE

The relationship between the central venous pressure (CVP) and the pulmonary capillary wedge pressure (PCWP) can be used to distinguish left from right-sided heart failure. The following criteria have been proposed:[3,4]

Right Heart Failure: CVP above 10 mm Hg, and

CVP greater than PCWP or

CVP = PCWP

Left Heart Failure: PCWP above 12 mm Hg, and

PCWP greater than CVP

One-third of patients with acute right heart failure will not satisfy these criteria.[4] In this situation, the response to volume infusion can unmask the problem.[4,5] In right heart failure, volume infusion will increase the CVP more than the PCWP, while in left heart failure, the increase in PCWP will exceed the increase in CVP.

One of the problems with the CVP and PCWP for identifying right heart failure is the interaction between the right and left sides of the heart. This is illustrated in Figure 14–3. Both ventricles share the same septum, so that enlargement of the right ventricle will push the septum to the left and compromise the left ventricular chamber. This interaction between right and left ventricles is called "interventricular interdependence," and it can confuse the interpretation of ventricular filling pressures. In fact, as indicated by the diastolic pressures in Figure 14–3, the

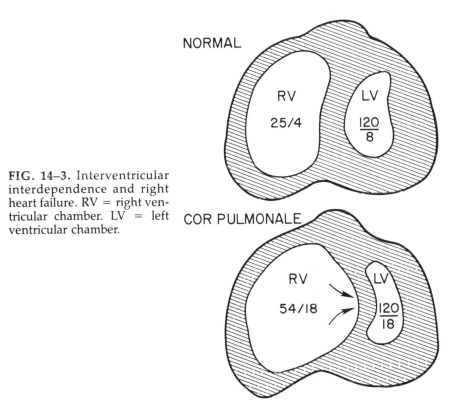

NORMAL

RV
25/4

LV
$\frac{120}{8}$

COR PULMONALE

RV
54/18

LV
$\frac{120}{18}$

FIG. 14–3. Interventricular interdependence and right heart failure. RV = right ventricular chamber. LV = left ventricular chamber.

hemodynamic consequences of right heart failure can look much like the hemodynamics of pericardial tamponade.

Echocardiography can be useful at the bedside for differentiating right from left heart failure. Three findings typical of right heart failure are: (1) an increase in right ventricular chamber size, (2) segmental wall motion abnormalities on the right, and (3) paradoxical motion of the interventricular septum.[4]

SYSTOLIC VERSUS DIASTOLIC FAILURE

Heart failure is no longer synonymous with contractile failure during systole. As many as 30 to 40% of patients with recent onset heart failure have normal systolic function.[6,7] The problem in these patients is a decrease in the distensibility of the ventricle during diastole (diastolic heart failure). This form of heart failure is most often caused by ventricular hypertrophy, myocardial ischemia, pericardial effusions, and positive-pressure ventilation.[6] All of these conditions are common in the adult ICU patient population. The distinction between systolic and diastolic dysfunction is important because therapy for each condition differs considerably.

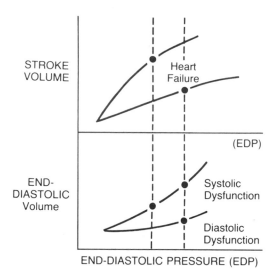

STROKE VOLUME

END-DIASTOLIC Volume

END-DIASTOLIC PRESSURE (EDP)

FIG. 14–4. The influence of systolic and diastolic dysfunction on end-diastolic pressure (EDP) and end-diastolic volume (EDV).

Hemodynamic Assessment. The ability of invasive hemodynamic monitoring to identify diastolic or systolic heart failure is limited. The problem is that end-diastolic pressure (EDP) is used as an index of preload instead of end-diastolic volume (EDV). This is illustrated in Figure 14–4. The curves in the lower graph describe the relationship between EDP and EDV in both types of heart failure. The curve defining diastolic dysfunction has a reduced slope because the compliance is reduced in diastolic heart failure (see Chapter 1 for a discussion of compliance curves). The EDP increases in both types of heart failure, but the EDV changes in opposite directions. The upper graph in the figure indicates that the increase in EDP measured at the bedside can be the same in both types of heart failure, and therefore is of no value in identifying the type of heart failure.

End-Diastolic Volume. The end-diastolic volume can be estimated using radionuclide ventriculography[8] to measure the "ejection fraction" (EF), and combining this with a thermodilution cardiac output. The stroke volume from thermodilution is related to the EDV by the ejection fraction; i.e., the stroke volume is a fraction (EF) of the end-diastolic volume:

$$EDV = SV/EF \times 100$$

When patients have an indwelling pulmonary artery catheter, the EF can be measured at the bedside with portable gamma camera. If a portable camera is not available at your hospital, cardiac ultrasound may be useful in some patients. Ultrasound is reliable for estimating EF when the heart size is normal, but is unreliable when heart size or geometry is abnormal.[6]

TABLE 14–1. DRUG THERAPY FOR HEART FAILURE		
Drug	Adult Dose Range	Actions
Dobutamine	5–20 mcg/kg/min	Positive Inotrope
Dopamine	1–10 mcg/kg/min	Inodilator*
	over 10 mcg/kg/min	Vasoconstrictor
Amrinone	5–10 mcg/kg/min	Inodilator
Nitroglycerin	1–50 mcg/min	Venodilator
	over 50 mcg/min	Vasodilator
Nitroprusside	0.5–2 mcg/kg/min	Vasodilator

*Inodilator is an inotropic agent and a vasodilator

MANAGEMENT STRATEGIES

The following two goals apply to any type of heart failure:
1. Decrease venous (capillary) pressure to prevent edema formation
2. Increase forward flow

The strategies presented here are designed to achieve both of these goals. Table 14–1 lists the drugs used in this approach, along with the recommended dose ranges. These drugs are presented in more detail in Chapter 20.

LEFT HEART FAILURE

The approach to left heart failure centers on the pulmonary capillary wedge pressure (PCWP), and is outlined in Figure 14–5. Three major categories are separated based on the PCWP (low, normal, or high).

Low Filling Pressure. Inadequate filling pressures must be corrected because the other hemodynamic drugs will be ineffective if the ventricle does not fill adequately during diastole.

Condition	Therapy
Low PCWP	Volume infusion to optimal PCWP

Optimal Filling Pressure. The optimal filling pressure is the highest pressure that will augment cardiac output without producing pulmonary edema. This is shown in Figure 14–6. The optimal filling pressure in the lower (heart failure) curve is the highest point on the curve that does not enter the hatched "pulmonary edema" zone. In this case, the optimal PCWP is 20 mm Hg, which is the optimal pressure reported in patients with chronic congestive heart failure.[9] The optimal PCWP may differ widely in individual patients because of differences in the colloid osmotic pressure (COP) of blood. Therefore, the optimal PCWP must be defined by the plasma COP in each patient. This topic is discussed in more detail in Chapter 23.

When the wedge pressure is optimal, therapy is dictated by the blood pressure (BP). The hemodynamic drugs included here are given by con-

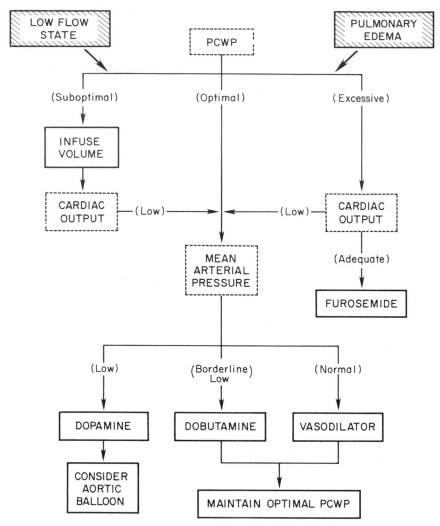

FIG. 14–5. Treatment strategies for acute left heart failure.

tinuous IV infusion only. These agents are discussed in detail in Chapter 20.

Condition	Therapy
Optimal PCWP, Low BP..............	Dopamine; Dobutamine

Dopamine stimulates both beta receptors in the heart and alpha receptors in peripheral arteries. The beta stimulation increases cardiac output while the alpha stimulation produces vasoconstriction to elevate the blood pressure. Dobutamine will increase cardiac output but may not increase the blood pressure because the systemic vascular resistance will drop in response to the increased cardiac output.[10,11]

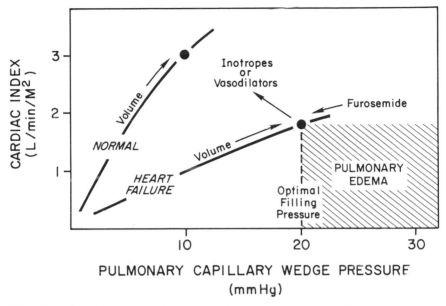

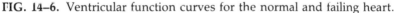

FIG. 14–6. Ventricular function curves for the normal and failing heart.

Condition	Therapy
Optimal PCWP, Normal BP ...	Dobutamine and/or Amrinone

Dobutamine is the inotropic agent of choice for the acute management of systolic heart failure.[11] Amrinone was introduced as a combined vasodilator and positive inotropic agent but the current opinion is that the drug is a vasodilator with minimal inotropic activity.[12] Combination therapy with dobutamine and amrinone has been more effective than dobutamine alone in patients with severe heart failure.[13]

Condition	Therapy
Optimal PCWP, High BP ...	Nitroprusside, etc.

Several vasodilators are available that can be given by continuous infusion.[13] Nitroprusside is the traditional vasodilator given by continuous infusion and this agent is still the most popular in most settings. However, cyanide can accumulate in certain patient populations (see Chapter 20), and this risk must temper the use of nitroprusside. Labetalol (a combined alpha-beta blocker), esmolol (a short-acting beta blocker), and trimethaphan (a ganglionic blocker) are all effective vasodilators but these agents can drop cardiac output and may not be safe in patients with severe ventricular dysfunction. Trimethaphan and esmolol are popular in the treatment of aortic dissection.

Pulmonary Edema. If the wedge pressure is excessive and the patient is in hydrostatic pulmonary edema, the therapy is determined by the cardiac output (CO).

Condition	Therapy
High PCWP, Low CO ...	Dobutamine and/or Amrinone

Dobutamine is the preferred agent for acute management of low cardiac output states accompanied by pulmonary edema. Amrinone will also improve cardiac output and reduce the wedge pressure. As mentioned, combination therapy with dobutamine and amrinone can add to therapy with either agent alone.[13] This combination of effects is the optimal goal of managing heart failure. Dopamine should be avoided in this situation if possible because dopamine increases the PCWP,[16] possibly by constricting pulmonary veins. Vasodilator therapy can be detrimental in pulmonary edema because vasodilators increase shunt fraction and can aggravate hypoxemia.[14]

Condition	Therapy
High PCWP, Normal CO	Nitroglycerin/(?) IV Furosemide

A normal cardiac output in the face of pulmonary edema suggests diastolic heart failure. Aggressive diuresis is not recommended as the first line of therapy in this setting because the high filling pressures are helping to maintain the cardiac output. Intravenous nitroglycerin (less than 100 mcg/kg/min) should be useful here because this agent will reduce the wedge pressure while also reducing the arterial resistance to maintain cardiac output.[14] Sublingual nitroglycerin can be given for immediate results. In the setting of pulmonary edema, nitroglycerin can increase shunt fraction and decrease the arterial Po_2. Therefore, monitor arterial gases carefully when using nitroglycerin in the face of pulmonary edema. If nitroglycerin does not produce the desired results, low-dose dobutamine (5 mcg/kg/min) can be started even though the results should not be dramatic if the problem is diastolic failure. An increase in heart rate during dobutamine infusion suggests inadequate filling (diastolic failure) and should prompt discontinuation of the drug.

Intravenous furosemide can be given if the wedge pressure remains elevated after the initial drug therapy. However, diuretics must be given cautiously in this setting because of the possibility of diastolic heart failure. In addition, **intravenous furosemide can cause an acute decrease in cardiac output**[15] due to venodilatation and peripheral vasoconstriction. This effect is transient but undesirable for as long as it lasts.

RIGHT HEART FAILURE

Therapeutic strategies for right heart failure are similar in principle to those just described. The strategies below pertain only to primary right heart failure (e.g., acute MI), and not to right heart failure secondary to chronic obstructive lung disease or to left heart failure. The PCWP will again be used as the focal point of the approach.

1. If PCWP is below 15 mm Hg, infuse volume until the PCWP or CVP increases by 5 mm Hg or either one reaches 20 mm Hg.[5]

2. If PCWP is above 15 mm Hg, infuse dobutamine.

The response to volume infusion is not consistent in right heart failure. The volume may completely correct the hemodynamic problem, or it may have no effect on cardiac output.[5] In fact, aggressive volume in-

TABLE 14–2. INFLUENCE OF DIFFERENT TREATMENT MODALITIES ON MYOCARDIAL ENERGY BALANCE			
Myocardial O$_2$ Balance	**Dobutamine**	**Vasodilators**	**IABP**
Preload	↓	↓	↓
Contractility	↑ ↑	→	→
Afterload	↓	↓ ↓	↓
Heart Rate	→ ↑	→	→
Myocardial O$_2$ Consumption	↑ (→)	↓	↓
Coronary Blood Flow	↑	↑ ↓	↑ →

fusion can further reduce cardiac output[4,5] because of interventricular interdependence explained earlier.

Dobutamine has proven efficacy in right heart failure from acute MI[5] and from acute pulmonary embolus. Vasodilators that reduce venous return to the right heart are not recommended, because they could further reduce the cardiac output. Nitroprusside has been used in right heart failure, but it is not as effective as dobutamine.[5]

Ischemia of the AV node is common in patients with right ventricular infarction[4] because the AV node is often supplied by the right coronary artery. This can result in AV dissociation or complete heart block that is resistant to atropine. Sequential AV pacing is usually required in this setting,[4] while ventricular pacing is to be avoided because it is ineffective and can be deleterious.[4]

MYOCARDIAL ENERGY BALANCE

In patients with active coronary artery disease, the aim of therapy should be to increase coronary flow (cardiac output) while reducing the workload placed on the heart. This will optimize the balance between O$_2$ supply (coronary flow) and O$_2$ consumption (myocardial stroke work).

The workload of the heart is determined by four factors: preload, afterload, contractility and heart rate. An increase in any one of these will increase myocardial work. Table 14–2 summarizes the effects of different treatment modalities on these variables, and their influence on coronary flow. The inotropic agent dobutamine will reliably increase coronary flow (cardiac output), but the benefit may be offset by an increase in cardiac work (by increasing contractility and heart rate). The vasodilators will reduce myocardial work, but the benefit can be offset by a reduction in coronary flow (if aortic diastolic pressure is drastically reduced). The intraaortic balloon pump will reduce myocardial stroke work, and should increase coronary flow. The latter effect is not a consistent observation,[17,20] but the energy balance of the myocardium should not be adversely affected, even if coronary flow is not enhanced.

INTRA-AORTIC BALLOON COUNTERPULSATION

The intraaortic balloon was introduced over 25 years ago, and is presently the only accepted method of mechanical circulatory assistance.[17–20] The intraaortic balloon is a 30 cm long polyurethane balloon attached to one end of a large-bore catheter. The balloon is wrapped tightly around the catheter, and the entire device is inserted in the femoral artery at the groin either percutaneously or via arteriotomy. The balloon is advanced up the aorta until the tip of the device lies just beyond the origin of the left subclavian artery. Correct placement does not require fluoroscopy, although fluoroscopic guidance assures more precise placement.

Once in place, the balloon is inflated with helium (35 to 40 ml capacity) at the onset of ventricular diastole, when the aortic valve closes. Rapid deflation occurs just before the aortic valve opens at the beginning of ventricular systole.

HEMODYNAMIC EFFECTS

Inflation of the balloon produces two changes in the arterial pressure waveform, as illustrated in Figure 14–7.

1. Balloon inflation displaces blood from the aorta towards the periphery, resulting in an increase in peak diastolic pressure. The diastolic pressure augmentation increases the mean arterial pressure, which is the principal determinant of peripheral blood flow. Coronary flow should increase because the bulk of coronary blood flow occurs during diastole, however the response is variable. It seems that the IABP increases coronary flow only when patients are hypotensive,[20] and does not promote coronary flow in normotensive patients.

2. The balloon inflation also reduces the end-diastolic pressure, which reduces the impedance to flow when the aortic valve opens at the onset of systole. This promotes ventricular stroke output.

INDICATIONS

The goal of balloon assistance is to provide temporary support for the left ventricle when corrective surgery or spontaneous recovery is anticipated. The most common indications for the IABP include:

1. Cardiopulmonary bypass (pre and post)
2. Acute MI with cardiogenic shock
3. Acute mitral insufficiency
4. Unstable angina

Almost half of all balloon insertions occur in the immediate postoperative period after cardiopulmonary bypass.[18] The next most common situation is cardiogenic shock from acute MI (23%) and the next is prophylaxis before bypass surgery (20%).

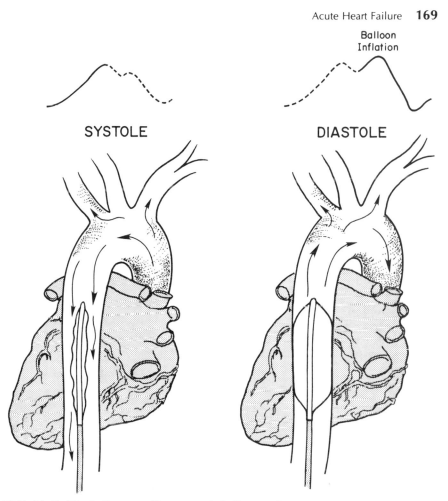

Balloon
Inflation

SYSTOLE

DIASTOLE

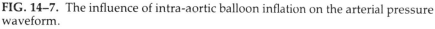

FIG. 14–7. The influence of intra-aortic balloon inflation on the arterial pressure waveform.

CONTRAINDICATIONS

The one contraindication to IABP is aortic regurgitation, because balloon inflation will aggravate the regurgitant flow.

COMPLICATIONS

Serious and even fatal complications have been reported.[17–20] The most common complication is leg ischemia, with a reported incidence of 30%.[18] Other complications include aortic perforation, renal insufficiency, and thrombocytopenia. The leg ischemia can occur in the ipsilateral or contralateral leg, and can appear either with the device in place or soon after it is removed. When distal pulses disappear while the balloon is in place, removal is frequently sufficient to restore flow without any further therapy. About 10% of patients will require additional therapy for ischemia after the balloon is removed,[17] and leg amputation has been necessary on occasion.[19]

WEANING

The balloon assist is usually withdrawn gradually by decreasing the frequency of balloon inflations per cardiac cycle (1:2, 1:3, etc.). Another method is to reduce the inflation volume of the balloon in steps of 25% of the maximal volume.[18] The choice of method is a matter of individual preference because neither one has proven superior to the other. The period of weaning is also determined by individual preference. One suggestion is a 6-hour wean period for every 24 hours on the pump,[18] but this seems excessive for patients who have received several days of balloon assistance.

CARDIAC SURGERY

The immediate period after cardiopulmonary bypass surgery is often marked by hemodynamic instability. Several factors are involved, and the major ones are outlined in the following paragraphs.

CARDIAC TAMPONADE

Cardiac tamponade occurs in 3 to 6% of patients undergoing open heart surgery.[20] It often appears in the first few hours after surgery, but can occur at a later time when the pacemaker wires are removed. The pericardium is open after cardiac surgery and this prevents fluid from accumulating evenly around the heart. The most common cause of tamponade after surgery is a blood clot compressing the right heart.

Presentation. The clinical presentation is often atypical and diagnosis may not be possible on clinical grounds alone. The following statements summarize some of the pertinent observations:

1. Pulsus paradoxus (drop in systolic blood pressure of at least 10 mmHg) is masked in patients receiving mechanical ventilation.[21] This is because of the increase in systolic pressure during positive-pressure lung inflation; a phenomenon called "reverse pulsus paradoxus." This increases baseline systolic pressure so that a pulsus paradoxus can be present without an inspiratory drop in pressure.

2. Diastolic equalization of pressures (CVP, PA diastolic pressure, PCWP) may not be a feature of tamponade when a clot is compressing the right atrium. In this situation, the pressure in the superior vena cava (CVP) will increase while the downstream pressures across the right heart will decrease.

Diagnosis and Therapy. Bedside echocardiography can sometimes locate a compressive clot.[22] However, the method is technically difficult in the immediate postoperative period and diagnosis often requires thoracotomy. Pericardiocentesis is not safe after bypass surgery because of the risk of injuring the grafts and thoracotomy is required to evacuate blood clots and ligate bleeding sites. Aggressive volume infusion is warranted in the early period when diagnosis is suspect.

POST-BYPASS HEMODYNAMICS

The rewarming period after cardiopulmonary bypass is associated with a decrease in the compliance of the ventricles.[23] Etiology is not clear, but myocardial edema from cooling and reperfusion may play a role. The peripheral vascular resistance can either increase or decrease in the immediate postoperative period. Vasoconstriction is believed to be the result of catecholamine excess[25] and vasodilatation is due to unknown factors.[23] Systolic function is variable in the immediate postoperative period, but seems to be well maintained in most patients.[23] Acute MI can appear when vein grafts are clotted or as a result of hypotension when bypass is discontinued.

Therapy. The decrease in ventricular compliance after surgery causes a decrease in end-diastolic volume (preload) at any given end-diastolic pressure (PCWP). This means that a normal PCWP in the immediate postoperative period represents a low end-diastolic volume. Therefore, when cardiac output is low and the PCWP is not elevated, infuse volume until the PCWP is in the range of 15 to 20 mmHg. The colloid osmotic pressure (COP) of plasma can be reduced following bypass surgery, presumably because of dilutional hypoproteinemia.[24] Therefore, it is wise to monitor plasma COP after surgery to guide volume therapy.

Drug therapy can be selected according to the systemic vascular resistance (SVR). The following scheme may be helpful:

SVR	Blood Pressure	Agent
High	High	Nitroprusside*
High	Normal	Dobutamine
High	Low	Dopamine, IABP
Normal	Normal	Dobutamine
Normal	Low	Dopamine, IABP
Low	Normal	Dobutamine
Low	Low	Dopamine, Epinephrine

BIBLIOGRAPHY

Weber K ed. Heart failure: Current concepts and management. Cardiol Clin 1989; 7:1–204.
Ewer MS, Nicarelli GV eds. Cardiac critical care. Crit Care Clin 1989; 5:415–706.
Quaal SJ ed. Comprehensive intra-aortic balloon pumping. St. Lous: C.V. Mosby, 1984.

---

*Nitroprusside infusion in the post-bypass period can carry an increased risk for cyanide toxicity (see Chapter 20) and therapy should be continued for only a few hours. Nitroglycerin has also been used successfully.[25]

REFERENCES

REVIEWS

1. Passmore JM, Goldstein RA. Acute recognition and management of congestive heart failure. Crit Care Clin 1989; 5:497–532.
2. McElroy PA, Shroff SG, Weber K. Pathophysiology of the failing heart. Cardiol Clin 1989; 7:25–38.

RIGHT HEART FAILURE

3. Cohn JN, Gulha NH, Broder MI, et al. Right ventricular infarction: clinical and hemodynamic features. Am J Cardiol 1974; 33:209–214.
4. Isner JM. Right ventricular myocardial infarction. JAMA 1988; 259:712–718.
5. Dell'Italia LJ, Starling MR, Blumhardt R, et al. Comparative effects of volume loading, dobutamine and nitroprusside in patients with predominant right ventricular infarction. Circulation 1986; 72:1327–1335.

DIASTOLIC HEART FAILURE

6. Harinzi AC, Bianco JA, Alpert JS. Diastolic function of the heart in clinical cardiology. Arch Intern Med 1988; 148:99–109.
7. Kessler KM. Heart failure with normal systolic function (editorial). Arch Intern Med 1988; 148:2109–2111.
8. Konstam MA, Wynne J. Radionuclide ventriculography. In: Conn PF, Wynne J eds. Diagnostic methods in clinical cardiology. Boston: Little, Brown and Co., 1982:165–198.

SPECIFIC THERAPIES

9. Franciosa JA. Optimal left heart filling pressure during nitroprusside infusion for congestive heart failure. Am J Med 1983; 74:457–464.
10. Leier CV, Unverferth DV. Dobutamine. Ann Intern Med 1983; 99:490–496.
11. Mackawa K, Liang C, Hood WP. Comparison of dobutamine and dopamine in acute myocardial infarction. Circulation 1983; 67:750–758.
12. Franciosa JA. Intravenous amrinone: An advance or a wrong step? Ann Intern Med 1985; 102:399–400.
13. Uretsky LF, Lawless CE, Verbalis JG, et al. Combined therapy with dobutamine and amrinone in severe heart failure. Chest 1987; 92:657–662.
14. Milero RR, Fenwell WH, Young JB, et al. Differential systemic arterial and venous actions and consequent cardiac effects of vasodilator drugs. Prog Cardiovasc Dis 1982; 24:353–374.
15. Francis GS, Siegel RM, Goldsmith SR, et al. Acute vasoconstrictor response to intravenous furosemide in patients with chronic congestive heart failure. Ann Intern Med 1986; 103:1–6.
16. Molloy WD, Dobson K, Girling L, et al. Effects of dopamine on cardiopulmonary function and left ventricular volume in patients with acute respiratory failure. Am Rev Respir Dis 1984; 130:396–399.

INTRA-AORTIC BALLOON PUMP

17. Bregman D, Kaskel P. Advances in intra-aortic balloon pumping. In: Bregman D ed. New techniques in mechanical cardiac support. Crit Care Clin 1986; 2:221–236.
18. Balooki H. Current status of circulatory support with an intra-aortic balloon pump. Cardiol Clin 1985; 3:123–133.
19. Corral CH, Vaughn CC. Intra-aortic balloon counterpulsation: An eleven-year review and analysis of determinants of survival. Tex Heart Inst J 1986; 13:39–44.
20. Williams DO, Korr KS, Gewirtz H, Most AS. The effect of intra-aortic balloon counterpulsation on regional myocardial blood flow and oxygen consumption in the presence of coronary artery stenosis with unstable angina. Circulation 1982; 3:593–597.

CARDIAC SURGERY

21. Weeks KR, Chatterjee K, Block S, et al. Bedside hemodynamic monitoring. Its value in the diagnosis of tamponade complicating cardiac surgery. J Thorac Cardiovasc Surg 1976; 71:250–252.
22. D'Cruz IA, Callaghan WE. Atypical cardiac tamponade: Clinical and echocardiographic features. Internal Med Specialist 1988; 9:68–78.
23. Ivanov J, Weisel RD, Mickelborough LL, et al. Rewarming hypovolemia after aorto-coronary bypass surgery. Crit Care Med 1984; 12:1049–1054.
24. Klancke KA, Assey ME, Kratz JM, Crawford MA. Postoperative pulmonary edema in postcoronary bypass graft patients. Chest 1983; 84:529–534.
25. Flaherty JT, Magee PA, Gardner TL, et al. Comparison of intravenous nitroglycerin and sodium nitroprusside for treatment of acute hypertension developing after coronary artery bypass surgery. Circulation 1982; 65:1072–1077.

c h a p t e r

15

SEPTIC SHOCK AND RELATED SYNDROMES

One of the early discoveries you will make in the ICU is the prevalence of sepsis and the role it plays in the mortality associated with critical illness. The next discovery you will make is the inability of aggressive antibiotic therapy to eradicate severe infections. The growing army of antibiotics is proving to be no match for serious infections, as shown in the following statistic: **the mortality in septic shock was 41% in 1909 and 40% in 1985.**[1]

THE SEPSIS SYNDROME

The sepsis syndrome is a constellation of clinical findings that identifies an inflammatory process with systemic involvement.[2] The emphasis here is on the difference between inflammation and infection. The sepsis syndrome does not require absolute documentation of infection or isolation of a specific pathogen. The clinical features of this syndrome include:
1. Fever or hypothermia
2. Leukocytosis or leukopenia
3. Tachypnea and tachycardia
4. Organ dysfunction
   a. Altered mental status
   b. Hypoxemia
   c. Oliguria

These clinical findings represent a systemic response to inflammation[3] and the assumption is that the inflammation represents an infection. The systemic manifestations include dysfunction in several organ systems, most notably the central nervous system, lungs, and kidneys. The organ dysfunction can be progressive, culminating in a lethal condition known as "multiple systems organ failure."[4]

> The purpose of the sepsis syndrome is not to identify a specific infection or pathogen but to identify patients at risk for developing multiorgan failure.

The goal here is to initiate antibiotic therapy and other therapeutic measures (e.g., hemodynamic monitoring) that might help in halting the progression to multiorgan failure.

MEDIATORS

The systemic manifestations of sepsis are caused by proteins called "cytokines" that are released by macrophages and circulating monocytes in response to infection.[3] One of the products of infection that can stimulate the release of cytokines is **endotoxin,** which is a lipopolysaccharide contained in the cell wall of gram negative bacteria. Two of the cytokines that have been isolated are called **interleukin-1** and **tumor necrosis factor** (also called cachectin). Both are released into the systemic circulation during infection and both participate in the multitude of systemic manifestations of sepsis. Fever is produced by direct effects on the hypothalamus. Widespread endothelial damage is mediated by cytokine-induced activation of circulating neutrophils. The endothelial damage from activated neutrophils produces a variety of organ dysfunction syndromes like the "adult respiratory distress syndrome" (ARDS). Widespread endothelial damage is responsible for the multiorgan failure syndrome that characterizes the terminal stages of sepsis.

SEPTICEMIA

The systemic involvement in sepsis is due to inflammatory mediators and does not require spread of pathogens in the bloodstream. This is used to explain the prevalence of negative blood cultures in the sepsis syndrome.

> Blood cultures are sterile in roughly 50% of patients with the sepsis syndrome.[2]

The lack of documented invasion of the bloodstream does not exclude septicemia but may indicate intermittent seeding of the bloodstream that can be missed in random blood samples. Whatever the situation, the fact remains that positive blood cultures are not necessary for the diagnosis of sepsis syndrome.

When pathogens are isolated by blood cultures, the isolates are, in part, determined by the specific site of dissemination. Staphylococci and gram negative enteric pathogens are the predominant isolates in nosocomial (hospital-acquired) infections. Candida is also isolated from the blood in select patients (i.e., immunocompromised patients and those who have received multiple antibiotics). Chapters 43 through 46 contain the specific pathogens isolated in nosocomial infections.

SYSTEMIC SIGNS

Fever is considered the most common clinical finding in sepsis.[2] The febrile response is caused by cytokine-mediated prostaglandin production in the hypothalamus.[3] The fever is beneficial if judged by clinical outcome because mortality is higher in septic patients who do not generate a fever.[2] The difference in mortality is reason for discouraging the routine use of antipyretics or other measures aimed at suppressing the febrile response in sepsis. The benefits and drawbacks of fever are discussed briefly in Chapter 43.

Leukocytosis is also an expected finding in sepsis. The characteristic response to bacterial infections is a granulocytosis with an increase in immature forms (leftward shift). The absence of leukocytosis (including leukopenia) increases mortality significantly.[2]

MULTIORGAN FAILURE

The inevitable consequence of uncontrolled sepsis is progressive dysfunction in multiple organs including the lungs, kidneys, liver, and central nervous system. Involvement of two or more organs is defined as the "multiple organ failure" (MOF) syndrome.[4] This is an expression of the terminal stages of sepsis and indicates failure to thrive. Some of the individual organ dysfunction syndromes are in the following paragraphs.

Septic Encephalopathy

The central nervous system (CNS) dysfunction in sepsis presents as a depressed sensorium and the severity can vary from somnolence to frank coma. This "septic encephalopathy" has been attributed to the same metabolic abnormalities that characterize hepatic encephalopathy.[5] This theory claims that aromatic amino acids that are normally cleared by the liver will accumulate in sepsis while branched chain amino acids are diminished in circulating blood because they are used as energy substrates. The branched chain AAs normally prevent the aromatic AAs from crossing the blood-brain barrier. Therefore, the decrease in circulating branched chain AAs in sepsis allows aromatic AAs to cross the blood-brain barrier. The CNS metabolism of aromatic AAs then produces false neurotransmitters and these are responsible for the clinical syndrome of septic encephalopathy.

ADULT RESPIRATORY DISTRESS SYNDROME

Approximately 1 in every 4 patients with the sepsis syndrome will develop the "adult respiratory distress syndrome" (ARDS) as a result of endothelial damage to the pulmonary capillaries.[2] This illness appears similar to the pulmonary edema of heart failure but carries a mortality in excess of 50%. The diagnosis and management of ARDS is described in Chapter 23.

ACUTE RENAL FAILURE

Acute renal failure is probably caused by several factors, including systemic vasodilatation and hypotension, endotoxin-induced renal artery vasoconstriction and nephrotoxic drugs.[6] Despite the advent of acute hemodialysis, the mortality in acute renal failure remains in excess of 50%,[6] which means that the acute renal failure is not a cause of death (but is a manifestation of a larger ongoing process).

ISCHEMIC HEPATITIS

One of the earliest signs of disseminated sepsis can be an increase in liver transaminases and intrahepatic cholestasis.[7] The mechanism is believed to be a selective reduction in hepatic blood flow and endotoxin-mediated cholestasis, although some studies point to an increase in liver blood flow in sepsis.[7] Whatever the mechanism, the clinical presentation is usually one of unexplained jaundice and a rapid rise in liver transaminases. The liver enzymes can reach extremely high levels but tend to subside in a few days. This clinical picture was called "ischemic hepatitis."

HEMODYNAMICS OF THE SEPTIC STATE

The major hemodynamic changes in sepsis and septic shock are illustrated in Figure 15–1.[2] The septic state is associated with several different hemodynamic patterns, depending on the severity of the shock.[3] These patterns are shown below. (PCWP: pulmonary capillary wedge pressure, CO: cardiac output, and SVR: systemic vascular resistance)

Hemodynamic Patterns

Early Sepsis:	Low PCWP / High CO / Low SVR
Late Sepsis:	High PCWP / Normal CO / Normal SVR
Terminal Stage:	High PCWP / Low CO / High SVR

The early stage is a hyperdynamic pattern characterized by tachycardia and vasodilatation.[8] Both arteries and veins are dilated, producing the decrease in SVR and PCWP. The high cardiac output (CO) is due to tachycardia, not to increased contractility. In fact, the systolic and dia-

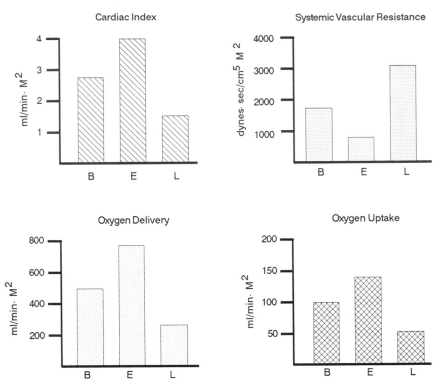

FIG. 15–1. The hemodynamic alterations in septic shock. B = baseline; E = early sepsis; L = late stage.

stolic function of the ventricles is often depressed in sepsis despite the high cardiac output.[9]

As the shock state progresses, the cardiac function deteriorates further, and the cardiac output begins to decrease. This marks the beginning of the decompensated phase of septic shock. In the terminal stages, the hemodynamic pattern resembles cardiogenic shock.

OXYGEN TRANSPORT

The hyperdynamic state of sepsis is associated with an increase in O_2 delivery ($\dot{D}O_2$) as well as an increase in O_2 uptake ($\dot{V}O_2$).[10] The increase in $\dot{V}O_2$ is less than the increase in $\dot{D}O_2$, indicating a decrease in oxygen extraction at the periphery (remember that the $\dot{V}O_2$ measures oxygen uptake from the capillaries, not the metabolic consumption of oxygen). The oxygen transport pattern in sepsis, therefore, looks like the following:[10]

High $\dot{D}O_2$ / High $\dot{V}O_2$ / Low O_2 Extraction

The etiology of the defect in O_2 extraction is unclear. The prevailing

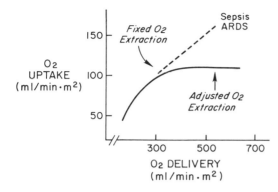

FIG. 15–2. Oxygen delivery versus oxygen uptake in health (solid line) and in sepsis.

opinion is that there are vascular shunts that open, diverting blood away from metabolizing tissues.

THE $\dot{D}O_2$-$\dot{V}O_2$ LINK IN SEPSIS

The relationship between $\dot{D}O_2$ and $\dot{V}O_2$ in sepsis is shown in Figure 15–2.[10-13] Unlike the normal curve where $\dot{V}O_2$ is constant over a wide range of changes in $\dot{D}O_2$ (see Chapter 2), the relationship between $\dot{V}O_2$ and $\dot{D}O_2$ in sepsis is linear. In other words, the $\dot{V}O_2$ is flow-dependent (i.e., dependent on the cardiac output) in sepsis, so that increases in cardiac output will result in increases in O_2 uptake.

The link between $\dot{V}O_2$ and $\dot{D}O_2$ in sepsis means that O_2 uptake from the peripheral capillaries may not be linked to the metabolic rate. In other words, if the $\dot{V}O_2$ is linked to $\dot{D}O_2$, it can't be linked to the metabolic rate. This means that the metabolic rate can exceed the $\dot{V}O_2$ in sepsis even when the $\dot{V}O_2$ is elevated. This can result in inadequate tissue oxygenation and ischemia. In this situation, lactic acid will begin to accumulate (see next section).

USING THE $\dot{V}O_2$ IN SEPSIS

The $\dot{V}O_2$ can prove valuable in a number of ways for the patient in septic shock.

$\dot{V}O_2$ as Early Marker. Serial measurements of $\dot{V}O_2$ can be valuable as an early marker of shock in selected patients at risk. The $\dot{V}O_2$ can decrease 8 to 12 hours before the blood pressure decreases,[13] and early measures to correct this problem will also minimize ongoing tissue ischemia that might otherwise go unnoticed.

$\dot{V}O_2$ as End-Point. The $\dot{V}O_2$ should be kept above normal to meet the needs of the hypermetabolic state. The specific goal for $\dot{V}O_2$, suggested by Shoemaker,[11,12] is shown in Table 15–1. A normal $\dot{V}O_2$ may be inadequate in active sepsis and should be elevated to supranormal levels whenever possible.

TABLE 15–1. MANAGEMENT GOALS IN SEPTIC SHOCK			
Variable	Normal*	Optimal*	
Cardiac Index	2.8–3.6	>4.5	
Oxygen Delivery	500–600	>600	
Oxygen Uptake	110–160	>170	
Blood Volume	2.7	>3.0	Males
(ml/m²)	2.3	>2.8	Females

*From Shoemaker WC. Intensive Care Med 1987; 13:230–243.
Transport Variables = ml/min·m²

$\dot{V}O_2$ **and Disease Severity.** The severity of the septic state is directly proportional to the defect in O_2 uptake at the periphery. Therefore, a low $\dot{V}O_2$ carries a poor prognosis in septic shock.[10–12] The discovery of a low $\dot{V}O_2$ should prompt aggressive measures to increase $\dot{V}O_2$ to normal (or supranormal) levels.

LACTIC ACID

The lactic acid in circulating blood should provide an index of the balance between $\dot{V}O_2$ and metabolic rate in sepsis (or any state of shock). Serum lactate levels have shown to be a reliable measure of inadequate tissue oxygenation and can be valuable as a prognostic index for survival in sepsis.[15,16]

Normal serum lactate levels are usually 2 mM/L or less. Arterial lactate levels in excess of 2 mM/L are associated with increased mortality.[16] Although the liver clears most lactate, significant lactic acidosis in patients with liver disease usually indicates a circulatory abnormality like shock.[10]

MANAGEMENT GOALS

The management of septic shock has two general goals: (1) restore the hemodynamic abnormalities to acceptable levels and (2) eradicate the infection.

HEMODYNAMIC MANAGEMENT

The goals of hemodynamic management are listed in Table 15–1. The idea here is to aim for supranormal levels of oxygen supply ($\dot{D}O_2$ and $\dot{V}O_2$) because the metabolic rate is supranormal. The real goal is to keep the $\dot{V}O_2$ high enough to match the hypermetabolism of sepsis. The $\dot{V}O_2$ is kept at a supranormal level by manipulating the cardiac output, which is possible because the $\dot{V}O_2$ is dependent on the $\dot{D}O_2$ in sepsis.[17] The cardiac index in this case is kept at a level that is 50% higher than normal.

When the $\dot{V}O_2$ is at the desired level, serum lactate should be measured to assess the balance between $\dot{V}O_2$ and the metabolic rate. The final goal is to maintain a serum lactate below 2 mM/L.

VOLUME INFUSION

Fluid loading is probably the single most effective therapy in sepsis for increasing the $\dot{V}O_2$. Colloid fluids are more effective than crystalloids for improving cardiac output and O_2 delivery.[6] Colloids have been shown to improve $\dot{V}O_2$ only in patients who have elevated serum lactate levels.[18,19] When the serum lactate levels are normal, colloid infusion has no influence on $\dot{V}O_2$. As explained in Chapter 14, volume infusion should be gauged by the plasma colloid osmotic pressure (COP) and the PCWP, that is, the PCWP should not exceed the plasma COP.

VASOACTIVE AGENTS

Vasoconstrictor agents are usually needed to help reverse the peripheral vasodilatation and to restore the blood pressure. However, unwanted vasoconstriction can be deleterious for the following reasons:

1. Vasoconstrictors can produce lactic acidosis, presumably because of excessive constriction in small peripheral arterioles.[20]

2. Catecholamines can elevate the metabolic rate and this will offset the benefit of any increase in cardiac output.[19]

3. Epinephrine infusion can increase serum lactate levels to 4 mEq/L as a result of glycogenolysis.[21] The following drugs may or may not prove valuable in septic shock. Chapter 20 contains a more detailed description of each drug.

1. DOBUTAMINE

Dose: 2 to 20 μgr/kg/min

When combined with volume infusion, dobutamine is superior to dopamine for increasing $\dot{V}O_2$.[22] It is also effective in some patients who are resistant to dopamine.[23] Dobutamine usually does not elevate blood pressure but has been noted to increase blood pressure in septic shock.

2. DOPAMINE

Dose: 5 to 20 μgr/kg/min (moderate dose)

Dopamine will increase the blood pressure without producing excessive vasoconstriction. Dopamine also promotes renal blood flow and this may help to minimize the renal consequences of sepsis.[25]

3. STEROIDS

High-dose intravenous steroids enjoyed an undeserved popularity in septic shock,[25] but two multicenter trials have failed to document an improved outcome in sepsis or septic shock with high-dose steroid therapy.[26,27] As a result, steroids are no longer recommended as a therapy for septic shock.

4. GLUCOSE-INSULIN-POTASSIUM (GIK)

Dose: D50 at 1 gr/kg; Insulin at 1.5 U/kg;
Potassium chloride, 10 mM

Infusion of this glucose-insulin-potassium mixture has improved the hemodynamic status in patients with septic shock but only when the cardiac index was low (below 4 L/min·M²).[28] GIK has positive inotropic effects, although the cellular mechanisms are not clear. Lactate levels can also increase, but the significance of this is unclear.[22] At present, GIK is recommended only when cardiac output is low and does not respond to conventional vasoactive drugs.

5. NALOXONE

The endogenous opioids have been implicated in the hemodynamic changes of septic shock.[29-32] Naloxone (an opiate antagonist) has been evaluated in septic shock in both animal models and human studies but the response has been variable. An increase in blood pressure has been observed with doses as low as 0.4 mg,[30] while doses up to 1.6 mg/kg have been ineffective in raising blood pressure.[31] Unfortunately, there are no clinical factors that predict response to naloxone.

Naloxone has proven safe in most situations[29] but adverse effects are reported occasionally.[31] Naloxone should be avoided in the postoperative state because it can enhance pain sensation and can cause severe hypercatecholamine reactions.

Recommendations: Naloxone can be considered in patients with septic shock refractory to other vasoactive agents. Start with a dose of 2.0 mg (5 ampules) as an intravenous bolus. The response should be evident in 3 to 5 minutes. The dose can be doubled every 15 minutes until a bolus dose of 10 mg is reached.[32] If there is a response to an intravenous bolus of naloxone, a continuous infusion should be started using two thirds the bolus dose infused every hour.[32] We have used continuous infusion naloxone since 1981 without apparent toxicity.

ANTIBIOTICS

Antibiotic therapy is mandatory in septic shock although the value of antibiotics in severe infections is not as clear as you might think. One study failed to show any difference in survival in patients receiving appropriate or inappropriate antibiotics.[33] Another showed that early antibiotic selection for the first 24 hours did not influence survival, regardless of the appropriateness of the antibiotics selected.[34] However, this latter study showed improved survival in patients receiving appropriate antibiotics after the first day of therapy.

The consensus recommendation is to begin intravenous antibiotics as soon as possible after the onset of clinically evident sepsis. The selection of antibiotics is beyond the scope of this chapter. Broad-spectrum coverage with bactericidal agents is recommended for empiric therapy. The following regimen is one recommendation for empiric therapy when the source of infection is unknown.[35]

EMPIRIC ANTIBIOTIC THERAPY

1. Neutropenic patients: Ticarcillin plus Aminoglycoside.
2. **Origin below diaphragm:** Clindamycin plus an aminoglycoside.
3. **All others:** Cefazolin plus an aminoglycoside.
4. **If methicillin-resistant *Staphylococcus aureus* is possible:** Add vancomycin to the above regimens.

The combination therapy in granulocytopenic patients (granulocyte count below 1,000/mm^3) is aimed at synergistic coverage for pseudomonas organisms. When the infection arises from the GI tract, clindamycin is used to cover *Bacteroides fragilis*, the predominant anaerobic organism in the gut. If the biliary tract is suspect, ampicillin or cefazolin plus an aminoglycoside is appropriate because anaerobes are not usually involved in biliary tract infections. See Chapter 47 for a detailed discussion of antibiotics used in the ICU.

TOXIC SHOCK SYNDROME

Toxic shock is a clinical syndrome characterized by fever, hypotension, rash, and multiorgan failure.[36] An exotoxin from *Staphylococcus aureus* produces the syndrome. The toxin-producing pathogens are usually in mucocutaneous locations (e.g., skin or vagina), and remain localized while the toxin is absorbed into the systemic circulation. Predisposing conditions are tampon use in menstruating females (the tampon may disrupt the vaginal mucosa), childbirth, pelvic infections, and sinusitis. Virtually any staphylococcal infection can produce the syndrome if the strain secretes the toxin.[37]

CLINICAL PRESENTATION

The onset is non-specific, with fever, headache, and diarrhea predominating.[36] Within 24 to 48 hours of onset, there is rapid deterioration to hypotension and multiorgan failure. The hallmarks of the disease are rash and multiorgan failure. The major criteria for diagnosis are:

1. Fever
2. Hypotension
3. Erythematous rash (diffuse)
4. Involvement of three organ systems

Note that early rash is erythematous (like a sunburn) and blanches. Another rash that has received more attention is a desquamative rash that involves the palms and soles, but this rash appears later (1 to 2 weeks), during the convalescent phase of the illness.[36] The multiorgan involvement can include renal failure, rhabdomyolysis, hepatitis, encephalopathy, and noncardiac pulmonary edema. The diagnosis is based on the clinical presentation, since blood cultures are frequently unrevealing.

Invasive hemodynamic monitoring is usually performed because of the hypotension.

Early changes resemble early septic shock:[32]

$$\text{Low PCWP / High CO / Low SVR}$$

THERAPY

1. **Aggressive volume infusion** is the initial therapy of choice.
2. **Dopamine** may be required for hypotension that does not respond to volume.
3. **Dobutamine** is effective when cardiac failure develops.[38]
4. **Antibiotic therapy** with antistaphylococcal agents has little impact on the acute illness (since disseminated infection is uncommon) but reduces the incidence of recurrence that occurs in one third of menstruating cases.[30] Vancomycin, nafcillin, or first-generation cephalosporins (e.g., cephalothin) are all effective.
5. **Immediate tampon removal** is mandatory. Vaginal douches to clear local toxin are of unproven value.

Although the acute illness can be devastating, mortality is only 5% or less.[36]

ANAPHYLACTIC SHOCK

The incidence of anaphylaxis in hospitalized patients is 1:10,000 and 10% of the reactions can be fatal. The common precipitating agents are drugs, contrast material, and plasma products. Virtually any drug is capable of producing anaphylaxis, even steroids.[39]

CLINICAL PRESENTATION

Reactions to intravenous drugs are rapid and are usually evident within 3 minutes. The major reactions include hypotension and cardi-

TABLE 15–2. MANAGEMENT OF ANAPHYLAXIS	
Primary Therapy	Dose
1. Epinephrine	Load: 3–5 ml (1:10,000) IV Maintenance: 2–4 mcg/min
2. 5% Albumin	250 ml aliquots
Secondary Therapy	
1. Aminophylline	Load: 6 mg/kg over 20 min Maintenance: 0.5 mg/kg/h
2. Hydrocortisone	100–200 mg IV q 4–6 hr
3. Diphenhydramine	25–50 mg IV q 4–6 hr

ovascular collapse, laryngeal edema, bronchospasm, and angioedema. Urticaria is a minor reaction and may not accompany the severe anaphylactic reactions.[39]

The predominant hemodynamic changes are peripheral vasodilatation and hypovolemia.[40] The latter is primarily the result of increased capillary permeability, which promotes fluid loss from the vascular space.

THERAPY

Prompt and aggressive management is most important in anaphylaxis. The specific components of the approach are shown in Table 15–2 and are outlined below.[39] Treatment is separated into primary and secondary modalities.

Primary Therapy

1. **Intubation** must be considered immediately for any signs of airway compromise. Inspiratory stridor indicates laryngeal edema, which is a life-threatening condition. Remember that stridor may not appear until over 80% of the upper airway is obstructed, so the absence of stridor means little.

2. **Epinephrine** is the agent of choice for severe reactions because it specifically blocks mediator release from mast cells and basophils. Give the initial dose as an intravenous bolus and follow with a maintenance infusion. The IV route is always preferred to the subcutaneous route when the patient is hypotensive. However, the endotracheal tube can be used to deliver the drug when IV access is not immediately available.[39]

3. **Volume Infusion** is one of the most important aspects of therapy because fluid loss from the vascular space can be profound in anaphylaxis. Colloid fluids (e.g., 5% albumin) are preferred to crystalloids because of the more rapid volume expansion achieved with colloids (see Chapter 17). Remember that short peripheral catheters permit more rapid flow than the longer central venous catheters (see Chapter 13) and, therefore, you do not have to spend unnecessary time trying to insert a central venous line at the outset.

Secondary Therapy. The following treatment has no proven value in improving outcome but may help alleviate the severity of the illness.[39]

1. **Aminophylline** is reserved for patients with persistent bronchospasm after epinephrine is administered. This drug may aggravate arrhythmias when given with epinephrine and should be used only when necessary.

2. **Steroids** are often used despite their unproven benefit. Hydrocortisone is favored by some because of mineralocorticoid effects but has no proven benefit over methylprednisolone. Remember that steroids can take hours to show an effect.

3. **Antihistamines** are used more as a matter of tradition than as a reliable remedy. Diphenhydramine (Benadryl) is the agent most recommended.

BIBLIOGRAPHY

Balk RA, Bone RC eds. Septic shock. Crit Care Clin 1989; 5:1–190.

Pinsky MR, Matuschak GM eds. Multiple systems organ failure. Crit Care Clin 1989; 5:195–410.

Root RK, Sande MA eds. Septic shock. Contemp Issues Infect Dis 1985; 4:1–277.

Sibbald WJ, Sprung C eds. Perspectives on sepsis and septic shock. Fullerton: Society of Critical Care Medicine, 1986.

REFERENCES

THE SEPSIS SYNDROME

1. Sanford J. Epidemiology and overview of the problem. In: Root RK, Sande MA eds. Septic shock. Contemp Issues Infect Dis 1985; 4:1–12.

2. Balk RA, Bone RC. The septic syndrome: Definition and clinical implications. Crit Care Clin 1989; 5:1–8.

3. Jacobs, RF, Tabor DR. Immune cellular interactions during sepsis and septic injury. Crit Care Clin 1989; 5:9–26.

4. Pinsky MR, Matuschak GM. Multiple systems organ failure: Failure of host defense mechanisms. Crit Care Clin 1989; 5:199–220.

5. Hasselgran PO, Fischer JE. Septic encephalopathy. Etiology and management. Intensive Care Med 1986; 12:13–16.

6. Cameron JS. Acute renal failure in the intensive care unit today. Intensive Care Med 1986; 12:64–71.

7. Gimson AES. Hepatic dysfunction during bacterial sepsis. Intensive Care Med 1987; 13:162–166.

HEMODYNAMICS OF SEPSIS

8. Hess ML, Nastillo A, Greenfield LJ. Spectrum of cardiovascular function during gram-negative sepsis. Prog Cardiovasc Dis 1981; 4:279–298.

9. Parker MM, Shelhammer JH, Bacharach SL, et al. Profound but reversible myocardial depression in patients with septic shock. Ann Intern Med 1984; 100:403–490.

OXYGEN TRANSPORT

10. Rackow EC, Astiz ME, Weil MH. Cellular oxygen metabolism during sepsis and shock. JAMA 1988; 259:1989–1993.
11. Shoemaker WC. Relation of oxygen transport patterns to the pathophysiology and therapy of shock states. Intensive Care Med 1987; 13:230–243.
12. Shoemaker WC. Hemodynamic and oxygen transport patterns in septic shock: Physiologic mechanisms and therapeutic implications. In: Sibbald WJ, Sprung CL eds. Perspectives on sepsis and septic shock. Fullerton: Society of Critical Care Medicine, 1986:203–234.
13. Abraham E, Bland RD, Cobo JC, et al. Sequential cardiorespiratory patterns associated with outcome in septic shock. Chest 1980; 85:75–80.
14. Abraham E, Shoemaker WC, Bland RD, et al. Sequential cardiorespiratory patterns in septic shock. Crit Care Med 1983; 11:799–803.
15. Waxman K, Nolan LS, Shoemaker WC. Sequential perioperative lactate determinations. Crit Care Med 1982; 10:96–99.
16. Kruse JA, Zaidi SAJ, Carlson RW. Significance of blood lactate levels in critically ill patients with liver disease. Am J Med 1987; 83:77–82.

HEMODYNAMIC MANAGEMENT

17. Wolf YG, Cotev S, Perel A, et al. Dependence of oxygen consumption on cardiac output in sepsis. Crit Care Med 1987; 15:198–203.
18. Haupt MT, Gilbert EM, Carlson RW. Fluid loading increases oxygen consumption in septic patients with lactic acidosis. Am Rev Respir Dis 1985; 131:912–916.
19. Gilbert AM, Haupt MT, Mandanas RY, et al. The effect of fluid loading, blood transfusion and catecholamine infusion on oxygen delivery and consumption in patients with sepsis. Rev Respir Dis 1986; 134:873–878.
20. Hardaway RM. Metabolic acidosis produced by vasopressors. Surg Gynecol Obstet 1980; 151:203–204.
21. Haljmae H. Lactate metabolism. Intensive Care World 1987; 4:118–121.
22. Vincent JL, Van der Linden P, Domb M, et al. Dopamine compared with dobutamine in experimental septic shock: Relevance to fluid administration. Anesth Analg 1987; 66:565–571.
23. Tell B, Majerus TC, Flancbaum L. Dobutamine in elderly septic shock patients refractory to dopamine. Intensive Care Med 1987; 13:14–18.
24. De La Cal MA, Miravalles E, Pascual T, et al. Dose-related hemodynamic and renal effects of dopamine in septic shock. Crit Care Med 1984; 12:22–25.

STEROIDS

25. Schumer W. Steroids in the treatment of clinical septic shock. Ann Surg 1978; 184:333–341.
26. Bone RC, Fisher CJ, Clemmer, TP. A controlled clinical trial of high-dose methylprednisolone in the treatment of severe sepsis and septic shock. N Engl J Med 1987; 317:653–658.
27. VA Systemic Sepsis Cooperative Study Group. Effect of high-dose glucocorticoid therapy on mortality in patients with clinical signs of systemic sepsis. N Engl J Med 1987; 317:659–665.

GLUCOSE-INSULIN-POTASSIUM

28. Bronsveld W, Vanden Bos GC, Thjs LG. Use of glucose-insulin-potassium (GIK) in human septic shock. Crit Care Med 1985; 13:566–570.

NALOXONE

29. Holaday JW. Opioid antagonists in septic shock. In: Root RK, Sande MA, eds. Septic Shock. Contemp Issues Infect Dis 1985; 4:117–134.
30. Peters WP, Friedman PA, Johnson MW, et al. Pressor effect of naloxone in septic shock. Lancet 1981; 1:529–531.
31. Rock P, Silverman H, Plump D, et al. Efficacy and safety of naloxone in septic shock. Crit Care Med 1985; 13:28–33.
32. Goldfarb L, Weisman RS, Errick JK, et al. Dosing nomogram for continuous infusion of intravenous naloxone. Ann Emerg Med 1986; 15:566–570.

ANTIBIOTIC THERAPY

33. Bryant RE, Hood AF, Hood CE, et al. Factors affecting mortality of gram-negative bacteremia. Arch Intern Med 1971; 127:120–125.
34. Bryan CS, Reynolds KL, Brenner ER. Analysis of 1186 episodes of gram-negative bacteremia in non-university hospitals: The effects of antimicrobial therapy. Rev Infect Dis 1983; 5:629–635.
35. Sheagren JN. Controversies in the management of sepsis and septic shock: Empiric antimicrobial therapy. In: Sibbald WJ, Sprung CL eds. Perspectives on Sepsis and Septic Shock. Fullerton: Society of Critical Care Medicine, 1986:257–274.

TOXIC SHOCK

36. Ciesielski CA, Broome CV. Toxic shock syndrome: Still in the differential. J Crit Illness 1986; 1:26–40.
37. Sperber SJ, Francis JB. Toxic shock syndrome during an influenza outbreak. JAMA 1987: 257:1086–1088.
38. Fisher CJ, Horowitz, BZ, Albertson TE. Cardiorespiratory failure in toxic shock syndrome: Effect of dobutamine. Crit Care Med 1985; 13:160–165.

ANAPHYLAXIS

39. Fisher M. Anaphylaxis. Vol. 8. Disease-A-Month Chicago: Year Book Medical Publishers, 1987.
40. Silverman HJ, Van Hook C, Haponik EF. Hemodynamic changes in human anaphylaxis. Am J Med 1984; 77:341–344.

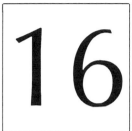

CARDIAC ARREST AND CEREBRAL IMPAIRMENT

A man's dying is more the survivor's affair than his own.
Thomas Mann

Of the estimated 200,000 cardiac arrest victims who receive cardio-pulmonary resuscitation (CPR) each year, about 70,000 (30%) survive the ordeal.[4] However, only 10% of the survivors (3.5% of the total population) are able to resume their former lifestyle.[1] The poor outcome in the survivors results primarily from neurologic damage sustained during the arrest and resuscitation period. This chapter will present the factors that contribute to neurologic damage during and after CPR, and will suggest some guidelines for predicting neurologic outcome in the survivors.

The techniques of basic and advanced cardiac life support are not covered here, but can be found in the first three references listed at the end of the chapter. Reference 2 contains the recent recommendations of the National Conference on Cardiopulmonary Resuscitation and Emergency Cardiac Care.

THE TRAGEDY OF INDECISION

Modern medicine is plagued by a fear of legal reprisals. As a result, there is a growing tendency to shun decisions relating to the dying process. The damage produced by lack of physician input into the dying process is illustrated in the following case. This is what fear and indecision did to Paul Brophy and his family.

THE BROPHY CASE

Paul Brophy was an emergency medical technician who underwent neurosurgery to repair a basilar artery aneurysm in April, 1983. Just before surgery, Mr. Brophy clearly stated to one of his daughters that he did not want to be kept alive in a vegetative state.[5] Paul Brophy never regained consciousness after the surgery.[5] The following chronicle highlights the events that followed.

4/83: Mr. Brophy does not regain consciousness.

9/83: He is transferred to a convalescent facility in a persistent vegetative state.

12/83: A feeding gastrostomy is performed.

2/85: Mrs. Brophy requests removal of the feeding tube, to allow her husband to die with dignity, as he wished. The physicians decline to honor the request.

9/86: The feed tube is removed by order of the Massachusetts State Supreme Court.

10/86: Paul Brophy dies by accepted medical criteria.

Total time of vegetative existence: *3.5 years*

The final vegetative years of Paul Brophy's life may be the predominant memory that lingers with his wife and daughters, and this is a tragedy of indecision.

RESUSCITATION PHYSIOLOGY

The goal of cardiopulmonary resuscitation (CPR) is to provide temporary support to the coronary and cerebral circulation. Unfortunately, the present methods of CPR are far from attaining this goal, as illustrated by Figure 16–1.

THE CEREBRAL CIRCULATION

The central nervous system (CNS) receives 15% of the cardiac output, even though it accounts for only 2% of the total body mass. Cerebral perfusion is maintained in the face of decreasing perfusion pressures down to a mean pressure of 60 mmHg.[6] This is achieved by a process called "autoregulation," which protects the CNS during periods of reduced oxygen delivery. When autoregulation is no longer able to maintain normal flowrates, cerebral function is sustained until the cerebral flow falls to 25 to 30% of normal levels.[7,8]

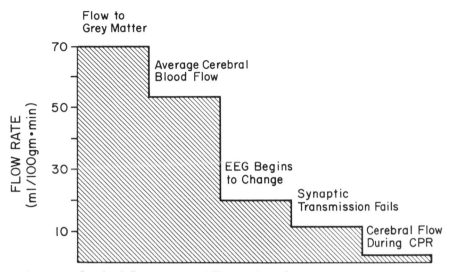

FIG. 16–1. Cerebral flowrates in different clinical situations. Note that flows achieved with CPR are less than the minimum flow for synaptic transmission.

CPR AND CEREBRAL PERFUSION

Manual chest compressions are far from effective in supporting cerebral blood flow.

Manual chest compressions achieve only 5% of the normal cerebral flowrates,[7] which is less than the minimum flow needed to maintain cerebral metabolism.

Open chest cardiac massage can achieve normal or supranormal cerebral flows,[7] but this technique is not feasible in most clinical situations (the exception being the immediate period following cardiopulmonary bypass surgery). The inability of closed chest CPR to maintain adequate levels of cerebral blood flow is the principal reason for the low survival rates and poor neurologic recovery.

THE THORACIC PUMP MODEL

The traditional view was that chest compressions propelled blood forward by compressing the heart between the sternum and the bony spine. This "cardiac pump" theory fell from favor when it was discovered that cough-induced increases in intrathoracic pressure could produce adequate levels of cerebral blood flow for brief periods of time.[10] This is called "cough CPR" and it led to the "thoracic pump" theory, which claims that the entire thorax acts as a pump to propel blood forward.

Manual chest compression produces a positive intrathoracic pressure and this will enhance systolic emptying of the heart, possibly by reducing the afterload of the left ventricle.

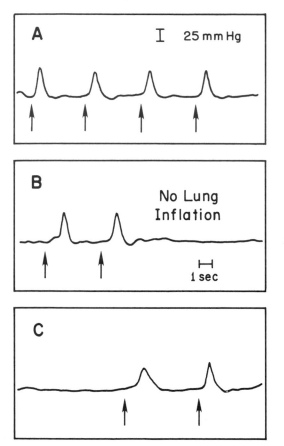

FIG. 16–2. The influence of positive intrathoracic pressure on systemic blood pressure. The arrows indicate lung inflations from an Ambu bag without sternal compressions. Pressure recorded from the radial artery.

Remember that, in Chapter 1, afterload was defined as peak systolic *transmural* pressure. Positive pressure outside the heart will reduce transmural pressure and thereby reduce afterload. The pressure tracings in Figure 16–2 illustrate the ability of positive intrathoracic pressure to generate a systemic blood pressure. The tracings in the figure were recorded from the radial artery in a patient with refractory asystole. The phasic pressure tracings were produced by repeated lung inflations from an anesthesia bag. When the lung inflations were temporarily stopped, the phasic pressures disappeared. This proves that positive intrathoracic pressure is capable of producing a systemic blood pressure and this supports the thoracic pump model of CPR.[11]

THE NEW CPR

The thoracic pump model created additional maneuvers aimed at creating positive intrathoracic pressures during CPR. These maneuvers are called "New CPR."[11,12] The most promising maneuver involves simultaneous lung inflation and sternal compression. This is associated with higher intrathoracic pressures than conventional CPR, but the influence on cerebral blood flow has been variable.[9,11,12] Another maneuver for creating more positive intrathoracic pressures is to bind the abdomen and limit diaphragm excursion. However, this maneuver has not been promising to date.[13]

POST-RESUSCITATION INJURY

Ischemic damage to organs can continue after the resuscitation period, despite restoration of a normal (or baseline) blood pressure. These "post-resuscitation ischemic syndromes" were presented in Chapter 12 and will be reviewed briefly because of their potential impact on recovery following CPR.

NO REFLOW

The "no reflow" phenomenon is a state of persistent vasoconstriction that follows a period of hypotension (see reference 3 for a detailed discussion of this phenomenon). Remember the following statement after an apparently successful resuscitation.

> Blood flow to several organs can actually decrease further after CPR despite restoration of the blood pressure and this hypoperfusion can last for 18 hours.[16]

Postresuscitation hypoperfusion is most prominent in the cerebral and splanchnic circulations.[7,14,16] The proposed mechanism is vasoconstriction from calcium that moves into damaged vascular smooth muscle.[14] The principal evidence for the calcium hypothesis is the observation that calcium channel blockers such as verapamil and magnesium can abolish the postarrest cerebral hypoperfusion in animal models.[17]

REPERFUSION INJURY

The other proposed mechanism for postresuscitation injury involves the toxic products of oxygen metabolism (the same ones implicated in pulmonary oxygen toxicity). These metabolites accumulate during the ischemic period and are disseminated during the reperfusion period to produce widespread organ damage.[15] This theory differs from the no reflow theory in that there is adequate blood flow after the resuscitation. At present, the participation of oxygen metabolites in postresuscitation injury is under investigation.

CEREBRAL PRESERVATION

The low rates of neurologic recovery after CPR are due to the combination of ischemic injury during CPR and persistent injury after CPR.

The following measures are designed to counteract these processes in an attempt to reduce the incidence of neurologic impairment. These maneuvers are unproven at the present time.

RESUSCITATION MEASURES

The following maneuvers are designed to promote cerebral blood flow **during** the resuscitation period.

New CPR. The CPR maneuvers designed to increase intrathoracic pressure have not been adopted in the most most recent guidelines for CPR.[2] The following statement is the position on "new CPR" reported in 1986.

"At this time there is no documented evidence that the use of any of these techniques during resuscitation improves survival of the cardiac arrest victim. Thus, their **routine** use is not recommended, but further research is encouraged."[6]

This is a noncommittal statement, as shown by the phrase "routine use". I use the simultaneous lung inflation-chest compression method (without abdominal binding) in patients who do not have a condition that predisposes to intracranial hypertension. **These maneuvers are contraindicated in patients with head injury and elevated intracranial pressure** because the high intrathoracic pressures can increase intracranial pressure.

Restrict Calcium. The ability of calcium to augment cardiac contraction led to the popularity of calcium for asystole and electromechanical dissociation.[18] However, the possible participation of calcium in the no-reflow phenomenon led to a re-evaluation of the merits of calcium therapy during CPR. In 1986, the recommendations for calcium infusion were limited to the following:[18] (1) hyperkalemia, (2) hypocalcemia, and (3) overdose with calcium-channel blockers. Remember that **Ringer's lactate solution contains calcium (3 mEq/L) and can promote vasoconstriction.** This must be considered a contraindication to its use during CPR (my recommendation only) until its safety is proven.

Avoid Dextrose. Dextrose infusion is common during CPR, either as a constituent of the routine intravenous solutions or as therapy for life-threatening hyperkalemia. Recent evidence in animals shows that dextrose infusion during CPR increases mortality.[19] The prevailing theory is that glucose enters ischemic areas in the CNS and is metabolized anaerobically to produce lactic acid. The local accumulation of lactic acid then accelerates tissue damage.

The significance of carbohydrate infusion during CPR has not been adequately studied in humans. However, until the issue is studied in more detail, **it is not wise to infuse glucose during CPR unless absolutely necessary.**

THE POST-RESUSCITATION PERIOD

Measures aimed at preventing post-CPR cerebral injury are appealing in theory, but unproven. Two of the more prominent approaches that have been suggested are outlined below.

Calcium Blockade. The role of calcium in producing no-reflow created a flurry of interest in calcium blockade in the early 1980s,[14,17] however, there seems to be little continuing interest in this concept. Both calcium-blocking drugs (verapamil, 0.1 mg/kg IV and magnesium infusion 100 mg/kg) have proven to be effective in maintaining cerebral blood flow after CPR in animal studies,[11,14] but their effectiveness in humans is unknown. Intravenous magnesium has been used safely in humans but the influence on outcome has not been reported.[17]

Unfortunately, many patients require blood pressure support with vasoconstrictors after CPR, which is a contraindication to calcium blockade. In selected patients who do not require vasoconstrictor support, calcium blockade is a consideration. As mentioned in Chapter 12, the oxygen uptake ($\dot{V}O_2$) might be helpful after resuscitation in that **a low $\dot{V}O_2$ after CPR suggests persistent ischemia and might be reason to consider calcium blockade** when it is safe to do so. In selected patients who do not require vasoconstrictors and do not have a history of renal failure, I infuse magnesium (2 grams elemental Mg or 4 ml 50% $MgSO4$ over 20 minutes) as soon as possible after CPR.

Steroids and Barbiturates. Both steroids and barbiturates were considered for cerebral protection by virtue of their ability to reduce edema (steroids) and to diminish the metabolic requirement for oxygen (barbiturates). However, clinical trials have failed to show any benefit from either type of agent,[7] and their use has been abandoned in the postresuscitation period.

NEUROLOGIC SEQUELAE

As mentioned earlier, only 10% of the survivors of cardiac arrest will be able to resume their former lifestyles.[4] Most of the disability in the survivors results from some form of neurologic impairment.[4,8]

IMPAIRED AWARENESS

The most feared consequence in survivors of cardiac arrest is the inability to regain an independent lifestyle. The following definitions are used to describe the spectrum of impaired awareness syndromes.

1. **Coma**—An unconscious state characterized by the lack of spontaneous eye opening, failure to localize to noxious stimuli, and absence of verbal communication.

2. **Vegetative State**—Similar to coma, but includes spontaneous eye opening. Approximately 20% of survivors of cardiac arrest will remain in a persistent vegetative state.[7]

3. **Stupor**—A state of deep sleep arousable only by vigorous stimulation.

4. **Obtundation**—A state of apathy or decreased interest in the surroundings, with frequent periods of sleep.

5. **Amnesia**—An awake state with selective loss of memory for events

prior to the arrest (retrograde amnesia) or impaired ability to retain new memories (anterograde amnesia).

Brain death is not included in the above because fewer than 2% of patients who survive cardiac arrest will meet the criteria for brain death.[6]

CORTICAL BLINDNESS

This type of blindness is associated with intact retina and optic nerves. The pupillary light reflexes are intact but the patient does not blink in response to visual threats. Some patients may even deny being blind (Anton's syndrome). In many cases, this condition is temporary and younger patients have a better prognosis for full recovery.[8] Unfortunately, there are no clinical markers for predicting recovery in the individual patient.[8]

SEIZURES

Seizures can be expected in about one-third of patients who do not regain consciousness immediately after CPR.[20] The most common are partial seizures (elementary or complex) and myoclonus. Generalized (grand-mal) seizures are least common. The types of seizures are described as follows:

1. **Elementary Partial Seizures**—Characterized by repetitive clonic movements localized to a specific region of the body (e.g., a limb).

2. **Complex Partial Seizures**—Characterized by lip smacking, chewing, or swallowing, and may include psychotic behavior with visual or auditory hallucinations.

3. **Myoclonus**—An irregular jerking-type motion (unlike clonic movements, which are regular in amplitude and frequency). Can be localized or generalized.

Seizures usually occur in the first 24 hours but can appear after 1 to 2 weeks.[6,20] More than one type of seizure may appear in the same patient. Partial seizures do not influence prognosis but myoclonus carries a poor prognosis.[6] Most seizures following CPR (particularly myoclonus) are resistant to anticonvulsant therapy. Fortunately, they do not commonly recur and fewer than 2% of patients discharged from the hospital will experience recurrent seizures.[6]

Anticonvulsant therapy for the immediate management of seizures is outlined in the Appendix. Prophylactic therapy is not necessary.

PREDICTING NEUROLOGIC RECOVERY

This may be one of the most important aspects of your care of the patient who survives cardiac arrest. In particular, you must provide guidance to the families of patients who do not regain consciousness soon after CPR. The following guidelines may help you to predict the chances for neurologic recovery.

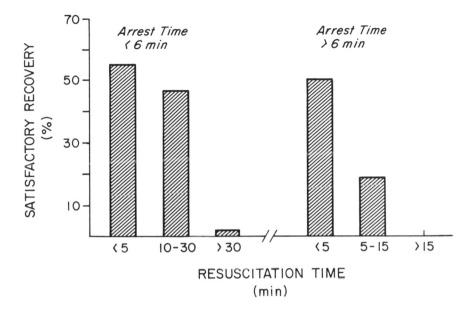

FIG. 16–3. Neurologic outcome versus the duration of cerebral ischemia. From the Brain Resuscitation Clinical Trial I Study Group. Crit Care Med 1985; 13:930–931.

ISCHEMIC TIME

The ischemic time includes the time from onset of the arrest to the start of CPR (arrest time), plus the time required for successful resuscitation (CPR time). Figure 16–3 illustrates the influence of the ischemic time on neurologic outcome reported in one large multicenter study.[21]

If the arrest time was less than 6 minutes and the CPR time did not exceed 30 minutes, 50% of the patients achieved a satisfactory neurologic recovery. However, if the arrest time exceeded 6 minutes, there were no survivors when the CPR time exceeded 15 minutes.

COMA

Postresuscitation coma can carry a poor prognosis but only after some time has elapsed.

Coma in the immediate postresuscitation period has no predictive value, because as many as 30% of these patients can eventually regain consciousness.[6]

However, coma that persists beyond a few hours after CPR carries a poor prognosis for satisfactory cerebral recovery. The longer the coma persists, the less is the likelihood of awakening. This is shown in Figure 16–4, which represents the results of a study that evaluated 500 patients

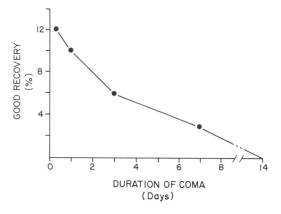

FIG. 16–4. Neurologic outcome versus the duration of coma. Redrawn with permission from Levy DE, et al. Prognosis in nontraumatic coma. Ann Intern Med 94:293–301, 1981.

with nontraumatic coma from diverse causes.[22] The prognosis was poor at 6 to 12 hours and declined further if the coma persisted for longer than 1 to 2 days.

> Coma that persists after 24 to 48 hours carries only a 2 to 7% chance of favorable neurologic recovery.[22,25]

After 48 hours, the chances for satisfactory recovery are extremely poor and are virtually nil if the coma persists for 7 days. Therefore, the 48-hour period can be used to gather prognostic information for the families.

Coma Scores. Scoring systems can be used to document the depth of coma and to follow the clinical course of the neurologic deficit. The most popular system is the Glascow Coma Scale (GCS), which was developed for patients with head injury. The Pittsburgh Brain Stem Score (PBSS) has been developed to complement the GCS in patients with nontraumatic coma.[3] Each of the scoring methods is shown in the Appendix.

The GCS has recently been shown to be valuable in predicting outcome in patients with cardiac arrest occurring outside the hospital.[26] Neurologic outcome was correctly predicted on day 2 in most patients. If the best score was 10 or higher (best possible score: 15), the patients recovered satisfactorily. However, if the best score was only 4 or lower by the second day, the chances for satisfactory recovery were poor. This represents only one study and must be interpreted as such. However, it adds another guideline that can be used to supplement the other prognostic signs.

BRAINSTEM REFLEXES

In patients who do not regain consciousness soon after the resuscitation period, the following reflexes can provide some prognostic information: (1) pupillary light reflex; (2) corneal touch reflex; (3) oculocephalic reflex and (4) oculovestibular reflex.

The Ocular Reflexes. The ocular reflexes are demonstrated in Figure 16–5. The **oculocephalic reflex** is elicited by rotating the head from side to side, first slowly then briskly. When the brainstem is intact but the

Brainstem Intact

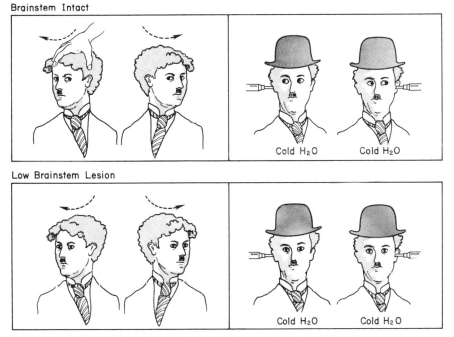

FIG. 16–5. The ocular reflexes. See text for explanation.

cerebral hemispheres are impaired, the eyes will deviate away from the direction of rotation (if the head is rotated to the right, the eyes will deviate to the left). When the brainstem is damaged or when the patient is awake, there is no eye deviation (the eyes will follow the direction of head rotation). The popular term **doll's eyes** was originally used to describe the reflex opening of the eyelids that is occasionally observed when the neck is flexed. However, this term is now used to indicate a positive oculocephalic reflex (brainstem intact).

The **oculovestibular reflex** (cold calorics) is elicited by injecting 30 ml of iced saline in the external auditory canal using a syringe and a short (2 inch) plastic catheter. When the brainstem is intact, the response involves conjugate eye deviation towards the irrigated ear. If the hemispheres are intact, there will also be a few minutes of nystagmus with the rapid component away from the irrigated ear. This nystagmus is not expected when the cerebral hemispheres are impaired.

Prognostic Signs. Brainstem reflexes can be absent immediately after CPR but they should return within 1 hour in patients who will have a satisfactory neurologic recovery.[6] More prolonged loss of these reflexes (particularly the pupillary and corneal reflexes) carries a poor prognosis.

> Absence of the pupillary or corneal reflexes at 6 to 24 hours after cardiac arrest has a dismal prognosis for cerebral recovery.[22,27]

In one often quoted study,[27] no patient with an absent pupillary or corneal reflex 24 hours after CPR regained an independent lifestyle. The oculocephalic reflex adds nothing to your evaluation if the pupillary or corneal reflexes are absent.[27] When the brainstem reflexes are preserved, they have little prognostic value.

REFERENCES

1. Jacobson S ed. Resuscitation. Clinics in emergency medicine. Vol. 2. Churchill Livingstone: New York, 1983.
2. National Conference on Cardiopulmonary Resuscitation and Emergency Cardiac Care. Standards and Guidelines for Cardiopulmonary Resuscitation (CPR) and Emergency Cardiac Care. JAMA 1986; 255:2905–2989.
3. Safar P, Bircher NG. Cardiopulmonary cerebral resuscitation. 3rd ed. W.B. Saunders: Philadelphia, 1988.
4. Maiese K, Caronna JJ. Coma following cardiac arrest: A review of the clinical features, management, and prognosis. J Intensive Care Med 1988; 3:153–163.
5. Steinbrook R, Lo B. Artificial feeding—solid ground, not a slippery slope. N Engl J Med 1988; 318:286–290.
6. Bruns FJ, Fraley DS, Haigh J, et al. Control of organ blood flow. In: Snyder JV, Pinsky MR eds. Oxygen transport in the critically ill. Chicago: Year Book Medical Publishers, 1987: 87–124.
7. Koehler RC, Michael JR. Cardiopulmonary resuscitation, brain blood flow, and neurologic recovery. Crit Care Clin 1985; 1:205–222.
8. Kirsch JR, Dean JM, Rogers MC. Current concepts in brain resuscitation. Arch Intern Med 1986; 146:1413–1419.
9. Arai T, Kentaro D, Tsukahara I, et al. Cerebral blood flow during conventional, new and open chest cardio-pulmonary resuscitation in dogs. Resuscitation 1984; 12:147–154.
10. Babbs CF. New vs. old theories of blood flow during CPR. Crit Care Med 1980; 8:191–195.
11. Ducas J, Roussos C, Karsadis C, Magder S. Thoracoabdominal mechanics during resuscitation maneuvers. Chest 1983; 84:446–451.
12. White JD. The New CPR. In: Jacobsen S ed. Resuscitation. New York: Churchill Livingstone, 1983:27–37.
13. Howard M, Carubba C, Foss F, Janiak B, Hogan B, Guinness M. Interposed abdominal compression—CPR: Its effects on parameters of coronary perfusion in human subjects. Ann Emerg Med 1987; 16:253–259.
14. White BC, Winegar CD, Wilson RF, Hochner PJ, Trombley JH. Possible role of calcium blockers in cerebral resuscitation: A review of the literature and synthesis for future studies. Crit Care Med 1983; 11:202–207.
15. Babbs F. Reperfusion injury of postischemic tissues. Ann Emerg Med 1988; 17:1148–1157.
16. McNamara JJ, Suehiro GT, Suehiro A, Jewett B. Resuscitation from hemorrhagic shock. J Trauma 1983; 23:552–558.
17. White BC, Winegar CD, Wilson F, Krause GS. Calcium blockers in cerebral resuscitation. J Trauma 1983; 23:788–794.
18. Hughes WG, Ruedy JR. Should calcium be used in cardiac arrest? Am J Med 1986; 81:285–296.
19. Yatsu FM, McKenzie JD, Lockwood AH. Cardiopulmonary arrest and intravenous glucose. [Editorial] J Crit Care 1987; 2:1–3.
20. Snyder BD, Hauser WA, Lowenson RB, Leppik IE, Ramirez-Lassepas M, Gumnit RJ. Neurologic prognosis after cardiopulmonary arrest: III Seizure activity. Neurology 1980; 30:1292–1297.
21. Brain Resuscitation Clinical Trial I Study Group. Neurologic recovery after cardiac arrest: Effect of duration of ischemia. Crit Care Med 1985; 13:930–931.

22. Levy DE, Bates D, Caronna JJ, et al. Prognosis in nontraumatic coma. Ann Int Med 1981; *94*:293–301.
23. Bedell SE, Delbanco TL, Cook EF, Epstein FH. Survival after cardiopulmonary resuscitation in the hospital. N Engl J Med 1983; *309*:569–576.
24. Snyder BD, Loewenson RB, Gumnit RJ, Hauser WA, Leppik IE, Ramirez-Lassepas M. Neurologic prognosis after cardiopulmonary arrest: II Level of consciousness. Neurology 1980; *30*:52–59.
25. Longstreth WT Jr. The neurologic sequelae of cardiac arrest. West J Med 1987; *147*:175–180.
26. Cerebral Resuscitation Study Group of the Belgian Society for Intensive Care: Predictive value of Glascow coma score for awakening after out-of-hospital cardiac arrest. Lancet 1988; 1:137–140.
27. Levy DE, Caronna JJ, Singer BH, Lapinski RH, Grydman H, Plum F. Predicting outcome from hypoxia-ischemic coma. JAMA 1985; *253*:1420–1426.

section V
RESUSCITATION PRACTICES

"It is common sense to take a method and try it: If it fails, admit it frankly and try another. But above all, try something."

Franklin D. Roosevelt

c h a p t e r

COLLOID AND CRYSTALLOID RESUSCITATION

The introduction to volume resuscitation in Chapter 13 is the background for the next two chapters on replacement fluids. This chapter focuses on colloid and crystalloid fluid therapy and the next chapter looks at blood transfusion therapy. See the reviews[1-8] at the end of the chapter for further information on asanguinous fluid therapy.

CRYSTALLOID RESUSCITATION

Crystalloid fluids are mixtures of sodium chloride and other physiologically active solutes. Sodium is the major component of crystalloid fluids and the distribution of sodium determines the distribution of infused crystalloid fluids. Sodium is the major solute in the extracellular space and 80% of the extracellular space is extravascular.[9] Therefore, infused sodium will reside primarily outside the vascular compartment.

> Crystalloid (sodium-containing) fluids are designed to expand the interstitial space, not the vascular space. Only 20% of infused sodium chloride solutions will remain in the vascular space.[1-3]

The influence of crystalloid fluids on blood volume is shown in Figure 17–1.[8] Infusion of 1 L of Ringer's lactate would cause a 200 ml increment in blood volume in an average sized adult (1.7 m²), which is consistent with the expected distribution of sodium in the body fluid compartments.

205

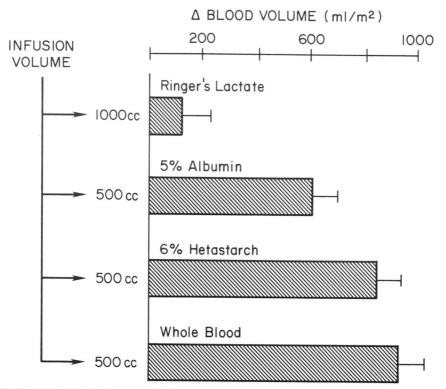

FIG. 17–1. The influence of colloid and crystalloid infusion on blood volume in critically ill adults. Redrawn from Shippy CR, Appel PR, Shoemaker WC. Crit Care Med 1984; *12*:107–112.

RATIONALE FOR CRYSTALLOIDS

Crystalloid fluids are well suited for the replacement of extracellular fluid losses (dehydration) but they are also used to replace blood volume loss. This latter practice is based on the notion that acute hemorrhage (or hypovolemia) leaves an interstitial fluid deficit that must be replenished (see Chapter 13). This was used to explain the results in animal studies of hemorrhagic shock showing improved survival when salt solutions (which should replace the interstitial fluid deficits) were added to blood replacement.[10] The significance of the interstitial fluid deficit in acute hemorrhage has since been questioned.[11] Nevertheless, crystalloid fluids have proven effective in the resuscitation of patients with acute hemorrhage[1,3,4,6,12,28,29] and they continue to be popular resuscitation fluids for trauma victims.

CRYSTALLOID FLUIDS

The prototype crystalloid fluids are shown in Table 17–1. Many other fluids are available for clinical use, but most are variations on the fluids in this table.

TABLE 17–1. CRYSTALLOID SOLUTIONS					
	Plasma*	0.9% Saline	Ringer's Lactate	Normosol	
Na	141	154	130	140	
CL	103	154	109	98	
K	4–5	—	4	5	mEq/L
Ca/Mg	5/2	—	3/0	0/3	
Buffer	Bicarbonate (26)	—	Lactate (28)	Acetate (27) Gluconate (23)	
pH	7.4	5.7	6.7	7.4	
Osmolality (mosm/kg)	289	308	273	295	

*Plasma values from Brenner BM, Rector FC Jr. eds. The Kidney. Philadelphia: W.B. Saunders. 1981:95.

Isotonic Saline. Isotonic saline is the standard crystalloid fluid and contains 9 grams of sodium chloride per L (a 0.9% solution). It is also called "normal" saline, which is an incorrect term (a 1N NaCl solution would have 58 grams of NaCl, which is the combined molecular weights of sodium and chloride).

FEATURES:
1. Slightly hypertonic to plasma.
2. Has an acid pH.

RISKS:
1. May produce a hyperchloremic metabolic acidosis, although this is rare.[13]

Ringer's Lactate. Ringer's lactate is a "balanced" electrolyte solution that substitutes potassium and calcium for some of the sodium in isotonic saline.[14] Lactate is added as a buffer. This fluid is popular in trauma resuscitation for unknown reasons.

FEATURES:
1. Isotonic to plasma.
2. The lactate is converted to bicarbonate in the liver and acts as a buffer.

There is no evidence that Ringer's lactate provides any real benefit over isotonic saline. In particular, there is no evidence that lactate provides any buffering capacity in shock states.

RISKS:
1. The added potassium can be detrimental in patients with adrenal insufficiency or renal failure.
2. The calcium seems risky in hypovolemic patients because of the

TABLE 17–2. INCOMPATIBLE MEDICATIONS WITH LACTATED RINGER'S SOLUTION*			
Definitely Incompatible	Partially Incompatible	Possibly Incompatible	
Cefamandole	Ampicillin	Amikacin	Penicillin
Amicar	Vibramycin	Azlocillin	Procainamide
Amphotericin	Minocycline	Bretylium	Propranolol
Ethyl Alcohol		Cleocin	Cyclosporin
Pentothal		Levophed	Trimethaprim sulfa
Metaraminol		Mannitol	Vancomycin
		SoluMedrol	Vasopressin
		Nitroglycerin	Urokinase
		Nitroprusside	

*From Griffith CA. J Natl Intravenous Therap Assoc 1986; 9:480–483.

ability for calcium to promote the "no-reflow" phenomenon after resuscitation from hemorrhagic shock (see Chapter 12).

3. In addition to blood products, there are several drugs that are incompatible with Ringer's lactate because of calcium binding. These drugs are listed in Table 17–2.

Normosol. This fluid is highly buffered, with about twice the buffer capacity of Ringer's lactate.

FEATURES:

1. The pH is equivalent to plasma.
2. Contains magnesium instead of calcium.

The major benefit of normosol is the adjusted pH. The magnesium is potentially beneficial because it blocks calcium-induced vasoconstriction and may help to limit the no-reflow phenomenon if it exists (see Chapter 12).

RISKS:

1. Magnesium is a vasodilator and could interfere with the compensatory vasoconstriction that maintains the blood pressure in hypovolemia.

DEXTROSE SOLUTIONS

Dextrose is available as a 5% solution (50 g per L) in saline, water, or Ringer's solutions. Dextrose was originally added to intravenous fluids to supply carbohydrate substrate for the central nervous system during brief periods of fasting (protein-sparing effect). However, the advent of full parenteral nutrition has made this use of 5% dextrose solutions obsolete.

FEATURES:

1. Dextrose provides 3.4 kcal/g or 170 kcal/L for a 5% dextrose solution.
2. Each 50 g of dextrose contributes 278 mOsm to a solution.

Dextrose is more of an osmotic load than a caloric source. The increase in osmolality of the standard crystalloid solutions produced by dextrose is shown below:

Solution	mOsm/L
0.9% Saline	308
5% Dextrose in 0.9% saline	586
Ringer's lactate	273
5% Dextrose in Ringer's lactate	527

The addition of 50 g dextrose to saline or lactated Ringer's solution will raise the osmolality of the fluid to roughly twice that of plasma. This can produce significant changes in serum osmolality when large volumes of fluid are infused. The tendency for critically ill patients to receive a multitude of drips increases the risk for hypertonicity if dextrose solutions are used routinely.

RISKS:

1. Dextrose infusion can fuel the production of lactic acid in ischemic organs, particularly the central nervous system.

Dextrose and Cerebral Ischemia. The ability of carbohydrates to promote ischemic damage in the central nervous system is not new but seems forgotten.[15] The central nervous system relies on glucose for much of its energy needs. When cerebral ischemia develops, the infusion of glucose will fuel anaerobic glycolysis and produce large quantities of lactic acid. The lactic acid that accumulates locally can reduce flow even further and add to the problem. This explains some of the animal experiments showing that dextrose infusion during cardiopulmonary resuscitation can be associated with a much higher mortality.[16] Until more information is gathered on this topic, the routine infusion of glucose is not recommended in patients at risk for cerebral insufficiency.

COLLOID RESUSCITATION

Colloids are large molecular weight substances that do not pass readily across capillary walls. The particles retained in the vascular space will exert an osmotic force (the "colloid osmotic pressure") that keeps fluid in the blood vessels. Figure 17–1 illustrates the change in blood volume from infusion of 500 ml of colloid solution.[8]

RATIONALE FOR COLLOIDS

The most life-threatening aspect of acute hemorrhage is hypovolemia. Because colloids are more effective than crystalloids for increasing vascular volume, colloid resuscitation should be preferred in patients with brisk bleeding. Most volume resuscitation protocols combine colloid and crystalloid fluids to expand both vascular and interstitial volume.

TABLE 17–3. COLLOID SOLUTIONS				
	25% Albumin	**5% Albumin**	**6% Hetastarch**	**Dextran-40**
COP (mm Hg)	70	20	30	40
Unit Size	50 ml	250 or 500 ml	500 ml	250 ml
*Potency	4:1	1.3:1	1.3:1	2:1
Bleeding	—	0.001	0.010	0.010
†Unit Cost	$19.22 per 50 ml	$19.22 per 500 ml	$43.50 per 500 ml	$20.00 per 500 ml

*Potency expressed as increase in vascular volume (mls) per milliliter of infused colloid.
†Manufacturer's cost at our hospital as of March 1, 1989.

COLLOID SOLUTIONS

The colloid solutions available for clinical use are shown in Table 17–3.
Human Serum Albumin. Albumin is responsible for about 80% of the colloid osmotic pressure of plasma and is an effective colloid. In addition, albumin serves as an important transport protein for drugs (e.g., antibiotics) and ions (e.g., calcium and magnesium). The albumin used commercially is prepared by heating human serum to denature any viral particles. This preparation is available as a 5% solution (50 g per L) or a 25% solution (250 g per L) in isotonic saline. The 25% solution is referred to as "salt-poor" albumin because it is given in small volumes (usually 50 to 100 ml) and represents a small salt load.
FEATURES:
1. The 5% solution has a colloid osmotic pressure (COP) of 20 mmHg,[18,19] which is equivalent to plasma COP.
2. The 25% solution has a COP of 70 mmHg.[20]
3. Infusion of 5% albumin will expand the vascular volume by an amount slightly in excess of the infused volume.[8]
4. Infusion of 100 ml of 25% albumin will expand the plasma volume by about 500 ml.[32]
5. The effect lasts for 24 to 36 hours.[30]
Contrary to popular belief, over 50% of the albumin in the body resides outside the vascular space. The infused albumin eventually passes into the interstitial space and is either returned to the bloodstream via the lymph or is metabolized for energy.
DISADVANTAGES:
1. Can produce a dilutional coagulopathy in large volumes.[7]
2. Can transmit viral hepatitis, but this is rare.[7]
3. Allergic reactions occur, but rarely.[7,21]

Hydroxyethyl Starch. Hetastarch is a synthetic starch that was introduced as an inexpensive alternative to albumin. A 6% solution (60 g per L) in isotonic saline is available for clinical use.
FEATURES:
1. The 6% solution has a COP of 30 mmHg.[18,19]
2. The acute volume expansion from hetastarch is equivalent to that produced by 5% albumin.[18,19,22]
3. Has a longer serum half-life than albumin, with 50% of the osmotic effects persisting at 24 hours.[23]

Unlike albumin, hetastarch is cleared primarily by the kidneys. The starch polymers are variable in size and are constantly cleaved by serum amylases until they are small enough to be cleared by the kidneys. The largest particles can take weeks to be cleared.[23]
DISADVANTAGES:
1. Serum amylase levels rise to two or three times normal during hetastarch infusion[24] and this can persist for 5 days. The hyperamylasemia is a normal response to degrade the hetastarch and does not indicate pancreatitis. Serum lipase must be used to diagnose and follow pancreatitis when hetastarch is used.
2. Early concerns about a specific coagulopathy from hetastarch have not been confirmed,[25] and large volumes of hetastarch have been used without clinical bleeding.[26]
3. Allergic reactions occur, but are rare.[7,21]

Hetastarch is not a protein and can produce a dilutional decrease in serum protein concentrations. Because the total protein concentration is used to calculate the colloid osmotic pressure (see Chapter 23), the COP must be measured and not calculated when using hetastarch as a plasma expander.

The Dextrans. The dextrans are polysaccharides obtained from the juice of sugar beets. The available preparations are dextran-40 (average molecular weight of 40,000) and dextran-70 (average molecular weight of 70,000).
FEATURES:
1. Dextran-40 is available as a 10% solution with a COP of 40 mmHg.[18]
2. The acute volume expansion from dextran-40 is roughly twice the infused volume[18] but more than 50% is cleared after just 6 hours.[7,18]
DISADVANTAGES:
1. Dextrans can produce a bleeding tendency by inhibiting platelet aggregation, reducing activation of Factor VIII, and promoting fibrinolysis.[21] However, large doses (1.5 gr/kg/day) are required to produce the anticoagulant effect.[7,21]
2. Anaphylactic reactions can occur in up to 1% of patients.[7] This can be prevented by preinjection of a dextran hapten that blocks the binding sites of the dextran antibodies.
3. Dextrans coat the surface of red blood cells and interfere with the ability to crossmatch blood. The red cell concentrates must be washed to eliminate this problem.
4. Dextran has been implicated as a cause of acute renal failure.[27] The proposed mechanism is a hyperosmolar state in the glomerular blood leading to a decrease in effective filtration pressure.

THE COLLOID-CRYSTALLOID WARS

The appropriate resuscitation fluid is more than a topic of debate, it is a passionately fought war. The following is a brief summary of the salient arguments in the debate. Like all wars, the truth is somewhere in the middle.

EXPENSE

Colloids are much more expensive than crystalloids. This is evident in Table 17–3 (the prices in this table are the manufacturer's cost at our hospital in March 1989). The crystalloid soldiers estimate the annual cost differential for colloid and crystalloid resuscitation is 500 million dollars.[4] The colloid soldiers maintain that the cost per patient more than justifies the benefit to be gained.

HEMODYNAMIC EFFECTS

When rapid expansion of plasma volume is desirable, colloids are clearly superior to crystalloids.

> The resuscitation volume will be 2 to 4 times larger with crystalloids than with colloids to produce the same increment in plasma volume,[30] and the resuscitation time with crystalloids can be twice that of colloids.[31]

Colloids are also superior to crystalloids in their ability to improve cardiac output and oxygen transport.[32,33] This is illustrated in Figure 17–2 for an adult ICU patient population.[2] Note that the Ringer's solution is administered in twice the volume of the 5% albumin, and ten times the volume of the 25% albumin. This ability of colloids to improve cardiac output and oxygen transport is an obvious bonus in patients with severe or life-threatening cardiovascular compromise. In patients with less severe degrees of hypovolemia, crystalloid infusion will suffice.

RISK FOR PULMONARY EDEMA

Pulmonary edema should not pose a problem with either type of fluid if proper hemodynamic monitoring is employed and the pulmonary capillary pressure is kept below 20 mmHg.[34,35] Although crystalloids should produce edema more readily than colloids, the risk for producing pulmonary edema with crystalloids appears to be small, even when large volumes are infused.[4,17]

When the permeability of pulmonary capillaries is increased, colloid fluids could leak out of the vascular space and become "trapped" in the interstitium, thereby promoting increased edema formation. However, the present evidence shows that colloids do not cause more pulmonary edema than crystalloids when the pulmonary capillaries are dam-

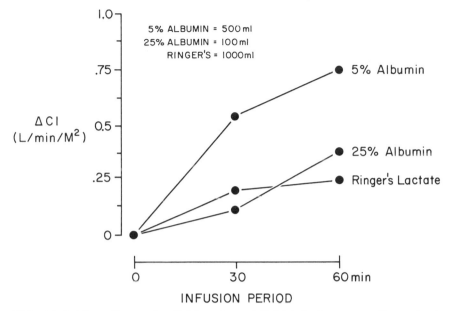

5% ALBUMIN = 500 ml
25% ALBUMIN = 100 ml
RINGER'S = 1000ml

5% Albumin

25% Albumin

Ringer's Lactate

ΔCI
$(L/min/M^2)$

INFUSION PERIOD

FIG. 17–2. The effects of colloid and crystalloid infusion on cardiac output. Redrawn from Shoemaker WC. Intensive Care Med 1987; 13:230–243.

aged.[36,37] In fact, one study has shown that crystalloid fluids cause more pulmonary edema when the capillaries become leaky.[37]

CLINICAL OUTCOME

The final, and possibly the most important, issue in this controversy is the clinical outcome.

> The survival in hypovolemic shock is no different when using colloid or crystalloid fluids for the resuscitation.[1,28,29]

Although there may be a subset of patients with severe hemorrhagic shock who would benefit from rapid volume expansion with colloids, it seems that most patients fare the same regardless of the fluid that is infused.

SUMMARY

The **hole-in-the-bucket analogy** may help to explain my approach to fluid resuscitation. If you want to fill a bucket, you would prefer not to have a hole in the bottom of the bucket. If the bucket is the vascular space, the resuscitation with crystalloid instead of colloid is analogous to creating a hole in the bucket because you can still fill the bucket but it will take more volume and more time to achieve your goal. In other words, if the goal is to expand the plasma volume, colloid solutions seem to be the logical choice. If the goal is to replenish the entire extra-

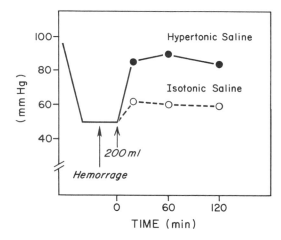

FIG. 17–3. The effect of hypertonic saline resuscitation. From Kramer GC, Perron PR, Lindsey P. Surgery 1986; 100:239–246.

cellular space, then crystalloid fluids are the fluids of choice. This approach is simple: first identify your goal (which body fluid compartment needs to be filled) then match the goal to the appropriate fluid.

HYPERTONIC RESUSCITATION: THE FUTURE

The use of concentrated resuscitation fluids is an appealing concept because of the reduced volumes of fluid that are required. This will decrease the risk of producing edema and will improve the ability to deliver effective volume resuscitation in the field. The present "scoop and run" approach to trauma victims in the field is less than optimal, because the mortality in civilian trauma is greatest in the first hour after the event.[38] The military is particularly interested in the hypertonic method because small volumes of resuscitation fluid can be carried by soldiers into remote areas of combat.

Hypertonic saline solutions have proven effective in hemorrhagic shock in animal studies and clinical trials.[39,40] A common regimen is as follows:

Fluid:	7.5% sodium chloride
Osmolality:	2400 mOsm/kg
Volume:	4 ml/kg over 2 minutes
Onset of Response:	1 to 2 minutes
Duration of Response:	1 to 2 hours

The major drawback of hypertonic saline resuscitation is the short duration of response. Combining saline with a colloid like 6% dextran-70 has prolonged the response considerably.[41]

An example of the blood pressure response to hypertonic resuscitation is shown in Figure 17–3. This figure is taken from a study where animals were subjected to controlled hemorrhage until the mean arterial pressure was lowered to 50 mmHg.[41] After the hypotension was maintained for 3 hours, the animals were given a bolus of either normal saline or a hypertonic fluid (a mixture of 7.5% saline and 6% dextran-70). Nothing further was given for the next 30 minutes (to simulate the time period needed to transport trauma victims to the hospital), after which resuscitation was continued with Ringer's lactate infusion. Note the prompt increase in blood pressure after the hypertonic fluid was given, and the relative lack of response to isotonic saline.

The principal concern with hypertonic resuscitation is the possibility of producing a hypertonic state, but this seems to be minimal if small volumes are used.[39] At present, hypertonic resuscitation is a promising area that needs more clinical investigation.

REFERENCES

REVIEWS

1. Moss GS, Gould SA. Plasma expanders. Am J Surg 1988; 155:425–434.
2. Shoemaker WC. Relation of oxygen transport patterns to the pathophysiology and therapy of shock states. Intensive Care Med 1987; 13:230–243.
3. Dodge C, Glass DD. Crystalloid and colloid therapy. Semin Anesth 1982; 1:293–301.
4. Tranbaugh RF, Lewis FR. Crystalloid fluid. In: Dailey RH, Callaham M eds. Controversies in trauma management. Clinics in emergency medicine. Churchill Livingstone, 1985; 121–133.
5. Dawson RB, Cowley RA. Colloid Fluid. In: Dailey RH, Callaham M eds. Controversies in trauma management. Clinics in emergency medicine. Vol. 6. New York: Churchill Livingstone, 1985; 135–146.
6. Shackford SR. Fluid resuscitation of the trauma victim. In: Shackford SR, Perel A eds. Trauma. Problems in critical care. Philadelphia: J.B. Lippincott. Vol. 1. 1987; 576–587.
7. Messmer KFW. The use of plasma substitutes with special attention to their side effects. World J Surg 1987; 11:69–74.
8. Shippy CR, Appel PL, Shoemaker WC. Reliability of clinical monitoring to assess blood volume in critically ill patients. Crit Care Med 1984; 12:107–112.

BODY FLUIDS AND HEMORRHAGE

9. Edelman IS, Leibman J. Anatomy of body water and electrolytes. Am J Med 1959; 27:256–263.
10. Shires T, Carrico J, Lightfoot S. Fluid therapy in hemorrhagic shock. Arch Surg 1964; 88:688–693.
11. Elwyn DH, Bryan-Brown CW, Quigley L, et al. Nutritional aspects of body water dislocations in postoperative and depleted patients. Ann Surg 1975; 182:76–82.

CRYSTALLOID RESUSCITATION

12. Horton J, Landreau R, Tuggle T. Cardiac response to fluid resuscitation from hemorrhagic shock. Surg Gynecol Obstet 1985; 160:444–452.
13. Lowery BD, Cloutier CT, Carey LC. Electrolyte solutions in resuscitation in human hemorrhagic shock. Surg Gynecol Obstet 1971; 131:273–279.
14. Griffith CA. The family of Ringer's solutions. J Natl Intravenous Therap Assoc 1986; 9:480–483.

15. Voll CL, Auer RN. The effect of postischemic blood glucose levels on ischemic brain damage in the rat. Ann Neurol 1988; 24:638–646.
16. Lundy EF, Kuhn JE, Kwon JM, et al. Infusion of 5% dextrose increases mortality and morbidity following six minutes of cardiac arrest in resuscitated dogs. J Crit Care 1987; 2:4–14.
17. Gallagher TJ, Banner MJ, Barnes PA. Large volume crystalloid resuscitation does not increase extravascular lung water. Anesth Analg 1985; 64:323–326.

COLLOID RESUSCITATION

18. Singh S, Schaeffer RC, Valdes S, et al. Cardiorespiratory effects of volume overload with colloidal fluids in dogs. Crit Care Med 1983; 11:585–590.
19. Puri VK, Howard M, Paidapaty BB, et al. Resuscitation of hypovolemia and shock: A prospective study of hydroxyethyl starch and albumin. Crit Care Med 1983; 11:518–523.
20. Albright AL, Latchaw RE, Robinson AG. Intracranial and systemic effects of hetastarch in experimental cerebral edema. Crit Care Med 1984; 12:496–500.
21. Munoz E. Costs of alternative colloid solutions (dextran, starch, albumin). Intensive Care World 1987; 4:12–17.
22. Moggio RA, Rha CC, Somberg ED, et al. Hemodynamic comparison of albumin and hydroxyethyl starch in the postoperative cardiac surgery patient. Crit Care Med 1983; 11:943–945.
23. Belcher P, Lennox SC. Avoidance of blood transfusion in coronary artery surgery: A trial of hydroxyethyl starch. Ann Thorac Surg 1984; 37:365–370.
24. Condit D, Freeman K, Brodman R. Hyperamylasemia in cardiac surgical patients receiving hydroxyethyl starch. J Crit Care 1987; 2:36–38.
25. Falk JL, Rackow EC, Astiz ME, et al. Effects of hetastarch and albumin on coagulation in patients with septic shock. J Clin Pharmacol 1988; 28:412–415.
26. Shatney CH, Deepika K, Militello PR, et al. Efficacy of hetastarch in the resuscitation of patients with multisystem trauma and shock. Arch Surg 1983; 118:804–809.
27. Feest TG. Low molecular weight dextran: A continuing cause of acute renal failure. Br Med J 1976; 2:1300–1303.

COMPARATIVE STUDIES

28. Lowe RJ, Moss GS, Jilek J, et al. Crystalloid vs. colloid in the etiology of pulmonary failure after trauma: A randomized trial in man. Surgery 1979; 81:676–683.
29. Virgilio RW, Rice CL, Smithe DE, et al. Crystalloid vs. colloid resuscitation. Is one better? Surgery 1979; 85:129–139.
30. Rackow EC, Falk JL, Fein IA, et al. Fluid resuscitation in circulatory shock: a comparison of the cardiorespiratory effects of albumin, hetastarch, and saline solutions in patients with hypovolemic and septic shock. Crit Care Med 1983; 11:839–850.
31. Shoemaker WC, Schluchter M, Hopkins JA, et al. Comparison of the relative effectiveness of colloids and crystalloids in emergency resuscitation. Am J Surg 1981; 142:73–84.
32. Hauser CJ, Shoemaker WC, Turpin I, et al. Oxygen transport responses to colloids and crystalloids in critically ill surgical patients. Surg Gynecol Obstet 1980; 150:811–816.
33. Appel PL, Shoemaker WC. Evaluation of fluid therapy in adult respiratory distress syndrome. Crit Care Med 1981; 9:862–869.
34. Schaeffer RC, Reeiewicz RA, Chilton SW, et al. Effects of colloid or crystalloid solutions on edemagenesis in normal and thrombomicroembolized lungs. Crit Care Med 1987; 15:1110–1115.
35. Karanko MS, Klossner JA, Laaksonen VO. Restoration of volume by crystalloid versus

colloid after coronary artery bypass: Hemodynamics, lung water, oxygenation, and outcome. Crit Care Med 1987; *15*:559–566.

36. Finch JS, Reid C, Bandy K, et al. Compared effects of selected colloids on extravascular lung water in dogs after oleic acid-induced lung injury and severe hemorrhage. Crit Care Med 1983; *11*:267–270.

37. Pearl RG, Halperin BD, Mihm FG, et al. Pulmonary effects of crystalloid and colloid resuscitation from hemorrhagic shock in the presence of oleic acid-induced pulmonary capillary injury in the dog. Anesthesiology 1988; *68*:12–20.

HYPERTONIC RESUSCITATION

38. Trunkey DD. Trauma Sci Am 1983; *249*:28–35.

39. Maningas PA. Hypertonic sodium chloride solutions for the prehospital management of traumatic hemorrhagic shock: A possible improvement in the standard of care? Ann Emerg Med 1986; *1*:1411–1414.

40. Auler JOC, Periera MHC, Gomide-Amaral RV, et al. Hemodynamic effects of hypertonic sodium chloride during surgical treatment of aortic aneurysms. Surgery 1987; *101*:594–601.

41. Kramer GC, Perron PR, Lindsey C, et al. Small-volume resuscitation with hypertonic saline dextran solution. Surgery 1986; *100*:239–246.

chapter

PRINCIPLES OF TRANSFUSION THERAPY

Blood transfusion therapy is far from a rational practice in the hospital and there is a real need to develop guidelines for blood transfusion. This is particularly true given the recent discoveries about the immune suppression associated with blood transfusion. This chapter will introduce you to the different types of blood products that are available. A section on transfusion reactions is included, as is a brief description of massive transfusion.

BLOOD COMPONENT THERAPY

The introduction of closed blood collection systems in the 1960's allowed whole blood to be separated into its constituents without risk of contamination. The use of whole blood components allows transfusion therapy to be tailored to specific needs and allows each unit of whole blood to be used for several purposes. The following is a brief description of whole blood and its components. Several comprehensive reviews of this topic are listed at the end of this chapter.[1-5]

WHOLE BLOOD

Whole blood is collected directly into a storage bag at the bedside. The standard "unit" of whole blood contains 450 ml of blood added to 50 to 60 ml of a liquid anticoagulant-preservative. Citrate acts as the anticoagulant because it binds calcium. Dextrose is used as a fuel source for the erythrocytes and phosphate is added to keep the pH close to normal (which retards the breakdown of 2,3 diphosphoglycerate). Whole blood is stored at 1 to 6°C.

FEATURES:
1. The shelf life of whole blood is 21 days, but the platelets lose their viability after 1 to 2 days.
2. Potassium is continually leaking from the red blood cells, and can reach extremely high levels by 21 days.

INDICATIONS:
1. Active hemorrhage.

Whole blood is usually separated into its components within hours after collection although it is still considered by many to be the replacement fluid of choice for active bleeding. Prolonged storage of whole blood carries a risk for producing a coagulopathy because it is devoid of functional platelets after 24 to 48 hours.

ERYTHROCYTE PRODUCTS

Red Cell Concentrates. Red blood cell concentrates are prepared by centrifuging whole blood and removing two-thirds of the plasma supernatant. These concentrates are called "packed red cells".

FEATURES:
1. Contains 200 ml of cells (both red cells and white cells) and 100 ml of plasma.
2. Hematocrit varies from 60 to 90% and hemoglobin ranges from 23 to 27 gm/dL.
3. Viscosity increases exponentially when hemoglobin rises above 20 gm/dL.[4]
4. Newer preservatives can reduce the viscosity to that of whole blood.[1]

INDICATIONS:
1. Anemia

Packed red cells are used as a source of hemoglobin and not as a source of volume. Consider packed cells a "viscous load" and not a volume load. The sluggish flow of packed cells is shown in Table 18–1. Viscosity is improved by infusing the packed cells with isotonic saline.

"Leukocyte-Poor" Red Cells. Removal of the white blood cells from erythrocyte concentrates is necessary for transfusing patients who have antileukocyte antibodies. The white blood cells can be separated in a variety of ways (e.g., centrifugation and filters) although no technique can achieve complete separation.

FEATURES:
1. Contains only 10 to 30% of the leukocytes present in red cell concentrates.
2. The hematocrit is 10 to 30% lower than in packed red cells.

INDICATIONS:
1. For patients with a history of febrile, nonhemolytic transfusion reaction.

The most common cause of febrile transfusion reactions is antibodies directed at leukocytes in donor blood. Removal of the donor white cells helps to minimize this febrile reaction. This is discussed later in the chapter.

Washed Red Blood Cells. Red cell concentrates are washed with isotonic saline to remove leukocytes and plasma. Removing plasma will reduce the risk of allergic reactions to blood transfusion.

FEATURES:

1. Devoid of plasma proteins and most leukocytes.
2. The hematocrit is lower than packed red cells (similar to leukocyte-poor red cells).
3. Can be stored for only 24 hours.

INDICATIONS:

1. For transfusing patients with a history of allergic transfusion reactions.
2. Patients with IgA deficiency.

Allergic reactions are the result of prior sensitization to plasma proteins in donor blood (see later in the chapter). IgA deficiency predisposes to allergic reactions without prior exposure.

PLASMA COMPONENTS

Fresh Frozen Plasma. When packed red blood cells are separated from whole blood, the remaining plasma fraction is stored at −18°C and is called "fresh frozen plasma" (FFP).

FEATURES:

1. One unit of FFP contains 200 to 250 ml of plasma.
2. FFP can be stored for up to 1 year.
3. After thawing, FFP must be given within 6 hours.

INDICATIONS:

1. To provide coagulation factors in selected patients with liver disease.
2. To reverse warfarin effects.
3. Should NOT be used as a plasma expander.[5]

Fresh frozen plasma can transmit hepatitis (estimated incidence of non-A non-B hepatitis is 1:100) and can produce allergic reactions in sensitized recipients. Because of these risks, FFP should never be used to expand the plasma volume if a colloid or crystalloid can be used.

Cryoprecipitate. Cryoprecipitate is a concentrated mixture of coagulation factors obtained by centrifuging fresh frozen plasma. It is freeze stored at −18°C, as is done with FFP. This precipitate is rich in fibrinogen and Factor VIII. It is prepared in "units" and 6 to 10 units are usually given in each transfusion. The major use is in hemophilia. It is seldom used in the ICU because it carries a high risk of hepatitis (non-A non-B) and it is costly.

FEATURES:

1. Contains the following:
   Fibrinogen (250 mg/unit)
   Factor VIII
   Fibronectin
   von Willebrand's Factor
   Antithrombin III

2. Each unit carries the same hepatitis risk as one unit of whole blood.
INDICATIONS:
1. In rare instances when clotting factors are needed for patients who are volume overloaded and NOT massively bleeding.
2. Refractory bleeding in uremia or following cardiopulmonary by-pass.

The von Willebrand's Factor in cryoprecipitate is instrumental in reversing the platelet abnormality in uremia and cardiopulmonary bypass. However, the clinical value of this is not clear (see Chapter 19).

Fibronectin. Cryoprecipitate is also rich in fibronectin, an opsonin that promotes phagocytosis of encapsulated gram-positive bacteria (e.g., staphylococci) by neutrophils. Circulating fibronectin is often reduced in critically ill patients,[2] and this generated some enthusiasm about possible benefits from replenishing the fibronectin with cryoprecipitate infusion. However, clinical trials have failed to show an improved outcome from cryoprecipitate infusions in serious infections caused by susceptible bacteria.[2]

PLATELET CONCENTRATES

Platelet transfusion therapy is the subject of Chapter 19, and will not be covered here.

INFUSION STRATEGIES

The infusion strategies in this section are aimed at promoting the infusion rate of blood products and minimizing some of the complications of the infusion. Many of the maneuvers in this section are included in the blood transfusion system shown in Figure 18–1. The strategies for improving infusion rate are similar to those presented in Chapter 13 for fluid replacement therapy. Each maneuver is dictated by one of the determinants of flow ($\dot{Q}$) defined by the Hagen-Poisseulle equation.

$$\dot{Q} = \Delta P \left(\frac{\pi\, r^4}{8\mu L} \right)$$

This equation predicts that transfusion rate can be enhanced by increasing the pressure head (ΔP) along the infusion set, using wide (r) and/or short (L) intravenous catheters, and reducing the viscosity (μ) of the blood product.

REDUCING VISCOSITY

The viscosity of red cell products plays a major role in limiting infusion rates. The influence of viscosity on flowrates is illustrated in Table 18–1.[7,8]

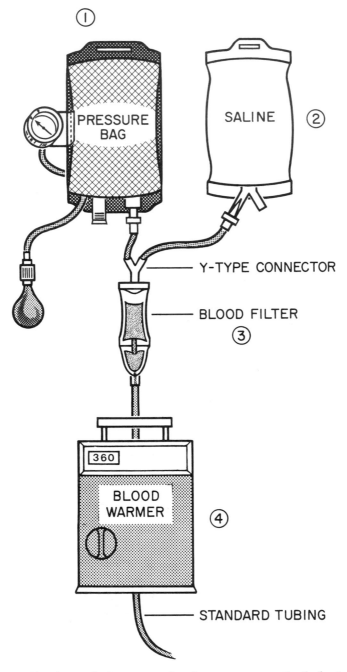

FIG. 18–1. Blood transfusion setup showing common methods for improving infusion rate and reducing adverse effects.

TABLE 18–1. THE INFLUENCE OF CELL DENSITY AND PRESSURE CUFF ON INFUSION RATE*		
Fluid	Gravity	Pressure Cuff (200 mmHg)
Tap Water	100 ml/min	285 ml/min
Whole Blood	65	185
Packed Cells	20	70
Diluted Packed Cells	—	210

*16-gauge catheter, 2 inches long
From Dula DJ, et al. Flowrate variance of commonly used IV infusion techniques. J Trauma 1981; 21:480–482.

The fluids in the table were passed through a 16-gauge catheter used for peripheral venous infusions (2 inches in length). At gravity flow, the infusion rate is greatest with tap water (negligible viscosity), and slowest with the packed cell preparation (highest viscosity). Note that the dilution of packed cells (with 200 ml of normal saline in this case) increases the infusion rate to a level comparable to that of whole blood.

Saline Dilution. Special Y-configured tubing is available that permits packed cells to be diluted with an equal volume of isotonic saline (see Figure 18–1). This maneuver will triple the flowrate of packed cells.[8] Only isotonic saline should be used for this purpose, because Ringer's lactate contains calcium and can promote clotting in the blood sample.

Blood Warmers. Warming reduces the viscosity of refrigerated blood by 2½ times,[7] and this can speed infusion. A simple method for warming blood is to immerse the storage bags in hot water prior to transfusion. However, it may take 30 minutes to achieve the desired temperatures using this method and inability to control for overheating can lead to hemolysis. Controlled warming devices are available that consist of coiled tubing immersed in a water bath whose temperature is controlled by electrical heating elements. Blood flowing through these coils will reach temperatures about 32°C at flows up to 150 ml/min.[10]

Although warming blood can improve infusion rates, the major indication for blood warmers is to minimize the risk of hypothermia from massive infusion of refrigerated blood. The recommended minimum temperature for blood transfusion is 35°C, although troublesome ventricular arrhythmias are not usually seen until core temperature falls below 28°C. At present, there is no documented benefit from blood warming devices.

PRESSURIZED INFUSIONS

Inflatable cuffs like the ones used to take blood pressures can be used to increase the infusion pressure. As illustrated in Figure 18–1, the cuff is placed over the plastic blood storage bags and is inflated to 200 mmHg.

This usually increases flow by 2 to 3 times baseline (gravity) flow.[7] The influence of pressure cuffs on flowrate is evident in Table 18–1.

Hand-compressed chambers called blood "pumps" can also be used to speed infusion, but pressure cuffs are preferred because they cause less trauma to donor cells.

CATHETER DIMENSIONS

The influence of catheter dimensions on flow was covered in some detail in Chapter 13 (see Table 13–2). Some reminders are mentioned below.
1. Flow through a 2-inch catheter is more than 50% faster than the flow through an 8-inch catheter of similar diameter.
2. Flow through a 14-gauge catheter is almost 75% greater than flow through a 16-gauge catheter of similar length.[9]

The fastest flows can be achieved with large-bore introducer sheaths as shown in Table 13–2.

BLOOD FILTERS

Each blood administration set contains a filter to trap debris that can accumulate in stored blood. This debris consists of decomposed platelets and white blood cells covered with a coat of fibrin. Filters should be replaced after every 3 to 4 units of blood,[7,10] because they can become filled and impede the rate of infusion. The standard filters allow the smaller microaggregates to pass freely, and these microaggregates can become lodged in the pulmonary capillaries and create abnormalities in gas exchange. Special microaggregate filters are available, and have been recommended for use when more than a few units of blood are transfused. However, the value of these filters in preventing pulmonary complications has not been proven.[1]

MASSIVE TRANSFUSION

Massive transfusion is defined as the replacement of an entire blood volume in 24 hours (or 10 units of whole blood in an average-sized adult). Several early misconceptions about massive transfusion have been clarified over the past few years, and the more important ones are listed below.
1. Coagulation abnormalities are common but there is no relationship between the volume of blood infused and the risk for coagulopathy.[1,11]
2. Infusion of platelets and fresh frozen plasma at fixed intervals during massive transfusion does not reduce the incidence of coagulopathy.[1,12]
3. Dilutional thrombocytopenia should not develop until 1.5 times the blood volume is replaced.[1,11]

TABLE 18–2. TRANSFUSION REACTIONS		
Reaction	Incidence	Source
Fever	1:50–1:100	Antibodies to Donor Leukocytes
Urticaria	1:100	Sensitization to Donor Plasma
Acute Lung Injury	1:5,000	Leukoagglutinins in Donor Blood
Acute Hemolysis	1:6,000	ABO Antibodies to Donor Red Cells
Fatal Hemolysis	1:100,000	ABO Antibodies to Donor Red Cells

4. Excessive infusion of citrate can bind calcium in the recipient's blood and produce hypocalcemia but the significance of this is not clear. However, the conversion of citrate to bicarbonate can produce a severe metabolic alkalosis.[1]
5. Hyperkalemia is uncommon in massive transfusion, but hypokalemia can occur when there is a severe metabolic alkalosis.[1]
6. Blood warming devices and microaggregate filters are recommended in massive transfusion but without proof of benefit.[1]

ACUTE TRANSFUSION REACTIONS

Approximately 10% of blood recipients will experience some form of adverse reaction. The transfusion reactions that develop acutely are listed in Table 18–2 along with their reported incidence.[6] Delayed reactions like hepatitis will not be considered.

ACUTE HEMOLYTIC REACTIONS

Major transfusion reactions are uncommon and are usually not life-threatening. These reactions are produced by antibodies in the recipient that react with ABO surface antigens on the donor erythrocytes. These antibodies fix complement and can produce rapid lysis. One unit of packed red blood cells can be completely lysed in less than 1 hour.[13]

Clinical Features. Severe reactions require only 10 to 50 ml of donor blood and are usually evident within a few minutes after the transfusion is started.[13] Fever, dyspnea, chest pain, and low back pain are common. Hypotension can appear suddenly and may be the only sign in comatose patients. Disseminated intravascular coagulation is characteristic of severe cases. Mortality is the result of irreversible shock and multiorgan failure.

Bedside Strategies. The approach listed below should be used for any patient who develops transfusion-associated fever.
1. STOP the transfusion immediately. This is probably the most crucial aspect of the approach to fever because morbidity and **mortality in hemolytic reactions is a function of the volume of incompatible blood tranfused**[13]

2. Immediately check blood pressure and respiratory status. If the blood pressure is dropping:
   a. Start volume resuscitation as soon as possible. Colloids may be preferred because of their ability to acutely increase blood volume.
   b. Dopamine (start at 5 mcg/kg/min) may be preferred for blood pressure control because of its renal vasodilating effects. Renal failure is often stated as a poor prognostic sign but the incidence of this is not clear.

Once the patient is stabilized:

3. Obtain a blood sample and inspect the plasma for the pink-red color of hemoglobin.
4. Obtain a first-voided urine specimen for hemoglobin (a dipstick test for blood will suffice if there are no red cells in the urine).
5. Send the blood sample for a direct Coombs' test. A positive test is confirmatory but negative reactions can occur if most of the cells are already hemolysed.
6. Laboratory tests for DIC are usually recommended but have little value in acute bedside management.

FEBRILE NONHEMOLYTIC REACTIONS

Febrile reactions occur in 1 to 4% of transfusions,[3] and are caused by antileukocyte antibodies in the recipient that are produced in response to prior transfusions or prior pregnancies. This is by far the most common cause of transfusion-associated fever.

Clinical Features. The fever usually appears 1 to 6 hours after starting the transfusion and is not accompanied by other signs of systemic illness. However, severe reactions do occur and can appear similar to an acute hemolytic reaction.

Bedside Strategies. The initial approach is the same as outlined for acute hemolytic reactions. A transfusion history is valuable to identify prior blood recipients. The diagnosis is made by exclusion of hemolysis. Bacterial contamination of blood products is the other potential cause of fever but this is rare. However, some recommend routine culture of donor and recipient blood for any fever associated with systemic symptoms.

Recommendations. These reactions recur in less than 50% of patients and no precautions are necessary for future transfusions. If a second episode of fever appears, leukocyte-poor red cell preparations should be used for further transfusions.

ALLERGIC REACTIONS

Allergic reactions occur in 1 to 3% of recipients and are the result of sensitization to plasma proteins in prior transfusions.[3] Patients with IgA deficiency seem prone to developing severe reactions, without prior exposure to plasma products.[3]

Clinical Features. The usual manifestation is mild urticaria and pruritus that develops during transfusion. Fever may also be present. Severe anaphylaxis (e.g., hypotension and wheezing) is uncommon, but does occur.

Bedside Strategies. It is not mandatory to stop the transfusion if the reaction is mild and there is no fever. The transfusion is usually interrupted while antihistamines are given and then resumed. Diphenhydramine (25 to 50 mg IM) may or may not relieve the pruritus. This agent can also be given as a premedication prior to any future transfusions in a susceptible patient. Anaphylaxis is treated in the conventional manner, with aggressive volume infusion (colloids are preferred here) and epinephrine (0.1 ml of 1:1000 IV for hypotension, otherwise 0.3 to 0.5 ml subcutaneously). Anaphylaxis is discussed in Chapter 15.

Recommendations. Future transfusions should be avoided if at all possible for patients with anaphylaxis. Otherwise, washed red blood cells can be used. A special preparation of frozen deglycerolized red cells can be used for highly sensitized subjects. All transfusions should be supervised and approved by the blood bank physician. All patients who develop anaphylaxis should be evaluated for possible IgA deficiency.

ACUTE LUNG INJURY

Acute respiratory failure is an often talked about but rare consequence of blood transfusion, with an estimated incidence of only 1 per 5,000 transfusions.[14] This reaction has been observed after a single transfusion of either whole blood or packed RBCs.[14] The prevailing theory involves antileukocyte antibodies in donor blood that bind to circulating granulocytes in the recipient. The white cells form aggregates that become trapped in the lung, where the cells release toxic substances that can damage the pulmonary capillaries. The result is a "leaky capillary" pulmonary edema that resembles the "adult respiratory distress syndrome" (ARDS). However, this transfusion reaction is unlike ARDS because it almost always resolves, whereas ARDS has a high mortality. At present, the exact nature of this reaction is not known.

Clinical Features. Signs of respiratory failure usually develop within 1 to 2 hours after the transfusion begins. Fever is common and hypotension has been reported.[14] The chest x-ray reveals a pulmonary edema pattern and the pulmonary capillary pressure is usuallly normal. The acute syndrome can be severe but the pulmonary process usually resolves in 4 to 5 days, with no permanent lung damage.

Bedside Management. The transfusion should be stopped (if still running) at the first sign of respiratory problems. The remainder of the management is directed at the respiratory failure (see Chapter 23). There is no specific therapy to speed the resolution of this lung injury.

Recommendations. There are no firm recommendations for future transfusions. Some advocate the use of washed RBCs (to remove the plasma from the sample), while others caution against any future transfusion unless absolutely necessary.[14]

UNCROSSMATCHED BLOOD

A major crossmatch is performed to determine the likelihood for an acute hemolytic transfusion reaction. This procedure involves incubating donor cells with recipient plasma and it can take 45 minutes or longer to complete.[15] If blood is needed before the crossmatch is completed, two types of uncrossmatched blood can be infused.

UNIVERSAL DONOR

The traditional blood type for uncrossmatched emergency transfusion is type O negative, called "universal donor" blood. This blood type has no ABO or Rh antigens on the surface of the blood cells so a major hemolytic transfusion reaction (recipient plasma against donor cells) is not possible. However, the donor serum has anti-A and anti-B antibodies and will precipitate a minor transfusion reaction (donor serum against recipient blood cells) if given to patients with A, B, or AB blood types. These reactions are usually of no consequence but they can be severe if enough antibody is present. Following massive transfusion of O negative blood, the recipient will have anti-A and anti-B antibodies in sufficient quantities to run the risk of a major hemolytic reaction if they are given their own blood (unless it is O negative). The problems with universal donor blood has led to the adoption of "type-specific" uncrossmatched blood for emergency transfusion.

TYPE-SPECIFIC BLOOD

Using type-specific uncrossmatched blood will circumvent the problems with universal donor blood. The ABO and Rh typing procedure takes only 5 minutes and will not delay transfusion time. The safety of type-specific uncrossmatched blood is proven in one report involving close to 4,000 transfusions.[16]

INDICATIONS FOR RED CELL TRANSFUSIONS

The modern practices regarding red cell transfusions are guided more by dogma than by reason. The goal of blood transfusion should be to maintain an adequate level of tissue oxygenation but the focus in clinical medicine has been on the serum hemoglobin or hematocrit.

OPTIMAL HEMATOCRIT

The optimal hematocrit is one that is high enough to support aerobic metabolism but is low enough to reduce viscosity and improve peripheral blood flow. This level is assumed to be a hematocrit of 30%.[17] The same concept is applied to hemoglobin but the analogy seems invalid because hemoglobin will not influence viscosity like the hematocrit. Nevertheless, an optimal serum hemoglobin level of 10 gm/dl has been proposed.[17] A recent Consensus Conference on Perioperative Blood Transfusions concluded that

> "The available evidence does not support the 10/30 (hemoglobin/hematocrit) rule."[6]

The evidence against maintaining a hemoglobin of 10 gm/dl in all patients is summarized below.

1. Patients with chronic renal failure tolerate hemoglobin levels less than 10 gm/dl without apparent ill effects.[6]
2. The body does not recognize anemia until the hemoglobin falls to below 7 gm/dl.[18]
3. In anesthetized animals, serum hemoglobin levels as low as 3 gm/dl are tolerated as long as the blood volume is adequate.[19]
4. Major surgery on Jehovah's Witnesses is successful without blood transfusions when hemoglobin levels fall to below 10 gm/dl.[20]
5. Orthopedic surgery has been performed successfully in adults with hemodilution to a hematocrit of 20%.[21]

Patients with active coronary artery disease do not apply to the statements above. These patients may require earlier transfusion than other patients, particularly if they have fixed coronary stenosis.[22]

The decision to transfuse a patient should not necessarily be based solely on the arterial oxygen carrying capacity. A more logical choice of end-point would be some measure of tissue oxygenation like the "oxygen uptake" ($\dot{V}O_2$) from the Fick equation. This is presented in Chapter 13 and will not be repeated here (see Figure 13–4).

REFERENCES

REVIEWS

1. Kruskall MS, Bergen JJ, Klein HG, et al. Transfusion therapy in emergency medicine. Ann Emerg Med 1988; 17:327–335.
2. Hogman CF, Bagge L, Thoren L. The use of blood components in surgical transfusion therapy. World J Surg 1987; 11:2–13.
3. Nusbacher J. Transfusion of Red Cell Products. In: Peltz LD, Swisher SN eds. Clinical practice of blood transfusion. New York: Churchill Livingstone, 1981; 289.
4. Sheldon GF, Watkins GM, Glover JL, et al. Panel: Present use of blood and blood products. J Trauma 1981; 21:1005–1012.

CONSENSUS CONFERENCE REPORTS

5. Fresh frozen plasma. Report of consensus development conference on fresh frozen plasma. JAMA 1985; 253:551–553.
6. Perioperative red blood cell transfusion. Report of consensus development conference on perioperative red cell transfusion. JAMA 1988; 260:2700–2703.

INFUSION TECHNIQUES

7. Dula DJ, Muller A, Donovan SW. Flow rate of commonly used IV infusion techniques. J Trauma 1981; 21:480–482.
8. Mateer JR, Thompson BM, Aprahamian C, et al. Rapid fluid resuscitation with central venous catheters. Ann Emerg Med 1983; 12:149–152.
9. Aeder MI, Crowe JP, Rhodes RS, et al. Technical limitations in the rapid infusion of intravenous fluids. Ann Emerg Med 1985; 14:307–310.
10. Gianino N. Equipment used for transfusion. In: Rutman RC, Miller WV eds. Transfusion Therapy. Rockville: Aspen Publishers, 1981; 131–150.

MASSIVE TRANSFUSION

11. Reiner A, Kickler TS, Bell W. How to administer massive transfusions effectively. J Crit Illness 1987; 2:15–24.
12. Phillips TF, Soulier G, Wilson RF. Outcome of massive transfusion exceeding two blood volumes in trauma and emergency surgery. J Trauma 1987; 27:903–909.

TRANSFUSION REACTIONS

13. Seyfried H, Walewska I. Immune hemolytic transfusion reactions. World J Surg 1987; 11:25–29.
14. Gans ROB, Duurkens VAM, van Zundert AA, et al. Transfusion-related acute lung injury. Intensive Care Med 1988; 14:654–657.

UNCROSSMATCHED BLOOD

15. Petz LD, Swisher SN eds. Clinical practice of transfusion medicine. 2nd ed, New York: Churchill Livingstone, 1989; 213–222.
16. Gervin AS, Fischer RP. Resuscitation of trauma patients with type-specific uncrossmatched blood. J Trauma 1984; 24:327–331.

INDICATIONS FOR TRANSFUSION

17. Messmer KFW. Acceptable hematocrit levels in surgical patients. World J Surg 1987; 11:41–46.
18. Duke M, Abelmann WH. The hemodynamic response to chronic anemia. Circulation, 1969; 39:503–515.
19. Takaori M, Safar P. Treatment of massive hemorrhage with colloid and crystalloid solutions. JAMA 1967; 199:297–302.
20. Henling CE, Carmichael MJ, Keats AS, et al. Cardiac operation for congenital heart disease in children of Jehovah's witnesses. J Thorac Cardiovasc Surg 1985; 89:914–921.

21. Laks H, Pilon RN, Klovekorn WP, et al. Acute hemodilution: Its effect of hemodynamics and oxygen transport in anesthetized man. Ann Surg 1974; *180*:103–109.
22. Martin E, Hansen E, Peter K. Acute limited normovolemic hemodilution: A method
for avoiding homologous transfusion. World J Surg 1987; *11*:53–59.
23. Blumberg N, Heal J, Chuang C, et al. Further evidence supporting a cause and effect
relationship between blood transfusion and early cancer recurrence. Ann Surg 1988;
207:410–415.
24. Stephan RN, Kisala JM, Dean RE, et al. Effect of blood transfusion on antigen presentation function and on interleukin-2 generation. Arch Surg 1988; *123*:235–240.

chapter

PLATELETS IN CRITICAL ILLNESS

Platelet transfusions more than doubled from 1980 to 1985,[1] and the consumption continues to increase 10 to 15% each year. Recent evidence suggests that platelet transfusions may be more inappropriate than suspected.[2,5] This chapter presents some guidelines that can be used for platelet transfusions as well as some specific platelet disorders that you may encounter in the ICU.

PLATELET HEMOSTASIS

The platelet count is overemphasized as a test of platelet hemostatic ability, while the "bleeding time" is often neglected. A normal bleeding time ensures adequate platelet hemostasis, a normal platelet count does not.

THE PLATELET COUNT

The traditional method of determining platelet counts is by visual inspection of a blood smear on a hemocytometer grid. This method is the gold standard but it has been replaced by time-saving electronic particle counters that use light scatter or electrical impedance to detect small particle collections the size of platelets. This method is influenced by platelet clumping, and the platelet count can be falsely lowered by clotting in the test tube. Fragmented pieces of red cells and white cells can be confused with platelets, thereby producing a false elevation in the platelet count above actual levels.

Thrombocytopenia is defined as a platelet count below 150,000 per mm³, however, the ability to form a hemostatic plug is retained until the platelet count falls below 100,000/mm³.[3] When platelet adhesiveness is abnormal, hemostasis can be abnormal despite a platelet count in excess of 100,000/mm³. Therefore, the platelet count will not detect a bleeding tendency from defective platelet adhesion. This is the main drawback of the platelet count.

TEMPLATE BLEEDING TIME

The bleeding time measures the ability of platelets to form a hemostatic plug. A specially designed template is placed on the forearm just below the antecubital fossa and two identical incisions are created by a scalpel device on the template. A blood pressure cuff on the upper arm is inflated to 40 mmHg to facilitate capillary bleeding and the cuts are blotted with filter paper every 30 seconds until the bleeding stops. The bleeding time is then reported as the average of the time for both cuts to stop bleeding.

Normal bleeding time: 4.5 ± 1.5 minutes

The bleeding time is prolonged when: (1) the circulating platelet count is less than 100,000/mm³ or (2) platelet adhesiveness is abnormal.[3]

INDICATIONS FOR TRANSFUSION

The guidelines for platelet transfusions need to be defined much more rigidly. For example, in a university hospital, only 27% of the platelet transfusions were given for the appropriate reasons.[5] The following guidelines are taken mostly from The Consensus Conference on Platelet Transfusion Therapy, convened in 1987 in response to the lack of rational guidelines for platelet transfusions.[2]

ACTIVE BLEEDING

The following statements apply to all active bleeding except ecchymotic or petechial bleeding.

1. Platelet transfusion is appropriate when circulating platelet counts fall below 50,000/mm³.

2. Platelet transfusion will probably not benefit patients with platelet counts above 50,000/mm³ and normal platelet function.[2]

3. When platelet function is abnormal, a template bleeding time greater than twice the upper limit of the normal range can be used as an indication for platelet transfusion.

4. When platelet function is abnormal and there is another coagulation disorder, any increase in the bleeding time can be used as an indication for platelet transfusion.

MASSIVE TRANSFUSION

Whole blood loses most of its viable platelets after just one day of storage at 4°C. Since whole blood is not rich in platelets, massive blood transfusion can result in a dilutional thrombocytopenia.

1. After replacing one blood volume in an average-sized adult, the platelet count can be expected to decrease from 250,000/mm[3] to 80,000/mm[3],[4] but this should be enough to promote clotting if platelet function is normal.

2. Clinically significant thrombocytopenia should not occur in adults until the blood transfusion reaches 1.5 to 2 times the blood volume or 15 to 20 units of whole blood.[6]

This means that routine infusion of platelets during massive transfusion is not necessary and serial platelet counts should be monitored to determine the need for platelets.[2]

PROPHYLAXIS

The traditional practice is to infuse platelets to prevent spontaneous bleeding when the circulating platelet count is below 20,000/mm[3].[2] However, levels as low as 5,000/mm[3] may be tolerated without bleeding.[4]

1. The traditional cutoff level of 20,000/mm[3] should not be considered an absolute indication for platelet transfusion in every patient.[2]

2. To prepare for invisible procedures or surgery, use the bleeding time to determine the need for platelet transfusion. A platelet count above 80,000/mm[3] should be sufficient for hemostasis when platelet function is normal.[3]

3. Platelet transfusions are not indicated as a routine prophylactic measure for patients undergoing open heart surgery.[2]

4. Platelet transfusions should not be given prophylactically when the thrombocytopenia is the result of an immune process.

PLATELET TRANSFUSIONS

Platelet concentrates are prepared by centrifuging fresh whole blood and suspending the platelet pellet in a small volume of plasma. Each concentrate contains about 5.5 billion platelets,[3] and the concentrates from several donors (usually 8 to 10) are pooled together and suspended in 50 to 70 ml of plasma. Platelets can be stored for as long as 7 days but viability may begin to decline after 3 days.[3]

MONITORING PLATELET COUNTS

In the average-sized adult, each platelet concentrate should raise the circulating platelet count by 5,000 to 10,000/mm[3] and the infused cells should last about 8 days.[3,4] These criteria are sometimes used to evaluate the efficacy of platelet transfusions. A baseline platelet count is followed by infusion of one platelet pack and repeat platelet counts are obtained at 1, 6, and 24 hours after the infusion. The problem with this method is that it does not take into account ongoing platelet losses or abnormalities in platelet function. For this reason, the bleeding time is favored as the test for gauging the effect of platelet transfusions.

COMPLICATIONS

Platelet transfusions are composed of platelet concentrates from several donors. These pooled concentrates carry the same risk for hepatitis transmission and transmission of human immunodeficiency virus. Febrile and anaphylactic reactions can also be seen with platelet transfusions from sensitization to the proteins in the plasma suspension.

Platelet membranes have ABO antigens but major incompatibility reactions do not occur.[3] However, recipients will develop antiplatelet antibodies after multiple transfusions and these antibodies will limit the effectiveness of subsequent transfusions. When this becomes a problem, platelets can be harvested by plateletpheresis from a single HLA-matched donor.

SPECIFIC PLATELET DISORDERS

The platelet abnormalities encountered in the ICU are shown in Figure 19-1.

HEPARIN AND THROMBOCYTOPENIA

Thrombocytopenia develops in about 10% of patients receiving heparin, regardless of the dose or route of administration.[7] Heparin doses as small as those used to flush catheters can produce the phenomenon. The mechanism is unclear but may be the result of heparin-induced antibodies that promote platelet aggregation. The major complication is thrombosis (usually arterial) and not bleeding. Major complications develop in only 10 to 15% of affected patients.

Many of the affected patients are those receiving heparin for the first time. However, any patient can be affected. The thrombocytopenia usually develops within 2 weeks after heparin is started and platelet counts can fall below 50,000/mm³ in 50% of patients. Other coagulation studies are usually normal and there is no leukocytosis. Since heparin flushes are a common practice in the ICU:

> Heparin must be considered in virtually every case of isolated thrombocytopenia in patients with intravascular catheters.

Any patient to be given heparin should have a baseline platelet count drawn before heparin is administered and this should be repeated every 3 to 4 days for the first few weeks of therapy. If thrombocytopenia develops but is mild, the heparin can be continued if absolutely nec-

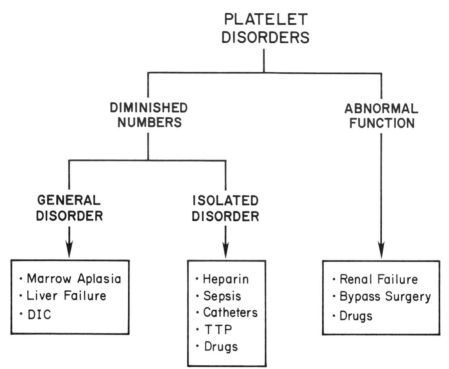

FIG. 19–1. Common causes of platelet abnormalities in the ICU.

essary while Coumadin is started. Heparin must be stopped at once if the platelet count falls below 20,000/mm³ or if a complication (usually thrombosis) develops. **Remember to stop heparin flushes also.** When heparin must be stopped abruptly, dextran-40 (500 mL/day) can be used as a temporary anticoagulant until Coumadin therapy is established. Thrombolytic therapy should be considered for any acute thrombosis unless there is a specific contraindication.

The thrombocytopenia recurs in only one-third of patients who receive the drug again. Therefore, affected patients are candidates for future therapy with heparin if it is absolutely necessary (e.g., cardiopulmonary bypass). Some advocate switching to another heparin preparation if the original heparin source is known (beef or pig intestine) but the value of this practice is presently unproven.

SEPSIS[8]

Thrombocytopenia is almost universal in serious bacterial infections associated with bacteremia and is usually the result of increased platelet consumption. The reduced platelet count may be an isolated finding or may be associated with a generalized coagulopathy like "disseminated intravascular coagulation" (DIC). The thrombocytopenia usually occurs early and **can be an early indication of bacteremia.** Either gram-positive or gram-negative organisms can be involved.

PULMONARY ARTERY CATHETERS[9]

Platelets can adhere to the surface of pulmonary artery catheters and produce a mild decrease in circulating platelets (to 150,000) in the first 1 to 2 days after catheter insertion. Bleeding is not a problem but thrombus formation around the catheters can occlude the central veins. Pulmonary embolism from detached thrombi is uncommon.[10]

THROMBOTIC THROMBOCYTOPENIA PURPURA[11]

This is an uncommon illness but is critical to recognize early because it can be rapidly fatal. Young adults are usually affected (predominantly women), particularly after a non-specific illness. The "pentad" of presenting features are:
1. Fever
2. Neurologic changes
3. Acute renal failure
4. Thrombocytopenia
5. Microangiopathic hemolytic anemia

Multiple organ failure can develop rapidly from massive platelet aggregation (presumably immunologic) and small vessel occlusion. The thrombocytopenia is not associated with other coagulation abnormalities, which can differentiate this disorder from DIC. The diagnosis is confirmed by the presence of schistocytes in the blood smear (indicating a microangiopathic hemolytic anemia). Immediate plasmapheresis or exchange transfusion may be the only effective measures for severe cases. Platelet transfusions can contribute to the problem (fuels the fire) and are not to be given.

DRUGS

Isolated thrombocytopenia has been a rare consequence of therapy with antibiotics, diuretics, and histamine (H2) blockers. Oral amrinone (used for heart failure) was a frequent offender before it was discontinued, but intravenous amrinone is considered safe.

GENERALIZED HEMATOLOGIC DISORDERS

Thrombocytopenia can be one component of a more generalized hematologic derangement, like the pancytopenia associated with bone marrow aplasia or the diffuse coagulopathy associated with liver failure and disseminated intravascular coagulation (DIC). The recognition of these processes depends on the pattern of hematologic abnormalities. The coagulopathy of liver failure and DIC can be similar (including elevated fibrin split products). Distinguishing tests include the thrombin time for fibrinolysis (abnormal in DIC and normal in liver failure) and the serum factor VIII level (decreased in DIC and normal in liver failure).

DEFECTIVE PLATELET ADHESION

RENAL FAILURE[6]

Acute and chronic renal failure are well-known causes of platelet dysfunction and this may be responsible for the bleeding tendency seen in renal failure. The platelet defect varies from patient to patient and is improved with dialysis. The bleeding time can be used to identify the problem if necessary. Aggressive hemodialysis or peritoneal dialysis is effective in correcting the defect but less involved measures can also be useful (discussed further later in this section).

CARDIOPULMONARY BYPASS[12]

Platelet function is altered through unknown mechanisms when blood passes through the oxygenator apparatus during cardiopulmonary bypass. The severity of the abnormality is determined by the duration of bypass. In most cases, the defect resolves within a few hours after bypass is completed. However, platelet dysfunction may contribute to the troublesome mediastinal bleeding that is seen in 3% of the patients in the immediate postoperative period.

DRUGS

The agents you may encounter that alter platelet function are aspirin, dipyridamole, nonsteroidal anti-inflammatory agents, semisynthetic penicillins, and dextran solutions. Intravenous nitroglycerin can also prolong the bleeding time but the mechanism is not known.[13] Drug-associated bleeding is usually not a problem, since 80% of the platelets must be affected to alter hemostasis.

Aspirin may be important in emergency surgery. The platelet effect occurs at low doses (one 325 mg tablet) and lasts for the life of the platelets (9 to 10 days). Aspirin should be stopped at least one week prior to surgery or other procedures prone to bleeding. When this is not possible, the bleeding time can be of value. A bleeding time of 10 to 12 seconds or greater indicates a bleeding tendency. This can be corrected by the infusion of 0.5 to 1 platelet concentrates for every 1 kg (2.2 lbs) of body weight.[6]

ACUTE THERAPY

A synthetic analog of vasopressin called DDAVP (Deamino-D Arginine Vasopressin) has been used to promote platelet aggregation in patients with renal failure and following cardiac bypass surgery.[14,15] This agent releases a substance (von Willebrand factor) into the bloodstream that increases platelet adhesiveness. A dose of 0.3 μ/kg given intravenously over 30 minutes can normalize the bleeding time for 4 hours in adults.[14] Unlike vasopressin, DDAVP has no vasoconstrictor effects. This agent should only be used as an acute measure to limit bleeding because repeated administration reduces or eliminates the effect (probably by depleting the platelet-aggregating substance that is released). Cryoprecipitate can be used when DDAVP is ineffective, because it contains substances that promote platelet aggregation.

At our hospital, DDAVP is used empirically in all patients with troublesome bleeding in the immediate postoperative period after cardiac bypass surgery. In patients with renal failure who are bleeding, DDAVP is given if the bleeding time is prolonged and the circulating platelet count is over 100,000/m³. However, the value of this practice is unknown. In fact, the value of DDAVP in the management of hemorrhage associated with platelet function abnormalities remains to be proven.

BIBLIOGRAPHY

Hardaway RM, Adams WH eds. Blood problems in critical care. Prob in Critical Care 1989; (Jan–Mar)3:108–138.

REFERENCES

REPORTS

1. Blood services operations report. Washington, D.C.: American Red Cross. 1980–1985.
2. Platelet Transfusion Therapy. Consensus Conference on Platelet Transfusion Therapy. JAMA 1987; 257:1777–1780.

PLATELET TRANSFUSIONS

3. Lee VS, Tarassenko LL, Bellhouse BJ. Platelet transfusion therapy: Platelet concentrate preparation and storage. J Lab Clin Med 1988; 111:371–383.
4. Slichter SJ. Indications for platelet transfusions. Plasma Ther Transfus Tech 1982; 3:259–264.
5. McCullough J, Steeper TA, Connelly DP, et al. Platelet utilization in a university hospital. JAMA 1988; 259:2414–2418.
6. Tomasulo PA. Platelet transfusions for nonmalignant disease. In: Petz LD, Swisher SN eds. Clinical practice of blood transfusion. New York: Churchill Livingstone, 1981; 527–544.

PLATELET DISORDERS

7. Bell WR. Heparin-associated thrombocytopenia and thrombosis. J Lab Clin Med 1988; *111*:600–605.

8. Poskitt TR, Poskitt PKF. Thrombocytopenia of sepsis. The role of circulating IgG-containing immune complexes. Arch Intern Med 1985; *145*:891–894.

9. Kim YL, Richman KA, Marshall BE. Thrombocytopenia associated with Swan-Ganz catheterization in patients. Anesthesiology 1980; *53*:261–262.

10. Chastre J, Cornud F, Bouchama A, et al. Thrombosis as a complication of pulmonary artery catheterization via the internal jugular vein. N Engl J Med 1982; *306*:278–282.

11. Ridolfi R, Bell W. Thrombotic thrombocytopenic purpura. Medicine 1981; *60*:413–428.

12. Harker LA: Bleeding after cardiopulmonary bypass. [Editorial] N Engl J Med 1986; *314*:1446–1447.

13. Lichtenthal PR, Rossi EC, Louis G, et al. Dose-related prolongation of the bleeding time by intravenous nitroglycerin. Anesth Analg 1985; *64*:30–33.

14. Mannucci PM, Remuzzi G, Pusineri F, et al. Deamino-8-D-arginine vasopressin shortens the bleeding time in uremia. N Engl J Med 1983; *308*:8–12.

15. Salzman EW, Weinstein MJ, Weintraub RM, et al. Treatment with desmopressin acetate to reduce blood loss after cardiac surgery. N Engl J Med 1986; *314*:1402–1406.

20

HEMODYNAMIC DRUGS

Particular facts are never scientific; only generalization can establish science.
Claude Bernard

This chapter contains information on ten of the more common drugs used to support the circulation. Only intravenous therapy is described and most of the drugs can only be given via the intravenous route. Each drug is presented in alphabetical order, as listed below. An asterisk indicates that a dosing chart is available for the drug in the Appendix (see rear of the text).

1. Amrinone
*2. Dobutamine
*3. Dopamine
4. Epinephrine
5. Furosemide
6. Labetalol
*7. Nitroglycerin
*8. Nitroprusside
*9. Norepinephrine
10. Trimethaphan

Three texts are listed at the end of the chapter for a more comprehensive list of hemodynamic drugs and their characteristics.

DRUG DOSING

The effective dose of most drugs is determined in animal studies. The jump from the laboratory to the bedside is often difficult because the laboratory animals are lean and healthy, whereas the patients in the ICU are far from that norm. The statement by Claude Bernard applies

```
┌─────────────────────────────────────────────────────────────┐
│        TABLE 20–1.   CALCULATING DRUG INFUSION RATES          │
├─────────────────────────────────────────────────────────────┤
│       IF: The diluent volume = 250 ml                         │
│                                                               │
│       AND: The infusion rate = 15 gtts/min                    │
│                                                               │
│       THEN: The desired dose = Amount of drug to add          │
│              (in mcg/min)                    (in mg)          │
│                              ─────────────────────────        │
│                                                               │
│       IF: You want to infuse a drug at ___X___ mcg/min        │
│                                                               │
│            THEN: ADD: X mg of the Drug                        │
│                                                               │
│                 TO: 250 ml of Diluent                         │
│                                                               │
│            INFUSE: @ 15 gtts/min                              │
└─────────────────────────────────────────────────────────────┘
```

to this situation; the specific actions and doses for each drug are not as important as understanding the broader actions of each drug and the clinical applications. The recommended doses should only be used as general guidelines; the rest is determined by the judgement you will develop at the bedside.

CALCULATING INFUSION RATES

When you select a drug and the appropriate dose for a specific task, the next step is to select the proper mixture and infusion rate. This involves knowing the "unit dose" (the quantity of drug in a standard vial) and how much to add to a standard volume of diluent to achieve the desired drug infusion rate. This is usually done by the nurse or by a computer program but the method presented below will be useful if you should ever find yourself without a nurse or a computer.

CONSTANT INFUSION METHOD

This method is outlined in Table 20–1.[6] There are two requirements: (1) volume of the diluent solution: 250 ml, and (2) infusion rate: 15 microdrops/min (1 ml = 60 microdrops or gtts). The rules are stated in algorithm form (IF:THEN).

IF you want to infuse a drug at ___X___ mcg/min, THEN add ___X___ mg of the drug to 250 ml of saline and run the drip at 15 microdrops/min.

Note that the drug must be given in mcg/min and not in mcg/kg/min (the latter infusion rate is more common for specifying drug doses). If a drug dose is given in mcg/kg/min, don't forget to multiply the dose by the ideal body weight when using this method.

AMRINONE

Amrinone is a phosphodiesterase inhibitor (like theophylline) that was introduced as a combined inotropic agent and vasodilator.[7-9] The inotropic actions are inconsistent and the predominant action of the drug is vasodilatation.[8] The oral form was discontinued by the FDA because of troublesome thrombocytopenia.[9] Acute therapy with intravenous amrinone should not pose a problem.

ACTIONS

1. Dilates arteries and veins through a direct action. It can increase contractility in select patients.
2. The overall response should decrease myocardial stroke work.

INDICATIONS

1. The main indication is acute therapy of left ventricular failure when the blood pressure is normal or adequate.

PREPARATION

Available in 20 ml vials containing 100 mg of the drug. Mixed with saline to a final concentration of 1 to 3 mg/ml. Amrinone should not be diluted with glucose, and the final mixture should not be exposed to light.

INTRAVENOUS DOSING

1. Start with an IV bolus of 0.75 to 1.5 mg/kg given over 3 to 5 minutes, and follow with infusion of 5 to 10 μgr/kg/min.[9]
2. A second bolus of 0.75 mg/kg can be given 15 to 30 minutes after the initial bolus.[7]

ADVERSE EFFECTS

1. **Thrombocytopenia** (usually not less than $70,000/mm^3$) occurs in 2 to 3% of patients receiving acute intravenous therapy.[9] The mechanism is nonimmunogenic platelet destruction.
2. **Ventricular Ectopy** is reported in 3% of patients.[9] Amrinone can also enhance the ventricular response to atrial flutter or fibrillation.
3. Other uncommon (less than 2%) side effects include hypotension, nausea, vomiting, and a flu-like syndrome.[8,9]

CONTRAINDICATIONS

1. Thrombocytopenia. The other contraindications apply to all vasodilators (e.g., hypertrophic cardiomyopathy).

DOBUTAMINE

Dobutamine is a synthetic catecholamine that was introduced in 1978.
It has become the preferred inotropic agent for acute therapy of septalic
heart failure (but not cardiogenic shock).

ACTIONS

1. A selective beta-1 agonist (cardiac stimulation), with mild beta-2
stimulation (peripheral vasodilatation).
2. Produces a dose-related increase in cardiac output up to an infusion
rate of 40 μgr/kg/min.[13] Systemic vascular resistance decreases through
reflex mechanisms,[10] while preload decreases from the improved cardiac
performance. The heart rate is usually unchanged, but tachycardia can
be prominent when patients are hypovolemic.
3. The change in cardiac output and peripheral resistance are equal
and opposite, leaving the blood pressure unchanged.
4. Compared to dopamine, dobutamine produces more of an increase
in cardiac output and is less arrhythmogenic.[11] The greater increment
in cardiac output is the result of the absence of vasoconstriction with
dobutamine.
5. Short periods of dobutamine infusion can be associated with long-
term (4 weeks) improvement in cardiac performance.[12] The mechanism
is not clear.

INDICATIONS

1. The inotropic agent of choice for acute management of heart failure
(either left or right).
2. May not improve blood pressure in cardiogenic shock because of
equal and opposite effects on cardiac output and systemic vascular
resistance.
3. Can be combined with amrinone in the therapy of low cardiac
output states.[14]

PREPARATION

Available in 250 mg vials that can be diluted in 250 ml of saline, to
yield a final concentration of approximately 1 mg/ml.

TABLE 20–2. DOBUTAMINE DOSE CHART							
Preparation							
	Mix:	250 mg in 250 ml Normal Saline					
	Concentration:	1000 mcg/ml					
	Usual Dose:	5 to 15 mcg/kg/min					
Patient Profile							
	Patient:	50 kg (110 lb) Female					
	Desired Dose:	10 mcg/kg/min					
	Drip Rate:	30 gtts/min					
Administration							

Infusion Rate
(gtts/min)

Weight (kg)	40	50	60	70	80	90	100
Dose (mcg/kg/min)							
5	12	15	18	21	24	27	30
10	24	30	36	42	48	54	60
15	36	45	54	63	72	81	90
20	48	60	72	84	96	108	120
40	96	120	144	168	192	216	240

INTRAVENOUS DOSING

1. Usual dose range: 5 to 15 μgr/kg/min. Infusion rate can be increased to up to 40 μgr/kg/min if necessary with few ill effects.[13] Table 20–2 shows a sample dose chart for dobutamine in an average-sized adult.

ADVERSE EFFECTS

1. Tachycardia can be prominent in hypovolemic patients. Ventricular arrhythmias are seen on occasion.

CONTRAINDICATIONS

1. Hypertrophic cardiomyopathy.

DOPAMINE

Dopamine is part of the metabolic pathway that leads to norepinephrine synthesis. It has both alpha and beta effects depending on the dose employed. It is one of the most versatile hemodynamic drugs available at present.

ACTIONS

1. Stimulates adrenergic receptors both directly and through the release of norepinephrine.
2. Produces selective vasodilatation in the renal, splanchnic, and cerebral circulations via discrete dopaminergic receptors.
3. High doses produce vasoconstriction via peripheral alpha receptor stimulation.
4. Increases pulmonary capillary hydrostatic pressure through pulmonary venoconstriction.[10]
5. Increases renal sodium excretion, independent of effects on renal blood flow.

INDICATIONS

1. Cardiogenic shock and septic shock.
2. In the first few hours of oliguric renal failure, dopamine administered in dopaminergic doses can produce an increase in urine output.[15]

PREPARATION

Available in 200 mg vials, which can be added to 250 ml saline to yield a final concentration of 100 mcg/ml.

INTRAVENOUS DOSING

1. Start infusion at 1 μgr/kg/min and increase to desired effect. The usual dose range is 1 to 15 μgr/kg/min.
2. Range of effects:

Dopaminergic: 1 μgr/kg/min

Predominant beta: 3 to 10

Combined alpha-beta: 10 to 20

Predominant alpha: greater than 20

3. See Appendix for dose chart.

ADVERSE EFFECTS

1. Tachyarrhythmias are the most common adverse effects.
2. Can produce profound vasoconstriction in very high doses.

CONTRAINDICATIONS

1. Patients with existing arrhythmias where an alternative agent is available.

EPINEPHRINE

Epinephrine is the drug of choice in the treatment of anaphylaxis, otherwise it is reserved for hypotension resistant to conventional measures. Epinephrine may be valuable when venous access is not readily available because it may be administered via endotracheal tubes.

ACTIONS

1. A combined alpha-beta agonist. Predominant effect depends on the dose and regional circulation.
2. Can produce profound peripheral vasoconstriction, particularly in the splanchnic and renal beds.
3. Inhibits mediator release from mast cells and basophils in response to antigen-antibody complexes in anaphylactic reactions.
4. Metabolic effects include lactic acidosis,[16] ketoacid accumulation (because of lipolysis), and hyperglycemia (because of enhanced hepatic gluconeogenesis).

INDICATIONS

1. Anaphylaxis.
2. As a second line agent in resistant hypotension.

PREPARATION

Available as 1 ml of 1:1000 solution (0.1 mg/ml), which can be added to 250 ml saline to yield a concentration of 4 mcg/ml.

INTRAVENOUS DOSING

1. Anaphylaxis: 3 to 5 ml of 1:1,000 solution, followed with a continuous infusion of 2 to 4 μgr/min.
2. Refractory hypotension: Start at 2 μgr/min and titrate to desired effect.

3. Dose range:

Renal vasoconstriction: less than 1 μgr/min

Cardiac beta: 1 to 4 μgr/min

Increasing alpha: 5 to 20 μgr/min

Predominant alpha: greater than 20 μgr/min

ADVERSE EFFECTS

1. Acute MI, serious arrhythmias, and lactic acidosis are potential developments during epinephrine infusion.
2. Acute renal failure can occur at small doses (less than 1 μgr/min) and this risk should discourage widespread use of the drug.

FUROSEMIDE

Intravenous furosemide is included here because it has specific hemodynamic actions that are distinct from its actions as a diuretic. It can produce deleterious effects during the initial stages of therapy for acute heart failure. These are distinct from the diuretic effect. If acute decreases in pulmonary venous congestion are desirable, nitroglycerin is preferred to furosemide because nitroglycerin decreases venous pressures without producing a decrease in cardiac output.

ACTIONS

1. Intravenous furosemide (1 mg/kg) produces an acute increase in systemic vascular resistance and a decrease in cardiac output. Onset of the response is within 5 minutes and lasts 30 minutes. The vasoconstriction may be caused by activation of the renin system.[19]
2. Prior to the diuretic actions, ventricular filling pressures can either increase or decrease.[19,20]
3. Onset of diuresis begins at 20 minutes and lasts for 2 hours. The diuretic effect can persist with a GFR down to 10 ml/min.

PHARMACOKINETICS

1. Intravenous half-life is 1.5 hours.
2. Elimination half-life is 6 hours.

INDICATIONS

1. Edema associated with venous congestion, not edema from nephrotic syndrome.
2. Early oliguric renal failure.

INTRAVENOUS DOSING

1. To prevent ototoxicity, do not exceed 20 mg/min when renal function is normal and do not exceed 4 mg/min in renal failure.
2. For acute heart failure start at 40 mg; if no response is seen in 1 hour, double the next dose.
3. For acute renal failure, there are no firm recommendations. Doses as high as 20 mg/kg have been suggested.

ADVERSE EFFECTS

1. Ototoxicity can result from rapid infusion and is facilitated by concurrent administration of other ototoxic agents (e.g., aminoglycosides). The hearing impairment is usually reversible (but not always), and resolves within 24 hours.[21]
2. Well-known electrolyte abnormalities include hypokalemia, hypomagnesemia, hypochloremia, and metabolic alkalosis.
3. Non-steroidal anti-inflammatory agents like indomethacin can diminish or abolish the response to furosemide and other loop diuretics.[21]

CONTRAINDICATIONS

1. History of allergy to sulfa.
2. Edema from nephrotic syndrome.
3. Hepatorenal syndrome.

GLUCAGON

Intravenous glucagon has been used successfully as an inotropic agent in human subjects.[22] Its principal use at present is the reversal of beta-blocker overdose.[23,24]

ACTIONS

1. Increases heart rate and myocardial contractility. The inotropic response is not mediated by beta receptors.[22]
2. Selectively dilates the splanchnic circulation.

INDICATIONS

1. To reverse the inotropic effects of beta-blocker overdose.[23,24] Does not reverse the chronotropic effects.
2. Consider when electromechanical dissociation is refractory to conventional measures.

INTRAVENOUS DOSING

1. Start with an intravenous bolus of 1 to 5 mg, and follow with a continuous infusion of 1 to 20 mg/hr.[22]
2. The phenol diluent used for glucagon can be toxic and the glucagon should be mixed with 10 ml saline.[23]

ADVERSE EFFECTS

1. Nausea and vomiting can be common after large doses (5 mg).
2. Other adverse effects include hypokalemia (from enhanced insulin release), hyperglycemia, and enhanced anticoagulant effect with warfarin.[22]

CONTRAINDICATIONS

1. Not recommended for use in hypertension.

LABETALOL

Labetalol is a combined alpha-beta blocker introduced in 1984, and has considerable potential in acute management of hypertension, particularly postoperative hypertension caused by catecholamine excess.[25,26]

ACTIONS

1. More potent as a beta-blocker (7:1 beta:alpha blockade after intravenous use).
2. Only 25% as potent as propranolol as a beta-blocker.
3. Does not increase heart rate when given for severe hypertension. Cardiac output is usually unchanged but mild decreases in cardiac output have been reported.[25]

PHARMACOKINETICS

1. Primarily metabolized in the liver. Less than 5% is eliminated unchanged in the urine.

INDICATIONS

1. Hypertension.
2. Theoretically of benefit in pheochromocytoma but clinical studies are awaited.

INTRAVENOUS DOSING

Can be given by continuous intravenous infusion, or by repeated bolus injections.

1. For Continuous IV: Add 200 mg labetalol to 200 ml diluent, and start infusion at 2 mg/min (2 ml/min). Continue until desired effect is produced. Usually effective cumulative dose is 50 to 200 mg.

2. For Bolus Therapy: Add 20 mg labetalol over 3 to 4 minutes while the patient is in the recumbent position. Repeat doses of 40 to 80 mg can be given every 10 to 20 minutes until a maximum of 300 mg is reached.

ADVERSE EFFECTS

1. Nonspecific side effects (nausea, vomiting, and diarrhea) occur in 15% of patients. The remainder of side effects are the result of alpha blockade (orthostatic hypotension) and beta blockade (bradycardia and bronchospasm).[25]

DRUG INTERACTIONS

1. Hypotensive effects may be exaggerated during cimetidine therapy.[25]

2. Significant cardiac depression when combined with halothane anesthesia.[25]

NITROGLYCERIN

Nitroglycerin is a time-honored vasodilator for angina but recent evidence suggests that tachyphylaxis may develop within 24 hours.[27,29]

ACTIONS

1. Produces direct relaxation of arteries and veins. The venodilatation predominates at low doses (less than 50 µgr/min), while arterial vasodilatation is predominant at high doses (greater than 200 µgr/min).

2. Nitroglycerin increases coronary flow in borderline ischemic regions of the myocardium.[27]

INDICATIONS

1. Myocardial ischemia/infarction when blood pressure is adequate.
2. Pulmonary hypertension.
3. Has been used successfully in heart failure, particularly when it is associated with acute MI.

PREPARATIONS

1. Commercial preparations (e.g., Nitrostat and Nitro-Bid) vary from 5 mg/ml to 50 mg/ml. A 50 mg vial added to 500 ml saline yields a concentration of 0.1 mg/ml.
2. **Nitroglycerin binds to polyvinylchloride tubing.**[27] Because 80% of the drug may be removed in this fashion, polyethylene tubing may be preferred.[2] Glass bottles are also favored over plastic IV containers to limit drug binding.

INTRAVENOUS DOSING

1. Start infusion at 10 μgr/min and increase by 10 μgr/min every 5 minutes until desired effect is produced.
2. The usual dose range for angina is 50 to 200 μgr/min.[27]

ADVERSE EFFECTS

1. **Tolerance** to continuous infusion can occur in 24 to 48 hours because of depletion of sulfhydryl groups in vessel walls that bind nitroglycerin.[29] N-acetylcysteine (Mucomyst) can partially reverse tolerance at a dose of 200 mg/kg given orally.[29] Intermittent infusions of nitroglycerin (12 hours on, 12 hours off) does not produce tolerance.
2. **Methemoglobinemia** can occur, but is often clinically silent. The hallmark of this illness is cyanosis despite adequate arterial blood gases. Nitrites from nitroglycerin can convert hemoglobin (Hb) to methemoglobin (metHb), and the conversion of 70% of Hb to metHb can be fatal.[31] Up to 10% metHb (enough to produce cyanosis) can accumulate when nitroglycerin infusions reach 300 μgr/min.[31] MetHb levels can be measured *in vitro* using a co-oximeter.

> When metHb levels exceed 10% (1.5 g), methylene blue (2 mg/kg IV over 10 min) will promptly reduce metHb levels.[34]

3. **Hypoxemia** can result from nitroglycerin infusion in patients with pulmonary edema.[30] This is caused by increased shunt but hypoxemia is not a consistent finding.
4. **Ethanol Intoxication** can be seen at high doses because of the ethanol diluent that is used in the intravenous nitroglycerin preparations.[32]
5. **Heparin Resistance** can occur during simultaneous infusion of heparin and nitroglycerin.[33]

CONTRAINDICATIONS

1. Increased intracranial pressure.
2. Closed angle glaucoma.
3. General contraindications for vasodilators (e.g., hypovolemia and tamponade).

NITROPRUSSIDE

Nitroprusside is the standard intravenous vasodilator for hypertensive emergencies.[35] The major drawback is the risk for cyanide toxicity, which may be higher than suspected.[36]

ACTIONS

1. Dilates systemic arteries and veins through a direct action on the vessel wall.[35] Also produces pulmonary artery vasodilatation.
2. Produces an increase in stroke volume with no change in heart rate. Ventricular filling pressures decrease, partly because of venodilatation.[35]

INDICATIONS

1. Considered the best drug available for acute control in hypertensive emergencies not associated with aortic dissection.
2. Acute MI with septal rupture or papillary muscle rupture.
3. Acute left ventricular failure without hypotension.

PREPARATION

1. Add 1 vial (50 mg) to each 100 ml of diluent for a final concentration of 500 mg/L.
2. Shield from sunlight or artificial light if exposure exceeds 3 hours.[37]

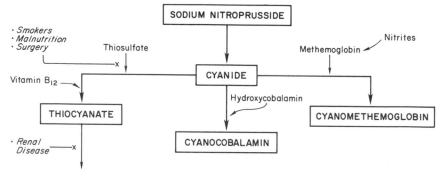

FIG. 20–1. The metabolism of nitroprusside.

INTRAVENOUS DOSING

Low cardiac output: Start at 0.2 μgr/kg/min

Hypertension: Start at 2 μgr/kg/min

Usual dose: 0.5 to 0 5 μgr/kg/min

Maximum dose: 2 to 3 μgr/kg/min for 72 hours

ADVERSE EFFECTS

The two major adverse effects are cyanide and thiocyanate accumulation.[36] Increased intracranial pressure has been reported on occasion.[38] Like other vasodilators, hypotension is common in patients who are hypovolemic.

The metabolism of nitroprusside yields cyanide and thiocyanate, as shown in Figure 20–1. The free cyanide combines with sulfur to form thiocyanate, which is eliminated by the kidneys. Thiosulfate is the sulfur donor, and the transfer of sulfur to cyanide requires vitamin B_{12}.

Cyanide Toxicity can be common because thiosulfate depletion is common in smokers, in the malnourished, and after coronary artery surgery.[36] We found cyanide levels (whole blood) of 5 to 7 times normal during usual doses of nitroprusside in postoperative patients who had coronary artery bypass surgery, and have abandoned the use of nitroprusside in this setting.

One important feature of cyanide toxicity is the fact that **lactic acidosis is often not present until the late stages of the illness.**[36-39] The more common clinical signs are: headache, nausea, and weakness, tolerance to nitroprusside, and progressive hypotension. **Increasing requirements**

for nitroprusside may be the most reliable sign of cyanide accumulation. Whole blood cyanide levels can be obtained (normal: less than 5 μgr/ml), but the results will not be available immediately. The diagnosis is, therefore, made on clinical grounds in most cases.

Preventive measures are being taken by mixing nitroprusside with a 1% thiosulfate solution to provide enough sulfur substrate to combine with excess cyanide. Vitamin B_{12} is also necessary for this reaction but B_{12} deficiency should not be common in the ICU population.

Thiocyanate toxicity is a different clinical syndrome and is often seen in the setting of renal insufficiency.[35] The clinical presentation usually involves mental status changes, including confusion, lethargy, and coma. Serum levels can be obtained (toxic levels are 10 mg/dl or greater), but the diagnosis is usually made on clinical grounds.

CONTRAINDICATIONS

1. Vitamin B_{12} deficiency.
2. Renal failure, when high doses (greater than 3 μgr/kg/min) are needed for over 72 hours.

NOREPINEPHRINE

Norepinephrine is a combined alpha-beta agonist that is used in septic shock.[1] The propensity for profound vasoconstriction from this drug should limit is use.

ACTIONS

1. Predominantly an alpha agonist, but can stimulate cardiac beta receptors in low doses (less than 2 μgr/min). Produces vasoconstriction in all vascular beds, including the renal circulation.[4] Addition of low-dose dopamine (1 μgr/kg/min) helps to preserve renal blood flow.[40]
2. Can be effective in septic shock refractory to dopamine infusion.[40]

INDICATIONS

1. Septic shock, when refractory to volume and dopamine therapy.

PREPARATION

1. Add 2 vials (4 mg/vial) of norepinephrine bitartrate to 500 ml normal saline: Final concentration: 16 μgr/ml. (See Appendix.)

INTRAVENOUS DOSING

1. Start infusion at 30 microdrops/min (or 0.5 ml/min), which is a dose of 8 μgr/min. Increase dose to desired effect.
2. The effective dose is variable, partly because vascular responsiveness may be diminished in severe septic shock. The effective dose in one human study was 0.5 to 1 μgr/kg/min or 30 to 70 μgr/min for an average-sized adult.[40]

ADVERSE EFFECTS

1. Renal failure and other manifestations of peripheral vasoconstriction.

CONTRAINDICATIONS

1. Hypotension associated with peripheral vasoconstriction (e.g., hypovolemic shock).

TRIMETHAPHAN

Trimethaphan camsylate (Arfonad) is a ganglionic blocker that is effective in hypertension, particularly in acute aortic dissection.[5]

ACTIONS

1. It blocks both sympathetic and parasympathetic ganglia and dilates both arteries and veins.
2. Onset of action is just 1 minute and the effect dissipates within 10 minutes.
4. Cardiac output can decrease but it may also increase in patients with hypertensive heart failure.[5]
5. The blood pressure reduction is more pronounced when the head of the bed is elevated.

INDICATIONS

1. Considered the drug of choice for acute aortic dissection.[5] Otherwise, it has no advantages over other vasodilators.

PREPARATION

1. Add one 10 ml ampule (50 mg) trimethaphan to 500 ml of saline to yield a final concentration of 100 μgr/ml.

INTRAVENOUS DOSING

1. Start infusion at 1 mg/min and increase every 3 to 5 minutes until the desired effect is achieved.[1]
2. The usual dose range is 1 to 15 mg/min.

ADVERSE EFFECTS

1. Paralytic ileus and urinary retention are common but not when the drug is used for less than 24 hours.[5]

CONTRAINDICATIONS

1. Hypovolemia, autonomic neuropathy, and bowel distention.

REFERENCES

GENERAL

1. Opie LH. Drugs for the heart. Orlando: Grune & Stratton, 1987; 93.
2. Khan MG. Manual of cardiac drug therapy. 2nd ed. Philadelphia: W.B. Saunders, 1988; 121.

REVIEWS

3. Chernow B, Rainey TG, Lake R. Endogenous and exogenous catecholamines in critical care medicine. Crit Care Med 1982; 10:409–416.
4. Higging TL, Chernow B. Pharmacotherapy of circulatory shock. Disease-a-month 1987; 33:314–360.
5. Ram CVS, Hyman D. Hypertensive Crisis. Intensive Care Med 1987; 2:151–162.
6. Tilden S, Hopkins RL. Calculation of infusion rates of vasoactive substances. Ann Emerg Med 1983; 12:697–699.

SPECIFIC AGENTS

AMRINONE

7. Mancini D, Lajemtel T, Sonnenblick E. Intravenous use of amrinone for the treatment of the failing heart. Am J Cardiol 1985; 56:8B–15B.
8. Franciosa JA. Intravenous amrinone: An advance or a wrong step. [Editorial] Ann Intern Med 1985; 102:399–400.
9. Treadway G. Clinical safety of intravenous amrinone—A review. Am J Cardiol 1985; 56:39B–40B.

DOBUTAMINE

10. Leier CV, Unverferth DV. Dobutamine. Ann Intern Med 1983; 99:490–496.
11. Leier CV, Heban PT, Huss P, et al. Comparative systemic and regional hemodynamic effects of dopamine and dobutamine in patients with cardiomyopathic heart failure. Circulation 1978; 58:466–475.
12. Liang CS, Sherman LG, Coherty JU, et al. Sustained improvement of cardiac function in patients with congestive heart failure after short-term infusion of dobutamine. Circulation 1984; 69:113–119.
13. Abdul-Rasool IH, Chamberlain JH, Swan PC, et al. Cardiorespiratory and metabolic effects of dopamine and dobutamine infusions in dogs. Crit Care Med 1987; 15:1044–1050.
14. Uretsky BF, Lawless CE, Verbalis JG, et al. Combined therapy with dobutamine and amrinone in severe heart failure. Chest 1987; 92:657–662.

DOPAMINE

15. Schwartz LB, Gewertz BL. The renal response to low dose dopamine. J Surg Res 1988; 45:574–588.

EPINEPHRINE

16. Barach EM, Nowack RM, Lee TG, et al. Epinephrine for treatment of anaphylactic shock. JAMA 1986; 251:2118–2122.
17. Balderman SC, Aldridge J. Pharmacologic support of the myocardium following aortocoronary bypass surgery: A comparative study. J Clin Pharmacol 1986; 26:175–183.
18. Hardaway RM. Metabolic acidosis produced by vasopressors. Surg Gynecol Obstet 1980; 151:203–204.

FUROSEMIDE

19. Francis GS, Siegel RM, Goldsmith SR, et al. Acute vasoconstrictor response to intravenous furosemide in patients with chronic congestive heart failure. Ann Intern Med 1985; 103:1–6.
20. Nelson GIC, Silke B, Forsyth DR, et al. Hemodynamic comparison of primary venous or arteriolar dilatation and the subsequent effect of furosemide in left ventricular failure after acute myocardial infarction. Am J Cardiol 1983; 52:1036–1040.
21. Opie LH, Kaplan NM. Diuretic therapy. In: Opie LH ed. Drugs for the heart. Orlando: Grune & Stratton, 1987; 111–130.

GLUCAGON

22. Hall-Boyer K, Zaloga GP, Chernow B. Glucagon: Hormone of therapeutic agent. Crit Care Med 1984; 12:584–588.
23. Mofenson HC, Caraccio TR, Laudano J. Glucagon for propranolol overdose. JAMA 1986; 255:2025.
24. Agura ED, Wexler LF, Witzburg RA. Massive propranolol overdose. Am J Med 1986; 80:755–758.

LABETALOL

25. Blakely B, Williams LL, Lopez LM, et al. Labetalol HCL: alpha- and beta-blocking properties may offer advantages over pure beta blockers. Hosp Form 1987; 22:864–869.
26. Frishman WH, Michelson EL. Labetalol: An alpha- and beta-adrenoceptor blocking drug. [Editorial] Ann Int Med 1983; 99:553–555.

NITROGLYCERIN

27. Herling IM. Intravenous nitroglycerin: Clinical pharmacology and therapeutic considerations. Am Heart J 1984; 108:141–149.
28. Abrams J. A reappraisal of nitrate therapy. JAMA 1988; 259:396–401.
29. Packer M, Lee WH, Kessler PD, et al. Prevention and reversal of nitrate tolerance in patients with congestive heart failure. N Engl J Med 1987; 317:799–804.
30. Hales CA, Westphal D. Hypoxemia following the administration of sublingual nitroglycerin. Am J Med 1978; 65:911–918.
31. Kaplan KJ, Taber M, Teagarden JR, et al. Association of methemoglobinemia and intravenous nitroglycerin administration.
32. Shook TL, Kirshenbaum JM, Hundley RF, et al. Ethanol intoxication complicating intravenous nitroglycerin therapy. Ann Int Med 1984; 101:498–499.
33. Habbab MA, Haft JI. Heparin resistance induced by intravenous nitroglycerin. Arch Int Med 1987; 147:857–860.
34. Gibson GR, Hunter JB, Raabe DS Jr. Methemoglobinemia produced by high-dose intravenous nitroglycerin. Ann Intern Med 1982; 96:615–616.

NITROPRUSSIDE

35. Cohn JN, Burke LP. Nitroprusside. Ann Intern Med 1979; 91:752–757.
36. Patel CB, Laboy V, Venus B, et al. Use of sodium nitroprusside in post-coronary bypass surgery: A plea for conservatism. Chest 1986; 89:663–667.
37. Vesey CJ, Batistoni GA. The determination and stability of sodium nitroprusside in aqueous solutions. J Clin Pharm 1977; 2:105–117.
38. Griswold WR, Riznik V, Mendoza SA. Nitroprusside-induced intracranial hypertension. JAMA 1981; 246:2679–2680.
39. Hall AH, Rumack BH. Clinical toxicology of cyanide. Ann Emerg Med 1986; 15:1067–1074.

NOREPINEPHRINE

40. Desjars P, Pinaud M, Potel G, et al. A reappraisal of norepinephrine therapy in human septic shock. Crit Care Med 1987; 15:134–137.

41. Schaer GL, Fink MP, Parillo JE. Norepinephrine alone versus norepinephrine plus low-dose dopamine: Enhanced renal blood flow with combination pressor therapy. Crit Care Med 1985; *13*:492–495.

TRIMETHAPHAN

42. Gonzales ER, Ornato JP. Cost-effective management of hypertensive emergencies. Clin Emerg Med 1986; *9*:97–113.

section VI

CARDIAC ARRHYTHMIAS

A localized change in the heart muscle cell may be sufficient to inaugurate a disturbance of the heartbeat. However, . . . these conditions in general are usually due to the peripheral sensitivities or hypersensitivities of the individual nervous patient.

George Herrmann, M.D.
1940

chapter

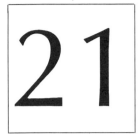

ACUTE MANAGEMENT OF TACHYARRHYTHMIAS

Acute arrhythmias are the gremlins of the ICU because they pop up unexpectedly, create some havoc, and are gone again in a flash. This chapter contains some management strategies for the most common and most troublesome arrhythmias in the ICU; the tachyarrhythmias. The focus is on the principles of acute management, not on recognition. Strategies for the common rhythm disturbances are presented as flow diagrams to organize the approach. The antiarrhythmic agents used in this chapter are presented in detail in Chapter 22.

RHYTHM STRIP CLASSIFICATION

Your first introduction to an arrhythmia is usually the moment when a nurse thrusts the rhythm strip in front of your eyes and informs you that the patient "just did this." The following system will allow you to quickly classify rhythms using the three "R"s: **Rate, Rhythm,** and **qRs duration**. This classification system is shown in Figure 21–1 for tachy-arrhythmias.[1,3,4,8]

First, the **heart rate** separates the bradycardias (rate below 60/min) from the tachycardias (rate above 100/min).

Next, a **QRS duration of 0.12 seconds** is used to localize the site of impulse generation in relation to the atrioventricular (AV) conduction system (above or below).

Finally, the **regularity of the R-R interval** (the duration between successive R waves) is used to identify the underlying mechanism (e.g., automaticity and circus movement).

263

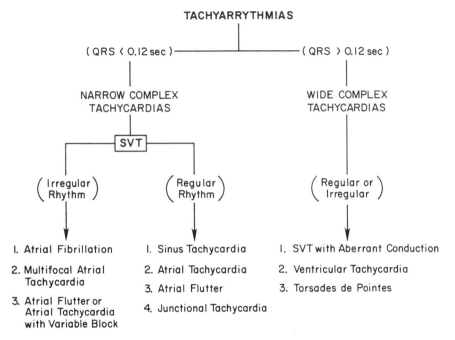

FIG. 21–1. Classification of the tachyarrhythmias.

HELPFUL CLUES

Several findings on the single-lead rhythm strip can help to identify the rhythm.

Rate and R-R Interval

a. Regular Rate above 200 bpm .... Sinus tachycardia unlikely
b. Regular Rate at 150 bpm .... Possible atrial flutter; 2:1 block
c. R-R markedly irregular .... Atrial fibrillation, MAT

Atrial Morphology

a. Uniform P waves .... Sinus tachycardia
b. Multiple P wave forms .... Multifocal atrial tachycardia
c. Inverted P Waves .... Junctional tachycardia
d. Sawtooth Waves .... Atrial flutter
e. No atrial activity .... Paroxysmal atrial tachycardia

When the rate is rapid, carotid sinus massage may help to slow the ventricular response and uncover the atrial activity.

Wide QRS Tachycardia. A wide QRS tachycardia can be ventricular tachycardia (VT) or a supraventricular tachycardia (SVT) with slow AV conduction. The following findings on the rhythm strip may help to differentiate between the two:[8]

A.

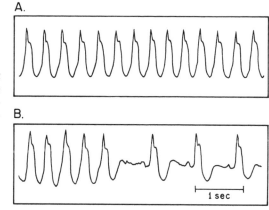

FIG. 21–2. SVT with aberrant conduction, appearing like venticular tachycardia. Courtesy of Dr. Richard M. Greenberg, M.D.

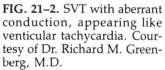

a. Pronounced R-R irregularity .... SVT
b. QRS longer than 0.14 seconds .... VT
c. Fusion beats .... VT
d. AV dissociation ....,,,.. VT

The last two signs are pathognomonic for VT.[8] In the absence of these, it is easy to be fooled. This is illustrated in Figure 21–2. The tracing in the upper panel shows a wide complex tachycardia that looks very much like VT with a QRS of longer than 0.14 seconds. However, the continuous tracing of the same arrhythmia in the lower panel shows that the QRS morphology did not change when the rhythm reverted to sinus, confirming that the tachycardia was a paroxysmal SVT superimposed on a bundle-branch block.

NARROW COMPLEX TACHYCARDIAS

The common tachycardias in this class are sinus tachycardia and atrial fibrillation. Paroxysmal atrial tachycardia (PAT) is prevalent in young, otherwise healthy subjects, but is not common in the ICU population.

SINUS TACHYCARDIA

Sinus tachycardia is identified by the following:
1. Gradual onset
2. Uniform P waves
3. Fixed PR Interval
4. Regular Rate

The rate is usually in the range of 100 to 180 beats per minute (bpm) in adults. Sinus tachycardia is a signal of another ongoing process and is not itself a clinical disorder.

Management Principles. The approach to sinus tachycardia is aimed at identifying the underlying cause, rather than direct intervention to slow the heart rate. Tachycardia decreases the diastolic period and reduces ventricular filling, but the heart rate must exceed 200 bpm in the normal heart before cardiac output begins to fall.[2] Since sinus rates usually do not exceed 180 bpm, there should be little hemodynamic compromise from sinus tachycardia when cardiac function is normal. When the ventricle becomes stiff and diastolic filling is compromised, small increases in heart rate can compromise cardiac output.

The major reason for slowing sinus tachycardia is ongoing myocardial ischemia/infarction. Beta blockers are the therapy of choice for reducing the sinus rate and Table 21–2 lists three of the many agents with proven efficacy.

ATRIAL FIBRILLATION AND FLUTTER

Atrial fibrillation and atrial flutter are indigenous to most adult ICUs and are particularly prominent in the first few days after cardiac surgery.[7] Although they can be identified by their atrial morphlogy, both have almost identical etiologies and treatment requirements. They are usually signs of underlying cardiac disease, but atrial fibrillation can be a manifestation of thyrotoxicosis in the elderly.[6]

MANAGEMENT STRATEGIES

Atrial fibrillation and atrial flutter (together abbreviated as AF) not only reduce the filling time, they eliminate the contribution of atrial contraction to the cardiac output. This is about 15 to 30% of the cardiac output under normal conditions,[6] and is likely to be higher when ventricular compliance decreases. The loss of atrial contraction in AF is well-tolerated if ventricular function is normal but not when the ventricle becomes stiff and noncompliant.

The acute therapy of AF is determined by the hemodynamic status of the patient. The goal in the hemodynamically stable patient (good ventricular function) is to reduce the heart rate to below 100 bpm, if necessary. Conversion to sinus rhythm is reserved for hemodynamically unstable patients (reduced ventricular compliance). The chronicity of the AF also dictates the need for cardioversion because chronic AF is difficult to convert and may not improve the cardiac output.[6]

The specific strategies used to treat AF are shown in Figure 21–3. The first step in the approach is to evaluate the hemodynamic status of the patient to determine the need for immediate cardioversion. Cardioversion is indicated for patients who show signs of hemodynamic compromise.

CARDIOVERSION

Atrial flutter can be converted by pacing the atria at a higher rate than the flutter rate.[3] Atrial fibrillation requires DC cardioversion. Rapid atrial pacing is usually impractical unless the patient has just received cardiac

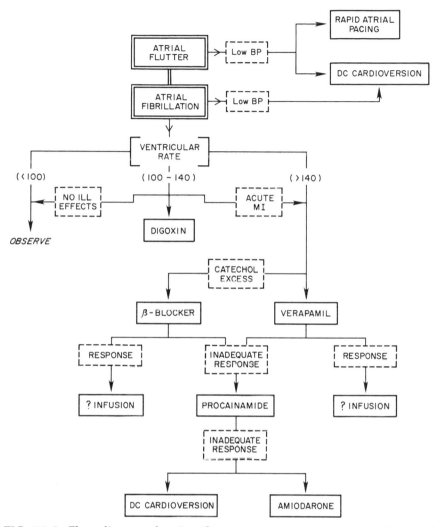

FIG. 21–3. Flow diagram showing the acute management strategies for atrial fibrillation and atrial flutter.

surgery and has atrial pacing wires in place. Otherwise, DC cardioversion is used for both flutter and fibrillation. Low energy levels (25 to 50 joules) are effective for flutter, but higher levels (start at 50 to 100 joules) will be necessary for fibrillation. Over 50% of patients will convert at energy levels of 200 joules or less.[5]

DRUG THERAPY

Acute therapy with intravenous agents is indicated if the ventricular rate is above 140 bpm, while less aggressive measures are used for a rate of 100 to 140. Below a rate of 100, there is usually no need to lower

TABLE 21–1. COMMONLY USED ANTIARRHYTHMIC AGENTS			
	SVT		
Drug	Narrow	Wide	VT
Beta Blockers	Yes	No	No
Verapamil	Yes	No	No
Digoxin	Yes	No	No
Procainamide	Yes	Yes	Yes
Lidocaine	No	Yes	Yes

the rate further. The actions of some of the more common antiarrhythmic agents are indicated in Table 21–1. The agents used for control of supraventricular tachycardias are listed in Table 21–2, along with the appropriate doses. The following is a brief description of the drugs that are used for acute control. Remember to consult Chapter 22 for more information.

Beta Blockers. These are indicated in hypercatecholamine states such as acute MI and the postoperative period. **Esmolol** is appealing because it has an elimination half-life of only 9 minutes and will disappear rapidly if it produces adverse effects.[10] This is a relatively new drug with limited clinical experience.

Verapamil. This calcium channel blocker is the preferred agent for immediate therapy because the response time is only 2 minutes in most cases.[3] The following IV doses are recommended:

Initial bolus: 0.075 mg/kg over 1 to 2 minutes.
Second bolus: 0.15 mg/kg, 15 minutes later if needed.
Maintenance infusion: .005 mg/kg/min.

It does not convert the rhythm but prolongs AV conduction and reduces the ventricular rate. Verapamil is particularly suited for patients with obstructive lung disease because it is a mild bronchodilator. The drug is eliminated by the liver and the dose should be reduced by 50% in patients with liver failure.

The major risk associated with verapamil is hypotension resulting from the vasodilating actions of the drug. This effect can be controlled with intravenous calcium, given either before or shortly after the blood pres-

TABLE 21–2. INTRAVENOUS Rx FOR SVT		
Agent	Loading Dose	Continuous Infusion
Verapamil	0.075–0.15 mg/kg	0.005 mg/kg/min
Propranolol	0.03 mg/kg	
Esmolol	500 mcg/kg	50–200 mcg/kg/min
Metoprolol	2.5 mg q 2 min (max = 15 mg)	
Digitalis	0.5 mg over 5 min, then 0.25 mg q 2 h × 4	
Procainamide	10 mg/kg (max = 50 mg/min)	1–6 mg/min

sure drops.[11,12] Verapamil is also a negative inotrope but the vasodilating action offsets this so that the cardiac output may not decrease.[13] Combining verapamil with beta blocker therapy can result in profound hypotension in patients with significant left ventricular dysfunction and these two drugs should not be given together in this patient population.[11]

Digitalis. Digitalis is similar to verapamil in that it slows the ventricular rate and does not convert the rhythm to a sinus rhythm.[1,3] The response to intravenous digoxin is not immediate and can take up to 2 hours to develop.[3] This delay limits the role of digoxin when immediate control of the ventricular rate is required. The drug is more valuable in the chronic management of AF, while verapamil can be added for acute control when needed. Digoxin is well suited for patients with AF and abnormal ventricular function (systolic function), when the negative inotropic actions of beta blockers and verapamil should be avoided.

Procainamide. Procainamide therapy is aimed at converting the rhythm after verapamil or other drugs have been used to control the ventricular rate. The recommended dosing for this drug is shown in Table 21–2. The drug is cleared by the liver but its metabolite N-acetyl-procainamide is cleared by the kidneys. Because the metabolite has its own toxicity, the dose of procainamide should be reduced in renal failure.

PAROXYSMAL ATRIAL TACHYCARDIA

Paroxysmal atrial tachycardia (PAT) is not common in the ICU, as previously mentioned. This rhythm has an abrupt onset with a regular rate and P waves that are hidden in the QRS. Treatment includes vagal maneuvers (e.g., carotid sinus massage) and intravenous verapamil. Unlike atrial fibrillation, PAT frequently reverts to sinus rhythm with verapamil.[3]

MULTIFOCAL ATRIAL TACHYCARDIA

Multifocal atrial tachycardia (MAT) is just what it says; a rhythm with multiple foci of atrial ectopic activity. The P waves vary in appearance, as do the PR intervals. MAT is most common in patients with chronic lung disease and it resolves in almost 50% of the patients when theophylline is discontinued.[14]

MANAGEMENT STRATEGIES

1. Stop theophylline if possible, regardless of the serum level. This should be tolerated well in most patients, since most patients with COPD do not benefit from theophylline therapy (see Chapter 26).

2. If the serum magnesium is not high, give IV magnesium according to the protocol used in Chapter 37. Magnesium has been used successfully to manage this rhythm.[15] The mechanism is unclear at present.

3. Finally, verapamil can be used if necessary.[16] Beta blockers (selective) have been used safely in patients with lung disease who do not have active bronchospasm,[17] but the risk does not seem necessary because of the alternative choice to use verapamil.

In summary, MAT can be difficult to control. Refraining from theophylline may be the best therapy available.

AV JUNCTIONAL TACHYCARDIA

This rhythm can be identified by the presence of AV dissociation with a narrow complex ventricular response of 70 to 130 bpm. Junctional rhythms can be seen in association with acute myocardial infarction, coronary bypass surgery, and digitalis toxicity. This rhythm is usually transient and well-tolerated, and does not require therapy. If immediate therapy is warranted, DC cardioversion can be effective. If digitalis toxicity is the cause, potassium infusion, magnesium infusion, or lidocaine may be effective.

WIDE COMPLEX TACHYCARDIAS

The wide complex tachycardias (QRS longer than 0.12 sec) represent either VT or SVT with aberrant conduction. A number of ECG features have been evaluated as possible clues,[8] including the following:

Rhythm strip—AV dissociation and fusion beats are evidence of ventricular tachycardia.

12-Lead ECG—Ventricular tachycardia is likely if there is a left axis deviation, a right bundle branch block plus a QRS longer than 0.14 seconds or a left bundle branch block plus a QRS longer than 0.16 seconds.[8]

This issue has been simplified recently by the observation that ventricular tachycardia may cause over 95% of wide-complex tachycardias in patients who have underlying cardiac disease.[9] Since most patients in the ICU have cardiac disease,

Ventricular tachycardia is the diagnosis until disproven for all wide complex tachycardias in the ICU patient population.

MANAGEMENT STRATEGIES

Procainamide can be used as single agent therapy for both VT and SVT (except torsades de pointes, as discussed later). However, intravenous procainamide cannot be given at a rate of more than 50 mg/min, therefore, it may not be possible to achieve immediate control with procainamide.

TABLE 21-3.   INTRAVENOUS Rx FOR VENTRICULAR ECTOPY
1. Lidocaine a. Bolus: 1.5 mg/kg IV over 5 minutes b. Drip Rate: 1 mg/min . . . . for elderly/CHF/liver failure $\quad\quad\quad\quad\quad\quad\quad$ 2 mg/min otherwise **If Necessary:** c. Repeat bolus of 0.75 mg/kg over 5 minutes d. Increase infusion to 4 mg/min and e. Draw serum level 30 minutes later **2. Procainamide** a. Bolus: 10 mg/kg (less than 50 mg/min) b. Drip Rate: 1-6 mg/min

VENTRICULAR ARRHYTHMIAS

The appearance of ventricular ectopics is often of little consequence unless there is active myocardial ischemia or infarction. This represents a unique situation with its own special set of rules for arrythmia suppression.

MYOCARDIAL INFARCTION

Ventricular arrhythmias appear in three distinct time periods following acute myocardial infarction (MI).[18]

The first period begins within minutes after the onset of the MI and peaks at 2 to 3 hours. Ventricular ectopics in this period can degenerate into VT and ventricular fibrillation (V-Fib) and are considered malignant rhythms.

The second period begins at 6 to 12 hours and persists for up to 72 hours. Reperfusion arrhythmias from thrombolytic therapy occur in this time period. The ectopy at this time is usually benign.

The final period occurs 3 to 7 days after the MI and the arrythmias tend to be benign. There is no recommended surveillance for patients in this time period.

Arrhythmia Suppression. Lidocaine is the drug of choice for prophylaxis and suppression of ventricular ectopy in the peri-infarction period. Although there is no evidence that prophylactic lidocaine in the immediate post-MI period improves outcome,[18]

Over 50% of patients who develop V-Fib in the immediate postinfarction period will do so without warning.[19]

The consensus then is that all patients at risk should receive routine prophylaxis with lidocaine starting as early after the onset of the MI as possible.[20] Some recommend withholding prophylactic lidocaine therapy in patients over the age of 70 because of the high incidence of lidocaine toxicity in the elderly.[20] Table 21-3 contains the dosing recommendations for lidocaine in this setting.

After the bolus dose, a continuous drip of 2 mg/min is started and continued for the next 48 hours. If this does not suppress the ectopy, a repeat bolus of 0.75 mg/kg is administered over 5 minutes and the infusion rate is increased to 4 mg/min. Serum lidocaine levels should be monitored routinely at this infusion rate (see Chapter 22 for more information on lidocaine toxicity).

Ventricular arrhythmias refractory to lidocaine are treated by adding procainamide (see Table 21–3 for recommended doses).

OTHER CONSIDERATIONS

Coronary artery disease is not the only cause for ventricular ectopy. The following factors must also be considered as possible causes of ectopy in individual patients.

1. Electrolyte Abnormalities

Hypokalemia and hypomagnesemia are well-known causes of ventricular ectopy, particularly in combination with digitalis. These electrolyte abnormalities are discussed in Chapters 36 and 37. Remember that magnesium depletion can be associated with normal serum levels because of its predominant intracellular location.

2. Drugs

Digitalis is always a likely offender because digitalis toxicity is common in hospitalized patients.[21] The "pro-arrhythmic" effects of antiarrhythmic agents like procainamide must also be kept in mind.

3. Acid-Base Disorders

Alkalosis (particularly respiratory alkalosis) can increase myocardial irritability, possibly through changes in ionized calcium.

VENTRICULAR TACHYCARDIA

Ventricular tachycardia is defined as a series of more than three ventricular ectopic impulses. It can subside in less than 30 seconds (nonsustained VT) or can continue unabated (sustained VT). This rhythm signals a severe problem, the most likely being myocardial ischemia. The general approach to ventricular tachycardia is shown in the flow diagram in Figure 21–4. The approach in this diagram is summarized in the following statements:[5]

1. Sustained VT should always be treated.

2. Nonsustained VT is treated only when it is associated with active cardiac disease.

3. If the patient is unstable, use DC countershocks, starting at 50 joules. Increase by 50 joules each time as needed.

4. If the patient is stable, start lidocaine as a bolus and a continuous infusion. If this is ineffective and the QT interval is normal, consider intravenous amiodarone. This has proven effective for refractory ar-

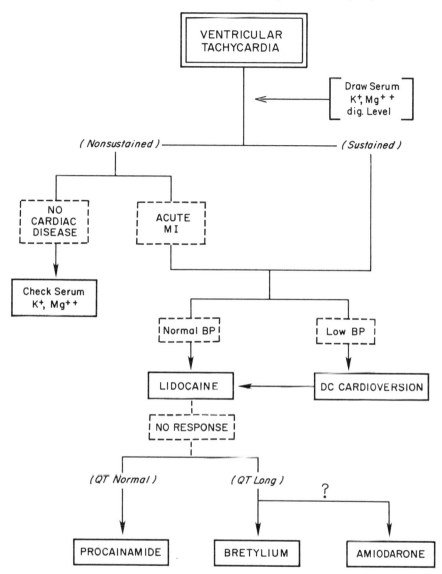

FIG. 21–4. Flow diagram showing the acute management strategies for ventricular tachycardia.

rythmias but the drug is presently not approved for intravenous use in this country.

TORSADES DE POINTES

This rhythm is characterized by phasic changes in the amplitude of the ventricular complexes as well as the polarity. This gives the ap-

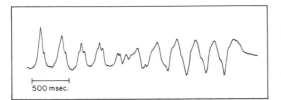

FIG. 21–5. Torsades de pointes. Note that the paper speed is twice normal. Courtesy of Dr. Richard M. Greenberg, M.D.

500 msec.

pearance that the complexes are "twisting around the (isoelectric) point." An example of this rhythm is shown in Figure 21–5.

Torsades is usually self-limited and only rarely degenerates into ventricular fibrillation.[21] However, it does tend to recur. It is almost always preceded by a prolonged QT interval, therefore, the factors that predispose to this rhythm also cause an increase in the QT interval.

Therapy is chosen according to the preceding QT interval.

1. If the QT interval is prolonged, all potential offending drugs should be discontinued. A serum sample should be obtained for magnesium, calcium, and potassium, and any decrease in the serum concentration of these ions should be corrected immediately. Therapy with traditional antiarrhythmic agents like lidocaine is not usually successful, and **therapy with agents that prolong the QT interval (e.g., pronestyl) is contraindicated.**

If the rhythm recurs, temporary ventricular pacing at a rate of 100 to 120 bpm is the treatment of choice. The goal here is to increase the heart rate and thereby decrease the QT interval. This can also be achieved with intravenous isoproterenol, however, this agent is not preferred to ventricular pacing because of the risk for arrhythmias and for myocardial ischemia.

2. If the preceding QT interval is normal, therapy with traditional antiarrhythmic agents including pronestyl and quinidine are safe.

DIGITALIS CARDIOTOXICITY

Digitalis toxicity is reported in 20% of hospitalized patients receiving the drug.[22] The conditions that promote digitalis toxicity (advanced age, abnormal renal function, heart disease, and hypokalemia) are common in critically ill patients, so digitalis toxicity should also be common in the ICU.

Digitalis toxicity can produce several types of arrhythmias. The more common ones are junctional tachycardia, first-degree AV block, type-I (Wenckebach) second-degree AV block, and complete AV block (with junctional escape) in patients with atrial fibrillation.[22] The latter process is responsible for one of the classic signs of digitalis toxicity during treatment for atrial fibrillation, that is, periods of regularization of the R-R interval.

Treatment. The treatment of digitalis toxicity should include the following:

1. Hypokalemia should be corrected as soon as possible to minimize the risk for digitalis-induced depression of the AV node,[22] and

aggressive potassium replacement is indicated for AV block from digitalis toxicity.

2. Magnesium depletion is more important than suspected because magnesium infusion can suppress digitalis-induced arrhythmias even when the serum magnesium levels are normal. Magnesium replacement is indicated for every patient with suspected digitalis toxicity who is not hypermagnesemic and who has normal renal function. The protocol for magnesium replacement is presented in Chapter 37.

3. Lidocaine is effective for suppressing ventricular ectopy from digitalis toxicity.

4. Life-threatening toxicity that is refractory to the usual measures can be treated with digoxin-specific antibodies given intravenously.[23] Once the arrhythmia is controlled, digitalis can be eliminated faster using oral activated charcoal in a dose of 25 gm every 4 hours for 40 hours.[24] or cholestyramine in a dose of 4 gr every 6 hours.[25]

REFERENCES

REVIEWS

1. Zipes DP. Genesis of Cardiac Arrythmias. In: Braunwald E ed, Heart disease. A textbook of cardiovascular medicine. 3rd ed. Philadelphia: W.B. Saunders, 1988.
2. Guyton AC. The relationship of cardiac output and arterial pressure control. Circulation 1981; 64:1079–1088.

SUPRAVENTRICULAR TACHYCARDIAS

3. Keefe DL, Miura D, Somberg JC. Supraventricular tachyarrhythmias: Their evaluation and therapy. Am Heart J 1986; 11:1150–1161.
4. Manolis AS, Estes AM III. Supraventricular tachycardia. Mechanisms and therapy. Arch Intern Med 1987; 147:1706–1716.
5. Walsh KA, Ezri MD, Denes P. Emergency treatment of tachyarrythmias. Med Clin North Am 1986; 70:791–811.
6. Morris DC, Hurst JW. Atrial fibrillation. Current problems in cardiology. Chicago: Year Book Medical Publishers, 1980:1–50.
7. Vecht RJ, Nicolaides EP, Ikweuke JK, et al. Incidence and prevention of supraventricular tachyarrhythmias after coronary bypass surgery. Int J Cardiol 1986; 13:125–134.

WIDE COMPLEX TACHYCARDIAS

8. Wellens HJJ, Bar FWHM, Lie KI. The value of the electrocardiogram in the differential diagnosis of tachycardia with a widened QRS complex. Am J Med 1978; 64:27–33.
9. Akhtar M, Shenasa M, Jazayeri M, et al. Wide QRS complex tachycardia. Ann Internal Med 1988; 109:905–912.

DRUG THERAPY

10. Turlapaty P, Laddu A, Murthy S, et al. Esmolol: A titratable short-acting intravenous beta blocker for acute critical care settings. Am Heart J 1987; *114*:866–885.
11. Henry M, Kay MM, Viccellio P. Cardiogenic shock associated with calcium-channel and beta blockers: Reversal with intravenous calcium chloride. Am J Emerg Med 1985; *3*:334–336.
12. Barnett JC, Touchon RC. Verapamil infusion with calcium pretreatment for acute control of supraventricular tachycardia. Crit Care Med 1989; *17*:S11.
13. Ferlinz J, Citron PD. Hemodynamic and myocardial performance characteristics after verapamil use in congestive heart failure. Am J Cardiol 1983; *51*:1339–1345.
14. Levine JH, Michael JR, Guarnieri T. Multifocal atrial tachycardia: A toxic effect of theophylline. Lancet 1985; *1*:1216.
15. Iseri LT, Fairshter RD, Hardeman JL, Brodsky MA. Magnesium and potassium therapy in multifocal atrial tachycardia. Am Heart J 1985; *110*:789–791.
16. Levine JH, Michael JR, Guarnieri T. Treatment of multifocal atrial tachycardia with verapamil. N Engl J Med 1985; *312*:21–26.
17. Arsura EL, Solar M, Lefkin AS, et al. Metoprolol in the treatment of multifocal atrial tachycardia. Crit Care Med 1987; *15*:591–594.
18. MacMahon S, Collins R, Peto R, et al. Effects of prophylactic lidocaine in suspected acute myocardial infarction. JAMA 1988; *260*:1910–1916.
19. Ahmad S, Giles TD. Managing ventricular arrhythmias during acute MI. J Crit Illness 1988; *3*:29–40.
20. Stamato NJ, Josephson ME. When and how to manage premature ventricular contractions. J Crit Illness 1986; *1*:41–48.
21. Stratmann HG, Kennedy HL. Torsades de pointes associated with drugs and toxins: Recognition and management. Am Heart J 1987; *113*:1470–1482.
22. Fisch C, Knoebel SB. Digitalis cardiotoxicity. J Am Coll Cardiol 1985; *5*:91A–98A.
23. Smith TW, Butler VP, Haber E, et al. Treatment of life-threatening digitalis intoxication with digoxin-specific Fab antibody fragments. N Engl J Med 1982; *307*:1357–1362.
24. Lalonde RL, Deshpande R, Hamilton PP, et al. Acceleration of digoxin clearance by activated charcoal. Clin Pharmacol Ther 1985; *37*:367–371.
25. Henderson RP, Solomon CP. Use of cholestyramine in the treatment of digoxin intoxication. Arch Intern Med 1988; *148*:745–746.

chapter

ANTIARRHYTHMIC AGENTS

This chapter contains information on eight drugs used for acute suppression of tachyarrythmias.[1-6] These agents are listed below and Table 22–1 contains the recommended doses and therapeutic serum levels when applicable. An asterisk (*) below indicates that a dosing chart is available for the drug in the Appendix.

The following drugs are listed alphabetically:

1. Amiodarone
2. Bretylium
3. Digitalis
4 Esmolol
*5. Lidocaine
*6. Procainamide
7. Propranolol
8. Verapamil

All suggested doses apply to the intravenous route only.

AMIODARONE

Amiodarone was introduced in 1967 as a coronary vasodilator. It is a highly effective agent for the therapy of both SVT and ventricular arrhythmias. However, its potential for serious toxicity (primarily pulmonary fibrosis) with chronic therapy has limited its use to arrhythmias that are unresponsive to conventional antiarrhythmic therapy. Although intravenous therapy is not presently FDA approved, it is presented here because of its potential future applications.

TABLE 22–1. INTRAVENOUS ANTIARRHYTHMIC AGENTS			
Agent	Loading Dose	Maintenance Dose	Serum Level
Amiodarone	5–10 mg/kg	12 mg/kg/day	0.7–3.5 μg/ml
Lidocaine	0.5–1 mg/kg	1–4 mg/min	1–6
Procainamide	10 mg/kg	1–6 mg/min	4–10
Bretylium	5–10 mg/kg	1–2 mg/min	0.5–1.5
Esmolol	500 μg/kg	50–200 μg/kg/min	
Verapamil	.075–0.15 mg/kg	0.005 mg/kg/min	

ACTIONS

1. Prolongs repolarization in the atria and the ventricles (class-III agent).
2. Prolongs the QT interval.
3. Produces mild alpha and beta blockade.

PHARMACOKINETICS

1. Lipid-soluble and achieves high concentrations in the liver and lungs.
2. Eliminated by biliary excretion.
3. Mean elimination half-life after oral administration is 25 days.

INDICATIONS

1. Ventricular arrhythmias unresponsive to conventional antiarrhythmic therapy.
2. Supraventricular arrhythmias (atrial flutter, fibrillation, and PAT) unresponsive to conventional therapy.

INTRAVENOUS DOSING

1. Loading Dose: 5 to 10 mg/kg over 20 to 30 minutes. Repeat the loading dose in 30 minutes if necessary.
2. Maintenance Dose: 10 to 12 mg/kg/day for 3 to 5 days.
3. Administer in dextrose-water solution, since the drug may precipitate in saline.
4. Therapeutic serum level: 0.75 to 3.5 μgr/ml.
5. IV administration presently not FDA approved.

ADVERSE EFFECTS

1. Chronic administration is associated with several adverse effects, including pulmonary fibrosis (which can be fatal), thyroid dysfunction, crystalline deposits in the cornea, elevated liver enzymes, and bluish skin discoloration.

2. Hypotension can result from combined alpha and beta blockade.

3. Can worsen ventricular arrhythmias through unclear mechanisms. Can induce torsades de pointes when given in the setting of a prolonged QT interval. May also facilitate arrhythmogenic potential of procainamide and quinidine (which also prolong the QT interval).

4. Can cause sinus bradycardia and AV block when used in combination with beta blockers or calcium antagonists.

DRUG INTERACTIONS

1. Increases serum levels of procainamide, quinidine, digoxin, and warfarin.[1] When amiodarone therapy is started, digoxin dosing should be reduced by 30%. Concurrent therapy with quinidine and procainamide is not recommended.

CONTRAINDICATIONS

1. Torsades de pointes associated with prolonged QT interval.

2. Ongoing therapy with drugs that prolong the QT interval.

BRETYLIUM TOSYLATE

Bretylium is an adrenergic blocker that was introduced in the 1950s as an antihypertensive agent.[5] Although it is an effective agent for ventricular arrhythmias, its value is limited by its ability to produce hypotension.

ACTIONS

1. Prolongs action potential duration and increases the refractory period in atrial and ventricular muscle (class-II agent).

2. Inhibits norepinephrine release from sympathetic nerve terminals.

PHARMACOKINETICS

1. Cleared almost exclusively by the kidneys.

2. Serum half-life is 9 hours in normal subjects, and 32 hours in patients with renal failure.

INDICATIONS

1. Ventricular arrhythmias unresponsive to lidocaine therapy.

INTRAVENOUS DOSING

1. Initial dose: 5 mg/kg. Give over 20 to 30 minutes if patients are hemodynamically stable. Otherwise, the initial dose can be given by rapid intravenous injection.
2. Maintenance dose: 1 to 2 mg/min.
3. Decrease the dose by at least 50% in patients with renal failure.
4. Therapy should not be continued for longer than 24 hours, if possible.

ADVERSE EFFECTS

1. Hypotension is common, particularly when bretylium is given for longer than 24 hours.
2. Transient hypertension can occur when therapy is started because of the release of norepinephrine from the sympathetic nerve terminals.
3. Nausea and vomiting are common after rapid intravenous administration.

DIGOXIN

Intravenous digoxin is a time-honored therapy for the management of certain SVTs (atrial flutter and fibrillation and PAT), however, it is being replaced by verapamil and esmolol for the acute control of these arrhythmias (see Chapter 21 for a discussion of this topic).[7] Nevertheless, digoxin continues to be valuable in long-term therapy of atrial flutter and fibrillation.

ACTIONS

1. Prolongs AV conduction.
2. Occasionally terminates atrial flutter and fibrillation.
3. Is a peripheral vasoconstrictor.[8]

PHARMACOKINETICS

1. Is widely distributed in body tissues, and has a long serum half-life of 44 hours.
2. Onset of action after intravenous administration usually occurs in 1 to 2 hours.
3. Clearance is primarily by renal excretion.

4. Biliary excretion can be responsible for 30% of drug clearance. Although much of the drug is reabsorbed in the GI tract, excretion in the stool can increase during renal failure.

INDICATIONS

1. Maintenance therapy for atrial flutter and atrial fibrillation.

INTRAVENOUS DOSING

1. Loading dose: 0.75 mg IV over 5 minutes, followed by 0.25 mg IV every 2 hours for 4 doses.
2. Maintenance dose: Start at 0.25 mg/day in patients without severe heart failure, renal failure, or in the absence of concurrent therapy with drugs that interfere with digoxin clearance. Otherwise start at 0.125 mg/day or less. Follow daily serum levels and keep serum levels below 2.0 ng/dl.

ADVERSE EFFECTS

1. Rapid IV administration can cause mesenteric ischemia in the elderly.[8]
2. Can sensitize carotid baroreceptors and promote vagal influences on the heart.
3. Digitalis toxicity can be associated with AV block, junctional rhythms, and ventricular arrhythmias.[9] Toxicity is particularly prevalent in patients with advanced age, low cardiac output, hypokalemia, hypomagnesemia, hypothyroidism, renal failure, and those receiving drugs known to retard digoxin clearance.

DRUG INTERACTIONS

1. Digoxin clearance is diminished by quinidine, calcium antagonists (verapamil), and amiodarone.[10]
2. A digitalis-like substance has been discovered in the serum of patients with chronic renal failure who require dialysis.[11,12] The meaning of this is not clear at present but should stress caution in interpreting digoxin levels in these patients.

CONTRAINDICATIONS

1. AV block.
2. Hypertrophic cardiomyopathy.
3. Severe hypokalemia or hypomagnesemia.

4. Sick sinus syndrome.
5. Wolff-Parkinson-White syndrome.

ESMOLOL

Esmolol is a newly introduced beta-blocker that may be particularly valuable for the acute management of SVT because of its short half-life (approximately 9 minutes) with intravenous administration.[13] Clinical experience with this agent is limited at present, however, the drug is tedious to use if a response is not obtained with the first dose (see below).

ACTIONS

1. A cardioselective beta-blocker with actions similar to other selective beta blockers (e.g., prolongs AV conduction, negative inotropic effects, peripheral vasodilatation).

PHARMACOKINETICS

1. Rapid onset of action. An effect is usually apparent within 2 minutes after the loading dose is given.
2. Metabolized by red blood cell esterases and is rapidly inactivated.
3. Elimination half-life is 9 minutes. Complete recovery from physiologic effects occurs 15 to 20 minutes after stopping the drug.

INDICATIONS

1. Acute control of ventricular rate in PAT, atrial flutter and fibrillation.

INTRAVENOUS DOSING

1. Loading dose: 500 μgr/kg given over 1 minute.
2. Maintenance dose: 50 to 200 μgr/kg/min. Start at a dose of 50 μgr/kg/min for 4 minutes. If desired effect is not achieved, repeat the loading dose and increase the maintenance dose to 100 μgr/kg/min for 4 minutes. If no effect, repeat the loading dose and increase maintenance infusion in increments of 50 μgr/kg/min to a dose of 200 μgr/kg/min. A loading dose should precede each increment in maintenance dose.

ADVERSE REACTIONS

1. Hypotension is reported in up to 50% of patients. This effect is dose-dependent and can resolve with a decrease in dose. Blood pressure

usually returns to baseline within 30 minutes after stopping drug administration.

2. Bronchospasm has been reported in asthmatics.[14]

3. Like all beta blockers, acute heart failure is a possibility. Heart failure has not been reported often with esmolol, but the patients studied have had normal ventricular function.

4. Can delay recovery from succinylcholine-induced neuromuscular blockade.

DRUG INTERACTIONS

1. Can increase serum digoxin levels.

CONTRAINDICATIONS

1. AV block.
2. Hypotension.
3. Severe myocardial dysfunction (systolic).
4. Asthma.

LIDOCAINE

Lidocaine was recognized in the early 1960s as an effective agent for the suppression of ventricular arrhythmias.[1] Since that time, lidocaine has become the most preferred agent for the acute control of life-threatening ventricular arrhythmias. Unlike most other antiarrhythmic agents, it is decidedly free of adverse cardiac effects in the usual doses.

ACTIONS

Depresses depolarization and shortens repolarization in ventricular fibers (class Ib agents).

PHARMACOKINETICS

1. Mean half-life: 1.5 to 2 hours.
2. Cleared by the liver.
3. Clearance decreased in low cardiac output states and significant hepatic dysfunction.
4. Prolonged administration of lidocaine reduces its own clearance, therefore, some recommend a steadily decreasing rate of infusion with prolonged use.[15]

INDICATIONS

Acute suppression of ventricular arrhythmias, particularly in association with acute MI and cardiac surgery.

INTRAVENOUS DOSING

1. In the absence of circulatory failure:
Loading dose: 1.0 to 1.5 mg/kg over 10 minutes, followed in 5 to 10 minutes by a booster dose of 0.75 to 1.0 mg/kg.
Maintenance dose: 10 μgr/kg/hr.
2. In patients with circulatory failure or hepatic failure:
Loading dose: 50 to 75 mg.
Maintenance dose: 10 μgr/kg/hr.
3. Therapeutic serum level: 1 to 6 μgr/ml.

ADVERSE EFFECTS

1. Major toxicity is central nervous system depression and seizures. Most common in elderly patients and in patients with low cardiac output.
2. Can precipitate complete heart block in patients with trifascicular block.

DRUG INTERACTIONS

1. Hepatic clearance decreased by cimetidine, propranolol, dopamine, and norepinephrine.

CONTRAINDICATIONS

1. Trifascicular block.

PROCAINAMIDE

ACTIONS

1. Depresses depolarization and prolongs repolarization in atrial and venticular muscle.[1,5]
2. Transiently facilitates AV conduction (vagolytic effect).
3. Prolongs QT interval.

PHARMACOKINETICS

1. 50% of the drug is excreted unchanged by the kidney, and 10 to 30% is eliminated by hepatic metabolism.
2. 15% is metabolized to N-acetyl procainamide (NAPA), which also has antiarrhythmic effects. NAPA is eliminated primarily by the kidneys.[16]
3. Clearance is decreased in the elderly and in patients with low cardiac output and renal insufficiency.

INDICATIONS

1. Acute suppression of ventricular arrhythmias when lidocaine is not effective.
2. Acute control (or termination) of atrial flutter and atrial fibrillation after initial therapy with drugs that block AV conduction (verapamil, beta-blockers, or digitalis).

INTRAVENOUS DOSING

1. Loading dose: 6 to 13 mg/kg given at a maximum rate of 50 mg/min.
2. Maintenance dose: 1–6 mg/min.
3. Reduce dose by 50% in elderly patients or patients with severe heart failure or renal insufficiency.
4. Therapeutic serum levels: 4 to 10 μgr/ml.

ADVERSE EFFECTS

1. Has negative inotropic effects. The clinical significance of this is not clear, but the drug should be used with caution in patients with severe ventricular dysfunction.
2. Hypotension can occur during rapid intravenous loading. The mechanism is not clear but may be secondary to peripheral vasodilatation.
3. Can predispose to ventricular arrhythmias by prolonging the QT interval.
4. NAPA can have the same toxicity as procainamide.[16]
5. Lupus syndrome not seen during acute administration.

DRUG INTERACTIONS

1. Renal clearance diminished by cimetidine.

CONTRAINDICATIONS

1. Torsades de pointes associated with a prolonged QT interval.
2. Therapy of atrial flutter and fibrillation without prior drug therapy to depress AV conduction.

PROPRANOLOL

Propranolol is the prototype beta blocker that has a long history in the acute management of certain supraventricular tachycardias.[17] Although it remains an effective agent, its use is declining with the advent of cardioselective beta blockers.

ACTIONS

1. A non-selective beta-blocker that blocks both beta-1 receptors in the heart and peripheral vasculature, and beta-2 receptors in the airways and skeletal muscles.
2. Decreases sinus rate and prolongs AV conduction.
3. Has negative inotropic effects.
4. Decreases automaticity in both atria and ventricles.
5. Causes peripheral vasodilatation.

PHARMACOKINETICS

1. Immediate onset of action (1 to 3 minutes) after intravenous administration.
2. Serum half-life: 3.5 to 6 hours.
3. Metabolized primarily in the liver to inactive metabolites that are excreted in the urine.

INDICATIONS

1. Acute control of the ventricular rate in PAT, atrial flutter, and atrial fibrillation, particularly when these rhythms are associated with hyper-catecholamine states (e.g., after cardiac surgery, pheochromocytoma, or ethanol withdrawal).
2. Acute control of sinus tachycardia associated with acute MI or angina.
3. Arrhythmias associated with thyroid storm.

INTRAVENOUS DOSING

1. Initial dose: 0.03 mg/kg given at a rate of 0.5 mg/min.
2. Repeat doses: If no effect from initial dose after 5 minutes, repeat

initial dose protocol and wait another 5 minutes. Continue this protocol until the desired effect is achieved or until the total dose reaches 0.1 mg/kg.

3. Maintenance doses: Start oral therapy if possible, or use IV therapy PRN.

ADVERSE EFFECTS

1. Hypotension is the most common adverse reaction to acute intravenous therapy.

2. Acute heart failure can occur in patients with severe ventricular dysfunction (systolic failure). This effect can be magnified when therapy is combined with verapamil.

3. Acute airways constriction may occur in patients wth asthma *and* COPD.[18] This is not reversed with beta-2 stimulants.

4. Bradycardia can occur with excessive doses because of AV block or sinus node depression.

DRUG INTERACTIONS

1. Decreases hepatic clearance of lidocaine.

2. Hepatic clearance of propranolol is reduced by cimetidine and enhanced by barbiturates.

CONTRAINDICATIONS

1. AV block.
2. Hypotension.
3. Asthma or COPD.
4. Sick sinus syndrome (unless a pacemaker is in place).
5. Severe myocardial failure (systolic failure) particularly when combined with verapamil.

VERAPAMIL

Verapamil is a calcium-channel blocker that was introduced in the late 1970s as a coronary vasodilator. However, its ability to prolong AV conduction has resulted in the drug being used primarily in the therapy of certain supraventricular tachycardias. Over the past few years it has replaced intravenous digitalis for acute control of atrial flutter and atrial fibrillation (see Chapter 21).[7]

ACTIONS

1. Prolongs AV conduction
2. Has negative inotropic effects.
3. Produces significant peripheral vasodilatation.

PHARMACOKINETICS

1. Rapid onset of action (1 to 2 minutes) after intravenous injection.
2. Cleared rapidly by the liver.

INTRAVENOUS DOSING

1. Initial dose: 0.075 mg/kg total body weight, followed in 15 minutes by an additional dose of 0.15 mg/kg.
2. Maintenance dose: 0.005 mg/kg/min.[19]
3. In hepatic failure, decrease IV doses by 50%.
4. Serum levels not monitored.

INDICATIONS

In the absence of hypotension, verapamil is recommended in the acute therapy of:
1. Paroxysmal atrial tachycardia that does not respond to vagal maneuvers.
2. Atrial flutter and atrial fibrillation.
3. Multifocal atrial tachycardia (not always effective).

ADVERSE EFFECTS

1. Hypotension secondary to peripheral vasodilatation. This can often be reversed with intravenous calcium infusion.
2. Can depress cardiac output in patients with severe dilated cardiomyopathy and systolic function, particularly when combined with beta-blockers.[20] However, negative inotropic effects are usually offset by vasodilatation, the net result being an increase in cardiac output.[21,22]

DRUG INTERACTIONS

1. Increases serum digoxin levels.

CONTRAINDICATIONS

1. AV block.
2. Hypotension.
3. Wolff-Parkinson-White syndrome.
4. Patients with severe ventricular dysfunction receiving beta-blocker therapy.

Verapamil can accelerate the ventricular response in patients with Wolff-Parkinson-White syndrome and atrial fibrillation due to shortening of the refractory period in accessory pathways.

BIBLIOGRAPHY

Opie H ed. Drugs for the heart. Orlando: Grune & Stratton, 1984.
Khan MG. Manual of cardiac drug therapy. 2nd ed. London: Balliere Tindall/W.B. Saunders, 1988.

REFERENCES

REVIEWS

1. Huang SK, Marcus SI. Antiarrhythmic drug therapy of ventricular arrhythmias. Curr Probl Cardiol 1986; 11:179–240.
2. Block PJ, Winkle RA. Hemodynamic effects of antiarrhythmic drugs. Am J Cardiol 1983; 62:14C–23C.
3. Campbell S. Pharmacologic principles of cardiovascular drug administration to the critically ill. Crit Care Clin 1985; 1:471–490.
4. Naccarelli GV, Rinkenberger RL, Dougherty AH, et al. Pharmacologic therapy of arrhythmias. Hosp Pract 1988, (Oct) 23:135–158.
5. Podrid PJ. Antiarrhythmic drug therapy (Part 1). Chest 1985; 88:452–460.
6. Zipes DP. Management of cardiac arrhythmias: Pharmacological, electrical, and surgical techniques. In: Braunwald E ed. Heart disease: A textbook of cardiovascular medicine. Philadelphia: W.B. Saunders, 1988.

DIGOXIN

7. Smith TW: Digitalis. Mechanisms of action and clinical use. N Engl J Med 1988; 318:358–365.
8. Longhurst JC, Ross, J. Extracardiac and coronary vascular effects of digitalis. J Am Coll Cardiol 1985; 5:99A–105A.
9. Moorman JR, Pritchett EL: The arrhythmias of digitalis intoxication. Arch Intern Med 1985; 145:1289–1292.
10. Marcus FI. Pharmacokinetic interactions between digoxin and other drugs. J Am Coll Cardiol 1985; 5:82A–90A.
11. Graves SW, Brown B, Valdes R. An endogenous digoxin-like substance in patients with renal impairment. Ann Intern Med 1983; 99:604–608.
12. Craver JL, Valdes RL. Anomalous serum digoxin concentrations in uremia. Ann Intern Med 1983; 98:483–484.

ESMOLOL

13. Turlapaty P, Laddu A, Murthy VS. Esmolol: A titratable short-acting intravenous beta blocker for acute critical care settings. Am Heart J 1987; *114*:866–885.
14. Sung RJ, Singh BH. Esmolol HCl: A short-acting beta-adrenergic blocker for the treatment of supraventricular tachyarrhythmias. Hosp Form 1988; *23*:352–356.

LIDOCAINE

15. Davidson R, Parker M, Atkinson AJ Jr. Excessive serum lidocaine levels during maintenance infusions: Mechanisms and prevention. Am Heart J 1982; *104*:203–208.

PROCAINAMIDE

16. Feld GK. N-acetylprocainamide (acecainide HCl): Electrophysiology and antiarrhythmic effects. Hosp Form 1987; *22*:1038–1046.

PROPRANOLOL

17. McBride JW, McCoy HG, Goldenberg IF: Supraventricular tachycardia treated with continuous infusions of propranolol. Clin Pharmacol Ther 1988; *44*:93–99.
18. Chester EH, Schwartz HJ, Fleming GM. Adverse effect of propranolol on airway function in nonasthmatic chronic obstructive lung disease. Chest 1981; *79*:540–544.

VERAPAMIL

19. Reiter MJ, Shand DG, Aanonsen LM. Pharmacokinetics of verapamil: Experience with a sustained intravenous infusion regimen. Am J Cardiol 1982; *50*:716–721.
20. Schwartz JB, Verapamil in atrial fibrillation, The expected, the unexpected, and the unknown. [Editorial] Am Heart J 1983; *106*:173–176.
21. Ferling J, Easthope JL, Aronow WS. Effects of verapamil on myocardial performance in coronary disease. Circulation 1979; *59*:313–319.
22. Ferling J, Citron D. Hemodynamic and myocardial performance characteristics after verapamil use in congestive heart failure. Am J Cardiol 1983; *51*:1339–1345.

section VII
ACUTE RESPIRATORY FAILURE

. . . the blood has its fountain, and storehouse, and the workshop of its last perfection in the heart and lungs.

William Harvey

chapter

LUNG INJURY AND PULMONARY EDEMA

"The cause of pulmonary edema is not altogether clear. The most acceptable view is that it is due to increased capillary tension accompanied, and in many instances preceded by, degenerative changes, toxic in character, in the capillary endothelium."
Landis HRM, Norris GW.
1920

The subject of this chapter is a pulmonary disorder similar to the one described by Landis and Norris. What is interesting about their description is that it was written almost half a century prior to the 1967 article cited as the first official description of this illness.[11]

The illness in question is known as the "adult respiratory distress syndrome" (commonly abbreviated ARDS) and it is estimated to cause 150,000 cases of respiratory failure each year.[3] Over 50% of the victims will not survive this illness, which places ARDS in the same class with lung cancer (100,000 deaths per year) as the most lethal pulmonary conditions of modern times.

The approach to ARDS that follows is based on the principles of edema formation. There is no specific therapy for ARDS; the approach involves general aspects of management that can be applied to any patient with respiratory failure, regardless of the etiology. The hemodynamic aspects of the approach are taken from the principles in Chapters 1, 2, and 9–11.

CAPILLARY FLUID EXCHANGE

Ernest Starling first described the forces that govern fluid exchange across capillaries almost 100 years ago. The popular equation that bears

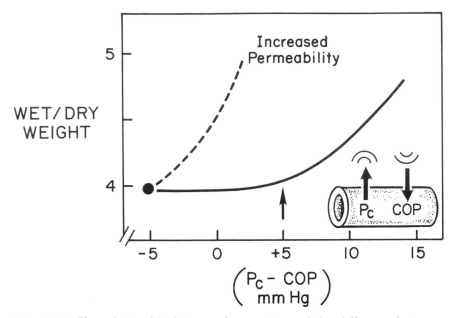

FIG. 23–1. The relationship between lung water and the difference between pulmonary capillary hydrostatic pressure (Pc) and serum colloid osmotic pressure (COP).

his name is shown here in an abbreviated form. Omitted are the components that cannot be measured in the clinical setting.

$$\dot{Q} = K\,(Pc - COP)$$

The equation states that the net fluid flow ($\dot{Q}$) across capillaries is proportional to the capillary permeability (K), and to the difference between the capillary hydrostatic pressure (Pc) and the colloid osmotic pressure (COP) of the plasma. The COP is the force created by large plasma proteins that do not pass freely out of the capillaries. This force draws fluid into the vascular space and opposes the hydrostatic pressure (Pc), which forces fluid out of the vascular space. The influence of these forces on lung water is shown in Figure 23–1. In the normal lung (solid line), fluid begins to accumulate when the Pc is 5 mmHg higher than the COP (arrow). However, when capillary permeability is increased (dashed line), fluid begins to accumulate when the Pc is lower than the COP and the rate of fluid accumulation (slope of the dotted line) increases more rapidly as Pc increases relative to COP. This graph demonstrates the role of capillary permeability in edema formation.

> An increase in capillary permeability reduces the threshold for edema formation and magnifies the influence of the capillary hydrostatic pressure on fluid accumulation in the extravascular space.

CAPILLARY HYDROSTATIC PRESSURE

The pulmonary capillary wedge pressure (PCWP) is used as the clinical measure of the pulmonary capillary hydrostatic pressure (Pc). However, as discussed in Chapter 10, the PCWP measures the left atrial pressure and not the capillary hydrostatic pressure. In fact, the PCWP (or left atrial pressure) cannot be the same as the Pc;

> If the wedge pressure (left atrial pressure) and the capillary hydrostatic pressure are identical, there will be no pressure gradient for flow across the pulmonary veins.

The difference between the PCWP and the hydrostatic pressure is explained in more detail in Chapter 10.

COLLOID OSMOTIC PRESSURE (COP)

The colloid osmotic pressure is mostly produced by serum albumin (60 to 80%), with fibrinogen and the globulins accounting for the remainder.[6] The normal plasma COP varies with body position:[6]

$$\text{Upright COP} = 25 \text{ mm Hg} \quad (\text{mean values})$$

$$\text{Supine COP} = 20 \text{ mm Hg}$$

The normal range of COP in the upright position ranges from 22 to 29 mmHg. The decrease in COP in the supine position takes about 4 hours to develop and is attributed to mobilization of protein-free fluid from dependent tissues into the central circulation.[6]

The COP can be measured with an electronic instrument called an oncometer or it can be estimated using the total protein concentration (TP) in grams per deciliter (gm/dL).[3,6,9]

$$\text{COP} = 2.1 \, (\text{TP}) + 0.16 \, (\text{TP}^2) + 0.009 \, (\text{TP}^3) \text{ mmHg}$$

Before you get discouraged, note that the last two terms contribute little to the overall value of the COP, so they can be eliminated without sacrificing accuracy. The reliability of this calculation has varied somewhat but it should provide an adequate approximation of the COP.[9] One source of error arises when nonprotein colloids are used as plasma expanders. These colloids will dilute the serum proteins and decrease the calculated COP while they maintain the actual COP. This means that the COP should be measured and not calculated when nonprotein colloids (hetastarch or the dextrans) are used for volume expansion.

CLASSIFICATION OF PULMONARY EDEMA

The determinants of fluid movement in the Starling equation are used to classify pulmonary edema:

1. Hydrostatic pulmonary edema: $(Pc - COP) >> 0$
2. Increased permeability edema: $(Pc - COP) << 0$

Hydrostatic edema is the familiar type of edema produced by left heart failure. The high permeability edema is the result of capillary damage from a diverse collection of disease entities and is more of an inflammatory infiltration than the watery edema of heart failure.

ADULT RESPIRATORY DISTRESS SYNDROME (ARDS)

This syndrome was first reported in 1967 (?) for 12 patients with diffuse pulmonary infiltrates and hypoxemia resistant to supplemental oxygen.[11] Autopsy in 7 patients revealed dense consolidation and alveolar hemorrhage with hyaline membranes.

It was given the name "adult respiratory distress syndrome" because of similarities to the "infant respiratory distress syndrome."

PATHOGENESIS

There are a multitude of conditions that predispose to ARDS and the list grows continuously. The common predisposing conditions are indicated on the body map in Figure 23–2. Sepsis is the leading offender and gram-negative bacteremia (endotoxemia) is particularly prominent. The link between the conditions in Figure 23–2 and ARDS is not clear, but the leading candidate at present is complement activation. The theory is that activated complement attracts neutrophils to the pulmonary microcirculation and the neutrophils adhere to the capillary endothelium and release toxic substances that damage the endothelium.[12,13] Figure 23–3 is an electron micrograph showing leukocytes adhering to the endothelium of a small pulmonary arteriole (PA) in an experimental model of ARDS. The lighter cell in the middle is a lymphocyte and the darker cells with the large cytoplasmic granules are neutrophils (N). Note that one of the neutrophils is beginning to squeeze through the endothelium (diapedesis) to gain access to the lung parenchyma. The dark granules in the neutrophils contain proteolytic enzymes and toxic oxygen metabolites that are capable of damaging the capillary endothelium and lung parenchyma.[12,13]

CLINICAL PRESENTATION

The onset of the clinical syndrome usually occurs within hours of the inciting event. The early course is characterized by severe hypoxemia,

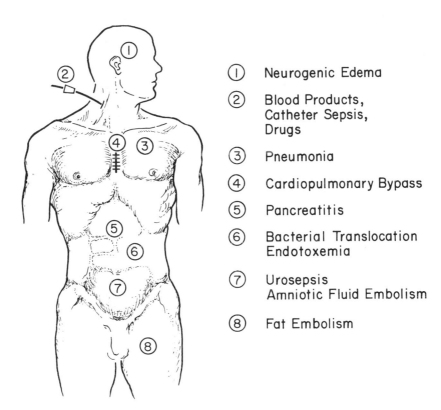

①	Neurogenic Edema
②	Blood Products, Catheter Sepsis, Drugs
③	Pneumonia
④	Cardiopulmonary Bypass
⑤	Pancreatitis
⑥	Bacterial Translocation Endotoxemia
⑦	Urosepsis Amniotic Fluid Embolism
⑧	Fat Embolism

FIG. 23–2. The body map indicating the common causes of adult respiratory distress syndrome (ARDS).

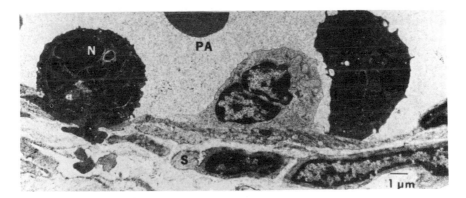

FIG. 23–3. Transmission electron micrograph of leukocytes adhering to the endothelium of a pulmonary arteriole (PA). N = neutrophil; S = smooth muscle (From Albertine KH. Ultrastructural abnormalities in increased-permeability edema. Clin Chest Med 1985; 6:345–370.)

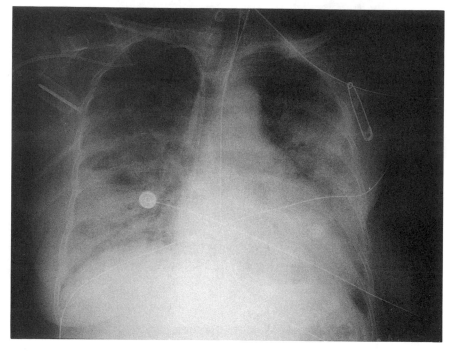

FIG. 23–4. Portable chest x-ray of a 46-year-old female with dyspnea. Is this hydrostatic pulmonary edema or adult respiratory distress syndrome? See text for details.

while the chest x-ray may show remarkably few changes.[9] The hypoxemia is particularly refractory to oxygen and the inspired oxygen requirement usually rises rapidly. The chest x-ray eventually begins to show diffuse infiltration and progresses rapidly over the next 24 to 48 hours to look like the chest film shown in Figure 23–4. The patients usually require ventilatory assistance within the first 48 hours of the illness.

DIAGNOSTIC APPROACH

The diagnostic approach to patients with diffuse pulmonary infiltrates is usually aimed at differentiating acute left heart failure from ARDS. As shown in the following sections, this may not be a simple task.

PHYSICAL EXAM

Physical findings are often non-specific in patients with diffuse pulmonary infiltrates. Rales will not differentiate inflammation from edema and neck vein distension or peripheral edema will not differentiate primary heart failure from ARDS with pulmonary hypertension. The lim-

TABLE 23–1. CLINICAL FEATURES OF THE PULMONARY EDEMA SYNDROMES		
Feature	Leaky-Capillary Edema	Hydrostatic Edema
Hypoxemia	Early	Late
Radiographic Appearance	Diffuse infiltrates, Peripheral prominence, No Kerley B lines, Clear lung bases	Patchy infiltrates, Perihilar prominence, Kerley B lines, Obscured lung bases
PCWP	< COP	> COP
Protein Ratio (Edema/Serum)	> 0.7	< 0.5
Clinical Setting	Sepsis, Trauma, Multiple organ failure	Acute MI, Severe hypertension, Renal failure

ited value of the physical exam is shown by a clinical study where physicians were correct in the diagnosis of diffuse pulmonary infiltrates only 40% of the time when the physical exam was the sole diagnostic test.[13]

DEGREE OF HYPOXEMIA

The severity of the hypoxemia can sometimes help to differentiate hydrostatic edema from ARDS. Unlike the severe, refractory hypoxemia of early ARDS, the hypoxemia from cardiogenic pulmonary edema is usually mild until the final stages of the illness.[3] The following general rule can be applied to the diagnostic workup of diffuse pulmonary infiltrates.

In early ARDS, the hypoxemia is more pronounced than the chest x-ray abnormalities while in early cardiogenic edema, the chest x-ray abnormalities are more pronounced than the hypoxemia.

There will be exceptions to this rule but severe hypoxemia in the face of minor abnormalities on chest x-ray points to ARDS (or pulmonary embolism) as the most likely underlying process.

THE CHEST X-RAY

The radiographic features of ARDS and hydrostatic pulmonary edema are listed in Table 23–1 for comparison.[14–20]

The hallmark of ARDS is a diffuse pattern with peripheral predominance and clear lung bases. Hydrostatic edema shows perihilar predominance, Kerley's B lines, and obscured lung bases from pleural fluid.

Unfortunately, there is a great deal of overlap in the radiographic appearance of ARDS and hydrostatic pulmonary edema. This is illustrated in the chest x-rays in Figures 23–4 and 23–5. The chest film in Figure 23–4 shows characteristic features of ARDS (peripheral infiltrates

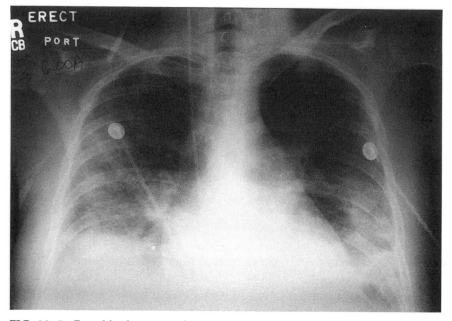

FIG. 23–5. Portable chest x-ray from a 36-year-old female with fever. The patient expired 3 days after this film was obtained. See text for explanations.

and clear lung bases) but this x-ray represents acute left heart failure. This patient was a 46-year-old female who presented to the emergency room with acute onset of dyspnea and an ECG with ST elevations in the anterior precordial leads. The diagnosis of acute myocardial infarction was subsequently confirmed by serial enzyme analysis. Pulmonary artery catheterization revealed a wedge pressure of 26 mmHg, confirming the diagnosis of hydrostatic pulmonary edema.

The chest film in Figure 23–5 has many of the features of cardiogenic pulmonary edema because of the basilar prominence of the infiltrates and the obscured lung bases. This patient was a 36-year-old female with a history of alcohol-related cirrhosis and ascites who was admitted with fever but no pulmonary symptoms. A pulmonary artery catheter revealed a pulmonary capillary wedge pressure of 12 mmHg and the measured serum colloid osmotic pressure was also 12 mmHg. Cultures of blood and peritoneal fluid grew *Escherichia coli* and the diagnosis of spontaneous bacterial peritonitis was considered. Despite adequate antibiotics by in vitro sensitivities, the patient became gradually worse after admission and died in refractory shock 3 days after the chest film in Figure 23–5 was obtained. Final diagnosis was sepsis with multiorgan failure and ARDS.

These two films point to the problems that can arise when you rely too heavily on the radiographic appearance of the chest x-ray to determine the etiology of diffuse pulmonary infiltrates.

CLINICAL SETTING

The clinical setting may be the single most predictive factor in the early stages of the evaluation. Look for the following conditions that would predispose the patient to ARDS:

1. Recent trauma, surgery, drugs, or blood transfusion
2. Sepsis from any site (look at the abdomen closely)
3. Gastric aspiration
4. Ileus, elevated liver enzymes, or rising creatinine
5. Pancreatitis

The sepsis may be occult and septicemia can be absent in over half the cases.[13] Occult sepsis syndrome can originate in the abdomen, particularly the bowel (translocation) and the biliary tree (acalculous cholecystitis). Acute MI with pulmonary edema does not ensure that hydrostatic edema is the culprit because acute MI has been reported to cause high permeability pulmonary edema.[15]

INVASIVE HEMODYNAMICS

The standard method for distinguishing ARDS from hydrostatic edema involves measuring the pulmonary capillary wedge pressure with a pulmonary artery catheter. Remember to use the "adjusted wedge pressure" (Pc), as discussed in Chapter 10:

$$Pc = PCWP + 0.4 (Pa - PCWP)$$

This adjustment is of little consequence in normal patients but there can be a wide discrepancy between PCWP and Pc in patients with severe ARDS and pulmonary hypertension. As shown in Chapter 10, the Pc can be twice the PCWP in severe ARDS.

The **colloid osmotic pressure** of the plasma should be measured or calculated in every patient because the average COP may be as low as 10 mmHg in ICU patients.[6] The COP can be particularly low in sepsis and other conditions that are associated with ARDS. **Although low COP alone does not produce pulmonary edema, a low COP will reduce the threshold for hydrostatic edema.**[5] This means that a wedge pressure of 15 mmHg with pulmonary edema will be called ARDS but if the COP is 12 mmHg, the diagnosis will change to hydrostatic edema (although both conditions can coexist).

The following rules are reasonable statements regarding the etiology of diffuse pulmonary infiltrates.[6]

1. If the PCWP is in the normal range (12 mmHg) and is at least 4 mmHg below the COP, the likely diagnosis is ARDS.

2. If the PCWP is greater than or equal to COP, hydrostatic edema is likely. However, high permeability edema cannot be ruled out as an additional problem.

RADIONUCLIDE SCANS

Labeled tracers and white cells have been used to identify the capillary leak in high permeability edema.[23] When the pulmonary capillaries are intact, the tracer stays in the vascular space and the activity over the heart and lungs is equivalent. When the pulmonary capillaries are damaged, the tracer passes into the lung parenchyma and the activity recorded over the lungs (activity in blood plus in lung parenchyma) will be greater than the activity over the heart (activity in blood only). The isotope method is unpopular at present, possibly because of the inconvenience of moving patients from the ICU to perform the test.

EDEMA FLUID PROTEIN

When edema fluid appears in the upper airways, the protein concentration in the fluid can be used to identify the underlying process. A serum protein level must be measured at the same time to determine the ratio of the protein in edema fluid to the serum protein. The following criteria have been suggested:[24]

Protein (edema/serum) < 0.5: Hydrostatic Edema

> 0.7: ARDS

This is the method I prefer because it can be done at the bedside with little risk or cost to the patient. The only shortcoming is the need for pure edema fluid in the upper airways uncontaminated by respiratory secretions. At least 3 ml of edema fluid is recommended for analysis.[24]

NORMAL CAPILLARY LEAK?

The high levels of protein in edema fluid from hydrostatic pulmonary edema (ratio up to 0.7 comparing edema protein to serum protein) is an interesting finding. This points to the fact that considerable amounts of protein cross the pulmonary capillaries normally. The pulmonary microcirculation is considered to be more leaky than other capillary beds, but the lymphatics in the lung are capable of clearing the fluid effectively. This creates some doubt about the characterization of an illness as having leaky capillaries (like ARDS) and also emphasizes the value of limiting any maneuvers that would decrease or impede lymphatic drainage from the lung (like positive-pressure ventilation).

MANAGEMENT GOALS IN ARDS

There are several experimental therapies under investigation for ARDS, including an investigation of antioxidant therapy that we are

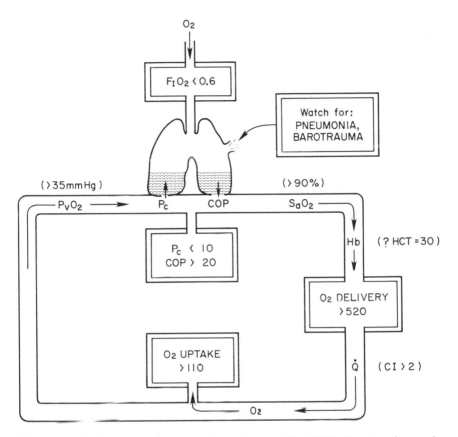

FIG. 23-6. Goals of management for patients with ARDS. See text for explanation. Oxygen delivery and oxygen uptake are expressed in ml/min/m². Pc and COP are expressed in mmHg.

conducting (Crit Care Med 1989; *17*:S153). However, at the present time, there is no therapy considered effective for reversing the capillary damage in ARDS. Management of these patients is based on the principles of edema formation and oxygen transport and can be applied to any patient with acute respiratory failure.

The specific goals of management for ARDS are illustrated in Figure 23-6. Four goals are identified.

1. Reduce edema
2. Maintain tissue oxygenation

3. Prevent oxygen toxicity
4. Prevent adverse occurrences

REDUCING LUNG WATER

As shown in Figure 23–1, an increase in capillary permeability will magnify the influence of capillary hydrostatic pressure (Pc) on fluid accumulation in the lung. Therefore, the strategy for reducing pulmonary edema is to decrease the Pc to as low a level as possible without compromising left ventricular filling and to maintain the colloid osmotic pressure (COP) in the normal range.

Diuretics. Diuretic therapy should be ideal for reducing edema because diuresis will decrease intravascular volume (decrease Pc) and will also concentrate the plasma proteins (increase COP). These two effects will optimize the forces that limit edema formation. However,

> Diuretic therapy has not proven effective for reducing the lung water in ARDS.[23]

This is not surprising because the infiltrates in ARDS are not the watery edema of heart failure but are dense collections of inflammatory cells. In other words, **ARDS is an acute inflammation of the lung and diuretics are not designed to reduce inflammation.** Intravenous furosemide can improve gas exchange in ARDS without decreasing lung water or producing a diuresis.[24] The mechanism may be an increase in pulmonary blood flow to better ventilated lung units. However, aggressive diuretic therapy with furosemide can be hazardous in patients with pulmonary hypertension by reducing the output of the right side of the heart[25] and diuretic therapy must be monitored carefully in patients with ARDS and pulmonary hypertension.

Other therapies aimed at reducing lung water, like the infusion of concentrated albumin, have not been successful.[26]

MAINTAINING TISSUE OXYGENATION

The ultimate goal in respiratory failure from any cause is to maintain oxygen delivery to metabolizing tissues. As mentioned in Chapter 15:

> Peripheral oxygen uptake ($\dot{V}O_2$) varies directly with changes in oxygen delivery ($\dot{D}O_2$) in ARDS[27] which means that the components of the $\dot{D}O_2$ (particularly the cardiac output) can be manipulated as a means of improving $\dot{V}O_2$ if necessary.

The management goals in Figure 23–6 show a $\dot{D}O_2$ above 520 ml/min/m² and a $\dot{V}O_2$ above 110 ml/min/m² as end-points but, as discussed in Chapter 15, supranormal levels of $\dot{D}O_2$ and $\dot{V}O_2$ may be necessary in patients who are hypermetabolic (see Table 15–1). Therefore, the optimal $\dot{D}O_2$ and $\dot{V}O_2$ must be determined for each individual patient. Serum lactate levels can be used to determine optimal values for oxygen transport in each patient.

The determinants of O_2 delivery ($\dot{D}O_2$) are the cardiac output ($\dot{Q}$), hemoglobin (Hb) and arterial O_2 saturation (SaO_2).

$$\dot{D}O_2 = \dot{Q} \times (1.3 \times Hb \times SaO_2) \text{ ml/min/m}^2$$

Although an increase in any one of these three variables will increase the $\dot{D}O_2$, they differ in their ability to increase the $\dot{V}O_2$ at the tissue level. The cardiac output has the greatest influence on the $\dot{V}O_2$ (see Fig. 13–5).

Cardiac Output. The cardiac output is often high in ARDS but if cardiac output is lower than satisfactory levels, intravenous **dobutamine** is an effective agent for increasing forward flow.[23] The usual dose is between 5 and 15 mcg/kg/min (see Chapter 20 for full dosing information on dobutamine). Avoid dopamine at moderate or high doses (above 10 mcg/kg/min) because it can constrict the pulmonary veins and increase the PCWP.[22,26] Also avoid vasodilators whenever possible because they can aggravate hypoxemia by increasing intrapulmonary shunt (hydralazine is an exception).

Blood Transfusion. Transfusion is often recommended to keep the Hb above 10 gm/dL but, as discussed in Chapter 13 and illustrated in Figure 13–5, **there is no evidence that blood transfusion improves tissue oxygenation.**[25] In fact, packed red cells can decrease cardiac output and increase intrapulmonary shunt,[4,11] because of the high viscosity of packed cells. Furthermore, the iron load from blood products can increase the production of toxic oxygen radicals in the lung, and this is not a desired endpoint in ARDS.

Arterial O_2 Saturation. The SaO_2 is usually kept above 90% to stay away from the bend in the oxyhemoglobin dissociation curve. Once the SaO_2 is on the flat part of the curve, there is little need to increase it further with supplemental oxygen.

PREVENTING O_2 TOXICITY

The fractional concentration of inspired oxygen (FIO_2) should be kept as low as possible or at least below 60%, to minimize the risk for oxygen toxicity. The SaO_2 is the measure of arterial oxygenation to monitor instead of the arterial PO_2 because the SaO_2 determines the oxygen content in arterial blood. An SaO_2 above 90% should be sufficient to maintain oxygen delivery to peripheral tissues. If the FIO_2 cannot be reduced to below 60%, external PEEP can be added to help reduce the FIO_2 to nontoxic levels. The topic of oxygen toxicity is presented in Chapter 25.

SPECIAL CONSIDERATIONS

Positive End-Expiratory Pressure. The major point to emphasize here is that **PEEP is not a therapy for ARDS** but it is simply a method for lowering the FIO_2 to safe levels when necessary. This is discussed in Chapter 28 but a few relevant points are listed below.

1. Application of PEEP to high-risk patients does not reduce the incidence of ARDS.[32]

2. PEEP does not decrease lung water in ARDS.[33] In fact, high levels of PEEP can increase lung water![30] The mechanism behind the latter effect may be a decrease in lymphatic drainage from the chest.

The observations above do not support the routine use of PEEP as a prophylactic or a therapeutic measure in ARDS. The use of PEEP should be reserved only for patients who require a toxic level of inspired oxygen.

Steroids. High-dose steroids were suggested to help diminish the inflammatory response in the lungs but recent studies are not supportive.

1. A multicenter trial of 99 patients randomized to receive either methylprednisolone (30 mg/kg every 6 hours for 4 doses) or placebo reported no difference between the steroid group and the control group in either mortality or the reversal of the ARDS.[34]

2. High-dose methylprednisolone given prophylactically to patients with septic shock did not decrease the incidence of ARDS.[35]

3. High-dose steroids for 24 hours have been associated with an increased incidence of secondary infections.[36]

As a result of these studies, steroid therapy is no longer recommended for ARDS and steroid use is being discouraged because of the possible risk for secondary infection.

REFERENCES

GENERAL WORKS

1. Fishman AP, Renkin EM eds. Pulmonary edema. Bethesda: American Physiological Society, 1979.
2. Klein EF ed. Acute respiratory failure. Probl Crit Care 1987; 1:345–524.
3. Weidemann HP, Matthay MA, Matthay RA eds. Acute lung injury. Crit Care Clin 1986; 2:377–667.

APPLIED PHYSIOLOGY

4. Michel CC. Fluid movement through capillary walls. In: Renkin EM, Michel CC, Geiger SR eds. The cardiovascular system. Vol 4. Microcirculation, Part 1. The Handbook of Physiology. Bethesda: American Physiological Society, 1984:375–410.
5. Staub NC. "State of the art" review. Pathogenesis of pulmonary edema. Am Rev Respir Dis 1974; 109:358–372.
6. Weil MH, Henning RJ. Colloid osmotic pressure. Significance, methods of measurement, and interpretation. In: Weil MH, Henning RJ eds. Handbook of critical care medicine. Chicago: Year Book Medical Publishers, 1979:73–81.
7. Allen SJ, Drake RE, Williams JP, et al. Recent advances in pulmonary edema. Crit Care Med 1987; 15:963–970.
8. Bernard GR, Brigham KL. Pulmonary edema. Pathophysiologic mechanisms and new approaches to therapy. Chest 1986; 89:594–600.
9. Sprung CL, Isikoff SK, Hauser M, Eisler BR. Comparison of measured and calculated colloid osmotic pressure of serum and pulmonary edema fluid in patients with pulmonary edema. Crit Care Med 1980; 8:613–615.

10. Klancke KA, Assey ME, Kratz JM, Crawford FA. Postoperative pulmonary edema in postcoronary artery bypass patients. Chest 1983; *84*:529–534.

ADULT RESPIRATORY DISTRESS SYNDROME

11. Ashbaugh DG, Bigelow DB, Petty TL, et al. Acute respiratory distress in adults. Lancet 1967; *2*:319–323.
12. Matthay MA. The adult respiratory distress syndrome. New insights into diagnosis, pathophysiology, and treatment. West J Med 1989; *150*:187–194.
13. Pepe PE. The clinical entity of adult respiratory distress syndrome. Crit Care Clin 1986; *2*:377–404.

CLINICAL DISTINCTIONS

14. Sibbald WJ, Cunningham DR, Chin DN. Non-cardiac or cardiac pulmonary edema? Chest 1983; *84*:452–461.
15. Richeson JF, Paulshock C, Yu PN. Non-hydrostatic pulmonary edema after coronary artery ligation in dogs. Circ Res 1980; *50*:301–309.
16. Connors AF, McCaffree DR, Gray BA. Evaluation of right heart catheterization in the critically ill patient without myocardial infarction. N Engl J Med 1983; *308*:263–267.
17. Sivak ED, Richmond BJ, O'Donovan PB, Borkowski GP. Value of extravascular lung water measurement vs. portable chest x-ray in the management of pulmonary edema. Crit Care Med 1983; *11*:498–501.
18. Halperin BD, Feeley TW, Mihm FG, et al. Evaluation of the portable chest roentgenogram for quantitating extravascular lung water in critically ill adults. Chest 1985; *88*:649–652.
19. Miniati M, Pistolesi M, Milne E, Giuntini C. Detection of lung edema. Crit Care Med 1987; *15*:1146–1155.
20. Zimmerman JE, Goodman LR, Shahvari MBG. Effect of mechanical ventilation and positive end-expiratory pressure (PEEP) on chest radiograph. Am J Radiol 1979; *133*:811–815.
21. Sugerman HJ, Strash AM, Hirsch JI, et al. Sensitivity of scintigraphy for detection of pulmonary capillary albumin leak in canine oleic acid ARDS. J Trauma 1981; *21*:520–527.
22. Sprung CL, Long Wm, Marcial EH, et al. Distribution of proteins in pulmonary edema. The value of fractional concentrations. Am Rev Respir Dis 1987; *136*:957–963.

MANAGEMENT

23. Broaddus VC, Berthiaume Y, Biondi JW, et al. Hemodynamic management of the adult respiratory distress syndrome. J Intensive Care Med 1987; *2*:190–213.
24. Ali J, Unruh H, Skoog C, Goldberg HS. The effect of lung edema on vasoreactivity of furosemide. J Surg Res 1983; *35*:383–390.
25. Mathur PN, Pugsley SO, Powles P, et al. Effect of diuretics on cardiopulmonary performance in severe chronic airflow obstruction. Arch Intern Med 1984; *144*:2154–2157.
26. Jing DL, Kohler JP, Rice CL, et al. Albumin therapy in permeability pulmonary edema. J Surg Res 1982; *33*:482–488.
27. Kariman K, Burns S. Regulation of tissue oxygen extraction is disturbed in adult respiratory distress syndrome. Am Rev Respir Dis 1985; *132*:109–114.

28. Conrad SA, Dietrich KA, Hebert CA, et al. Cardiopulmonary response to red blood cell transfusion in critically ill non-surgical patients. Crit Care Med 1989; 17:s20.

29. Molloy DW, Ducas J, Dobson K, et al. Hemodynamic management in clinical acute hypoxemic respiratory failure: dopamine vs dobutamine. Chest 1986; 89:636–640.

30. Demling RH, Staub NC, Edmunds LH. Effect of end-expiratory pressure on accumulation of extravascular lung water. J Appl Physiol 1975; 38:907–912.

31. Andrews CP, Coalson JJ, Smith JD, et al. Diagnosis of nosocomial bacterial pneumonia in acute diffuse lung injury. Chest 1980; 80:254–258.

32. Pepe PE, Hudson LD, Carrico J. Early application of positive end-expiratory pressure in patients at risk from the adult respiratory distress syndrome. N Engl J Med 1984; 311:281–286.

33. Helbert C, Paskanik A, Bredenberg CE. Effect of positive end-expiratory pressure on lung water in pulmonary edema caused by increased membrane permeability. Ann Thorac Surg 1984; 36:42–48.

34. Bernard GR, Luce JM, Sprung CL, et al. High-dose corticosteroids in patients with adult respiratory distress syndrome. N Engl J Med 1987; 31:1565–1570.

35. Luce JM, Montgomery AB, Marks JD, et al. Ineffectiveness of high-dose methylprednisolone in preventing parenchymal lung injury and improving mortality in patients with septic shock. Am Rev Respir Dis 1988; 138:62–68.

36. Bone RC, Fischer CJ Jr., Clemmer TP, et al. A controlled trial of high-dose methylprednisolone in the treatment of severe sepsis and septic shock. N Engl J Med 1987; 317:653–658.

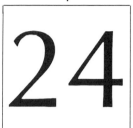

chapter

24

NONINVASIVE BLOOD GAS MONITORING

Several methods are now available for the noninvasive assessment of arterial blood gases. Although each has its own limitations, the developments in this field are the most useful advances in critical care monitoring in the last decade. Three methods are presented: oximetry, capnography, and transcutaneous blood gas monitoring.

OXIMETRY

Oximetry is an optical method for measuring oxygenated hemoglobin in blood. Ear oximeters were introduced in the early 1970s but it was not until lightweight "pulse" oximeters were introduced in the early 1980s that the methodology was considered acceptable. The popularity of pulse oximetry has grown so rapidly that, in 1987, the American Society of Anesthesiology recommended pulse oximetry as the standard of care for every patient receiving general anesthesia.[1]

PRINCIPLE

Oximetry is based on the ability of different forms of hemoglobin to absorb light of different wavelengths. Oxygenated hemoglobin (HbO_2) absorbs light in the red spectrum (hence the red color of oxygenated blood) and deoxygenated or reduced hemoglobin (RHb) absorbs light in the near-infrared spectrum. If a light beam composed of red and infrared wavelengths is passed through a blood vessel (Fig. 24–1), the transmission of each wavelength will be inversely proportional to the concentration of HbO_2 and RHb in the blood. The oxygen saturation

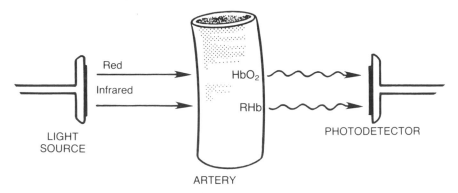

FIG. 24–1. The principle of pulse oximetry. See text for explanation.

(So_2) is then calculated as the ratio of HbO_2 to total Hb (HbO_2 plus RHb) in the sample:

$$So_2(\%) = \left(\frac{HbO_2}{HbO_2 + RHb} \right) \times 100$$

This calculation uses only two forms of hemoglobin and neglects methemoglobin and carboxyhemoglobin. The oximeters for in vitro use have four wavelengths of light and can detect all four forms of hemoglobin. The surface oximeters for continuous on-line monitoring have only two wavelengths of light and will miss methemoglobinemia and carboxyhemoglobinemia. However, these conditions are uncommon enough to justify the use of two wavelengths in most patients.

PULSE OXIMETRY

The original oximeters suffered from two limitations.[3] The first was interference from light absorption by pigments (e.g., bilirubin) and other tissue elements. The second and more formidable problem was the inability to differentiate hemoglobin in the arteries from that in veins. These problems were reduced or eliminated by oximeters that measure light transmission through pulsatile vessels only; these "pulse" oximeters are the major advance of the decade in ICU monitoring.

The principle of pulse oximetry is demonstrated in Figure 24–1. Arterial pulsations are caused by fluctuations in blood volume and these volume changes will cause fluctuations in light transmission. The photodetectors in pulse oximeters can sense an alternating light input from arterial pulsations and a steady light input from veins and other nonpulsatile elements. Only the alternating light input is selected for analysis (analogous to an AC amplifier) and this eliminates any contribution from the veins or any other nonpulsatile elements in the intervening tissue. This explains why pulse oximeters are not influenced by tissue thickness or pigments (including nail polish).

Accuracy. Pulse oximetry has been remarkably accurate in published reports.[1,2] Accuracy is reported to within 2 or 3% (standard deviation) of the oxyhemoglobin levels measured in vitro with multiwavelength oximeters.[1,2] The only requirement for accuracy is a patient who is not hemodynamically compromised and an arterial oxygen saturation (SaO_2) above 70%. Accuracy at SaO_2 levels below 70% is variable[4] but this range will not be encountered often (primarily because severe hypoxemia would not be allowed to continue).

Indications. The indications for pulse oximetry will be determined by the availability of oximeters because virtually every patient who requires supplemental oxygen could benefit from continuous monitoring with pulse oximetry unless they are hypotensive or have some other condition that could reduce the accuracy of the readings.

Limitations. The major limitation of pulse oximetry is the insensitivity of the arterial O_2 saturation for detecting changes in pulmonary gas exchange. This is due to the shape of the oxyhemoglobin dissociation curve (see next chapter, Figure 25–1). When the SaO_2 exceeds 90% and the PaO_2 is above 60 mmHg, the curve is flat and the arterial PO_2 can change considerably with little change in arterial SO_2. This means that the SaO_2 will be inadequate for sensing early changes in pulmonary gas exchange in the lungs. However, the significance of this limitation is not clear.

TRANSCUTANEOUS PO_2

Transcutaneous PO_2 electrodes were introduced in the early 1970s for neonates and have proven reliable for this population. However, the reliability in adults is variable and this has limited their popularity in adults. There is some recent interest in the use of transcutaneous oxygen electrodes for monitoring blood flow to the extremities but the experience is limited at present.

METHODOLOGY

Transcutaneous oxygen electrodes are designed to measure the PO_2 in the dermal capillary network just under the epidermis. The electrode itself is a miniaturized version of the Clark polarographic electrode (the one used for arterial blood gas measurements) that is secured to the skin surface with an adhesive ring. A heating element surrounds the electrode and is used to maintain the temperature of the underlying skin at 44° to 45°C. This improves the diffusion of oxygen across the epidermis and improves the accuracy of the measurement in adults (neonates have a thin epidermis and do not require surface heating). The electrodes are usually placed in the upper anterior thorax or the upper arms, where dermal blood flow is high. Electrode position must be changed every 4 hours to reduce any risk of burning the underlying skin.

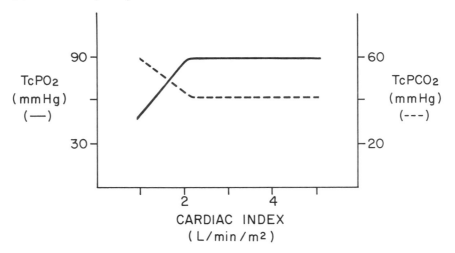

FIG. 24–2. The influence of cardiac output on transcutaneous blood gas measurements. Oxygen curve from Tremper KK, et al. Continuous transcutaneous oxygen monitoring during respiratory failure, cardiac decompensation, cardiac arrest, and CPR. Crit Care Med 1980; 8:377–381. Carbon dioxide curve from Tremper KK, et al. Effect of hypercarbia and shock on transcutaneous carbon dioxide at different electrode temperatures. Crit Care Med 1980; 8:608–612.

ACCURACY

The accuracy of transcutaneous P_{O_2} (TcP_{O_2}) is determined by the adequacy of the peripheral blood flow. When flow is normal, TcP_{O_2} is a reasonably reliable measure of Pa_{O_2}.[5,6] However, when flow to the periphery decreases, TcP_{O_2} can underestimate the arterial P_{O_2} (Pa_{O_2}). The influence of cardiac output on TcP_{O_2} is shown in Figure 24–2.[6] The TcP_{O_2} is independent of the cardiac index until the cardiac index falls to below 2 L/min/m² and then the TcP_{O_2} varies directly with the cardiac index.[6] At low flowrates, TcP_{O_2} may be a closer measure of the venous P_{O_2} than the arterial P_{O_2} because venous blood will dominate the underlying vessels when arterial inflow is reduced.

MONITORING BLOOD FLOW

The flow dependence of TcP_{O_2} has created another application for TcP_{O_2} as a means of assessing the adequacy of blood flow to a limb following trauma or arterial reconstruction surgery.[7] Figure 24–3 illustrates the use of TcP_{O_2} to monitor blood flow to the lower extremity. The tracing in the figure was recorded from an oxygen electrode placed on the left foot (dorsum) of a volunteer with no history of peripheral vascular disease. The femoral artery on the ipsilateral side was then occluded by applying pressure to the groin area. As indicated between the arrows, the TcP_{O_2} quickly fell during the period of arterial compression and returned to control levels when the compression was re-

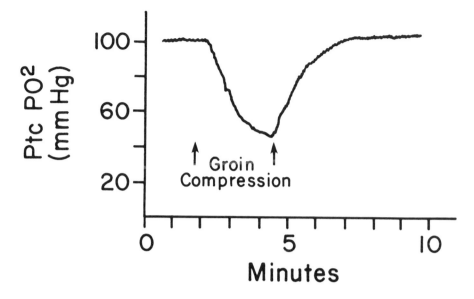

FIG. 24–3. Transcutaneous Po_2 during manual compression of a femoral artery. Oxygen electrode on dorsum of the foot.

leased. If another electrode had been placed in a control area, the limb TcPO₂ could have provided a marker of reduced blood flow.

CONJUNCTIVAL Po_2

The technique of monitoring conjunctival Po_2 takes advantage of the characteristics of the epithelium in this region.

PRINCIPLE

The adult skin is not the ideal monitoring surface because it is thick and relatively impermeable to oxygen unless heated artificially. The palpebral conjunctiva does not have these problems. The epithelial layer here is only 2 to 4 cells thick and the underlying capillary network is dense. Therefore, there is little or no gradient for O_2 diffusion across the epidermis and surface heating is not necessary. In addition, conjunctival Po_2 levels should reflect the Po_2 in the internal carotid artery, thereby providing an index of oxygen delivery to the central nervous system.

METHODOLOGY

The proposed advantages of conjunctival P_{O_2} has led to the development of a plastic eyepiece that contains a miniaturized Clark electrode.[8] The eyepiece is contoured to the surface of the eye, and contains a central opening to prevent damage to the cornea. The eyepiece is available for use in humans.

ACCURACY

Conjunctival P_{O_2} is an accurate reflection of arterial P_{O_2} in patients with normal cardiac output.[8] However, when cardiac output or peripheral oxygen delivery are diminished, the conjunctival P_{O_2} will decrease relative to arterial P_{O_2} (like the TcP_{O_2}).

TRANSCUTANEOUS P_{CO_2}

The principles and limitations of transcutaneous P_{CO_2} (TcP_{CO_2}) measurements are similar to those mentioned for TcP_{O_2}, in that accuracy is affected by age (being most accurate in neonates), skin thickness, and hemodynamic status. Heating the underlying skin has improved the accuracy of TcP_{CO_2} in adults by promoting CO_2 diffusion through the epidermis.[10]

METHODOLOGY

There are two types of cutaneous CO_2 electrodes. One measures P_{CO_2} by monitoring the change in pH of a bicarbonate-containing solution in contact with the skin (which is the electrode design used in blood gas machines). The other electrode uses infrared absorption through a gas collection chamber in contact with the skin.[8] Both electrodes use a heating element to improve accuracy and reduce response time.

ACCURACY

In adult subjects with a normal cardiac output and blood pressure, TcP_{CO_2} can provide a reasonably reliable measure of arterial P_{CO_2}.[9] However, when cardiac output is abnormally low, the TcP_{CO_2} increases relative to the Pa_{CO_2}. This is shown in Figure 24–2. The change in TcP_{CO_2} with reduced flow is opposite to the change in the TcP_{O_2} and is attributed to the decrease in CO_2 washout that occurs in low flow states. Because of this discrepancy, TcP_{CO_2} is presently not a popular method for noninvasive blood gas monitoring.

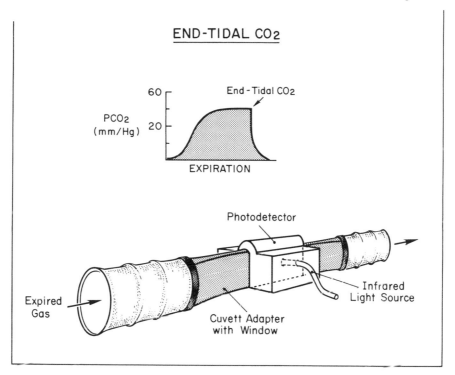

FIG. 24–4. Infrared device for monitoring CO_2 in exhaled gas. The graph is a schematic representation of the change in P_{CO_2} during exhalation. See text for details.

END-TIDAL CO_2

The carbon dioxide in exhaled gas can be used as a noninvasive measure of the arterial P_{CO_2} (Pa_{CO_2}) in select patients with tracheal tubes in place.[11,12]

PRINCIPLE

The normal pattern of CO_2 elimination in exhaled gas is illustrated in Figure 24–4. At the onset of expiration, the gas occupying the anatomic dead space in the upper airways is first to leave the lungs and the P_{CO_2} at the start of expiration is negligible. As expiration continues, alveolar gas begins to appear in the upper airways and the exhaled P_{CO_2} begins to rise. The P_{CO_2} rises steadily throughout expiration until it reaches a plateau near the end of expiration and then remains constant (or nearly so) until the onset of the next inspiration. When lung function is normal, the exhaled P_{CO_2} at the very end of expiration (called end-tidal CO_2 or ET_{CO_2}) is equivalent to the P_{CO_2} in end-capillary (arterial) blood.

METHODOLOGY

Infrared CO_2 analysers are placed in the path of exhalation, as shown in Figure 24–4. A light-emitting diode on one side of the electrode shines an infrared light beam across the exhaled gas and a phodetector diode on the other side measures the intensity of light transmission. These probes have a fast response and do not interfere in any way with gas flow.

THE Paco₂-ETco₂ RELATIONSHIP

Normally, the arterial PCO_2 and the end-tidal PCO_2 are within a few mmHg of each other.[11] In cardiopulmonary disorders, the $ETCO_2$ decreases relative to the arterial PCO_2. The following conditions are classified by the change in the $PaCO_2$-$ETCO_2$ gradient.

High Paco₂-ETco₂ Gradient. In this situation, the alveolar units with a high VD/VT are underperfused and the transfer of CO_2 from the pulmonary capillaries to the alveoli is impaired. This results in a decrease in exhaled PCO_2 relative to arterial PCO_2. The following situations can be the source of the problem:[10]

1. Low cardiac output
2. Excessive lung inflation (from PEEP)
3. High physiologic dead space (e.g., COPD)

Reverse Paco₂-ETco₂ Gradient. It is uncommon for the $ETCO_2$ to exceed the $PaCO_2$, but the following conditions can produce this situation:[11]

1. Excessive CO_2 production when inspiratory volumes are low
2. Alveoli that are overperfused
3. When high inspired oxygen levels are used CO_2 will be released from hemoglobin as it becomes saturated with oxygen

Since there are several factors that can influence the relationship between $ETCO_2$ and $PaCO_2$, it is wise to obtain arterial blood gases periodically to determine the accuracy of $ETCO_2$.

CLINICAL APPLICATIONS

The following applications for $ETCO_2$ have proven or potential value.

Ventilator Mishaps. The $ETCO_2$ monitors are equipped with alarms that can serve as a backup alarm system for the ventilators. A sudden drop in $ETCO_2$ can be a signal of patient disconnect or some other leak in the ventilator tubing system.[13]

Nosocomial Complications. There are several complications associated with prolonged mechanical ventilation and changes in $ETCO_2$ can be an early sign of these complications. A sudden drop in $ETCO_2$ associated with an increase in $PaCO_2$-$ETCO_2$ gradient is seen in acute pulmonary embolism, atelectasis, pneumonia, sepsis, and adult respiratory distress syndrome. Anxiety and nonpulmonary causes of agitation can decrease the $ETCO_2$ but should not change the $PaCO_2$-$ETCO_2$ gradient.

Postoperative Shivering. $ETCO_2$ can be valuable for monitoring patients in the immediate postoperative period following cardiopulmonary by-pass surgery. Shivering during the rewarming period can cause a com-bined respiratory acidosis and metabolic acidosis that can be severe and even life threatening. The respiratory acidosis is caused by increased CO_2 production in the face of poor ventilatory responsiveness because of residual anesthesia. The metabolic acidosis is caused by lactate pro-duction by skeletal muscle. Both processes will increase $ETCO_2$ and a sudden rise in $ETCO_2$ can herald the onset of problems and can prompt measures to correct the problem (e.g., paralysis or increased minute ventilation from the ventilator). The $ETCO_2$ is then used to gauge the efficacy of the corrective maneuvers.

Weaning. $ETCO_2$ can be valuable for monitoring patients during wean-ing from mechanical ventilation.[14] An increase in ETO_2 during the wean period may be an early sign of failure to wean. A constant $ETCO_2$ in the face of a rising minute ventilation can also be a sign of a failing wean. In this situation, the inability to decrease exhaled CO_2 as ventilation increases can be used as a sign of respiratory insufficiency (see Chapter 30).

Controlled Hyperventilation. $ETCO_2$ monitoring can help to maintain the desired level of hyperventilation for head injury patients or for any situation where hyperventilation is desired for control of intracranial pressure. The $PaCO_2$-$ETCO_2$ difference must be checked periodically in this setting and the gradient is used to select the $ETCO_2$ to maintain.

Cardiopulmonary Resuscitation. One of the recent applications of $ETCO_2$ has been to monitor the effectiveness of closed chest cardiac massage. The $ETCO_2$ will decrease as pulmonary blood flow decreases so $ETCO_2$ can be used as a noninasive index of blood flow during CPR. One study reported that no patient with an $ETCO_2$ less than 10 mmHg during the resuscitation went on to survive.[15] This application has several important implications and further studies are awaited.

BIBLIOGRAPHY

Payne JP, Severinghaus JW eds. Pulse oximetry. Berlin: Springer-Verlag, 1986.
Tremper KK, Barker SJ eds. Advances in Oxygen Monitoring. International Anesthesiology Clinics Vol 25, No. 3. Boston: Little, Brown and Company, 1987.

REFERENCES

OXIMETRY

1. Tremper KK, Barker SJ. Pulse oximetry. Anesthesiology 1989; 70:98–108.
2. Wukitsch MW, Petterson MT, Tobler DR, et al. Pulse oximetry: Analysis of theory, technology, and practice. J Clin Monit 1988; 4:290–301.

3. Chaudhary BA, Burki NK. Ear oximetry in clinical practice. Am Rev Respir Dis 1978; 17:173–175.
4. Sendak MJ, Harris AP, Donham RT. Accuracy of pulse oximetry during arterial oxyhemoglobin desaturation in dogs. Anesthesiology 1988; 68:111–114.

TRANSCUTANEOUS P_{O_2}

5. Tremper KK, Barker SJ. Transcutaneous oxygen measurement: Experimental studies and adult applications. Anesthesiol Clin 1987; 25:67–96.
6. Tremper KK, Waxman K, Bowman R, Shoemaker WC. Continuous transcutaneous oxygen monitoring during respiratory failure, cardiac decompensation, cardiac arrest, and CPR. Crit Care Med 1980: 8:377–381.
7. Moosa HH, Marakaroun MS, Peitzman AB, et al. TcP_{O_2} values in limb ischemia: Effects of blood flow and arterial oxygen tension. J Surg Res 1986; 40:482–487.

CONJUNCTIVAL P_{O_2}

8. Chapman KR, Liu FLW, Watson RM, Rebuck AS. Conjunctival oxygen tension and its relationship to arterial oxygen tension. J Clin Monit 1986; 2:100–104.

TRANSCUTANEOUS P_{CO_2}

9. Greenspan GH, Block AJ, Haldeman LW, Lindsey S, Martin CS. Transcutaneous noninvasive monitoring of carbon dioxide tension. Chest 1981; 80:422–446.
10. Tremper KK, Mentelos RA, Shoemaker WC. Effect of hypercarbia and shock on transcutaneous carbon dioxide at different electrode temperatures. Crit Care Med 1980; 8:608–612.

END-TIDAL CO_2

11. Snyder JV, Elliot L, Grenvik A. Capnography. Clin Crit Care Med 1982; 4:100–121.
12. Carlon GC, Ray C, Miodownik S, et al. Capnography in mechanically ventilated patients. Crit Care Med 1988; 16:550–556.
13. Murray IP, Modell JH. Early detection of endotracheal tube accidents by monitoring carbon dioxide concentration in respiratory gases. Anesthesiology 1983; 59:344–346.
14. Healey CJ, Fedullo AJ, Swinburne AJ, Wahl GW. Comparison of noninvasive measurements of carbon dioxide tension during withdrawal from mechanical ventilation. Crit Care Med 1987; 15:764–767.
15. Sanders AB, Kern KB, Otto CW, et al. End-tidal carbon dioxide monitoring during cardiopulmonary resuscitation. JAMA 1989; 262:1347–1351.

chapter

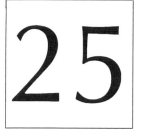

OXYGEN THERAPY

A moralist, at least, may say that the air which nature has provided for us is as good as we deserve.

Joseph Priestley

We have a peculiar relationship with oxygen because it is both a necessity and a danger.[1,2] As combustible engines, we rely on oxygen as an energy source to perform work. The problem is that the energy conversion process generates toxic byproducts. This creates a fine line for oxygen that separates necessity from harm. Priestley apparently realized this when he discovered the gas, as his statement intimates.

This chapter will present some practical aspects of oxygen therapy, including the indications and goals of oxygen therapy, the systems used to deliver oxygen, and the risks associated with concentrated mixtures of oxygen.

GOALS OF OXYGEN THERAPY

Virtually every patient in an ICU will receive supplemental oxygen, yet there are surprisingly few guidelines for oxygen therapy. In 1984, the American College of Chest Physicians and the National Heart, Lung, and Blood Institute published the following statement on the indications for oxygen therapy.[1]

"Supplemental oxygen therapy is *appropriate* in acute conditions when there is laboratory documentation of a Pa_{O_2} below 60 mmHg or when arterial saturation (Sa_{O_2}) is below 90%: tissue hypoxia is commonly *assumed* to be present at these laboratory values."

The uncertainty in this statement is shown in the words that are italicized (the italics are mine). "Appropriate" is used instead of "necessary" and "assumed" is chosen instead of "known". Now compare this statement with the conclusions of a clinical study reported 18 years before in the New England Journal of Medicine.[31]

"In the resting patient, even the most severe clinical hypoxemia due to pulmonary insufficiency does not itself lead to generalized tissue anaerobiasis . . . When present, anaerobic metabolism is related to a systemic *circulatory disorder*, with resultant inadequate tissue perfusion."

This study revealed that the arterial Po_2 could be as low as 22 mmHg without producing lactic acidosis as long as the cardiac output was maintained but when the cardiac output diminished, lactate promptly appeared. These results suggest that blood flow is the critical determinant of tissue oxygenation and that hemodynamic monitoring may be an integral part of monitoring the consequences of oxygen therapy.

OXYGEN CONTENT

As presented in Chapter 2, the content of oxygen in arterial blood (Cao_2) is determined by the serum hemoglobin concentration (Hb) and the percent saturation of hemoglobin with oxygen (Sao_2);

$$Cao_2 = (1.3 \times Hb \times Sao_2) + (0.003 \times Pao_2) \text{ ml/100 ml}$$

Note the small contribution made by the arterial Po_2 (Pao_2) to the total amount of oxygen in the blood. The Pao_2 is important only insofar as it influences the Sao_2. The relationship between the Pao_2 and the Sao_2 is defined by the oxyhemoglobin dissociation curve, which is shown in Figure 25–1. There is a linear relationship between Pao_2 and Sao_2 up to a Pao_2 of 60 mmHg and a Sao_2 of 90%. Above this level, the curve becomes flat, so that further increases in Pao_2 have little effect on the Sao_2. The shape of the curve has been used to recommend that the Sao_2 not be allowed to decline to 90% to stay away from the bend in the curve. Higher levels of inspired oxygen beyond this point will have little impact on oxygenation but can have serious adverse effects.

OXYGEN DELIVERY

An increase in arterial oxygenation during supplemental oxygen breathing does not ensure that tissue oxygenation is also improved because **oxygen breathing can depress myocardial function and decrease cardiac output.**[4] This is shown in the formula for oxygen delivery:

$$\overset{?}{} \qquad \overset{\downarrow}{} \qquad \overset{\uparrow}{} \qquad \overset{\uparrow\uparrow}{}$$

$$\text{Oxygen Delivery} = \dot{Q} \times (1.3 \times Hb \times Sao_2) + (.0031 \times Pao_2)$$

$$(\text{ml/min/m}^2)$$

The arrows indicate the direction and magnitude of change that could

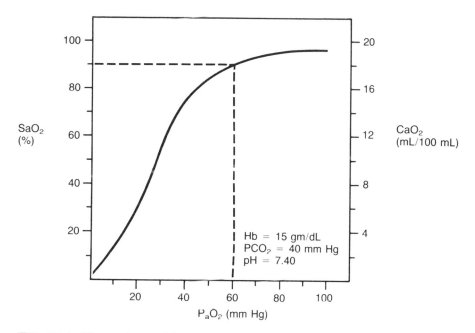

FIG. 25–1. The oxyhemoglobin dissociation curve. Pa_{O_2} is arterial P_{O_2}; Sa_{O_2} is percent saturation of hemoglobin with oxygen in arterial blood. Ca_{O_2} is the oxygen content in arterial blood.

occur in each of the variables during oxygen breathing. The Pa_{O_2} can increase considerably with only a small increase in the Sa_{O_2} and the cardiac output ($\dot{Q}$) can decrease. The final result may be a decrease in O_2 delivery despite the increases in arterial oxygenation.

> The ability of oxygen breathing to reduce cardiac output means that an increase in arterial oxygenation during supplemental oxygen administration does not mean that tissue oxygenation is also improved.[4,5]

The myocardial depression from oxygen is not predictable and can occur in patients with normal or abnormal cardiac function.[4] In one study of patients with acute exacerbation of COPD, over 50% of the patients showed a reduction in cardiac output during supplemental oxygen administration and these patients did not improve their oxygen delivery even though the arterial P_{O_2} increased in all cases.[4] This highlights the value of hemodynamic monitoring for patients with respiratory failure.[6]

OXYGEN ADMINISTRATION SYSTEMS

There are several ways to deliver supplemental oxygen to patients who are breathing spontaneously.[7] The common systems are described briefly in the following paragraphs.

TABLE 25–1. OXYGEN DELIVERY SYSTEMS*		
System	O$_2$ Flowrate (L/min)	FIO$_2$
Nasal Cannula	1	0.21–0.24
	2	0.24–0.28
	3	0.28–0.34
	4	0.31–0.38
	5	0.32–0.44
Simple Mask	8–15	0.40–0.60
Partial Rebreather	5–7	0.35–0.75
Nonrebreather	4–10	0.40–1.00
Venturi Masks	4–12	0.28–0.50
*Approximate values based on minute ventilation of 5–6 L/min		

NASAL CANNULAS

Nasal cannula systems deliver 100% oxygen at low flowrates (1 to 6 L/min). The value of nasal prongs is the high rate of patient acceptance. These cannulas are usually comfortable and are not as confining as face masks. Patients with a normal minute ventilation (5 to 6 L/min) are well-suited for low-flow systems and nasal cannulas can increase the fractional concentration of inspired oxygen (FIO$_2$) to 45% in these patients (see Table 25–1).

The problem with the low-flow systems is the inability to maintain an acceptable FIO$_2$ when patients have a high minute ventilation. That is, the final FIO$_2$ is determined by the relative contribution from the nasal prongs and the patient's inspiratory flowrate (or minute ventilation). As the patient's minute ventilation increases and exceeds the oxygen flowrate, the excess ventilation is drawn from the ambient air and the FIO$_2$ decreases. Therefore, nasal prongs are not recommended for patients who are in respiratory distress and are breathing rapidly.

STANDARD FACE MASKS

Standard face masks are equipped with open vents to allow exhaled gas to pass into the ambient air. However, these vents also allow ambient air to be inhaled when minute ventilation is excessive. Standard face mask systems can achieve higher rates of O$_2$ delivery than nasal cannula systems (up to 15 L/min), and therefore can attain higher levels of FIO$_2$ (up to 50 to 60%). However, these mask systems are also limited in patients with a high minute ventilation.[8]

RESERVOIR SYSTEMS

High levels of inspired O$_2$ (over 60%) can be achieved by placing a reservoir bag in the circuit, like the systems illustrated in Figure 25–2.

A. PARTIAL REBREATHING
SYSTEM

B. NON-REBREATHING
SYSTEM

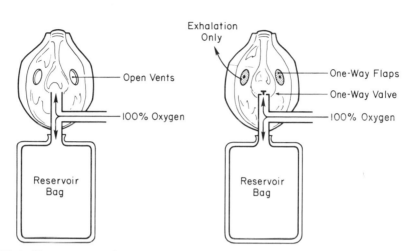

FIG. 25–2. Reservoir mask systems. The partial rebreathing system allows exhaled gas to enter the reservoir bag and this allows some rebreathing of carbon dioxide. Nonrebreathing systems use a one-way valve to prevent exhaled gas from returning back into the reservoir bag.

The oxygen flowrate is then adjusted to keep the reservoir bag continuously inflated. This insures that the patient will not "overbreathe" the oxygen delivery system and inhale ambient air. The system on the left of the figure is called a **partial rebreathing mask** system. This system has open vents on the mask that allow the exhaled gas to escape into the ambient air. However, some of the exhaled gas will enter the reservoir bag and become part of the next inhalation. This can decrease the final FIO_2. Partial rebreathing systems can achieve an FIO_2 of 70 to 80%.

The highest levels of inspired oxygen are achieved with a system like the one on the right in Figure 25–2. This is called a **non-rebreathing mask** system, and it uses a series of one-way valves to prevent exhaled gas from entering the reservoir bag, while also preventing any entrainment of ambient air. These systems can deliver an FIO_2 close to 100%.

CONTROLLED O_2 DELIVERY SYSTEMS

Strict control of the FIO_2 is sometimes necessary in patients with chronic CO_2 retention, to prevent further increases in arterial PCO_2. There are oxygen delivery systems for these patients that can maintain a constant FIO_2 despite changes in the oxygen flowrate. These systems are called Venturi systems or "Venti-mask" systems, even though the mechanism that keeps the FIO_2 constant is not the Venturi Principle. Figure 25–3 illustrates the mechanism behind controlled-flow systems.[9] The mixing tube in this system represents the tubing that delivers the desired FIO_2 to the patient. Pure oxygen passes into the mixing tube through a

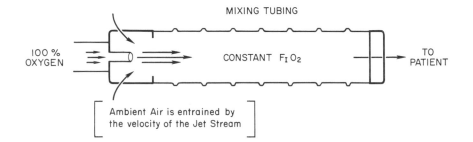

FIG. 25–3. Jet mixing principle for controlling the FIO_2.

nozzle equipped with a narrow exit port. This narrowing increases the velocity of the oxygen as it exits the nozzle and enters the mixing tubing (the Bernoulli Principle). The high velocity moving stream of oxygen drags the stationary air into the stream, producing a "jet-mixing" effect. When the flow of oxygen is increased, the velocity of the stream increases, and more air is drawn into the mixing tube. In this way, the FIO_2 delivered to the patient can be kept constant despite changes in the flow of oxygen. These systems can deliver an FIO_2 up to 50%, while maintaining the concentration within 1 to 2% of the desired level.[9]

OXYGEN TOXICITY

Oxygen is a relative newcomer to the atmosphere and was introduced about 3 billion years ago as a waste product of bacterial photosynthesis. Fortunately it is not a prominent gas in the atmosphere because it is toxic if inhaled in excessive quantities.[10]

PATHOGENESIS

Molecular oxygen is converted to water by cytochrome oxidase and the process generates intermediary metabolites that are toxic. The metabolic pathway for this conversion is shown in Figure 25–4. The oxygen is reduced by a series of single electron reductions so that each of the metabolites has a single unpaired electron in its outer orbital. This produces highly reactive metabolites that act as oxidants by accepting an electron from another molecule. The oxidant activity can damage cell membranes and denature cell proteins. The toxic metabolites identified in Figure 25–4 are the superoxide anion (O_2^-), hydrogen peroxide (H_2O_2), and the hydroxyl radical (OH^-).

One of the hallmarks of oxidant injury to cell membranes is the tendency to sustain itself.[10] This process is called lipid peroxidation and it is able to generate more oxidant species and set up a "chain reaction" that will magnify the original injury and can lead to widespread damage.

CELL DAMAGE

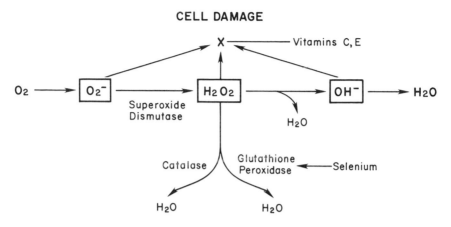

FIG. 25–4. The metabolic pathway for the conversion of oxygen to water by cytochrome oxidase. See text for details.

PROTECTIVE MECHANISMS

Protection from oxidant injury is mainly provided by a series of enzymes that speed the conversion of toxic metabolites to water. These enzymes are included in Figure 25–4. A second line of defense is provided by "scavengers" that block the action of the oxidants on membrane lipids. These are represented by vitamin C and vitamin E in Figure 25 4. These cell defenses can become overwhelmed in the presence of hyperoxia because of the volume of oxygen metabolites that are produced. This leads to cell damage and the syndrome of pulmonary oxygen toxicity.

CLINICAL FEATURES

Animal studies have shown that pure oxygen breathing can be fatal if continued for 3 to 5 days.[10] The illness is similar to the adult respiratory distress syndrome (ARDS) and it is believed to be the result of oxidant damage to the pulmonary capillaries. In fact, oxygen metabolites released from neutrophil granules are believed to be the cause of endothelial damage in ARDS.[11]

Very little is known about the clinical features of oxygen toxicity in humans because virtually all the experimental work has been performed on animals. This may be a relevant point because oxygen toxicity can be a species-specific phenomenon.[12] Two human studies deserve mention. The first is a study where healthy volunteers were given 100% oxygen to breathe for 6 hours.[13] All developed substernal chest pain and showed tracheal inflammation on endoscopy. Only one study has evaluated the prolonged effects of pure oxygen breathing in man.[14] This

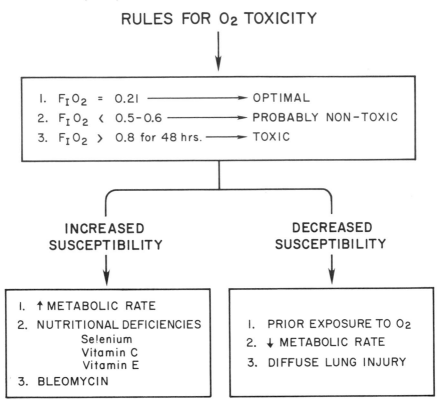

FIG. 25–5. Guidelines for preventing oxygen toxicity.

study involved 10 patients with severe, irreversible neurologic damage. Five of the patients were given 100% oxygen to breathe and these patients developed pulmonary infiltrates and hypoxemia at 40 hours. Unfortunately, this study group was small and it is not possible to extrapolate the results to larger patient cohorts.

PREVENTIVE STRATEGIES

The understanding of oxygen toxicity in humans is far from complete and this makes it difficult to create effective strategies to combat the problem. In fact, there is no specific test to diagnose the problem and the diagnosis is circumstantial only. Figure 25–5 contains some general rules based on our present understanding of the problem.

Inspired Oxygen. There is a persistent tendency to believe that there is an absolute threshold value for FIO_2 that applies to all patients and this FIO_2 is usually taken as 50% or 60%. Therefore, any patient with an FIO_2 that exceeds 60% is considered high risk for developing oxygen toxicity. The problem with this approach is that it negates the antioxidant defense system altogether. If this system is deficient or defective, oxygen toxicity will be produced at FIO_2 levels that are lower than expected. The uncertain status of the antioxidant system in individual patients makes the following the most reasonable recommendation:

The optimal FIO_2 for preventing pulmonary oxygen toxicity is the lowest FIO_2 (below 60%) that the patient will tolerate.

This assumes that any increase in inspired oxygen concentration above normal can be toxic, even if the level is below 60%.

An FIO_2 of 60% or greater should not be continued for more than 2 or 3 days because this poses a high risk for oxygen toxicity, even if antioxidant systems are functional. Patients who have received nontoxic levels of oxygen for the few days prior to the change may show less of a tendency to develop oxygen toxicity.[10] This is an empiric observation with no practical application.

Antioxidant Status. Evaluation of the antioxidant system is not entirely possible but selenium and vitamin E can be assayed in serum (see Appendix at the end of the book).

Selenium is a cofactor for glutathione peroxidase and participates in the reaction that converts hydrogen peroxide to water (see Fig. 25–4). Selenium deficiency may be common in critically ill patients,[15] and this could certainly increase susceptibility to oxygen toxicity. We frequently check selenium status in our medical and surgical ICU patients using the erythrocyte glutathione peroxidase activity test. Selenium is easy to replace intravenously as sodium selenite, and the maximum recommended daily dose is 200 micrograms (split into 4 doses).

Vitamin E is an important antioxidant that is often overlooked as a possible contributing factor in oxygen toxicity. Vitamin E deficiency may be common in hospitalized patients, as one study reported that 37% of hospitalized patients had abnormally low levels of vitamin E in random blood samples.[16] The incidence of vitamin E deficiency in critically ill patients is unknown at the present time, but is likely to be higher than the 37% incidence reported in the general patient population.

If you are concerned about oxygen toxicity in a particular patient, consider checking the status of vitamin E and selenium and supplementing these as needed. Remember that the daily requirements for trace elements and vitamins were developed in healthy volunteers and the hypermetabolic ICU patient may have much higher requirements. The Appendix section contains the assays and normal ranges for vitamins and trace elements.

REFERENCES

REPORTS

1. ACCP-NHLBI National Conference on Oxygen Therapy. Chest 1984; 86:234–247.

REVIEWS

2. Ryerson GG, Block AJ: Oxygen as a drug: Chemical properties, benefits and hazards of administration. In: Burton G, Hodgkin JE eds. Respiratory care. A guide to clinical practice. Philadelphia: J.B. Lippincott, 1984.

SELECTED REFERENCES

3. Eldridge F. Blood lactate and pyruvate in pulmonary insufficiency. N Engl J Med 1966; 274:878–882.
4. DeGaute JP, Demenighetti G, Naeije R, et al. Oxygen delivery in acute exacerbation of chronic obstructive pulmonary disease. Effects of controlled oxygen therapy. Am Rev Respir Dis 1981; 124:26–30.
5. Mithoefer JC, Holford FD, Keighley JFH. The effect of oxygen administration on mixed venous oxygenation in chronic obstructive pulmonary disease. Chest 1974; 62:122–130.
6. Danek SJ, Lynch JP, Weg JG, Dantzger DR. The dependence of oxygen uptake on oxygen delivery in the adult respiratory distress syndrome. Am Rev Respir Dis 1980; 122:387–396.
7. Fluk RB, Anthonisen NR. Administering oxygen effectively to critically ill patients. J Crit Illness 1986; 1:21–27.
8. Goldstein RS, Young J, Rebuck AS. Effect of breathing pattern on oxygen concentration received from standard face masks. Lancet 1982; 2:1188–1190.
9. Scacci R: Air entrainment masks: Jet mixing is how they work. The Bernoulli and Venturi Principles are how they don't. Resp Care 1979; 24:928–931.
10. Jenkinson SG: Oxygen toxicity. J Intensive Care Med 1988; 3:137–152.
11. Southorn PA, Powis G. Free radicals in medicine. II. Involvement in human disease. Mayo Clin Proc 1988; 63:390–408.
12. Fanburg BL. Oxygen toxicity: Why can't a human be more like a turtle? Intens Care Med 1988; 3:134–136. (editorial)
13. Sackner MA, Lauda J, Hirsch J, et al. Pulmonary effects of oxygen breathing: A 6-hour study in normal men. Ann Intern Med 1975; 82:40–48.
14. Barber RE, Hamilton WK. Oxygen toxicity in man. N Engl J Med 1970; 283:1478–1483.
15. Hesselvik F, Carlsson C, von Schenck H, Sorbo B. Low selenium plasma levels in surgical intensive care patients: Relation to infection. Clin Nutrition 1987; 6:279–283.
16. Dempsey DT, Mullen JL, Rombeau JL, et al. Treatment effects of parenteral vitamins in total parenteral nutrition patients. J Parent Ent Nutr 1987; 11:229–237.

c h a p t e r

26

THE PHARMACOTHERAPY OF RESPIRATORY FAILURE

The pharmacologic approach to respiratory failure includes drugs that improve airflow in the lungs (bronchodilators, steroids, and mucolytic agents), drugs that stimulate ventilation (progesterone and naloxone) and drugs that improve the balance between pulmonary gas exchange and the rate of metabolism (muscle relaxants and sedative-hypnotic agents). This chapter will present the benefits and drawbacks associated with each type of drug therapy in adults. Emphasis is placed on the use of bronchodilators and steroids in the ICU (not in the emergency room).

BRONCHODILATORS: AN OVERVIEW

Bronchodilator therapy has been disappointing in adults with acute respiratory failure (ARF). Bronchodilators and steroids are valuable in asthmatics but this illness is not common in adults with ARF. The common causes of ARF in adults are pneumonia, pulmonary edema, and chronic obstructive lung disease, and these illnesses do not respond dramatically to either bronchodilators or steroids. This is important to stress because these agents can have serious side effects and should not be used indiscriminantly. When considering bronchodilator therapy in ARF, every effort should be made to identify prior evidence of bronchodilator responsiveness on pulmonary function tests. If evidence is lacking or unavailable, the response to inhaled bronchodilators can be evaluated at the bedside using the methods described in the next section.

BEDSIDE TESTS FOR BRONCHODILATOR RESPONSE

The first point to emphasize is the limited value of the stethoscope in assessing the degree of airflow obstruction.

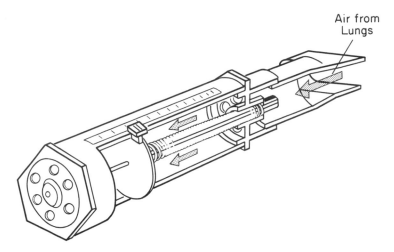

Air from
Lungs

FIG. 26–1. The principle of the peak flow meter. The piston is propelled by expired gas blown through the mouthpiece and pushes a marker that records the peak flow on a scale etched on the outer surface of the instrument.

Auscultation of the lungs is unreliable for evaluating bronchodilator response because the intensity of airway sounds does not correlate with the severity of the airway obstruction.[1]

Airway sounds may be particularly unreliable in ventilator-dependent patients because sounds produced by airflow in the ventilator tubing can be transmitted to the upper airways and will confuse the interpretation of adventitious sounds heard over the upper thorax. More objective measures of airway obstruction are required to evaluate airways obstruction at the bedside.

PEAK EXPIRATORY FLOWRATE

In spontaneously breathing patients, the peak flow in a forced exhalation can be used as an index of airways obstruction.[2] The peak expiratory flowrate (PEFR) can be measured at the bedside with an inexpensive hand-held instrument called a "peak flow meter" like the one shown in Figure 26–1. The patient inhales to total lung capacity and then exhales forcefully into the mouthpiece of the instrument. The exhalation propels the piston along the barrel of the instrument and the piston pushes a marker that records the peak flowrate on a scale that is etched on the upper surface of the device. The normal ranges for PEFR are usually supplied with the meter.

The PEFR is influenced by patient effort and is reliable only when the subject is alert and can perform a reliable forced expiration. The response to inhaled bronchodilators is evaluated by measuring the PEFR just before the drug is inhaled and again at the time when the peak effect is expected (see Table 26–1). An increase of 15% in the PEFR is taken as a positive response.[2] This test is performed by the respiratory therapy department on request and should be a routine test in patients receiving bronchodilators when there is no prior documentation of bronchodilator responsiveness.

PEAK INSPIRATORY PRESSURE

In patients receiving mechanical ventilation, the pressure in the proximal airways at the end of lung inflation is proportional to the flow resistance in the airways (see Figure 27–5). As the airways resistance decreases in response to a bronchodilator, the peak inspiratory pressure (PIP) will also decrease.[3] The PIP is monitored on the pressure gauge situated on the front panel of the ventilator. Bronchodilator responsiveness can be evaluated by recording the PIP just before the bronchodilator is inhaled and again at the time of expected peak response. There are no guidelines for the magnitude of change in PIP required for a positive response but any change greater than the baseline variability is likely to indicate a positive response (as long as other factors that influence the PIP are constant). The PIP measurement is discussed in more detail in the next chapter. The measurement is unreliable in patients who are agitated and breathing asynchronously with the ventilator.

AUTO-PEEP

The presence of positive pressure in the alveoli at end-expiration without externally-applied PEEP is called auto-PEEP (see Figure 29–7). The presence of auto-PEEP indicates that alveolar gas is still being expelled at the end of expiration. This is the result of an obstruction in the airways. When exhaled volume and the time for exhalation are constant, the level of auto-PEEP is proportional to the magnitude of airways obstruction. A decrease in airway resistance in response to a bronchodilator will therefore be associated with a decrease in the level of auto-PEEP. The principle of auto-PEEP and the measurement technique is presented in Chapter 29.

ADRENERGIC BRONCHODILATORS

The adrenergic agents stimulate beta receptors in smooth muscle and skeletal muscle. These beta receptors are subdivided according to their location as shown below.

	Location	Response
Beta-1:	Heart	Increased Rate & Contractility
	Blood Vessels	Vasodilatation
Beta-2:	Airways	Bronchodilatation
	Skeletal Muscle	Tremors

TABLE 26–1. SELECTIVE BETA AGENTS FOR INHALATIONAL USE			
		Response	
Drug	Usual Dose of Aerosol Solution*	Peak (minutes)	Duration (hours)
Isoetharine	0.3 ml of 1% solution (3 mg)	30	2
Metaproterenol	0.3 ml of 5% solution (15 mg)	45	3–6
Terbutaline	0.3 ml of 1% solution (3 mg)	60	4–6
Albuterol	0.1 ml of 5% solution (5 mg)	60	4–6
*Specified volumes are added to 2.5 ml saline and delivered via nebulizer			

The popular adrenergic bronchodilators stimulate beta-2 receptors preferentially and limit the undesirable effects from beta-1 activation and cardiac stimulation.

ISOPROTERENOL

Isoproterenol stimulates both types of beta receptors with equal potency. Although this drug is a powerful bronchodilator, beta-1 stimulation causes unwanted tachycardia and arrhythmias. The risk for cardiotoxicity has virtually eliminated isoproterenol as a bronchodilator in adults. This drug is contraindicated in patients with coronary artery disease or a history of tachyarrhythmias.

BETA-2 AGONISTS

A number of agents are available that selectively stimulate beta-2 receptors and minimize the risk for tachycardia and arrhythmias. The selective beta agents available for aerosol delivery are listed in Table 26–1 along with the recommended doses for each drug. Although these agents can be given orally, the inhaled route is more effective and produces fewer side effects.[4] The relative efficacy of the inhalational route for one of the beta-2 agonists is shown in Figure 26–2. This shows the change in expiratory flowrate produced by terbutaline when it is given as an inhaled aerosol, as an oral tablet, or by subcutaneous injection. The increase in flowrate is greatest when the drug is given by aerosol spray, indicating that the inhaled route produces the most effective bronchodilatation. This has been a consistent observation for all the beta-2 agonists, and has led to the recommendation that the inhaled route be used whenever possible.

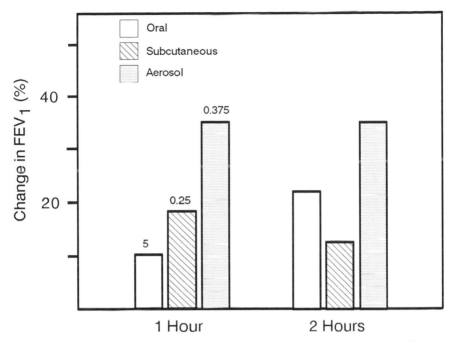

FIG. 26–2. The bronchodilator response to terbutaline given via three different routes in adults with acute exacerbation of asthma. The number at the top of each column on the left indicates the dose of the drug used in each route of delivery. (From Dulfano MJ, Glass P. Ann Allergy 37:357–366, 1976.)

The choice of beta agent to use is mostly a matter of personal preference because the drugs are considered to be comparable in many respects. Isoetharine is one exception because this drug has a shorter duration of action than the others. There is some evidence that albuterol may be slightly more effective and more selective than the other beta-2 agents[4,5] but the clinical significance of this difference is not proven.

TOXICITY

Selectivity is a dose-dependent phenomenon, so that beta-2 agonists can stimulate beta-1 receptors if given in high enough doses. The inhalation route will minimize but not eliminate the risk for beta-1 stimulation by delivering a lower dose of the drug. **Tachycardia** that develops from the aerosol spray usually subsides in 5 to 10 minutes and mandates a reduction in dosage. Other adverse effects include **muscle tremors** and a **decrease in serum potassium** (because of a shift of potassium into muscle cells). The reduction in serum potassium usually requires excessive doses of the inhaled agents but the effect can be magnified in patients receiving diuretics that promote hypokalemia.[5]

AEROSOL DELIVERY

Hospitalized patients should receive the beta agents by metered-dose inhaler or pressurized nebulizer. The latter route is the common route in the ICU population. A liquid preparation of the drug (see Table 26–1) is placed in the reservoir of the nebulizer and saline is added until the reservoir volume reaches 3 or 5 mls. The solution can be inhaled during spontaneous breathing or can be delivered through the inspiratory limb of a ventilator circuit. Only 10 to 15% of the solution actually reaches the upper airways, the remainder either condensing on the tubing or impacting on the oral mucosa.

Asthma. Aerosol therapy with beta-2 agents is the cornerstone of therapy in severe asthma and is used in combination with steroids for status asthmaticus. Addition of theophylline may not add much to the bronchodilatation produced by these agents (see later).

COPD. In patients with chronic bronchitis or emphysema the response to inhaled beta agents is variable,[7] therefore, the benefit of therapy must be determined on an individual basis. Prior tests of bronchodilator responsiveness should be reviewed whenever available to determine the need for therapy in individual patients.

THEOPHYLLINE

Theophylline is the most popular bronchodilator in the United States, but its value as a bronchodilator is now being questioned.[8,9] This drug is a methylxanthine (like caffeine) that inhibits the phosphodiesterase enzyme that breaks down cyclic AMP. The increase in cyclic AMP caused by the drug was considered to be the mechanism of action but recent evidence does not support this theory.[10] The mechanism of action of theophylline is presently unknown.

METABOLISM

Theophylline is metabolized in the liver and its clearance is influenced by several factors. There is a significant variability in the clearance rate in individual patients, and clearance rates can differ by as much as 50% in individual patients.[11] As a result, the serum half-life of theophylline can vary from 3 to 12 hours. There are a number of factors that may explain this interindividual variation in drug elimination. Clearance is enhanced by young age, smoking, and concomitant therapy with phenytoin, phenobarbital, and rifampin. Conversely, clearance is diminished by old age, liver disease, viral infections, heart failure, and therapy with allopurinol, cimetidine, erythromycin, or propranolol.[10]

TABLE 26–2. INTRAVENOUS AMINOPHYLLINE DOSING IN ACUTE ILLNESS*	
Condition	Dose†
A. Loading dose	
1. No prior Rx..........................6 mg/kg (ideal wt)	
2. Ongoing Rx..............................T_D–T_P/1.6‡	
3. Rate.................................<0.2 mg/kg/hr	
B. Infusion Rate	
1. Standard ....0.5 mg/kg/hr	
2. Low cardiac output.....................0.2 mg/kg/hr	
3. Smoker................................0.8 mg/kg/hr	

*From Powell JR, et al. Theophylline disposition in acutely ill hospitalized patients. Am Rev Respir Dis 1978; 118:229–238.
†The dose to achieve a serum theophylline level of 10 mg/L
‡T_D = desired serum theophylline level; T_P = present serum theophylline level

DOSE RECOMMENDATIONS

The variability in drug clearance in individual patients makes it difficult to predict serum theophylline levels in any individual patient using a fixed dose rate. For this reason, serum levels of the drug should be monitored routinely to guide therapy. The recommended therapeutic range is 10 to 20 mg/L.

Aminophylline (theophylline ethylenediamine) is usually given intravenously in patients with acute respiratory failure. A popular dosing regimen, designed to achieve serum levels of 10 mg/L, is shown in Table 26–2.[11] Remember that these dose recommendations may not achieve the desired serum level in any individual patient and serum levels are required to evaluate therapy.

SERUM LEVELS

In patients with respiratory failure, there is a tendency to maintain serum theophylline levels in the high therapeutic range (15 to 20 mg/L) to ensure optimal bronchodilator response. This practice originated from a study of six asthmatic patients that reported enhanced bronchodilatation when serum theophylline levels were increased from the lower to the upper therapeutic range.[12] However, the results of this study are misleading because the data was presented on a semilogarithmic graph. Figure 26–3 shows the same data plotted in a linear fashion.[13]

When the data is presented on a linear scale, the bronchodilator effects occur predominantly as the serum levels increase into the therapeutic range (10 to 12 mg/L) but there is little further response with further increases within the therapeutic range. This observation, combined with the risk for toxicity at higher serum levels, has led to the recommendation that the optimal serum theophylline level should be in the low end of the therapeutic range, or 10 to 15 mg/L.[10]

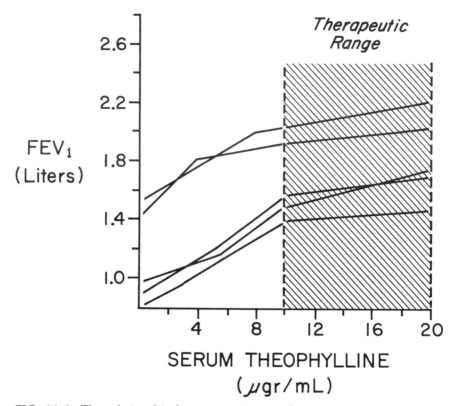

FIG. 26–3. The relationship between expiratory flowrates and serum theophylline concentration. FEV1 = Forced expiratory flow in one second. (From Rogers RM et al. Chest 1985; *87*:280–282.)

TOXICITY

Theophylline toxicity has a reported mortality of 10%.[14] The more serious reactions include seizures, arrhythmias, electrolyte abnormalities (e.g., hypokalemia), and hypotension.[14] These usually appear when serum theophylline levels exceed 20 mg/L. However, there may be no correlation between the height of the serum level and the appearance of serious reactions.[15] For this reason, serum levels should always be kept below 20 mg/L. As many as 40% of patients in the hospital can have serum theophylline levels in the toxic range[16] and regular monitoring of serum levels is therefore mandatory to limit drug toxicity.

When serious reactions appear during theophylline therapy, the drug should be stopped immediately and a blood sample obtained for a serum level. If theophylline toxicity is likely or proven, oral charcoal can be given to enhance clearance of the drug from the bloodstream. Charcoal in the bowel lumen will enhance drug clearance from the blood and is not used only to bind orally ingested forms of the drug.

Charcoal Dose: 20 grams PO every 2 hours to a total dose of 120 grams.[14]
Charcoal or resin hemoperfusion has been recommended for the most serious cases of theophylline toxicity but there is no evidence that this offers any advantage over oral charcoal.[14]

Specific therapy of a toxic reaction may also be necessary. Although seizures may not be recurrent, short-term therapy with anticonvulsants is often recommended until the serum theophylline levels are reduced to safe levels. Cardiac arrhythmias have been successfully treated with propranolol without aggravating bronchospasm,[14] however, a selective beta-1 blocker may be preferable. Hypotension may be refractory to conventional vasopressors and has been successfully treated with beta blockers.[14]

INDICATIONS

Intravenous aminophylline is commonplace in regimens used to treat acute respiratory failure from asthma and chronic obstructive pulmonary disease (COPD). However, the evidence that it is effective as a bronchodilator in this patient population is not convincing.

Asthma. Inhaled beta-2 agonists are considered the most effective bronchodilators in severe asthma, and aminophylline may add little or nothing to the effect produced by these agents.[5] This is shown in Figure 26–4 for adult asthmatics treated in an emergency room. As indicated, the addition of aminophylline added little to the bronchodilatation produced by the inhaled beta agonist in this group of patients. This kind of observation has led to a reappraisal of aminophylline in the management of acute asthma, and the consensus is that aminophylline is not the bronchodilator of choice for acute exacerbations of asthma and should not be used as sole therapy.[8]

COPD. The role of intravenous aminophylline in patients with severe COPD is also in question. Although some degree of bronchodilatation can be seen with high intravenous doses in some patients, there is no evidence that this provides any real clinical benefit.[9]

To summarize the reported experience with theophylline taken from references 8 through 10 at the end of the chapter:

> Aminophylline combines limited efficacy as a bronchodilator with the risk for serious toxicity and the cost of monitoring serum levels. This combination should discourage the use of this drug in the ICU unless there is objective evidence for a benefit in the individual patient.

I have refrained from this drug in the ICU for 10 years to eliminate unnecessary risks for unproven benefits. You might want to review references 8 through 10 cited at the end of the chapter to make your own decision about this drug.

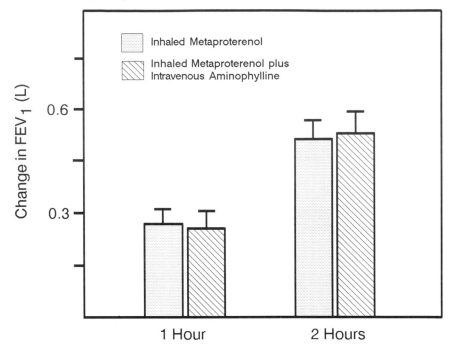

FIG. 26–4. The effects of adding intravenous aminophylline to inhaled meta-proterenol in the therapy of acute exacerbation of asthma. Cross bars represent the standard deviation from the mean for each group. (From Siegel D, et al. Am Rev Respir Dis *132*:283–286, 1985.)

ANTICHOLINERGIC AGENTS

The use of anticholinergic agents as bronchodilators is based on the observation that stimulation of the parasympathetic nerves that inner-vate the small airways causes bronchoconstriction. Although the para-sympathetic nervous system probably plays a minor role in most cases of obstructive lung disease, parasympathetic blockade with anticholin-ergic agents can result in significant bronchodilatation in certain situa-tions. The two anticholinergic agents used clinically are shown in Table 26–3.

Atropine is the prototype anticholinergic bronchodilator, and is avail-able in a liquid that can be given as an aerosol spray. The recommended dose for bronchodilator effects in adults is 0.025 to 0.075 mg/kg.[17] At-

TABLE 26–3. ANTICHOLINERGIC BRONCHODILATORS				
Agent	Inhalation Dose	Onset of Action	Peak Effect	Duration
Atropine Sulfate	0.025–0.075 mg/kg	15–30 minutes	30–170 minutes	3–5 hours
Ipatropium	0.02–0.03 mg/kg	3–30 minutes	90–120 minutes	3–6 hours

TABLE 26–4. COMPARATIVE PHARMACOLOGY OF STEROIDS			
Steroid	Equipotent Dose (mg)	Physiologic Half-Life (hours)	Comments
Hydrocortisone	20	8–12	Daily maintenance dose in adrenal failure is 25–37.5 mg
Prednisone	5	12–30	Must be converted in the liver to prednisolone
Methylprednisolone	4	15–30	No proven benefit over hydro-cortisone
Dexamethasone	0.75	36–54	No mineralocorticoid activity

ropine is readily absorbed from mucosal surfaces and is capable of producing systemic side effects (e.g., tachycardia). Ipatropium bromide is a synthetic derivative of atropine that produces fewer systemic side effects when given by inhalation. The drug is available in a metered-dose inhaler and a liquid preparation for nebulization. In patients with asthma, ipatropium is less effective than inhaled beta agents, but can enhance the response to beta agents when used in combination therapy.[15] In patients with acute exacerbation of COPD, ipatropium is as effective as inhaled beta agents, but does not cause enhanced bronchodilatation when combined with beta agents.[15]

INDICATIONS

The value of anticholinergic agents in patients with severe respiratory failure (those requiring mechanical ventilation) is not known because clinical trials have been performed on patients with less severe degrees of illness.

Asthma. Aerosolized atropine can add to the effects of other bronchodilators in patients with severe asthma, and it is occasionally effective when patients do not respond to conventional therapy.[17]

COPD. Anticholinergic agents do not add to the effects of conventional bronchodilators in severe COPD,[18] and it seems unlikely that these agents will have an impact on clinical outcome in this patient population.

STEROIDS

Steroids are considered the backbone of therapy for severe asthma, although you might be surprised at the paucity of clinical trials on the subject.[20,21] The mechanism of action is not known but they may enhance the responsiveness of beta receptors. Table 26–4 includes the common steroids used in clinical practice and some pharmacologic comparisons.

TABLE 26–5. CLINICAL EFFICACY OF STEROIDS	
Clinical Disorder	**Proven Benefit**
Asthma	Yes
COPD	No
ARDS	No
Septic Shock	No
Anaphylactic Shock	No
Diffuse Cerebral Edema	No
Aspiration Pneumonitis	No
Idiopathic Pulmonary Fibrosis	No

INDICATIONS

Steroids are far from the wonder drugs that some insist they are. Table 26–5 summarizes the clinical experience with these agents in various illnesses. Despite the lack of objective evidence for their benefit in most of the illnesses shown in the table, the steroid mystique continues to lure many followers.

Asthma. Steroids should be given to all patients with acute asthma who do not respond to initial bronchodilator therapy in the emergency room. Because the effect can take 6 to 12 hours to become evident,[20] therapy should begin as soon as possible. Either methylprednisolone (Solu-Medrol) or hydrocortisone (Solu-Cortef) can be given intravenously and there is no evidence that either agent is superior to the other. Suggested doses for severe asthma are:

Hydrocortisone: 2 mg/kg IV bolus. Follow with

0.5 mg/kg per hour [20]

Methylprednisolone: 40 to 125 mg IV every 6 hours[21]

Inhaled steroids have no role in the treatment of severe bronchospasm because the inhaled particles can irritate the airways and aggravate the bronchospasm.

COPD. Steroids have a limited role in patients with severe COPD. A few days of intravenous steroids may improve airflow in patients with acute exacerbation of COPD.[22] However, prolonged therapy with steroids does not improve lung function in most patients with COPD.[21]

Prolonged steroid therapy is not recommended for patients with severe COPD unless there is objective evidence of benefit in the individual patient.

In fact, chronic steroid administration can be hazardous in critically ill patients because of the susceptibility for infections associated with prolonged steroid use.

ARDS. Early steroid therapy has also been recommended for patients with adult respiratory distress syndrome (ARDS). However, intravenous steroid therapy has not been shown to improve outcome in ARDS.[23]

RESPIRATORY STIMULANTS

Respiratory stimulants can be used to counteract respiratory depression from general anesthesia or from the overzealous use of narcotic analgesics, and may provide some benefit in patients with respiratory failure resulting from alveolar hypoventilation syndromes (e.g., Pickwickian syndrome). These drugs should not be used in patients with respiratory failure caused by obstructive lung disease because these patients already have a high minute ventilation and further respiratory stimulation can be deleterious.

DOXAPRAM

Doxapram stimulates both peripheral chemoreceptors and brainstem respiratory centers. This drug has been used successfully in treating postoperative respiratory depression and in treating patients with alveolar hypoventilation syndromes.[24] The drug is given intravenously at a rate of 1 to 3 mg/min and can be continued to a maximal dose of 600 mg.[25] The risk for seizures is low unless the patient has a history of a seizure disorder. Doxapram can also stimulate the release of epinephrine from the adrenals, which may explain the cardiac arrhythmias and hypertension that can sometimes occur during doxapram infusion. For this reason, the drug is not recommended in patients with severe hypertension, pheochromocytoma, coronary artery disease, or in those with a history of life-threatening cardiac arrhythmias.

NALOXONE

Naloxone blocks the respiratory depression from exogenous and endogenous opiates by competing for specific opiate receptors in the brainstem. It is used primarily to reverse the central nervous system depression from exogenous opiates (morphine, methadone, and heroin) but has also been effective in overdoses from diazepam, propoxyphene, and ethanol.[25] The drug is given as an intravenous bolus, and the recommended dose for narcotic depression is 0.4 to 2.0 mg. However, a dose of 0.1 mg/kg may be necessary to reverse narcotic depression in selected cases.[26] Naloxone is a safe drug and administration of high doses has not been associated with untoward effects. The effect of naloxone can be short-lived, therefore, the initial dose should be followed by a continuous intravenous infusion when reversing a long-acting respiratory depressant such as methadone. The optimal dose for continuous infusion is not known. One recommendation, for adults, is to use the initial effective intravenous bolus dose and infuse this amount per hour for the next 12 to 24 hours.

PROGESTERONE

Progesterone is an effective respiratory stimulant in patients with obesity-hypoventilation (Pickwickian) syndrome. Sublingual progesterone is effective in outpatients with this syndrome and intramuscular administration (100 mg/day in a single injection) has proven effective in hospitalized patients.[24] The response is not immediate and maximum effects can take 2 to 3 weeks to develop. When using daily intramuscular injections, remember not to use the long-acting depot form of the drug. Administration of progesterone through feeding tubes is not recommended because absorption from the GI tract is antagonized by the presence of food.

THEOPHYLLINE

Theophylline has been shown to stimulate diaphragm contraction[28] and has been recommended as a possible aid in chronic ventilator patients who may have difficulty in weaning from the ventilator. However, the value of theophylline in this setting is unproven. First, the assumption that diaphragm weakness is responsible for the inability to wean in these patients may not be valid (see Chapter 26). In addition, the assumption that chronic stimulation of a weak or fatiguing muscle will increase muscle strength may not be sound. That is, the usual method of strengthening skeletal muscles is to combine periods of activity with periods of rest. If periods of rest are required to strengthen muscle, then chronic stimulation of a weak muscle could aggravate muscle fatigue. Until appropriate studies are performed, chronic stimulation of the diaphragm with theophylline should not be recommended routinely in patients who are unable to wean from mechanical ventilation.

MUSCLE RELAXANTS

The following agents are capable of paralyzing skeletal muscles by competing with acetylcholine at the motor end-plate. The "depolarizing" blockers act like acetylcholine and depolarize the muscle but, because the depolarization is persistent, the impulses are blocked. The "nondepolarizing" agents block the motor end-plate but cause no electrical change in the muscle membrane.

RISKS

There are several problems associated with paralysis, particularly if it is prolonged. The most noted shortcoming of paralysis is **inadequate sedation,** and the reports from patients who have been awake while paralyzed are frightening. Routine sedation is mandatory during paralysis, but the problem is gauging the extent of sedation, which is difficult if not impossible. The second problem with prolonged paralysis is the **inability to clear pulmonary secretions** because of the lack of cough. Routine tracheal suctioning is far from effective in clearing secretions from the lower airways, and the consequences can be life-threatening when pneumonia develops. Finally, **venous thrombosis** occurs with increased frequency in paralyzed patients, possibly because of a loss of the massaging action of the leg muscles on the deep veins, which normally promotes venous return from the leg.

INDICATIONS

The major indications for paralysis are listed below.[29]

1. Shivering after cardiopulmonary bypass surgery
2. Intubation when the patient is agitated, or trismus
3. *Temporary* control of agitated ventilator patient

The principal use of muscle paralysis in the ICU is for shivering during rewarming after cardiopulmonary bypass surgery.[29] In this situation, the shivering produces carbon dioxide and lactic acid, but the patient is incapable of responding to the combined metabolic and respiratory acidosis because of residual anesthesia. The result can be life-threatening acidosis. Temporary paralysis is well tolerated in this situation because the patient is under the influence of anesthesia.

The other indication for paralysis is a difficult intubation, either from generalized agitation or from trismus that occasionally occurs in the head-injured patient. The agitated patient on mechanical ventilation can be calmed with sedation in most cases. Asthmatics can pose a problem and often become agitated when first placed on a ventilator. Because paralysis is horrifying to a patient who feels short of breath, every effort should be made to sedate these patients heavily. Avoid large doses of morphine in asthmatics because of the risk for histamine release (although this has not been shown clinically). Halothane has proven effective in this situation because it combines central depression with its bronchodilating effects.[31] If paralysis is necessary, vecuronium may be preferred because it is least likely to stimulate histamine release.[29]

Flail chest is no longer a routine indication for intubation and paralysis, and paralysis for seizures is never appropriate unless there is continuous EEG monitoring to follow the seizure activity.

	Initial Dose (mg/kg)	Duration of Action (minutes)	Maintenance Dose	Side Effects
TABLE 26–6. NONDEPOLARIZING MUSCLE RELAXANTS*				
Agent				
Pancuronium	0.06–0.15	45–90	0.01–0.05 mg/kg q1 hr	Tachycardia
Atracurium	0.4–0.5	30	0.005–0.01 mg/kg min as continuous infusion	Histamine Release
Vecuronium	0.08–0.15	30	0.01–0.04 mg/kg q30 min 0.075–0.10 mg/kg hr as continuous infusion	None

*From Lumb PD. Sedatives and muscle relaxants in the intensive care unit. In: Fuhrman BP, Shoemaker WC eds. Fullerton, Society of Critical Care Medicine, 1989:145–172.

SUCCINYLCHOLINE

This is a depolarizing muscle relaxant that has little use in the ICU. It can be used to facilitate intubation because it is ultra-short acting. It is not to be used for prolonged paralysis because of the risk for life-threatening hyperkalemia from prolonged muscle depolarization.[29] The initial dose is 1 to 2 mg/kg.[30] Paralysis occurs within 1 to 2 minutes and disappears within 10 minutes.[30]

PANCURONIUM (PAVULON)

This nondepolarizing agent is the muscle relaxant traditionally used in the ICU. The recommended doses are shown in Table 26–6. The drug is eliminated via the renal and hepatic route, and dose adjustments are recommended for renal failure and hepatic failure.[26] The drug can accumulate when given by continuous infusion, therefore, intermittent bolus administration (usually every 1 to 2 hours) is recommended for prolonged paralysis. Pancuronium does not stimulate histamine release in the usual doses,[30] but it can occasionally cause significant tachycardia.[29] When this occurs, vecuronium may be preferred because of the low risk for cardiovascular side effects.[29]

ATRACURIUM (TRACRIUM)

This nondepolarizing agent is shorter acting than pancuronium but its popularity has been limited by reports that it causes histamine release in doses above 0.6 mg/kg.[29] Recommended doses for the drug are shown in Table 26–6.

VECURONIUM (NORCURON)

Vecuronium has been recommended as superior to pancuronium because it carries less risk for cardiovascular side effects.[29] However, this has yet to be shown in clinical trials. The dose recommendations for vecuronium are shown in Table 26–6. Bolus injection of the drug lasts approximately 30 minutes and it can be given by continuous infusion if necessary. This latter feature may prove an advantage over pancuronium for prolonged paralysis. However, there should be few instances where prolonged paralysis is necessary in the ICU.

REVERSAL

Anticholinesterase inhibitors will reverse the block from nondepolarizing agents and aggravate the block produced by depolarizing agents. The available agents are neostigmine (2.5 to 5.0 mg per 70kg), pyridostigmine (0.1 to 0.2 mg/kg to a maximum of 25 mg per 75 kg), and edrophonium (10 to 40 mg per 70 kg). Because these agents can produce bradycardia, pretreatment with atropine (0.6 to 1.5 mg per 70 kg) is advised.[29] The reversal can take at least 15 to 30 minutes, which may be equivalent to the time for the block to dissipate naturally. Prolonged blockade from pancuronium in renal or hepatic failure may be attenuated by these agents, but there is rarely a need for such intervention.

SEDATION

Agitation is common in acute respiratory failure and can further impair tissue oxygenation. Rapid breathing from the sense of dyspnea can produce auto-PEEP and further reduce O_2 delivery (see Chapter 29), while the increased metabolic rate from catecholamine excess will increase total body O_2 consumption. Sedation, therefore can play an important role in preventing further imbalance between O_2 delivery and O_2 consumption in patients with respiratory failure. The following anxiolytic agents have proven effective.

HALOPERIDOL (HALDOL)

Haloperidol is becoming the preferred anxiolytic agent in the ICU because it does not cause respiratory depression or hypotension.[32] Cardiovascular depression occurs only when the drug is given with propranolol[33] or when the patient is hypovolemic. The intravenous route has not yet received FDA approval, but this route has proven safe in clinical trials.[32,34] The recommended intravenous doses for haloperidol are shown in Table 26–7.[32]

Intravenous haloperidol has a prolonged distribution time (about 10 minutes) and therefore can be given by bolus injection.[32] The usual dose for mild-to-moderate agitation is 3 to 5 mg. If the desired response is

TABLE 26–7. INTRAVENOUS HALOPERIDOL FOR AGITATION	
Degree of Agitation	**Intravenous Dose***
Mild	0.5–2 mg
Moderate	5–10 mg
Severe	>10 mg

1. Give IV push
2. Allow 15 to 20 minutes for sedation
3. If first dose ineffective, double the dose
4. If second dose is not effective, switch to another agent

*From Tesar GE, Stern TA. Evaluation and treatment of agitation in the intensive care unit. J Intensive Care Med 1986; 1:137–148

not observed in 15 to 20 minutes, the dose can be doubled or a benzodiazepine can be added. The addition of a benzodiazepine is becoming popular because it limits the haloperidol dose and limits the risk for extrapyramidal reactions from haloperidol.[34] However, extrapyramidal side effects are uncommon when haloperidol is given intravenously.[32,34]

The most feared side effect of haloperidol is the **neuroleptic malignant syndrome** (NMS), a potentially fatal illness characterized by **hyperthermia, muscle rigidity, autonomic dysfunction, and mental confusion**.[35] The intense muscle rigidity can lead to myonecrosis and myoglobinuric renal failure. Early recognition of NMS is important to prevent progression of the illness while dantrolene (a skeletal muscle relaxant) has been effective in controlling the muscle rigidity.[35] This syndrome is similar to the malignant hyperthermia syndrome described in Chapter 43 (see Table 43–1). NMS has been reported rarely with intravenous haloperidol but we have seen two cases at our hospital (unpublished observation). NMS is an illness that you must always be aware of when using haloperidol regardless of the route of delivery.

BENZODIAZEPINES

The benzodiazepines are the traditional anxiolytics used in intensive care units. These agents can produce respiratory depression[36] and this has contributed to a diminished enthusiasm for these drugs in recent years. The benzodiazepines available for parenteral use are included in Table 26–8.

Diazepam (Valium). Diazepam is the prototype benzodiazepine and produces rapid sedation for immediate control of the severely agitated patient. The drug is metabolized in the liver and the metabolite is active as a sedative. This prolongs the elimination time of diazepam and the effects can accumulate when the drug is given repeatedly.[36]

TABLE 26–8. PARENTERAL BENZODIAZEPINES		
Drug	**IV Dose‡** **(Agitation Level)**	**Comments**
Diazepam* (Valium)	1–2 mg (mild) 2–5 mg (moderate) 5–10 mg (severe) Repeat in 3–4 h	1. Produces rapid sedation 2. Can cause phlebitis 3. Precipitates in IV fluids and ad- sorbs to IV tubing, so inject into or near the vein 4. Serum half–life: 24 hours 5. Accumulates with repeat dosing
Lorazepam* (Ativan)	0.04 mg/kg (mild) 0.05 mg/kg (severe) DO NOT exceed 2 mg/min	1. Allow 15 to 20 min for full effect 2. Dose interval must be individu- alized 3. Serum half–life: 16 hours 4. Has an amnesic effect
Midazolam† (Versed)	Start at 1 mg and repeat every 3 min PRN to to- tal dose of 0.15 mg/kg OR infuse at 0.4 mcg/min	1. Quickest onset and fastest elimination 2. Has an amnesic effect 3. Clinical experience limited

*From Drug facts and comparisons, 1985. St. Louis: J.B. Lippincott, 1985:935–939.
†From The medical letter 1986; 28:73–74.
‡All doses may need to be reduced when cimetidine is given, particularly diaz-
epam.

Lorazepam (Ativan). This has a shorter elimination half-life than diazepam (16 hours vs 24 hours) and has less of a tendency to accumulate.
Lorazepam also produces an amnesic effect that many consider to be an
advantage. The intravenous dose in adults is 2 mg or 0.04 mg/kg, which-
ever is smaller.[37] Dose intervals vary from patient to patient, and the
dose schedule must be individualized.

Midazolam (Versed). This is the newest parenteral benzodiazepine and
is characterized by a rapid onset and rapid elimination. The latter feature
makes it possible to give midazolam by continuous infusion. The bolus
dose is 1 to 2 mg (which is lower than the dose recommended by the
manufacturer) and the infusion rate is 0.4 micrograms per minute.[38] The
clinical experience with this drug is limited and there have been reports
of a variable elimination time in different patients.[39] More extensive
clinical experience is therefore needed before this drug can be recommended for continuous infusion in the ICU patient population.

MUCOLYTIC THERAPY

Mucolytic agents can reduce the viscosity of respiratory secretions and
can open airways that are obstructed by thick or tenacious secretions.
Airways obstruction from mucus plugs is well known in patients with

asthma and cystic fibrosis. However, the most common cause of tenacious secretions in the adult ICU population is infection.

HUMIDIFICATION OF INSPIRED GAS

There is a fear that intubation will dry secretions and produce airways obstruction because the normal humidification of inspired air that occurs in the nares and pharynx is bypassed with intubation. This fear has led to the regular use of humidification devices for adding water to the inspired gas delivered to intubated patients. However, adding water to secretions will not reduce their viscosity because the viscosity is caused by mucoproteins in the nonaqueous phase of the secretions and water will not enter this phase (by definition). Therefore, the often overzealous use of humidification for intubated patients has little support in theory. If there is a link between intubation and tenacious sputum, the culprit is more likely to be infection and not "dehydrated" sputum.

ACETYLCYSTEINE (MUCOMYST)

N-acetylcysteine (NAC) is an amino acid derivative that breaks disulfide links between mucoproteins and can produce rapid liquefaction of the respiratory mucus.[40] This agent is supplied in liquid form and can be delivered into the airways by inhaling an aerosol spray or by direct instillation through a bronchoscope. Both 10% and 20% solutions are available, and can be given in the following manner:[40]

Inhalation: 2.5 ml of 10% NAC solution plus

2.5 ml of normal saline

Deliver via nebulizer

Instillation: 2.0 ml of 20% NAC solution plus

2.0 ml normal saline or sodium bicarbonate

Deliver via syringe in 1 ml aliquots

Both concentrations are hyperosmolar and can irritate the airways. Bronchospasm has been produced by NAC in asthmatics[40,41] and the drug is not recommended in patients with reactive airways disease. The sodium bicarbonate vehicle is preferred by some because NAC is a reducing agent and works best at an alkaline pH (for you skeptics, the small volume of sodium bicarbonate will not produce pulmonary edema).

The only accepted indication for NAC is airways obstruction from tenacious secretions. The drug can be given for a limited time to patients with thick secretions who are at risk for airways obstruction. However, the irritation to the airways associated with repeated use limits the value of this practice when it is extended to more than a few days.

The liquid NAC can also be swallowed or infused intravenously. Both routes have proven effective for achieving adequate blood levels of NAC when the drug is used as an antidote for patients with acetaminophen overdose.[42] The risk for bronchospasm is not reduced by using the enteral or intravenous route.[41] Intravenous infusion of NAC is appealing because of the ability to deliver the drug to small airways when mucus plugs are beyond the reach of the bronchoscope. However, the intravenous route is not FDA approved at the present time.

REFERENCES

BEDSIDE EVALUATION

1. Shim CH, Williams MH Jr. Relationship of wheezing to the severity of obstruction in asthma. Arch Intern Med 1983; 143:890–892.
2. Williams MH. Expiratory flow rates: Their role in asthma therapy. Hosp Pract 1982; 95–110.
3. Gay PC, Rodarte JR, Tayyab M, Hubmayar RD. Evaluation of bronchodilator responsiveness in mechanically ventilated patients. Am Rev Respir Dis 1987; 136:880–885.

ADRENERGIC AGENTS

4. Herman JJ, Noah ZL, Moody RR. Use of intravenous isoproterenol for status asthmaticus in children. Crit Care Med 1983; 11:716–720.
5. Hendeles L. Asthma therapy: State of the art, 1988. J Respir Dis 1988; 9:82–109.
6. Popa V. Beta-adrenergic drugs. Clin Chest Med 1986; 7:313–329.
7. Anthonison NR, Wright EC, and the IPPB Trial Group. Bronchodilator response in chronic obstructive pulmonary disease. Am Rev Respir Dis 1986; 133:814–819.

THEOPHYLLINE

8. Littenberg B. Aminophylline treatment in severe, acute asthma. A meta analysis. JAMA 1988; 259:1678–1684.
9. Hill NS. The use of theophylline in "irreversible" chronic obstructive pulmonary disease. Arch Intern Med 1988; 148:2579–2584.
10. Bukowskyj M, Nakatsu K, Munt PW. Theophylline reassessed. Ann Intern Med 1984; 101:63–73.
11. Powell JR, Vozeh S, Hopewell P, et al. Theophylline disposition in acutely ill hospitalized patients. The effects of smoking, heart failure, severe airway obstruction, and pneumonia. Am Rev Respir Dis 1978; 118:229–238.
12. Mitenko PA, Ogilvie TI. Rational intravenous doses of theophylline. N Engl J Med 1973; 289:600–603.
13. Rogers RM, Owens GR, Pennock BE. The pendulum swings again. Toward a rational use of theophylline. Chest 1985; 87:280–282.
14. Paloucek FP, Rodvold KA. Evaluation of theophylline overdoses and toxicities. Ann Emerg Med 1988; 17:135–144.

15. Bertino JS, Walker JW. Reassessment of theophylline toxicity. Serum concentrations, clinical course, and treatment. Arch Intern Med 1987; *147:*757–760.
16. Jacobs MH, Senior RM, Kessler G. Clinical experience with theophylline. Relationship between dosage, serum concentration and toxicity. JAMA 1976; 2235:1983–1986.

ANTICHOLINERGIC AGENTS

17. Ziment I, Au JP. Anticholinergic agents. Clin Chest Med 1986; *7:*355–366.
18. Rebuck AS, Chapman KR, Abboud R, et al. Nebulized anticholinergic and sympathomimetic treatment of asthma and chronic obstructive airways disease in the emergency room. Am J Med 1987; *82:*59–64.
19. Bryant DH. Nebulized ipatropium bromide in the treatment of acute asthma. Chest 1985; *88:*24–29.

STEROIDS

20. Fanta CH, Rossing TH, McFadden ER. Glucocorticoids in acute asthma. A controlled clinical trial. Am J Med 1983; *74:*845–851.
21. Haskell RJ, Wong BM, Hansen JE. A double-blind, randomized clinical trial of methylprednisolone in status asthmaticus. Arch Intern Med 1983; *143:*1324–1327.
22. Albert RK, Martin TR, Lewis SW. Controlled clinical trial of methylprednisolone in patients with chronic bronchitis and acute respiratory insufficiency. Ann Intern Med 1980; *92:*753–758.
23. Bernard GR, Luce JM, Sprung CL: High-dose corticosteroids in patients with the adult respiratory distress syndrome. N Engl J Med 1987; *317:*1565–1570.

RESPIRATORY STIMULANTS

24. Lugliani R, Whipp BJ, Wasserman K. Doxapram hydrochloride: A respiratory stimulant for patients with primary alveolar hypoventilation. Chest 1979; *76:*414–419.
25. Martin RJ, Ballard RD: Respiratory stimulants. In: Cherniak RM ed. Drugs for the respiratory system. Orlando: Grune & Stratton, 1986:191–212.
26. Moore RA, Rumack BH, Connors CS, Peterson RG. Naloxone. Underdosage after narcotic poisoning. Am J Dis Child 1980; *134:*156–158.
27. Lyons HA, Huang CT. Therapeutic use of progesterone in alveolar hypoventilation associated with obesity. Am J Med 1968; *44:*881–888.
28. Aubier M, DeTroyer A, Sampson M, et al. Aminophylline improves diaphragmatic contractility. N Engl J Med 1981; *305:*249–252.

MUSCLE RELAXANTS

29. Lumb PD. Sedatives and muscle relaxants in the intensive care unit. In: Fuhrman BP, Shoemaker WC eds. Critical care. State of the art. Fullerton: Society of Critical Care Medicine 1989:145–172.
30. Drug facts and comparisons, 1985. St Louis: J.B. Lippincott, 1985:1112–1125.
31. Schwartz SH. Treatment of status asthmaticus with halothane. JAMA 1984; *251:*2688–2689.

SEDATIVE-HYPNOTIC AGENTS

32. Tesar GE, Stern TA. Evaluation and treatment of agitation in the intensive care unit. J Intensive Care Med 1986; 1:137–148.
33. Alexander HE, McCarty K, Giffen MB. Hypotension and cardiopulmonary arrest associated with concurrent haloperidol and propranolol therapy. JAMA 1984; 252:87–88.
34. Menza MA, Murray GB, Holmes VF, Rafuls WA. Controlled study of extrapyramidal reactions in the management of delirious, medically ill patients: Intravenous haloperidol versus intravenous haloperidol plus benzodiazepines. Heart Lung 1988; 17:238–241.
35. Rampertaap MP. Neuroleptic malignant syndrome. South Med J 1986; 79:331–336.
36. Altose MA, Hudgel DW. The pharmacology of respiratory depressants and stimulants. Clin Chest Med 1986; 7:481–494.
37. Drug facts and comparisons, 1985. St Louis: J.B. Lippincott, 1985:935.
38. Midazolam. The Medical Letter 1986; 28:73–74.
39. Oldenhof H, deJong M, Steenhoek A, Janknegt R. Clinical pharmacokinetics of midazolam in intensive care patients, a wide interpatient variability? Clin Pharmacol Ther 1988; 43:263–269.

MUCOLYTIC AGENTS

40. Ziment IW. Respiratory pharmacology and therapeutics. Philadelphia: W.B. Saunders, 1978; 60–104.
41. Ho SWC, Beilin LJ. Asthma associated with N-acetylcysteine infusion and paracetamol poisoning: Report of two cases. Br Med J 1983; 287:876–877.
42. Smilkstein MJ, Knapp GL, Kulig KW, Rumack BH. Efficacy of oral N-acetylcysteine in the treatment of acetaminophen overdose. N Engl J Med 1988; 319:1557–1562.

section VIII
MECHANICAL VENTILATION

All who drink of this remedy will recover . . . except those whom it does not help, who will die. Therefore, it is obvious that it fails only in incurable cases.

Galen

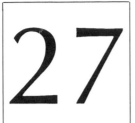

c h a p t e r

27

CONVENTIONAL MECHANICAL VENTILATION

" . . . an opening must be attempted in the trunk of the trachea, into which a tube of reed or cane should be put; you will then blow into this, so that the lung may rise again . . . . the lung will swell to the full extent of the thoracic cavity, and the heart becomes strong . . . "

Andreas Vesalius (1555)

Vesalius is credited with the first description of positive-pressure ventilation but it took exactly 400 years for his concept to be applied to clinical medicine on a widespread scale. The occasion was the polio epidemic of 1955, when the need for ventilators outgrew the supply of the popular negative-pressure tank ventilators (iron lungs). In Sweden, all medical schools shut down and medical students worked in 8-hour shifts as human ventilators, manually inflating the lungs of afflicted patients. In Boston, the nearby Emerson company put a prototype positive-pressure device to use at the Massachusetts General Hospital. The rest of the story involves the growth of positive-pressure mechanical ventilation and the birth of intensive care as a specialty.

VOLUME-CYCLED VENTILATION

The first positive-pressure ventilators were designed to inflate the lungs until a preset pressure was reached. These "pressure-cycled" ventilators fell out of favor because the inflation volume could not be kept constant unless the mechanical properties of the lungs were also kept constant. The newer "volume-cycled" ventilators can deliver a constant volume in the face of changing lung mechanics.[1-3] The waveforms produced by volume-cycled ventilation are shown in Figure 27–1. The in-

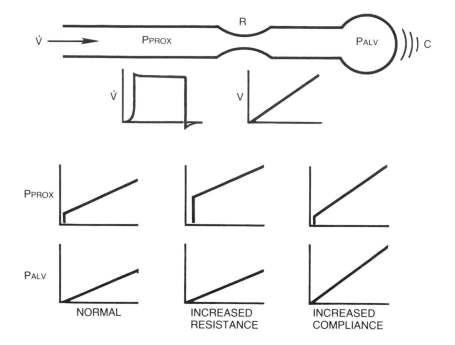

FIG. 27–1. Waveforms for volume-cycled ventilation. $\dot{V}$: inspiratory flowrate, V: inflation volume, R: airway resistance, Pprox: proximal airway pressure, Palv: alveolar pressure, C: lung compliance. Lower series of graphs illustrate the effects of lung mechanics on airway pressures.

spiratory flowrate ($\dot{V}$) is constant, producing a linear increase in lung volume (V) during inspiration (upper graphs). The pressure in the proximal airways (Pprox) increases abruptly at first and then rises more gradually through the remainder of the lung inflation. The pressure in the alveolus (Palv) shows only a gradual rise during all of inspiration. The early abrupt rise in the proximal airway pressure is produced by airways resistance between the proximal airways and the alveoli.

ABNORMAL LUNG MECHANICS

The series of graphs in the lower portion of Figure 27–1 show the changes in airways pressure in response to changes in lung mechanics. An increase in airways resistance (middle panel) augments the initial rise in proximal airways pressure but does not change the alveolar pressure. A decrease in lung compliance (graphs on the right) increases the rate of rise in both proximal and alveolar pressure. These patterns illustrate two points related to positive-pressure ventilation. First, when airways resistance is high, the proximal airways can buffer the alveoli from high inflation pressures. Second, when the lungs are stiff, the inflation pressure is easily transmitted to the alveoli and this can lead

NORMAL LUNG   PULMONARY EDEMA

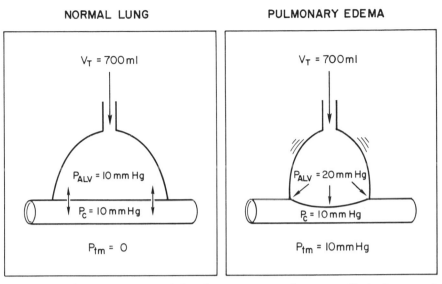

FIG. 27–2. The transmission of alveolar pressure to adjacent capillaries in normal and diseased lungs. Palv: alveolar pressure, Pc: capillary pressure, Ptm: transmural pressure across the alveolar-capillary interface, VT: tidal volume.

to compression of pulmonary capillaries and reduced left ventricular filling.

CARDIOVASCULAR INTERACTIONS

The influence of intermittent positive-pressure ventilation (IPPV) on the cardiovascular system is complex, and is determined by the balance between intravascular pressure and intrathoracic pressure.[4,5] The transmission of alveolar pressure to the surrounding vascular structures is the important variable because this will determine the change in transmural pressure (the physiologically important pressure).

TRANSMURAL PRESSURE

The influence of alveolar pressure on capillary transmural pressure is illustrated in Figure 27–2. Panel A represents a normal lung inflated with 700 ml from a positive-pressure source. The alveolar pressure equilibrates completely with the capillary pressure, resulting in a transmural pressure (Ptm) of zero. If the same conditions are imposed on a stiff lung (pulmonary edema), the alveolar pressure is not transmitted to the capillary, and the transmural pressure increases to 10 mmHg. Incomplete transmission of the positive-pressure in the alveoli will therefore tend to compress the heart and intrathoracic vessels, while complete equilibration of pressure has no influence on the diameter of the vascular structures.

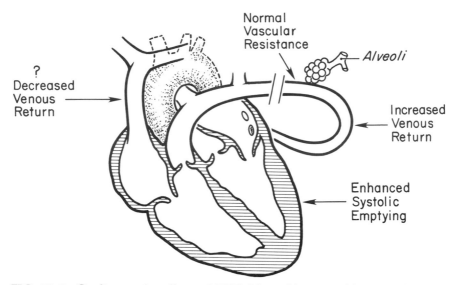

FIG. 27–3. Cardiovascular effects of IPPV: Normal lungs and low intrathoracic pressures.

CARDIAC PERFORMANCE

An increase in intrathoracic pressure can produce an increase in cardiac output when the intravascular volume is normal, but can decrease the cardiac output when intravascular volume is reduced.[4,5] The augmentation in cardiac output is the result of a decrease in left ventricular afterload and the decrease in cardiac output is the result of inadequate ventricular filling. The performance of the heart during IPPV, therefore, depends on the balance between the preload and afterload effects of positive intrathoracic pressure. The spectrum of changes in preload and afterload are illustrated in Figures 27–3 and 27–4.

Preload. Venous inflow into the chest decreases when the intrathoracic pressure exceeds the venous inflow pressure. This effect is magnified in hypovolemic patients, particularly when intrathoracic pressures are high. The venous inflow to the left ventricle is normally increased by positive intrathoracic pressure, because the positive pressure displaces blood from the pulmonary veins to the left atrium.[4] When thoracic pressures are excessive, left ventricular filling can decrease because of the increase in right ventricular afterload. This not only reduces the output of the right heart, it can produce right ventricular distension and push the interventricular septum toward the left to reduce left ventricular chamber size. This is illustrated in Figure 27–4 and is called "interventricular interdependence."

Afterload. The influence of IPPV on ventricular afterload differs for each side of the heart. Right ventricular afterload is unchanged during IPPV when the lungs are normal because the alveolar pressure equilibrates with the pulmonary vessels and the transmural pressure in the pulmonary arteries remains unchanged (see Fig. 27–2). When the lungs

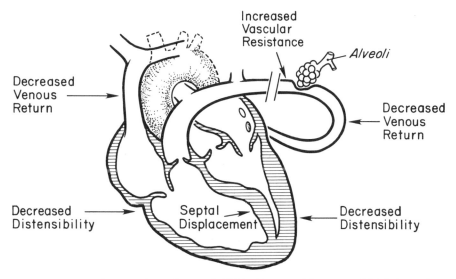

FIG. 27–4. Cardiovascular effects of IPPV: Abnormal lungs and high intrathoracic pressures.

are stiff from edema or pneumonia, the transmural pressure in the pulmonary arteries can increase during positive-pressure lung inflation and this will increase right-heart afterload.

The afterload of the left ventricle decreases during IPPV because the positive pleural pressure is transmitted to the outer surface of the ventricle and this "juxtacardiac pressure" decreases the transmural pressure across the ventricle during systole (remember from Chapter 1 that afterload is defined as the peak systolic transmural pressure). This will result in an increase in left ventricular stroke output as long as ventricular filling is maintained.

IPPV and CPR. The ability of positive intrathoracic pressure to reduce left ventricular afterload and promote cardiac output is illustrated by the phenomenon of "reverse pulsus paradoxus." This phenomenon is characterized by an increase in systolic blood pressure during positive-pressure lung inflation. An extreme example of this phenomenon is shown in Figure 16–2. The blood pressure tracing in Figure 16–2 was recorded from a patient with asystole that was refractory to standard resuscitative measures. The pressure swings in the tracing were produced *entirely* by manual lung inflation using an Ambu bag attached to the endotracheal tube. In the absence of lung inflation, the systemic pressure promptly falls to zero!

The principle of cardiac augmentation from positive intrathoracic pressure has become one of the explanations for the ability of closed chest cardiac compressions to promote systemic blood flow. This principle also explains "cough CPR," which is the application of sudden increases in intrathoracic pressure to promote blood flow during brief periods of hemodynamic instability from life-threatening arrhythmias. The role of positive intrathoracic pressure in cardiopulmonary resuscitation is presented in more detail in Chapter 16.

Summary. In summary, modest levels of positive pressure in the thorax can enhance cardiac output by reducing left ventricular afterload. However, excessive intrathoracic pressures eventually reduce the diastolic filling of both ventricles, and this counteracts the beneficial effects of IPPV on left ventricular afterload. This produces a decrease in cardiac output when intrathoracic pressures are high or intravascular volume is low.

INDICATIONS FOR MECHANICAL VENTILATION

The decision to intubate and place on assisted ventilation has always seemed to be more complex than it should be. Lists of criteria are not necessary. The following rules should suffice.

Rule 1: The indication for intubation and mechanical ventilation is thinking of it.

There is a real tendency to delay intubation as long as possible in the hopes that it will not be necessary. However, this can lead to problems if the intubation is done when the patient is severely ill. If a patient has a severe enough condition to make you consider intubation, it seems wise to proceed without delay.

Rule 2: Whenever in doubt, get control of the airways.

If you are vacillating and cannot make the decision, it is wise to get control of the situation first by intubating and starting mechanical ventilation. Once the patient is supported, you have time to evaluate the situation.

Rule 3: Endotracheal tubes are not a disease and ventilators are not addicting.

The concept of "once on a ventilator, always on a ventilator" implies that intubation and mechanical ventilation will promote the need for mechanical ventilation. Chronic ventilator patients require the ventilator because of their cardiopulmonary disease, not because they have been on a ventilator.

Rule 4: Intubating a patient does not reduce virility.

There is a tendency to view intubation as an act of cowardice and housestaff often apologize on morning rounds when they have intubated a patient that evening. You should never be criticized for intubating a patient but you will be criticized if there is an unnecessary delay in intubation that jeopardizes the patient.

INITIATING MECHANICAL VENTILATION

When mechanical ventilation is started, the respiratory therapist will ask for the following information: (1) Mode of ventilation, (2) Inflation volume, (3) Respiratory rate, and (4) Inspired oxygen level. These are presented briefly in this section.

MODE OF VENTILATION

The initial mode of ventilation that is selected is usually the "assist/control" mode. This allows the patient to initiate the mechanical breath by generating a small negative intrathoracic pressure (assist mode), and also provides adequate ventilation if the patient is unable to breathe at all (control mode). The one problem with the assist mode is the patient with a high respiratory rate who is triggering the ventilator with each breath. This can produce a severe respiratory alkalosis and can create auto-PEEP. In this situation, the options are to sedate the patient, or use a mode of ventilation called "intermittent mandatory ventilation" or IMV. This mode of ventilation is presented in the next chapter.

TIDAL VOLUME

The inflation volumes delivered during mechanical ventilation are excessive, as shown below.

$$\text{Normal } V_T = 5 \text{ to } 6 \text{ ml/kg} \quad \text{(ideal weight)}$$

$$\text{Ventilator } V_T = 12 \text{ to } 15 \text{ ml/kg}$$

The tidal volume (V_T) delivered by the ventilator is at least twice the volume of normal tidal breathing. The rationale for the large inflation volumes is a fear that prolonged mechanical ventilation will cause progressive alveolar collapse. Even larger volume "sighs" (one and one-half times the usual inflation volume) have been incorporated into most ventilators, despite the lack of evidence that sighs provide any benefit in patients with respiratory failure.[7] There is little to support the routine use of high inflation volumes in short-term mechanical ventilation, and this explains why respiratory alkalosis from overventilation is the most common cause of complications from mechanical ventilation.[8]

Patients who have undergone lung resection (particularly a pneumonectomy) will be at particular risk for barotrauma from excessive tidal volumes. In this situation, the inflation volume of 10 to 15 ml/kg should be reduced by the estimated percent loss in lung volume.

Connector Tubing. The connector tubing between the ventilator and the patient expands during positive-pressure inflation and this can result in loss of inflation volume. The volume lost is a function of the peak inflation pressure (Ppk) and the compliance of the tubing. The usual compliance of the tubing is 3 to 4 ml/cm H_2O, which means that 3 to 4 ml of volume is lost for every 1 cm H_2O increase in inflation volume.

The following examples will illustrate how this becomes important at high inspiratory pressures.
For a machine V_T of 700 ml and tube compliance of 4 ml/cm H_2O:

If Ppk = 20 cm H_2O, then actual V_T = 620 ml
If Ppk = 40 cm H_2O, then actual V_T = 540 ml
If Ppk = 80 cm H_2O, then actual V_T = 380 ml

At the highest Ppk, almost half the inflation volume is lost in the tubing and never reaches the patient. This can become a problem in patients with stiff lungs (e.g., pulmonary edema) and, therefore, newer ventilators can adjust for the lost volume to ensure that the patient is receiving the desired volume.

RESPIRATORY RATE

The machine rate is usually set at 12 to 14 breaths/minute. When patients are able to initiate the ventilator breaths, the machine rate serves only as a backup system in the event that the patient is no longer able to breathe adequately. The respiratory rate should be kept to a minimum at all times, if possible, to minimize the development of auto PEEP (see Chapter 29).

INSPIRED OXYGEN

The fraction of inspired oxygen (FIO_2) is usually set at 80% or higher initially and then decreased in steps of 10 to 20% until a safe level (below 60%) is reached. When significant lung disease is present, wait at least 20 minutes after the change in FIO_2 to allow the arterial PO_2 to reach a new steady-state level. If it is not possible to decrease the FIO_2 to nontoxic levels, consider using positive end-expiratory pressure (see Chapter 28).

MONITORING LUNG MECHANICS

During spontaneous breathing, the mechanical properties of the lungs (i.e., elastic recoil and airways resistance) can be monitored with pulmonary function tests. Lung volumes are used as a measure of elastic recoil and expiratory flowrates are used as a measure of airway resistance. However, these cannot be obtained routinely while patients are receiving mechanical ventilation. In this situation, the proximal airways pressures can be used to assess pulmonary function.[10]

PROXIMAL AIRWAY PRESSURES

Volume-cycled ventilators have pressure gauges that monitor the proximal airway pressure during each respiratory cycle. This pressure

INFLATION

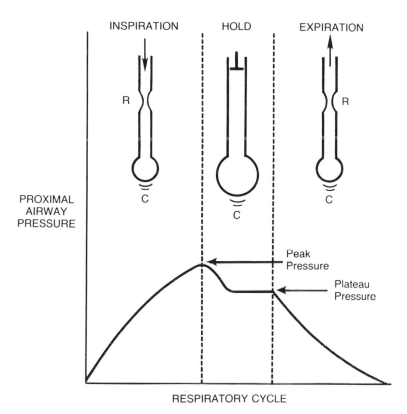

FIG. 27–5. Proximal airway pressure during an "inflation hold" maneuver. See text for explanation.

can be used to assess lung mechanics, as illustrated in Figure 27–5. The peak pressure at the end of inspiration is a function of the inflation volume, the resistance in the airways, and the compliance (distensibility) of the lungs and chest wall. At a constant inflation volume, the peak pressure (Ppk) is directly proportional to airway resistance (R), and inversely proportional to lung compliance (C):

$$Ppk \propto R + 1/C$$

Therefore, at constant lung volume, an increase in peak inflation pressure indicates either an increase in airway resistance or a decrease in compliance (or both).

The two elements of lung mechanics can be separated by occluding the expiratory tubing at the end of inspiration, as shown in Figure 27–5. When the tidal volume is held in the lungs, the proximal airway pressure decreases initially and then reaches a steady level and remains there until the occlusion is released and the lungs are allowed to deflate. The constant "plateau pressure" represents the elastic recoil pressure of the thorax (lungs and chest wall). Because compliance is the reciprocal of elastance, the relationship between plateau pressure (Ppl) and compliance (C) is:

$$Ppl \propto 1/C$$

Therefore, when lung volume is constant, an increase in the plateau pressure indicates a decrease in the compliance of the thorax, and vice-versa. Because the plateau pressure is measured in the absence of airflow, the difference between peak and plateau pressures is the pressure needed to overcome the resistance in the airways.

$$Ppk - Ppl \propto (R + 1/C) - 1/C$$

$$or\ Ppk - Ppl \propto R$$

Therefore, an increase in peak pressure with no change in plateau pressure indicates an increase in airways resistance. However, if both peak and plateau pressure increase, the problem is a decrease in lung (or chest wall) compliance.

MEASURING RESPIRATORY MECHANICS

The peak and plateau pressures can be used to generate a quantitative measurement of the mechanical properties of the respiratory system. It is important to point out that the proximal airway pressures represent transthoracic pressures (measured relative to atmospheric pressure) and not transpulmonary pressures (measured relative to pleural pressure). Therefore, the mechanical properties being measured are those of the lungs *and* the chest wall. For the remainder of the chapter, thorax will indicate the lungs and the chest wall.

COMPLIANCE

Compliance is defined in Chapter 1 as the change in volume associated with a change in pressure ($\Delta V/\Delta P$). The static (stationary) compliance of the thorax can be derived using the tidal volume from the ventilator

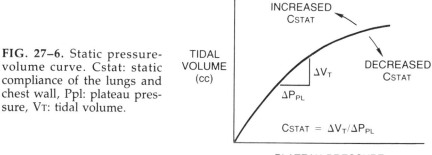

FIG. 27–6. Static pressure-volume curve. Cstat: static compliance of the lungs and chest wall, Ppl: plateau pressure, VT: tidal volume.

and the end-inspiratory plateau pressure at each tidal volume. For a tidal volume (VT) of 800 ml and the plateau pressure (Ppl) of 10 cm H_2O:

$$Cstat = VT / Ppl \ (L/cm \ H_2O)$$

$$= 0.8 / 10$$

$$= .08 \ L/cm \ H_2O \ (or \ 80 \ ml/cm \ H_2O)$$

$$Normal \ Range = .05 \ to \ .07 \ L/cm \ H_2O$$

The following considerations are important:
1. Measurements should be obtained with the patient at rest and breathing synchronously with the ventilator. Use of chest wall muscles will increase the contribution of the chest wall to the Cstat measurement.
2. The exhaled volume is used as the tidal volume to minimize errors from loss of inflation volume in connector tubing.

Because compliance is actually a **change** in volume and pressure, the more accurate method of determining compliance is to measure the plateau pressure at several tidal volumes,[10] and to generate a static pressure-volume curve like the one shown in Figure 27–6.
The slope of this curve is the static compliance of the respiratory system. A decrease in compliance will decrease the slope and shift the curve down and to the right, while an increase in compliance will increase the slope and shift the curve to the left. The use of pressure-volume curves to determine static compliance is tedious and there is no evidence that this method provides any clinical benefit over compliance determinations performed at a single tidal volume.
The Cstat in normal subjects during spontaneous breathing is over .09 L/cm H_2O,[11] while the value in intubated patients without lung disease is reported at .05 to .07 L/cm H_2O.[10,12] Most of the lung diseases that are responsible for acute respiratory failure will cause a decrease in lung compliance (e.g., pulmonary edema and pneumonia), while res-

olution of the disease will result in a return of the compliance to normal or baseline levels.

The major limitation in the compliance measurement is the uncertainty about the contribution of the chest wall to the measurement. One study showed that the elastic recoil pressure of the chest wall accounted for 35% of the total elastic recoil of the thorax (lungs and chest wall).[13] Factors such as contraction of the chest wall musculature and edema of the chest wall can increase the relative contribution of the chest wall to the compliance measurement. For this reason, a single measurement of respiratory compliance cannot be used to estimate lung compliance. Rather, changes in respiratory compliance can be used to indicate changes in lung compliance, but only when the mechanical properties of the chest wall have not changed.

RESISTANCE

The resistance to airflow during inspiration (Rinsp) can be determined by dividing the peak inspiratory flowrate (Vinsp) into the pressure needed to overcome the resistance to airflow (Ppk − Ppl). For example, if an inspiratory flowrate of 40 L/sec is associated with a peak pressure of 22 cm H_2O and a plateau pressure of 10 cm H_2O:

$$Rinsp = Ppk - Ppl / Vinsp$$

$$= 22 - 10/40$$

$$= 0.3 \text{ cm } H_2O/L/sec$$

This resistance represents the summed resistance of the connector tubing, the tracheal tube, and the airways. However, changes in Rinsp should represent changes in airways resistance as long as the inspiratory flowrate and the size of the tracheal tube and connector tubing is constant. In intubated patients without lung disease, Rinsp is 4 to 6 cm H_2O/L/sec.[12,14]

The major limitation in the resistance measurement may be the sensitivity of inspiratory resistance as an indication of resistance in the small airways. That is, airflow obstruction in the small airways is usually measured during expiration (particularly forced expiration) and the distending pressures delivered by the ventilator during inspiration may keep the small airways open. If this is the case, measurement of airflow resistance during inspiration may not be a sensitive measure of changes in small airways resistance.[15] However, measurement of airflow resistance during expiration cannot be performed routinely in a clinical setting; therefore, the inspiratory resistance measurement is the only index of airway resistance routinely available at the bedside.

PRACTICAL APPLICATIONS

The pressures in the proximal airways may be valuable in the following clinical situations:

TROUBLESHOOTING

When a ventilator patient develops sudden onset of respiratory distress or worsening blood gases, the proximal airway pressures can provide a simple and rapid method to help in identifying the problem at the bedside. The logic sequence for this is shown in Figure 27–7.

1. If the peak pressure is increased but the plateau pressure is unchanged, the problem is an increase in airways resistance. In this situation, the major concerns are obstruction of the tracheal tube, airway obstruction from secretions, and acute bronchospasm (e.g., anaphylaxis). Therefore, airways suctioning is indicated along with a search for an obstruction in the tracheal tube. Bronchodilators can be considered if the problem is suspected bronchospasm (which should be uncommon).

2. If the peak and plateau pressures are increased, the problem is a decrease in compliance of the lungs or chest wall, or auto-PEEP. In this situation, the major concerns are pneumothorax, lobar atelectasis, and pulmonary edema. Active contraction of the chest wall and increased abdominal pressure can also decrease the compliance of the thorax. In addition, any patient with obstructive lung disease who becomes tachypneic can develop auto-PEEP and this will increase the peak and plateau pressures (see Chapter 29).

3. If the peak pressure is decreased, the problem may be an air leak in the system (e.g., tubing disconnect or cuff leak). In this situation, manually inflate the lungs with an Ambu bag and listen for a cuff leak during lung inflation. A decrease in peak pressure can also be caused by hyperventilation when the patient is generating enough of a negative intrathoracic pressure to "pull" air into the lungs.

4. If there is no change in peak pressure, do not assume that there has been no change in lung mechanics. The sensitivity of the proximal airway pressures in detecting changes in lung mechanics is not known. When the pressures do not change, proceed with your evaluation as you would without the aid of the proximal pressures.

MONITORING CLINICAL COURSE

In patients with decreased lung compliance from conditions such as pulmonary edema and diffuse pneumonia, routine monitoring of plateau pressures may help in following the clinical course of the disease. Remember to make sure the tidal volume is constant when interpreting changes in plateau pressure.

In patients with airways disease from conditions such as asthma and COPD, the difference between peak and plateau pressures can be used

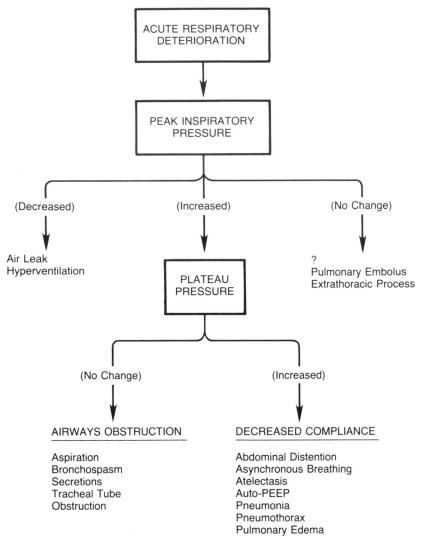

FIG. 27–7. Flow diagram for interpreting changes in peak and plateau pressures. See text for explanation.

to follow the resistance in the airways. Once again, the tidal volume should be constant when interpreting changes in these pressures.

ASSESSING RESPONSE TO BRONCHODILATORS

The routine administration of bronchodilators is a common practice in patients requiring mechanical ventilation although there is no clear documentation that this is beneficial for all patients. In any individual patient, the response to inhaled bronchodilators can be evaluated using the peak inspiratory pressure. Inhaled beta agonists both decrease airways resistance and increase lung compliance,[16] and either of these effects should decrease peak inspiratory pressures. Therefore, to determine if a nebulized bronchodilator is effective, monitor the peak pressure just before giving the agent and again 30 to 60 minutes later. A decrease in peak pressure can then be used as evidence that the bronchodilator is having an effect.

EVALUATING PEEP

As will be discussed in the next chapter, the application of PEEP should result in an increase in Cstat, so the plateau pressure should decrease. This can be seen almost immediately after PEEP is applied. The plateau pressure can then provide a simple and rapid assessment of the effects of PEEP on lung mechanics. As long as the plateau pressure decreases at each level of PEEP, it is safe to assume that PEEP is producing the desired effect on lung mechanics. Remember to subtract the amount of PEEP from the measured plateau pressure to arrive at the final pressure.

BIBLIOGRAPHY

Kirby RR, Smith RA, Desautels DA eds. Mechanical ventilation. New York: Churchill Livingstone, 1985.
Morganroth ML ed. Mechanical ventilation. Clin Chest Med 1988; 9(Mar).
Rattenborg CC, Via-Reque E eds. Clinical use of mechanical ventilation. Chicago: Year Book Medical Publishers, 1981.

REFERENCES

REVIEWS

1. Snyder JV, Carroll GC, Schuster DP, et al. Mechanical ventilation: Physiology and application. Curr Prob Surg 1984; 21(Mar).
2. Grum CM, Chauncey JB. Conventional mechanical ventilation. Clin Chest Med 1988; 9:37–54.

CARDIAC PERFORMANCE

3. Jardin F, Farcot JC, Gueret P, et al. Cyclic changes in arterial pulse during respiratory support. Circulation 1983; 68:266–274.
4. Biondi JW, Schulman DS, Matthay RA. Effects of mechanical ventilation on right and left ventricular function. Clin Chest Med 1988; 9:55–71.
5. Abel JG, Salerno TA, Panos A, et al. Cardiovascular effects of positive-pressure ventilation in humans. Ann Thorac Surg 1987; 43:198–206.

INITIATING MECHANICAL VENTILATION

6. Grum CM, Morganroth ML. Initiating mechanical ventilation. J Intensive Care Med 1988; 3:6–20.
7. Kacmarek RM, Venegas J. Mechanical ventilatory rates and tidal volumes. Respir Care 1987; 32:466-478.
8. Novak RA, Shumaker L, Snyder JV, Pinsky MR. Do periodic hyperinflations improve gas exchange in patients with hypoxemic respiratory failure? Crit Care Med 1987; 15:1081–1085.
9. Zwillich CW, Pierson DJ, Creagh CE, et al. Complications of assisted ventilation. Am J Med 1974; 57:161–170.

MONITORING LUNG MECHANICS

10. Bone RC. Diagnosis of causes for acute respiratory distress by pressure-volume curves. Chest 1976; 70:740–746.
11. Berger R, Burki NK. The effects of posture on total respiratory compliance. Am Rev Respir Dis 1982; 125:262–263.
12. Bergman NA. Measurement of respiratory resistance in anesthetized subjects. J Appl Physiol 1966; 21:1913–1917.
13. Katz JA, Zinn SE, Ozanne GM, Fairley BB. Pulmonary, chest wall and lung-thorax elastances in acute respiratory failure. Chest 1981; 80:304–311.
14. Gomez-Rubi JA, SanMartin A, Gonzalez-Diaz G, Apezteguia C, Torrez-Martinez G, Martin R. Assessment of total pulmonary airways resistance during mechanical ventilation. Crit Care Med 1980; 11:633–636.
15. Marino PL, Barkin P, Shaw D, et al. Bronchodilator effects on inspiratory and expiratory airflow resistance during mechanical ventilation. Am Rev Respir Dis 1983; 127:263.
16. DeTroyer A, Yernault JC, Rodenstein D. Influence of beta-2 agonist aerosols on pressure-volume characteristics of the lungs. Am Rev Respir Dis 1978; 118:987–995.

chapter

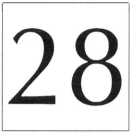

28

MODES OF VENTILATION

Mechanical ventilation was introduced in 1929 to "give all patients with respiratory paralysis the opportunity to recover normal breathing." (Drinker P, McKhann CF. JAMA 1929; 92:1658–1660.) This support role has evolved over the years as selective "modes" of ventilation have been developed for specific clinical situations. This chapter will present five of these specialized patterns of ventilation. There is a tendency to consider these as a therapy for the specific application. Remember that ventilators are not remote control devices that can make lung pathology vanish, and even the special modes of ventilation are meant to provide support only.

ASSISTED VENTILATION

The assist mode of ventilation allows the patient to set the breathing pattern and the respiratory rate. The patient initiates each machine breath by lowering the airway pressure (usually 1 to 2 cmH$_2$O) to open a unidirectional valve in the circuit. Once the valve is open, the lungs are inflated to the desired volume.

One of the major misconceptions about assisted ventilation is the notion that it permits the respiratory muscles to rest. On the contrary, the diaphragm does not stop contracting after the machine breath is initiated[1] because the activity in the phrenic nerve originates from the brainstem respiratory centers and these neurons fire automatically throughout life. In other words, the brainstem respiratory neurons do not know that the patient is on a ventilator or that a machine breath is being delivered. The inability to rest the diaphragm has some important implications in the methods used to wean patients from ventilators, as discussed in Chapter 30.

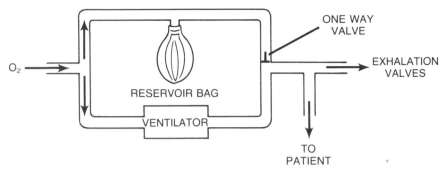

FIG. 28–1. Intermittent Mandatory Ventilation (IMV) circuit.

INTERMITTENT MANDATORY VENTILATION

Intermittent mandatory ventilation (IMV) intersperses spontaneous breaths with machine breaths. IMV was introduced in 1971 for neonates with respiratory distress syndrome because conventional ventilators were unable to deliver the rapid rates developed in this condition. The IMV mode was able to deliver an occasional machine breath while allowing the neonates to breathe at high rates between machine breaths.

Shortly after its introduction, IMV was proposed as an alternative method for weaning adults from mechanical ventilation.[2] Despite any evidence that it is superior to conventional methods of weaning,[3] IMV has become the most popular method of weaning in this country. This discussion will focus on IMV as a mode of ventilation, not a mode of weaning. The use of IMV in weaning is presented in Chapter 30.

THE IMV CIRCUIT

The IMV circuit is shown in Figure 28–1. The patient is connected to a common source of oxygen through two parallel circuits. One circuit contains a volume-cycled ventilator and the other contains a reservoir bag filled with the inhaled gas mixture. A unidirectional valve in the circuit allows the patient to breathe spontaneously from the reservoir bag when a ventilator breath is not being delivered. The pattern of breathing in IMV ventilation is shown in Figure 28–2. The upper panel shows the pattern obtained with the early IMV systems. Note that the mechanical breath (solid line) is delivered at the height of the spontaneous inspiration (dashed line). This random delivery pattern was poorly tolerated by patients and the system was modified so that machine breaths were delivered only when the patient first started to inhale. The newer IMV system produces a breathing pattern like the one shown in the middle panel of Figure 28–2. This is called "synchronized IMV" or SIMV and is standard on most of the newer ventilators. From here on, IMV and SIMV will be used interchangeably.

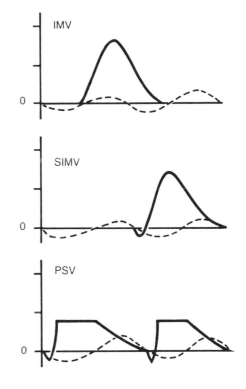

FIG. 28–2. Proximal airway pressure profiles for three methods of augmented ventilation. IMV: Intermittent Mandatory Ventilation; SIMV: Synchronized IMV; PSV: Pressure Support Ventilation (PSV). Augmented breaths shown as solid lines; spontaneous breaths shown as dashed lines. Proximal airway pressure on vertical axis.

USES AND MISUSES

IMV has both advantages and disadvantages when compared to conventional mechanical ventilation (CMV) and these are listed in Table 28–1. Few of the proposed advantages of IMV have been validated or tested in clinical studies.[3] The following is a brief description of what is known at present.

Respiratory Alkalosis. Respiratory alkalosis is the most common complication of CMV,[4] and this has led to the popularity of IMV in patients with rapid breathing rates. Although IMV is associated with less respiratory alkalosis than CMV, the mechanism is not a desirable one. That is, the increase in arterial PCO_2 associated with IMV ventilation is caused by an increase in the rate of CO_2 production and not a decrease in alveolar ventilation.[5] The enhanced CO_2 production indicates an increased work of breathing with IMV and this may not be desirable in some patients, particularly those prone to respiratory muscle fatigue. To summarize,

> The ability of IMV to correct respiratory alkalosis is because of an increase in the work of breathing and not a decrease in alveolar ventilation.

Cardiac Output. IMV is also considered less risky for adverse cardiac effects than CMV.[6] However, the cardiac output does not increase when IMV is substituted for CMV in individual patients.[7] In fact, the cardiac output can decrease when switching from CMV to IMV in patients with left ventricular dysfunction.[8]

TABLE 28–1. INTERMITTENT MANDATORY VENTILATION (IMV)
VERSUS CONVENTIONAL MECHANICAL VENTILATION (CMV)

Advantages of IMV versus CMV	Proven	Unproven
Less respiratory alkalosis	X	
Improves cardiac output		X
Prevents respiratory muscle atrophy		X
Disadvantages of IMV versus CMV		
Increases work of breathing	X	
Promotes respiratory muscle fatigue		X
Unresponsive to patient's ventilatory needs	X	

The Diaphragm. A popular notion is that the diaphragm becomes weak during prolonged mechanical ventilation because of disuse atrophy, much in the same way that other skeletal muscles become weak when immobilized. As such, IMV could maintain respiratory muscle strength by permitting continued contraction of the diaphragm. However, as stated earlier, the diaphragm does not rest during conventional mechanical ventilation, and there is no evidence at present to support the notion that the diaphragm is stronger with IMV compared to CMV.[3]

PRESSURE-SUPPORT VENTILATION

Pressure-support ventilation (PSV) is similar to IMV because it augments spontaneous breathing and it is similar to the assist mode because every breath is augmented. The airway pressure profile from PSV is illustrated in Figure 28–2 (lower panel). At the onset of each spontaneous breath, the negative pressure generated by the patient opens a valve that delivers the inspired gas at the desired pressure (usually 5 to 10 cmH_2O). This increases the tidal volume and reduces the work of breathing.[9]

The amount of pressure to use in PSV can be estimated with two methods.[10] The first involves the maximum inspiratory pressure (MIP) and the second involves the difference between the peak and plateau airway pressures (see Chapter 27).

$$Pressure = MIP/3$$

$$Pressure = Ppp - Ppl$$

The MIP method assumes that a patient will not be able to generate three times the MIP without becoming fatigued.[10] The proximal airway pressure method uses the notion that the difference between peak pressure (Ppk) and plateau pressures (Ppl) is the pressure needed to overcome resistance in the upper airways and tracheal tubes.

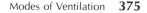

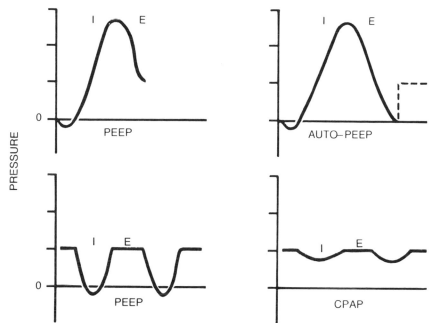

FIG. 28–3. Proximal airway pressure profiles for positive end-expiratory pressure (PEEP) and continuous positive airway pressure (CPAP). Upper panels show profiles from mechanical ventilation; lower panels are spontaneous breaths. Inhalation denoted as I, exhalation denoted as E.

INDICATIONS

At the present time the indications for PSV are not firm. It is designed to reduce the work of breathing and may be valuable in patients with high inspiratory flowrates to help overcome the inspiratory resistance from the artificial tubes. PSV is primarily used as a mode of weaning but there is no evidence that it is superior to conventional methods of weaning.[10] At the present time, there seems to be no clear benefit from this mode of ventilation over other more traditional modes.

POSITIVE END-EXPIRATORY PRESSURE

Mechanical ventilation with positive end-expiratory pressure (PEEP) is designed for any pulmonary condition associated with widespread alveolar collapse.[11-15] The airway pressure profile with PEEP ventilation is shown in Figure 28–3. A pressure-limiting valve in the expiratory tubing does not allow the pressure in the airways to return to atmospheric (zero) pressure at the end of expiration. The positive pressure in the alveoli at end-expiration helps to prevent alveolar collapse and promotes gas exchange across the alveolar-capillary interface.

TABLE 28–2. SPECTRUM OF PEEP EFFECTS ON OXYGEN TRANSPORT			
Arterial O_2 Sat	Cardiac Output	O_2 Delivery	Interpretation
A. ↑	→	↑	Benefit
B. ↑	↓	→	No Help
C. ↑	↓↓	↓	Harmful

THE PHYSIOLOGY OF PEEP

Pulmonary. PEEP increases the "functional residual capacity" (FRC); the end-expiratory lung volume. When applied to patients with the "adult respiratory distress syndrome" (ARDS), PEEP increases lung compliance and decreases intrapulmonary shunt fraction. This increases arterial PO_2 and allows the fractional concentration of inspired oxygen (FIO_2) to be lowered to less toxic levels. PEEP also increases dead space ventilation (VD/VT) by overdistending alveoli in normal lung regions. However, the improvement in shunt fraction should far exceed the increase in dead space ventilation if PEEP is used in the appropriate clinical situation.

Cardiac. The cardiac effects of PEEP are identical to the cardiac effects of positive-pressure ventilation described in Chapter 27.[12,14] Cardiac output is often increased when airway pressures are not excessive and the lungs are normal (see Fig. 27–3). When airway pressures are high and the lungs are stiff, PEEP often produces a decrease in cardiac output. The latter effect is primarily caused by a decrease in ventricular filling (see Fig. 27–4) but systolic function can also be depressed. The mechanism for the negative inotropic effects of PEEP include a reduction in coronary blood flow[13] and release of a negative inotropic substance from the lungs.[14]

Oxygen Delivery. The rate of oxygen delivery is determined by the cardiac output ($\dot{Q}$), the arterial hemoglobin concentration (Hb), and the percent saturation of hemoglobin with oxygen (SaO_2).

$$O_2 \text{ Delivery} = \dot{Q} \times Hb \times SaO_2$$

The influence of PEEP on oxygen delivery depends on the net balance between the changes in SaO_2 and cardiac output. This is demonstrated in Table 28–2. The three situations in this table represent equivalent increases in SaO_2. In situation A, there is an increase in oxygen delivery because the cardiac output does not decrease. In situation B, the increase in SaO_2 is offset by a decrease in cardiac output and O_2 delivery is unchanged. In situation C, the decrease in cardiac output exceeds the increase in SaO_2 and oxygen delivery is diminished. Therefore, there is no correlation between arterial oxygenation during PEEP and oxygen delivery rate.

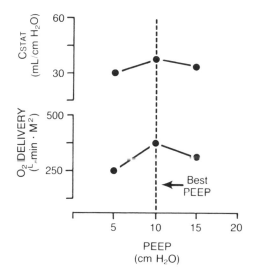

FIG. 28–4. The influence of incremental PEEP on oxygen delivery and static compliance of lungs and chest wall (Cstat). Best PEEP indicated by dashed line.

Best PEEP. Progressive increments in PEEP will eventually produce a decrease in both lung compliance and oxygen delivery. This is shown in Figure 28–4. The decrease in lung compliance from excessive PEEP may be caused by alveolar rupture or by an increase in lung water from reduced lymphatic drainage. The drop in oxygen delivery is the result of a decrease in cardiac output that exceeds the improvement in arterial oxygenation, as just described. The PEEP that is associated with the greatest improvement in either parameter is called "best PEEP".[15]

Monitoring. The ability for PEEP to produce deleterious effects on lung compliance and oxygen delivery is the reason for recommending routine monitoring of lung mechanics and oxygen transport during PEEP ventilation.

Static lung compliance is monitored with the end-inspiratory occlusion pressure or "plateau pressure", as described in the last chapter. The plateau pressure should decrease if PEEP is producing the desired effect, and the change should be evident within a few breaths. Remember to subtract the PEEP from the measured plateau pressure to obtain the actual lung recoil pressure.

Oxygen delivery is monitored in the usual fashion using pulmonary artery catheters (see Chapters 9 through 11). **The arterial oxygen levels should never be used alone to monitor the effects of PEEP** because of the ability for PEEP to reduce cardiac output.

USES AND MISUSES

PEEP is used in a variety of situations, even though the only real benefit from PEEP is in allowing the inspired oxygen level to be lowered to nontoxic levels. The following are some of the common situations where PEEP is used (and misused).

Pulmonary Edema. The major indication for PEEP is in patients with pulmonary edema (or any diffuse process that decreases FRC) who require toxic levels of inspired oxygen (FIO_2 greater than 60%) to maintain adequate arterial oxygenation. The increase in arterial PO_2 from PEEP in patients with pulmonary edema is not caused by a decrease in edema fluid.

> PEEP is not a therapy for pulmonary edema; i.e., it does not reduce the volume of edema.[16,17] In fact, positive intrathoracic pressures promote water accumulation in the lungs.[11]

The increase in extravascular lung water seen during positive-pressure ventilation is not often mentioned. The most likely explanation for this phenomenon is a reduction in lymphatic drainage from the lungs due to the increase in venous pressures produced by the positive intrathoracic pressure.[18]

Localized Lung Disease. When the pathologic process is confined to a portion of the lung (e.g., lobar pneumonia), PEEP can worsen the hypoxemia by overdistending normal lung and directing flow to the diseased segment.[19] When lung disease is localized, hypoxic vasoconstriction in the diseased area directs blood flow away from the area and toward normal areas of lung. This helps to preserve gas exchange. When PEEP is applied in this situation, it is distributed unevenly because it is applied more to normal lung areas. This overdistends the normal alveoli and redirects blood back to the diseased segments, counteracting the inherent tendencies to maintain ventilation-perfusion balance. Therefore, PEEP is not recommended for localized lung disease unless it is selectively applied to the diseased lung using differential lung inflation techniques.

Prophylactic PEEP. In patients at risk for developing ARDS (e.g., septic patients), early application of PEEP has been suggested as a means of preventing the syndrome from appearing. However,

> Prophylactic PEEP does not appear to reduce the incidence of ARDS in susceptible patients.[20]

Therefore, PEEP is not recommended as a preventive measure in patients at risk for ARDs.

Routine PEEP. The practice of applying PEEP to all patients who are intubated springs from the notion that glottic closure at the end of expiration creates low levels of PEEP (physiologic PEEP) in normal subjects. However,

> There is no evidence that adults produce PEEP from glottic closure or that routine use of PEEP for all patients provides any benefit.[21]

Therefore, the routine use of PEEP is not recommended at this time.

Mediastinal Bleeding. PEEP is commonly used to prevent or control mediastinal bleeding after coronary bypass surgery. This practice shows little understanding of the principle of transmural pressure, because **the transmission of PEEP into mediastinal blood vessels may not change transmural pressure and may not reduce the tendency for bleeding.** There is no convincing evidence that routine application of PEEP decreases the incidence of postoperative mediastinal bleeding,[22] or that PEEP helps to stop bleeding once it starts.[23]

COMPLICATIONS

The major complication of PEEP is the decrease in cardiac output described earlier. Some other complications are mentioned in the following paragraphs.

Barotrauma. Barotrauma from PEEP is a controversial area. Some studies report a higher incidence of pneumothorax with PEEP[24] while others observed no correlation between PEEP and barotrauma.[25] The variable correlation between PEEP and barotrauma is not surprising because peak inspiratory pressure may be the more important factor in determining risk for barotrauma.[24] The other important factor is the type of lung disease. Pulmonary barotrauma is discussed in more detail in the next chapter.

Fluid Retention. This is common with positive-pressure ventilation and with PEEP.[25] Several mechanisms have been proposed, including depression of atrial natriuretic factor (ANF) and stimulation of antidiuretic hormone (ADH). Compression of the atria from hyperinflated lungs is the proposed mechanism for the decrease in ANF and the increase in ADH.[26] Stimulation of the sympathetic nervous system may also be responsible for a redistribution of renal blood flow favoring perfusion of sodium-conserving nephrons.[25] The purpose of the fluid retention may be to promote cardiac output in the face of high intrathoracic pressures but the disadvantages of fluid overload are not to be overlooked.

Intracranial Hypertension. This is a variable finding when PEEP is administered to head-injured patients.[27] The mechanism is probably the increase in pressure in the superior vena cava associated with PEEP and the effect is more prominent in patients with reduced cerebral compliance. The variability of the response may be due to the lack of monitoring peak and mean intrathoracic pressures in the available studies. Intracranial pressure monitoring is advised when high intrathoracic pressures are present in head injury patients who are prone to increased intracranial pressure.

CONTINUOUS POSITIVE AIRWAYS PRESSURE

Continuous positive airways pressure (CPAP) is defined as "a pressure above atmospheric maintained at the airway opening throughout the respiratory cycle during spontaneous breathing."[28] The breathing pattern produced by CPAP is shown in Figure 28–3 along with the pattern produced by PEEP applied during spontaneous breathing (lower panel). Note that the end-expiratory pressure is the same with CPAP and PEEP, but that the pressure excursion during inspiration is much greater with PEEP than with CPAP. The larger excursion with PEEP will increase the work of breathing, and this is the fundamental difference between "spontaneous PEEP" and CPAP.

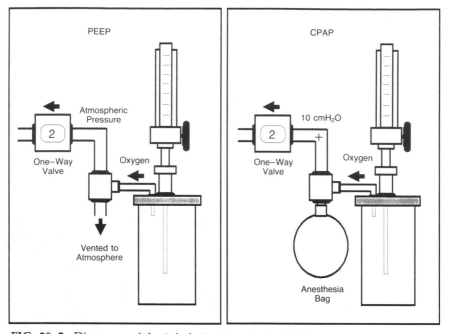

FIG. 28–5. Diagrams of the inhalation circuits for CPAP (right side) and "spontaneous PEEP." Unidirectional valve in each circuit opens when pressure differential reaches 2 cm H$_2$O. See text for explanation.

The difference in inspiratory pressure excursion between CPAP and PEEP is the result of differences in the pressure across a one-way valve in the circuits. This is shown in Figure 28–5. The valve in both circuits needs a pressure gradient of 2 cm H$_2$O to open. The valve in the PEEP circuit has atmospheric pressure on the side opposite the patient so the patient must generate a pressure equal to the PEEP plus 2 cm H$_2$O. The CPAP circuit uses an anesthesia bag to apply a positive pressure to the side of the valve opposite the patient so that the pressure generated by the patient to open the valve is reduced by the amount of positive pressure applied. This is how CPAP reduces the work of breathing.

INDICATIONS

The major use of CPAP at present is to postpone or prevent intubation in patients with ARDS and refractory hypoxemia. The CPAP is delivered via specially-designed masks equipped with pressure-limiting valves. These masks must be fitted tightly and cannot be removed to allow patients to eat. Because of poor patient tolerance, these masks are used as temporary measures only. CPAP can also be applied through artificial airways and was once popular for weaning patients from mechanical ventilation. However, CPAP weaning has largely been abandoned.

REFERENCES

ASSISTED VENTILATION

1. Marini JJ, Capps JS, Culver BH. The inspiratory work of breathing during assisted mechanical ventilation. Chest 1985; 87:612–618.

INTERMITTENT MANDATORY VENTILATION

2. Downs JB, Klein EF, Desautels D, et al. IMV: A new approach to weaning patients from mechanical ventilators. Chest 1973; 64:331–335.
3. Weisman IM, Rinaldo JE, Rogers RM, Sanders MH. Intermittent mandatory ventilation. Am Rev Respir Dis 1983; 127:641–647.
4. Zwillich CW, Pierson DJ, Creagh CE, et al. Complications of assisted ventilation. Am J Med 1974; 57:161–170.
5. Hudson LD, et al. Does intermittent mandatory ventilation correct respiratory alkalosis in patients receiving assisted mechanical ventilation? Am Rev Respir Dis 1985; 132:1071–1074.
6. Robotham JL, Scharf SM. Effects of positive and negative pressure ventilation on cardiac performance. Clin Chest Med 1983; 4:161–187.
7. Hastings PR, et al. Cardiorespiratory dynamics during weaning with IMV versus spontaneous ventilation in good-risk cardiac surgery patients. Anesthesiology 1980; 53:429–431.
8. Mathru M, et al. Hemodynamic response to changes in ventilatory patterns in patients with normal and poor left ventricular reserve. Crit Care Med 1982; 10:423–426.

PRESSURE SUPPORT VENTILATION

9. Macintyre NB. Pressure support ventilation: Effects on ventilatory reflexes and ventilatory muscle workloads. Respir Care 1987; 32:447–457.
10. Hughes CW, Popovich J, Jr. Uses and abuses of pressure support ventilation. J Crit Illness 1989; 4:25–32.

POSITIVE END-EXPIRATORY PRESSURE

11. Petty TL. The use, abuse and mystique of positive end-expiratory pressure. Am Rev Respir Dis 1988; 138:475–478.
12. Martin C, Saux P, Albanese J, et al. Right ventricular function during positive end-expiratory pressure. Chest 1987; 92:999–1004.
13. Tittley JG, Fremes SE, Weisel RD, et al. Hemodynamic and myocardial metabolic consequences of PEEP. Chest 1985; 88:496–502.
14. Pick RA, Handler JB, Friedman AS. The cardiovascular effects of positive end-expiratory pressure. Chest 1982; 82:345–350.
15. Suter PM, Fairley HB, Isenberg MD: Optimum end-expiratory pressure in patients with acute pulmonary failure. N Engl J Med 1975; 292:284–289.
16. Saul GM, Feeley TW, Mihm FG. Effect of graded administration of PEEP on lung water in noncardiogenic pulmonary edema. Crit Care Med 1982; 10:667–669.
17. Helbert C, Paskanik A, Bredenberg CE. Effect of positive end-expiratory pressure on lung water in pulmonary edema caused by increased membrane permeability. Ann Thorac Surg 1983; 36:42–48.

18. Pilon RN, Bittar DA. The effect of positive end-expiratory pressure on thoracic-duct lymph flow during controlled ventilation in anesthetized dogs. Anesthesiology 1973; 6:607–612.

19. Kanarek DJ, Shannon DC. Adverse effect of positive end-expiratory pressure on pulmonary perfusion and arterial oxygenation. Am Rev Respir Dis 1975; 112:457–459.

20. Pepe PE, Hudson LD, Carrico CJ. Early application of positive end-expiratory pressure to patients at risk for the adult respiratory distress syndrome. N Engl J Med 1984; 311:281–286.

21. Good JT, Wol JF, Anderson JT, et al. The routine use of positive end-expiratory pressure after open heart surgery. Chest 1979; 76:397–400.

22. Banasik JL, Tyler ML. The effect of prophylactic positive end-expiratory pressure on mediastinal bleeding after coronary revascularization surgery. Heart Lung 1986; 15:43–48.

23. Zurick AM, Urzua J, Ghattas M, et al. Failure of positive end-expiratory pressure to decrease postoperative bleeding after cardiac surgery. Ann Thorac Surg 1982; 34:608–611.

24. Petersen GW, Baier H. Incidence of pulmonary barotrauma in a medical ICU. Crit Care Med 1983; 11:67–69.

25. Pingleton SK. Complications of acute respiratory failure. Am Rev Respir Dis 1988; 137:1463–1493.

26. Leithner C, Frass M, Pacher R, et al. Mechanical ventilation with positive end-expiratory pressure decreases release of alpha-atrial natriuretic peptide. Crit Care Med 1987; 15:484–488.

27. Shapiro HM, Marshall LF. Intracranial pressure responses to PEEP in head-injured patients. J Trauma 1978; 18:254–256.

CONTINUOUS POSITIVE AIRWAY PRESSURE (CPAP)

28. Kirby RR, Taylor RW. PEEP and CPAP for respiratory failure: When, where, and why. J Crit Illness 1987; 2:42–52.

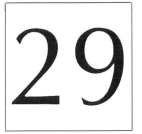

c h a p t e r

29

TUBES, BLOWOUTS, AND THE OCCULT

This chapter presents some of the prominent concerns associated with tracheal intubation and mechanical ventilation. The complications that are presented are only those directly related to tubes and ventilators. Other adverse occurrences in ventilator-dependent patients, like pneumonia, are related more to the patient population than the ventilatory apparatus, and are discussed elsewhere. The spectrum of complications that can arise in acute respiratory failure is the subject of an excellent review (with over 400 cited references), listed at the end of the chapter.[1]

ARTIFICIAL AIRWAYS

Intubation of the trachea with cuffed tubes is responsible for the birth of positive-pressure ventilation. The risks and benefits of tracheal intubation are determined by the route of entry, which is either translaryngeal (endotracheal) or transtracheal (tracheostomy).[1-10] The complications associated with both routes are shown in Figure 29-1. The asterisks mark the complications that are most prevalent or most feared. The following are some brief descriptions of issues that will surface each day for ventilator-dependent patients.

ENDOTRACHEAL INTUBATION

Endotracheal tubes are inserted through the nose or mouth. The nasal route is often preferred because the insertion technique is less involved and there is no risk for dental trauma. The oral route is usually reserved

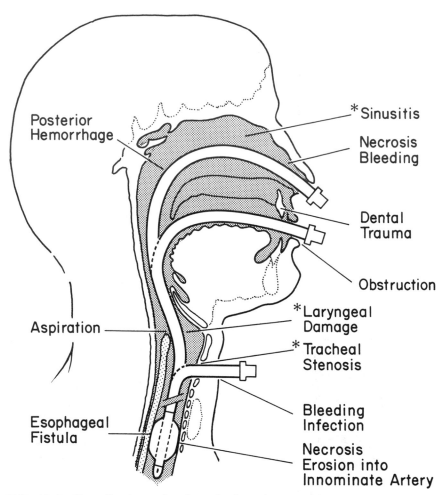

FIG. 29–1. Complications of endotracheal intubation and tracheostomy.

for comatose patients or for immediate intubation (e.g., cardiac arrest). Some comparative risks of each insertion route are listed below.

Risk Factor	Nasotracheal	Orotracheal
Intubation	Epistaxis	Dental Trauma
	Esophageal	Aspiration
	Intubation	
Tube in Place	Sinusitis	Tube Occlusion
	Retained	Laryngeal Damage
	Secretions	

The major problem with longterm nasal intubation is the risk of sinusitis and the major problem with oral intubation is the risk of tube occlusion in anxious or confused patients (who bite down on the tubes). The nasal tubes are also longer than the orotracheal tubes (see Appendix) and they can interfere with suctioning and reduce the ability to clear secretions.

TABLE 29–1. RADIOGRAPHIC LANDMARKS FOR ENDOTRACHEAL INTUBATION*			
		Radiographic Location	
Head Position	Carina	Mandible	Tip of Tube
Neutral	T5–T7	C5–C6	5–7 cm above carina
Flexion		Below T1	3–5 cm above carina
Extension		Above C4	7–9 cm above carina

*From Goodman LR, Putnam CE. Intensive care radiology. St. Louis: C.V. Mosby, 1978:29–55.

The longer tubes will also increase the work of breathing but the significance of this is probably minor. Orotracheal tubes may have a higher risk for laryngeal damage because of their greater mobility and because of the more acute angle taken by orotracheal tubes when they pass through the vocal cords.[4]

Selective Intubation. As many as 15% of intubations will result in accidental entry of one lung.[5] The right lung is entered much more commonly because the right mainstem bronchus runs a straight line down from the trachea. Tube migration into the right mainstem bronchus can occur at any time without warning and this is one of the reasons for recommending that chest films be obtained at regular intervals in intubated patients. The recommended tube positions are shown in Table 29–1.[6] The main carina should be located over the 5th to 7th thoracic vertebrae in 95% of adults[6] and the tip of the tubes should sit 5 to 7 cm above the carina when the head is in the neutral position. Note the distance that the tip can move when the head is flexed or extended.

The consequences of accidental intubation of one lung is shown in Figure 29–2. The tip of the tube is situated in the right mainstem bronchus (middle arrow). Note that the mediastinum is displaced to the left and the right lung appears to be herniating into the left hemithorax (large arrowheads). These findings are characteristic of a tension pneumothorax and this represents a life-threatening situation. Tension pneumothorax develops in 15% of right lung intubations,[5] and this is reason enough to obtain a chest x-ray after every intubation.

Sinusitis. Nasal tubes can obstruct the sinus ostia and produce a purulent sinusitis that can be life-threatening.[7,8] The maxillary sinus is almost always involved[7] and the diagnosis is often possible with portable sinus films (see Fig. 43–3). However, an air-fluid level in a sinus cavity does not mean infection, and the diagnosis of infection requires aspiration of the fluid for gram stain and culture. The incidence of sinusitis during nasotracheal intubation is not known, but it must always be considered in unexplained fever in intubated patients.[8] Chapter 43 contains a more detailed discussion of this problem.

Laryngeal Damage. Damage to the larynx is the most common and most feared complication of endotracheal intubation. However, this is not clinically evident until after the endotracheal tube is removed. The risk for laryngeal injury is the rationale for tracheostomy if prolonged

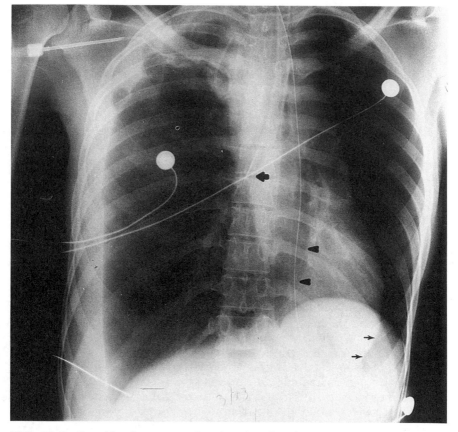

FIG. 29–2. Portable chest x-ray showing tip of endotracheal tube in the right mainstem bronchus (middle arrow) with tension pneumothorax.

intubation is anticipated. The risk factors for laryngeal injury include the route of intubation (orotracheal tubes cause more damage than nasotracheal tubes), the ease of intubation, tube diameter, the duration and number of intubations, and self-extubation with the cuff inflated.[3]

Visual evidence of laryngeal injury is almost always present when endotracheal tubes are removed,[10] but the incidence of serious complications is low.[9,10] Laryngeal edema may be evident immediately after extubation or it can become evident in the first few hours after extubation. In the latter situation, the lateral wall pressure exerted by the endotracheal tube in place prevents edema formation and the edema begins to form only when the tube is removed. Respiratory distress following extubation almost always indicates laryngeal obstruction and should prompt immediate reintubation. Inspiratory stridor is not a sensitive sign of laryngeal obstruction, particularly at low airflows, and the absence of stridor should not be interpreted as the absence of laryngeal obstruction.

The proper therapy for laryngeal edema from endotracheal tubes is to perform a tracheostomy and remove the endotracheal tube. Other therapies such as steroids or racemic epinephrine are of no proven value in this setting. These agents are used in allergic reactions, and should not benefit traumatic injury of the larynx.

Work of Breathing. Endotracheal intubation decreases the anatomic dead space but increases the resistance to airflow. The dead space in the mouth and upper airway is about 1 ml per kilogram[2] or 70 ml for an average-sized adult. The volume of most endotracheal tubes is 35 to 40 ml,[2] so the anatomic dead space is reduced by 50% with endotracheal intubation.

The resistance to airflow in a narrow tube is defined by the Poiseuille-Hagen equation described in Chapter 13. The tube diameter is the most important variable because resistance is proportional to the fourth power of the radius of the tube. Studies on the work of breathing through different size endotracheal tubes have revealed that tube diameter is not important at minute ventilations below 10 L/min (normal minute ventilation is 5 to 6 L/min). However, above 10 L/min, tubes of 7 mm (internal diameter) or less will create a significant increase in the work of breathing.[11] Therefore, when a tube of 7 mm or less is present in a patient who is not able to wean from the ventilator, it is wise to use a wider tube (at least 8 mm internal diameter), particularly if the patient develops a minute ventilation above 10 L/min during the wean.

TRACHEOSTOMY

Tracheostomy is preferred for patients who require prolonged mechanical ventilation. The advantages of tracheostomy over endotracheal intubation include patient comfort, more effective clearing of secretions, and absence of laryngeal injury.[2,3] Selected patients can also take food orally and can even converse with the aid of special tracheostomy tubes. The complications of tracheostomy are related to three factors: the surgical procedure, the tracheal stoma, and the patient population.

Surgical Complications. Tracheostomy is associated with serious complications in 5% of cases[3] and has a reported mortality of 2 to 3%![2] Immediate postoperative complications include pneumothorax (5%), stomal hemorrhage (5%), and accidental decannulation.[2,3]

Accidental decannulation in the first few days after surgery can be a serious problem because the tracheostomy tract closes quickly. Attempts to reinsert tubes can create false tracts. If a tracheostomy tube has to be replaced in the first week after surgery, a suction catheter (12 French) should be used as a guidewire to reduce the risk for a traumatic or unsuccessful reintubation.

Tracheal Stenosis. Tracheal stenosis usually occurs at the stoma site and not at the site where the cuff seals the trachea.[2,3,4,9] Tracheal stenosis is the most feared complication of tracheostomy but is a late complication and appears after the patient leaves the ICU.

General Complications. The complications from tracheostomy are more frequent than the complications from endotracheal intubation[4] but this may be due largely to the characteristics of the patients. That is, patients who require tracheostomy are usually sicker than patients who are in-

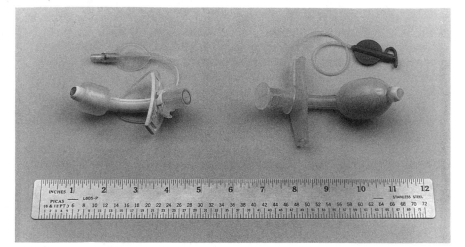

FIG. 29–3. Two tracheostomy tubes with cuffs inflated. Pilot balloons are situated beside each tube. The tube on the left requires cuff inflation with positive pressure; the tube on the right has a foam cuff that is normally inflated at atmospheric pressure.

tubated and they have been in the hospital longer. They also have been intubated prior to the tracheostomy. These factors must be weighed when considering complications like pneumonia, which is reported in 50% of patients with a tracheostomy.[3]

CUFF-RELATED PROBLEMS

All tracheal tubes for adults are equipped with an inflatable cuff at the distal end that seals the trachea and prevents air from escaping back through the larynx. Figure 29–3 shows two tracheostomy tubes equipped with inflated cuffs. The tube on the left has a standard design cuff attached to a pilot balloon with a narrow cannula called an inflating tube. The cuff is inflated by attaching a syringe to the pilot balloon and injecting air until the trachea is occluded (called a seal). Tracheal occlusion is documented by the absence of a leak around the balloon (see later). Once a seal is achieved, the syringe is removed and a one-way valve on the pilot balloon prevents the escape of air from the cuff.

Aspiration. There is a tendency to consider cuff inflation as insurance against aspiration of mouth secretions into the lower airways. Unfortunately, the soft, pliable cuffs designed to minimize pressure necrosis of the trachea have a drawback because of their ability to allow secretions to pass even when inflated.

> Inflation of the cuff on tracheal tubes does not eliminate the risk for aspiration of mouth secretions into the lower airways.

Aspiration of dye placed in the mouth has been documented in 20% of patients with endotracheal tubes[12] and 40% of patients with tracheostomy tubes[13] despite cuff inflation. The risk of aspiration decreases if cuff pressure is increased to 25 cm H_2O,[13] but this is the highest cuff pressure allowed to limit tracheal damage. The only defense against aspiration of mouth secretions is frequent suctioning and the patient's own defense mechanisms (e.g., cough).

Cuff Leaks. A leak is defined as air passing around the cuff and escaping out through the larynx. Cuff leaks are usually detected by hearing a sound during lung inflation that represents air passing over the vocal cords. The exhaled volume registered on the ventilator will be diminished and can be used to quantitate the volume of the leak.

The most common cause of a cuff leak is nonuniform contact between the cuff and the trachea. Another common source is the one-way valve on the pilot balloon. These valves can become faulty and allow air to escape from the cuff. Cuff leaks rarely result from disruption of the cuff itself.

When a leak is detected, separate the patient from the ventilator and manually inflate the lungs with an anesthesia bag to determine if the origin of the leak is at the cuff site. If a cuff leak is present, inflate the cuff with a few ml of air until the sound disappears. If the cuff pressure exceeds 25 cm H_2O, then replace the tracheal tube. If the cuff pressure is acceptable, then observe for return of the leak. If the leak returns quickly, the problem is likely to be in the pilot balloon valve, and the tube should be changed. If the valve is faulty, the inflation tube can be clamped to keep the cuff inflated until the tube is replaced.

Tracheal Injury. Pressure necrosis of the trachea from cuff inflation has decreased significantly since high compliance cuffs were developed in the early 1970s. The newer cuffs are larger and more elliptical, so the pressure is dispersed over a larger surface area. The systolic pressure in the mucosal vessels of the trachea is 20 to 25 mmHg,[3,13] and the cuff pressure is kept below 25 cm H_2O (18.4 mmHg) to prevent pressure necrosis of the trachea.

The tracheostomy tube on the right in Figure 29–3 has a large cuff filled with foam. The cuff on this tube is normally inflated and must be deflated by a syringe when the tube is inserted. Once the tube is in place, the balloon is allowed to inflate and seals the trachea at atmospheric (zero) pressure, thereby minimizing the risk for pressure necrosis of the trachea. This tube (called a Fome-Cuf) has been a personal preference for years and has performed well. The large size of the cuff is particularly appealing for maximizing surface contact to maintain a seal. The only disadvantage is that the tube is not fenestrated (like the Shiley tube on the left), and does not allow for a stepwise decannulation. However, the need for gradual decannulation is unproven.[3]

TIMING OF TRACHEOSTOMY

The optimal time for changing from endotracheal tube to tracheostomy is a time-honored controversy. The central issue in this decision involves the relative advantages and disadvantages of each method. These are summarized below:[3,4,11]

1. The proponents of early tracheostomy (3 to 7 days after intubation)

maintain that tracheostomy is more comfortable, provides less resistance to airflow, allows for more effective airways care, and permits oral feeding.

2. The advocates of prolonged endotracheal intubation (3 weeks or longer) maintain that tracheostomy is a costly surgical procedure with a high morbidity and an associated mortality rate. Moreover, the duration of intubation does not seem to determine the incidence or severity of complications (for at least 3 weeks).[4]

There is some validity in both arguments, but the decision to perform tracheostomy should be individualized. One approach that seems reasonable is as follows.

> Allow for 1 week of endotracheal intubation and then determine the likelihood for extubation. If extubation seems unlikely in the following week, consider tracheostomy.

In patients with a prior tracheostomy, it might be wise to wait longer than 1 or 2 weeks before considering tracheostomy because of the higher risk of tracheal stenosis with repeated tracheal incisions.

PULMONARY BAROTRAUMA

Pulmonary barotrauma occurs in 1 to 20% of patients receiving mechanical ventilation and the consequences can be devastating.[14,15]

PATHOGENESIS

Barotrauma means pressure-induced injury but the culprit in mechanical ventilation is overinflation (i.e., volume). When the air spaces rupture, air can dissect along tissue planes **(interstitial emphysema)** or can travel along the bronchovascular bundles into the mediastinium **(pneumomediastinium)** and up into the neck **(subcutaneous emphysema)**. The air can also rupture through the visceral pleura **(pneumothorax)** or can enter the peritoneal cavity **(pneumoperitoneum)**.

Predisposing factors include excessive inflation volume and high intrathoracic pressures. In one study, the incidence of barotrauma was 43% if the peak inflation pressure exceeded 70 cm H_2O while no patient experienced barotrauma if the inflation pressure remained below 40 cm H_2O.[16] Also important is the tendency of the lung to rupture, and predisposing illnesses include asthma, necrotizing pneumonia, and gastric acid aspiration. Asymmetric lung disease is not mentioned enough in pathogenesis.[14] In this situation, normal lung regions receive excessive volumes and pressures from the ventilator because the inflation volume from ventilators will preferentially travel to areas of least resistance and greatest distensibility. All pulmonary disorders are nonuniform to some degree and this mechanism is operative in all cases of barotrauma.

DIAGNOSIS

Vigilance and early recognition are the hallmarks of the approach to pneumothorax, as illustrated in the following statistic:

Delays in diagnosis can prove fatal in 1 of every 3 ventilator-dependent patients who develop a pneumothorax![13]

Clinical signs can be absent and, when present, are usually nonspecific. Common signs of pneumothorax in ventilator-dependent patients include tachycardia and sudden hypotension.[14] Breath sounds are unreliable for detecting pneumothorax in ventilator-dependent patients because sounds transmitted from the ventilator tubing can be mistaken for airway sounds and this can lead to missed diagnoses.

Subcutaneous Air. The presence of subcutaneous air in the neck or upper thorax is pathognomonic of pulmonary barotrauma. In one study, subcutaneous air was palpable in all 74 patients who developed a pneumothorax during mechanical ventilation.[17] This indicates that palpation for subcutaneous air in the neck and upper thorax may be the most valuable bedside test for the early diagnosis of pulmonary barotrauma in ventilator-dependent patients.

Chest Films. The problem is often detected on routine chest films before the clinical diagnosis is evident. The following are some radiographic features of barotrauma that are useful in the ICU patient population.

Interstitial Air. One of the early signs of barotrauma is called **pulmonary interstitial emphysema** (PIE), which appears as small parenchymal cysts or linear streaks projecting toward the hilum. This represents air that is dissecting along the pulmonary interstitium. In one study, 5 of 13 patients with radiographic evidence of PIE developed pneumothorax within the next 12 hours.[18] This indicates that PIE is not only an early sign of barotrauma, it can be a harbinger of pneumothorax.

Atypical Pneumothorax. Pneumothorax in the supine position has different radiographic features than pneumothorax in the upright position.[19]

In the supine position, pleural air collects in the anterior costophrenic sulcus at the base of the hemithorax. Therefore, searching for air at the apex of the hemithorax can lead to missed diagnoses of pneumothorax in supine patients.

Figure 29–4 shows some of the atypical patterns of pleural air collection in a supine patient. The hyperlucency outlined at the right lung base represents air extending from the anterior costophrenic recess. The sharp line outlining the descending aorta is produced by air trapped behind the inferior pulmonary ligament. The air outlined at the left lung base in Figure 29–2 also represents air in the anterior costophrenic sulcus (called the "deep sulcus sign").

Redundant Skin Folds. When the film cartridge used for portable chest x-rays is placed under the patient, the skin on the back can fold over on itself to produce a line that runs down the hemithorax and this line is often mistaken for a pneumothorax. Figure 29–5 shows a skin fold running down the left hemithorax. Note that there is a gradual increase

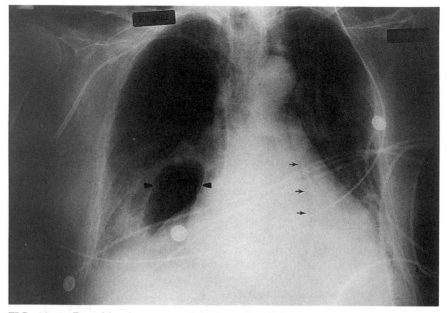

FIG. 29–4. Portable chest x-ray showing air collection extending from the anteromedial recess on the left (lower arrows). The sharp line delineating the descending thoracic aorta is air behind the inferior pulmonary ligament.

in radiodensity as the line is approached from the hilum and the line has a wavy appearance. The gradual increase in radiodensity is produced by skin that is folded back on itself. A pneumothorax would appear as a sharp white line with dark shadows (air) on both sides and the line would run parallel to the inner margin of the chest wall.

Skin folds are one of the gremlins that always seem to appear at night, when the support staff is minimal and you are left to your own talents for diagnosis and therapy. The radiographic features in Figure 29–5 should help to differentiate a skin fold from a pneumothorax and will also help you to sleep on your call nights.

CHEST TUBE THORACOSTOMY

Pneumothorax from positive-pressure ventilation always requires chest tube evacuation because tension pneumothorax is common in this setting.[2] Figure 29–6 shows the conventional 3-bottle system for evacuating the pleural space. Each bottle is placed in series between the pleural space and a suction device.

Collection Chamber. The purpose of Bottle I is to collect fluid from the pleural space while allowing air to pass through to the next bottle in the series. This "collection chamber" is able to collect fluid without imposing a back pressure on the pleural space (because the fluid is not communicating with the pleural space).

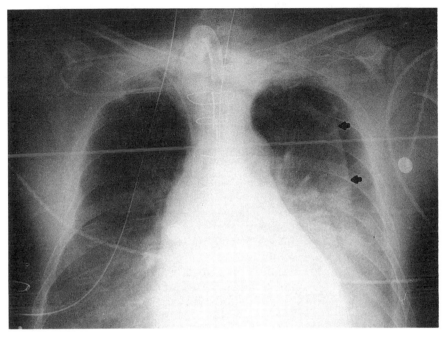

FIG. 29–5. Portable chest x-ray showing a wavy line in the left hemithorax. This is produced by a redundant skin fold and is not a pneumothorax.

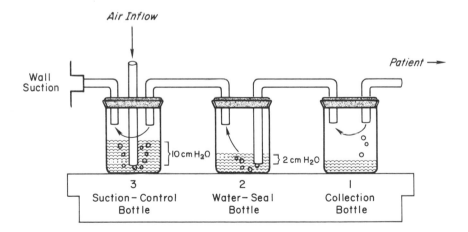

FIG. 29–6. Three-bottle system for evacuating air fluid from the pleural space. See text for explanation.

Water-Seal Chamber. The second bottle is used as a one-way valve so air can escape from the pleural space but atmospheric air cannot enter the pleural space. The inlet tube in this Bottle II is underwater and this imposes a back-pressure on the pleural space that is equal to the depth that the inlet tube is submerged. The water then "seals" the pleural space from the surrounding atmosphere because pleural air can be evacuated but atmospheric air cannot gain entry to the pleural space. The "water seal" pressure is usually 1 to 2 cmH$_2$O.

Air that is evacuated from the pleural space will pass through the water in the second bottle and create bubbles. The presence of bubbles in the water-seal chamber (called "bubbling") indicates an ongoing bronchopleural air leak.

Suction Control Chamber. The third bottle sets the limit on the negative pressure that is imposed on the pleural space. The maximum negative pressure is determined by the height of the water column in the inlet tube from the atmosphere. Negative pressure (from wall suction) will draw the water down the inlet tube and when the negative pressure exceeds the height of the water column, air is entrained from the atmosphere. This inflow of atmospheric air equalizes the pressure in the bottle so that it cannot become more negative. In other words, the negative pressure in the bottle cannot exceed the height of the water in the inlet tube because of the equilibration with atmospheric pressure. Therefore, the maximum suction that can be transmitted to the pleural space is equal to the height of the water in this "suction-control" device.

Why Use Suction? There seems to be a preoccupation with applying negative pressure to the pleural space. The goal of this practice is to draw the lung surface up to the chest wall and oppose the two pleural surfaces to seal the leak in the lung (bronchopleural fistula). However:

> Negative pressure in the pleural space will increase transpulmonary pressure, and this will increase the rate of airflow across a leak from the lung to the pleural space. This can keep a leak or bronchopleural fistula patent instead of helping it to close.

Ideally, the lungs should reinflate without the use of suction because the intrapleural pressure can still become negative when water-seal pressure (2 cm H$_2$O) is applied to the pleural space. If suction is used and the air leak persists, consider discontinuing the suction to reduce the transpulmonary pressure. If air accumulates in the pleural space without suction, it will be evacuated spontaneously when pleural pressure becomes more positive than water-seal pressure.

AUTO-PEEP

The concept of positive end-expiratory pressure (PEEP) was presented in Chapter 28. This section describes an "intrinsic PEEP" that is produced spontaneously (without added PEEP) during mechanical ventilation. The illustration in Figure 29–7 will help to explain this phenomenon.

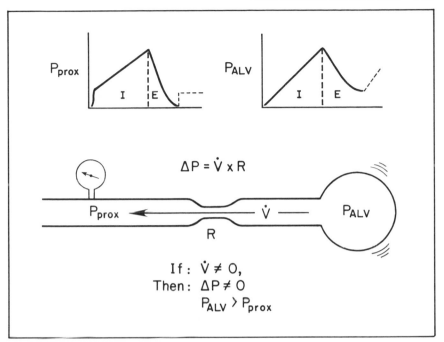

FIG. 29–7. The principle of auto-PEEP. $\dot{V}$ = airflow; R = resistance to flow in airways; Palv = alveolar pressure; Pprox = proximal airway pressure; I = inhalation; E = exhalation. The graph in the upper left shows proximal airways pressure after tube occlusion at end-expiration. Graph in upper right shows the proximal pressure profile with externally added PEEP.

PATHOGENESIS

In the normal lung, exhalation is complete and there is no airflow at the end of expiration. In the absence of airflow, alveolar pressure will equal proximal airway pressure (atmospheric pressure) at the end of expiration. Conversely, when there is an obstruction in the airways and exhalation is not complete, there will be airflow at the end of expiration. The presence of airflow will create a pressure difference between the alveoli and the proximal airways and the magnitude of this difference is determined by the resistance in the airways. Because alveolar pressure at end-expiration will be positive in this situation, it is called "auto-PEEP".[20]

Auto-PEEP can be produced by an increase in airway resistance (obstructive lung disease), by excessive inflation volumes (mechanical ventilation), or by a decrease in the time for exhalation (rapid breathing). All these factors are likely to play a role in producing auto-PEEP during mechanical ventilation.

DIAGNOSIS

Auto-PEEP may be universal in patients with obstructive lung disease who are receiving mechanical ventilation and it is particularly prominent in patients with status asthmaticus.[21] However, auto-PEEP is often overlooked because the proximal airway pressure (monitored on the front panel of the ventilator) often returns to zero at end-expiration in the presence of auto-PEEP. Because this PEEP is not evident by routine airway pressure monitoring, it is sometimes called "occult PEEP."

A special maneuver is needed to uncover this form of PEEP, and it is illustrated in the diagram in the upper left portion of Figure 29–7. The expiratory circuit is occluded at the end of expiration to eliminate airflow and the proximal airway pressure will then equal the alveolar pressure. If occult PEEP is present, it will then be uncovered.

> When the expiratory tubing is occluded at end-expiration, a sudden increase in the proximal airway pressure indicates the presence of occult PEEP.

Unfortunately, manual occlusion cannot be timed exactly to the very end of expiration, so the occlusion maneuver will not be reliable for determining the magnitude of occult PEEP.

WHY MONITOR OCCULT PEEP?

The consensus is that occult PEEP is widespread in ventilator-dependent patients with obstructive lung disease,[1] and it should be monitored routinely in this patient population. Other reasons to monitor this hidden PEEP are as follows:
1. It has the same consequences as external PEEP (e.g., reduced cardiac output).
2. It increases the proximal airway pressures (peak and plateau pressure) and can falsely lower the estimated lung compliance.
3. It can be used to measure the response to bronchodilators.
4. It can diminish the ability to wean by increasing the work of breathing.

Pressures in the Thorax. The peak inspiratory pressure and the end-inspiratory "plateau" pressure will both increase with PEEP. As presented in Chapter 27, the plateau pressure is taken as the static recoil pressure of the lungs and chest wall and static lung compliance (Cstat) is calculated as the tidal volume (V_T) divided by the plateau pressure (Ppl). When occult PEEP is present, the recoil pressure will be elevated and the calculated compliance of the thorax will be falsely lowered.[1] Therefore, the recoil pressure that is used in the compliance calculation should be the plateau pressure (Ppl) minus the occult PEEP.

$$Cstat = V_T \times (Ppl - PEEP) \quad L/cm\ H_2O$$

Occult PEEP can also be transmitted into the pulmonary circulation and can falsely elevate the pulmonary capillary wedge pressure (PCWP).

This can lead to errors in interpreting the PCWP and inappropriate therapeutic maneuvers.

Work of Breathing. The most discussed complication of occult PEEP is the increased work of breathing.[22] Two factors contribute to this greater workload. First, the hyperinflation produced by the PEEP places the patient on a flat part of the pressure-volume curve for the lungs so that a higher pressure is needed to move a given volume (take a deep breath and then try to breathe in further and you will appreciate this point). Second, the PEEP must be overcome before the patient can initiate a lung inflation and the higher the PEEP, the greater the pressure excursion needed for lung inflation. This increases the inspiratory work performed by the patient.

Management. One strategy for reducing this PEEP is to promote more complete exhalation. The maneuvers suggested for this purpose include: (1) decreasing the inflation volume; (2) increasing the inspiratory flowrate to increase the time for exhalation; and (3) decreasing the respiratory rate. None of these maneuvers has been effective in our hands.

The maneuver that has received the most attention is the use of external PEEP. The idea here is to reduce the pressure excursion needed to inflate the lungs and thereby decrease the work of breathing. If external PEEP is applied, the inspiratory pressure will decrease because alveolar pressure needs only to drop below the PEEP level (rather than below zero level) to initiate lung inflation.[22] The clinical impact of this is presently unclear because this will not reduce the level of occult PEEP.

REFERENCES

REVIEWS

1. Pingleton SK. State of the art. Complications of acute respiratory failure. Am Rev Respir Dis 1988; 137:1463–1493.
2. Consensus conference on artificial airways in patients receiving mechanical ventilation. Chest 1989; 96:178–193.
3. Heffner JE, Miller S, Sahn SA. Tracheostomy in the intensive care unit. Parts 1 and 2. Chest 1986; 90:269–274, 430–436.

ARTIFICIAL AIRWAYS

4. Stauffer JL, Olson DE, Petty TL. Complications and consequences of endotracheal intubation and tracheostomy. Am J Med 1981; 70:65–76.
5. Zwillich CW, Pierson DJ, Creagh CE, et al. Complications of assisted ventilation: A prospective study of 354 consecutive episodes. Am J Med 1974; 57:161–170.
6. Goodman LR. Pulmonary support and monitoring apparatus. In: Goodman LR, Putnam CE eds. Intensive care radiology. St. Louis: C.V. Mosby, 1978:29–90.
7. Gridlinger GA, Niehoff J, Hughes L, et al. Acute paranasal sinusitis related to nasotracheal intubation of head-injured patients. Crit Care Med 1987; 15:214–217.
8. Knodel AR, Beekman JF. Unexplained fevers in patients with nasotracheal intubation. JAMA 1982; 248:868–872.

9. Whited RE. A prospective study of laryngotracheal sequelae in long-term intubation. Laryngoscope 1984; *94*:367–377.

10. Dunham CM, LaMonica C. Prolonged tracheal intubation in the trauma patient. J Trauma 1984; *24*:120–124.

11. Shapiro M, Wilson RK, Cesar G, et al. Work of breathing through different sized endotracheal tubes. Crit Care Med 1986; *14*:1028–1031.

12. Spray SB, Zuidema GD, Cameron JL. Aspiration pneumonia. Am J Surg 1976; *13*:701–703.

13. Bernhard WN, Cottrell JE, Sivakumaran C, et al. Adjustment of intracuff pressure to prevent aspiration. Anesthesiology 1979; *50*:363–366.

BAROTRAUMA

14. Haake R, Schlichtig R, Ulstad DR, et al. Barotrauma. Pathophysiology, risk factors and prevention. Chest 1987; *91*:608–613.

15. Powner DJ. Pulmonary barotrauma in the intensive care unit. J Intensive Care Med 1988; *3*:224–232.

16. Petersen GW, Baier H. Incidence of pulmonary barotrauma in a medical ICU. Crit Care Med 1983; *11*:67–69.

17. Steir M, Ching N, Roberts EB, Nealon TF. Pneumothorax complicating continuous ventilatory support. J Thorac Cardiovasc Surg 1974; *67*:17–23.

18. Woodring JH. Pulmonary interstitial emphysema in the adult respiratory distress syndrome. Crit Care Med 1985; *13*:786–791.

19. Chiles C, Ravin CE. Radiographic appearance of pneumothorax in the intensive care unit. Crit Care Med 1986; *14*:677–680.

AUTO-PEEP

20. Pepe PE, Marini JJ. Occult positive end-expiratory pressure in mechanically ventilated patients with airflow obstruction. Am Rev Respir Dis 1982; *126*:166–170.

21. Qvist J, Pemberton M, Bennike KA. High-level PEEP in severe asthma. N Engl J Med 1982; *307*:1347. (Letter)

22. Tobin M, Lodato RF. PEEP, auto-PEEP, and waterfalls. Chest 1989; *96*:449–451.

chapter

30

THE PRACTICE OF WEANING FROM MECHANICAL VENTILATION

"All who drink of this remedy will recover . . . except those whom it does not help, who will die. Therefore it is obvious that it fails only in incurable diseases."

Galen

The patient who requires chronic ventilator support becomes the target of an exercise called weaning. This practice usually appears after several days of rounding on a ventilator-dependent patient who has no active process to treat and nothing new to report on rounds. The wean involves a variety of protocols aimed at gradually removing ventilatory support. These protocols have a number of functions. First, they furnish daily rounds with a topic of discussion. Second, they give the ICU staff a sense of doing something for the patient. Finally, they occasionally remove the patient from the ventilator.

The description of weaning above is more sardonic than scientific, but there is a tendency to view the weaning process as a form of therapy that will help to remove patients from the ventilator. Weaning seems more like Galen's description of a remedy; it will fail unless the underlying illness is treated or cured. In this sense, the focus of weaning should be to correct the underlying illness and not to concentrate on the weaning process.

VENTILATORS AND RESPIRATORY MUSCLES

The need for gradual weaning implies that the respiratory muscles must be strengthened gradually over a period of time before spontaneous breathing is tolerated. This assumes that the respiratory muscles

399

TABLE 30–1. BEDSIDE CRITERIA FOR WEANING		
Parameter	Required to Wean	Reference
$PaO_2 - FIO_2$	>60 mmHg $- <0.60$	
Tidal Volume	>5 ml/kg	4
Vital Capacity	>10 ml/kg	4
Minute Ventilation	<10 L/min	5
Negative Inspiratory Pressure	> -30 mmHg	7

become atrophic during mechanical ventilation much like the muscles of an arm become atrophic when the arm is placed in a cast. The "arm-in-a-cast" analogy is not entirely valid, at least not for the diaphragm.

Disuse atrophy is unlikely in the diaphragm because this muscle is not a voluntary muscle and it continues to contract regularly during mechanical ventilation.

The diaphragm receives a periodic input during inspiration from the automatic brainstem respiratory centers and it cannot be silenced or immobilized during mechanical ventilation (see first section in Chapter 28).

THE BEDSIDE ASSESSMENT

The concerns involved in removing a patient from the ventilator depend on the patient population. In the routine postoperative patient, the ventilator can be removed as soon as the patient awakens from anesthesia. In the patient with severe lung disease and chronic ventilator support, a number of decisions are involved in the wean process.[1-3] The list in Table 30–1 contains the traditional criteria used to determine ability to wean. Accompanying each parameter is the reference that first cited the parameter.[4-8] The following is a brief description of the conditions that must be satisfied for a successful wean attempt.

GAS EXCHANGE

The arterial PO_2 should be above 60 mmHg when the fractional concentration of inspired oxygen is below the toxic level (FIO_2 less than 0.6) and little or no PEEP is being used.

The tidal volumes delivered during mechanical ventilation are excessive (10 to 15 ml/kg) compared to spontaneous breathing (5 to 6 ml/kg), and alveolar ventilation will decrease when the patient is removed from the ventilator.[16] As such, there should be room to increase the FIO_2 during the wean without reaching toxic levels of inspired oxygen. Because an FIO_2 above 60% is considered toxic (see Chapter 25), the FIO_2 should be 50% with satisfactory levels of arterial PO_2 before considering a wean trial.

The patient should not require PEEP to maintain adequate oxygenation. Although it is possible to wean using spontaneous PEEP, the patient who requires PEEP during mechanical ventilation is unlikely to wean and should not be extubated.

LUNG VOLUMES

The spontaneous tidal volume should be at least 5 ml/kg and the vital capacity 10 ml/kg.[4] The minute volume should not exceed 10 L/min.[5]

These volume criteria are applicable to postoperative patients or those with neuromuscular weakness but not to patients with severe lung disease. In the latter condition, the problem is not the inability to move air but an inability to exchange oxygen and carbon dioxide across the alveolar-capillary interface. In other words, the benefit of inspiratory lung volumes will be minimal if the alveoli and capillaries are not speaking to each other.

RESPIRATORY MUSCLE STRENGTH

The bedside evaluation of respiratory muscle strength involves the following measures.

Abdominal Movements. The movement of the abdomen during quiet breathing can provide information about the functional status of the diaphragm.[3] This is illustrated in Figure 30–1. When the diaphragm contracts during inspiration, it descends into the abdomen and increases the abdominal pressure. This pushes the anterior abdominal wall outward during inspiration, as shown in the upper panel of Figure 30–1. When the diaphragm is paralyzed, the negative inspiratory pressure in the thorax pulls the diaphragm into the thorax. This upward displacement decreases the abdominal pressure and causes an inward displacement of the anterior abdominal surface during inspiration.

Summary. During quiet breathing in the supine position, outward movement of the abdomen during inspiration indicates a functioning diaphragm and inward movement indicates a nonfunctioning diaphragm. The inward movement of the abdomen during inspiration is called "abdominal paradox" and it is a reliable sign only during quiet breathing. When breathing is labored, the contractions of the accessory muscles can overcome the diaphragm and pull a functioning diaphragm upward during inspiration, resulting in abdominal paradox with a functioning diaphragm.

Inspiratory Pressure. The strength of the diaphragm and the other muscles of inspiration can be evaluated by having the patient exhale fully and then inhale as forcefully as possible against a closed valve. The pressure generated is called the "maximum inspiratory pressure" (PImax). Table 30–2 shows the normal ranges for this pressure in adults of different ages. The minimum acceptable level of PImax for weaning is -30 cmH$_2$O (see Table 30–1), which is far below the normal range

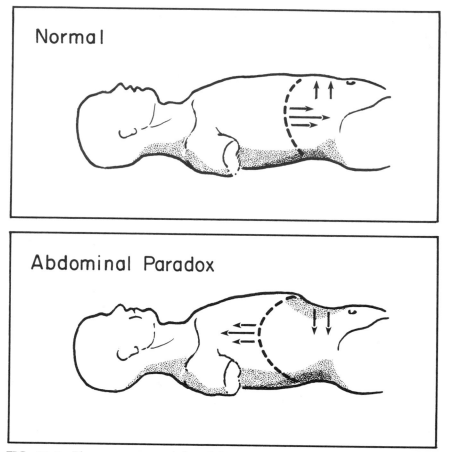

FIG. 30–1. The movement of the abdomen during inhalation in the supine position, as an index of diaphragm function. Upper panel: normal subject. Lower panel: bilateral diaphragm weakness or paralysis. See text for explanation.

TABLE 30–2. MAXIMUM INSPIRATORY PRESSURE*		
	Age Range (yrs)	**PI max (cm H₂O)**
Female	19–49	-91 ± 25
	50–70	-77 ± 18
	>70	-66 ± 18
Male	19–49	-127 ± 28
	50–70	-112 ± 20
	>70	-76 ± 27
Minimum for Weaning		-30
*From Rochester DF, Arora NS. Respiratory muscle failure. Med Clin North Am 1983; 67:573–598.		

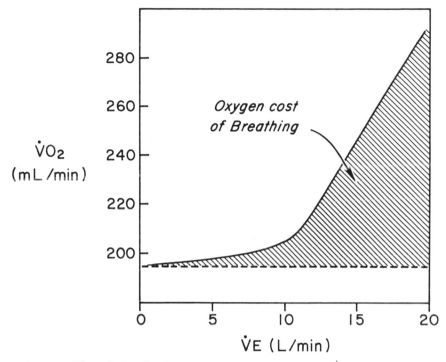

FIG. 30–2. The relationship between oxygen consumption ($\dot{V}O_2$) and the minute ventilation. See text for explanation.

for adults. This is the level that produces CO_2 retention in patients with neuromuscular weakness.[3]

RELIABILITY OF WEAN CRITERIA

The parameters listed in Table 30–1 will not correlate with ability to wean in roughly one-third of patients.[8] This means that one-third of patients with adequate parameters will not wean and one-third with inadequate parameters will wean successfully. These parameters are not to be used solely to predict ability to wean but also can be used to indicate how closely to monitor the individual patient during the wean period.

THE OXYGEN COST OF BREATHING

In the normal adult, the act of quiet breathing consumes only 5% of the total oxygen consumption ($\dot{V}O_2$) in the adult.[9,10] When breathing is labored, the relative proportion of oxygen consumed by the respiratory muscles increases considerably. The influence of minute ventilation on the $\dot{V}O_2$ is shown in Figure 30–2. As the minute ventilation increases above 10 L per minute, the $\dot{V}O_2$ begins to increase geometrically. This increase in $\dot{V}O_2$ is called the "oxygen cost of breathing" and it represents the oxygen consumed by the respiratory muscles in performing the work of breathing.[9,10] This is a measure of the "efficiency" of breathing, or the relationship between the work performed and the energy needed to perform the work. At a given workload, an efficient engine consumes less energy than an inefficient engine.

This principle has been applied to the evaluation of patients for weaning. The $\dot{V}O_2$ is measured at the bedside using a metabolic cart or the pulmonary artery catheter. The measurement is first obtained while the patient is resting on the ventilator, and again shortly after removal from the ventilator. The difference in $\dot{V}O_2$ in the two conditions is the O_2 cost of breathing. If the $\dot{V}O_2$ increases less than 10% after removal from the ventilator, the patient should wean successfully. If the $\dot{V}O_2$ increases more than 20% after removal, the wean is likely to be unsuccessful.[10]

METHODS OF WEANING

There are two methods of weaning and each is analogous to an electrical switch: one is abrupt like an on-off toggle switch, while the other is gradual like a rheostat. The abrupt method is called the "T-piece" method because of the shape of the tubing in the circuit and the gradual method is the mode of ventilation called "intermittent mandatory ventilation" (IMV) that was described in Chapter 28. A survey of ICU directors reported in 1987 shows that IMV is by far the most popular method of weaning in this country.[11] As we will see, there is little to justify this popularity.

THE T-PIECE METHOD

The circuit design shown in Figure 30–3 has an adaptor that is shaped like the letter "T" and this circuit is called a "T-piece." Oxygen-rich gas is delivered at constant flow from the inlet arm of the apparatus and flows past the patient to exit the circuit at the other end. When the patient takes a breath, the gas is drawn into the lungs from the inlet side only. A rapid flow of gas along the upper arm of the circuit prevents the patient from entraining room air. When the patient exhales, this high gas flow also carries the exhaled gas out of the circuit so the patient cannot rebreathe the exhaled gas.

The CPAP Mode. The original T-piece circuit was not connected to the ventilator, which made it difficult to monitor tidal volume and respiratory rate during the wean. The newer ventilators are equipped with circuits that allow a T-piece wean while monitoring tidal volume and rate on the ventilator. This is done by using the "continuous positive airways pressure" (CPAP) mode of ventilation. When no pressure is applied in the CPAP mode, the patient will receive the inspired O_2 concentration from the ventilator at constant flow. The only drawback to the CPAP circuit is that a valve must be opened by the patient to receive the inhaled gas and the pressure needed to open the valve can increase the work of breathing. For normal subjects, this increase in

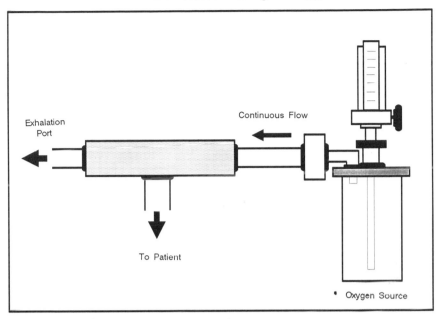

FIG. 30–3. A schematic representation of the T-shaped circuit used for weaning. A continuous flow of gas passes along the horizontal arm of the T-circuit to prevent the patient from entraining room air or rebreathing exhaled gas.

work would not be deleterious. However, in a patient with borderline respiratory function, the added workload can be enough to eventually fatigue the patient and prevent extubation. Therefore, when a difficult wean is anticipated, the stand-alone circuit is preferred.

The Protocol. When starting a T-piece wean trial, the patient is first allowed to stay off the ventilator as long as tolerated. If it is not possible for the patient to wean at this point, then a wean schedule can be started using trials of shorter duration (to prevent any further muscle fatigue) alternating with periods of total ventilatory support.

INTERMITTENT MANDATORY VENTILATION

The pattern of breathing with IMV is described in Chapter 28 and illustrated in Figure 28–2. The IMV method provides a "backup" level of ventilation for the patient while also allowing the patient to breathe spontaneously between ventilator breaths. The backup rate is usually started at 8 to 10 breaths/min and is then gradually reduced in increments of 1 to 2 breaths/minute, until there is no input from the ventilator. The period of time over which the IMV rate is tapered is extremely variable, and is determined by the condition of the patient.

False Security of IMV. There is a tendency to view IMV as safer than the T-piece method because IMV provides a ventilator backup. This produces a false sense of security with IMV weaning that can be dangerous. The ventilator backup is misleading because the IMV circuit is not a closed-loop feedback system. That is, the ventilator is unable to sense changes in the patient's ventilatory demands and adjust the backup rate. If the patient's minute ventilation decreases, the ventilator will not increase ventilatory input to keep overall minute ventilation constant. Therefore, the patient can get into trouble with IMV despite the presence of backup ventilator breaths. This can be dangerous because patients weaned with IMV tend to be unattended more than those weaned with the T-piece method.

T-PIECE VERSUS IMV WEANING

Neither method of weaning has proven superior to the other,[12,13] so the method selected is largely one of personal preference. I prefer T-piece trials for the following reasons:

1. IMV can prolong weaning in patients who will be easily weaned and extubated (e.g., postoperative patients). Because IMV ends up as a T-piece trial, the time needed to taper the IMV rate is wasted time for patients who will wean easily.

2. The T-piece method forces the physician to watch the patient more closely during the wean, therefore providing a safer environment for weaning.

3. T-piece weaning is superior to IMV for increasing muscle strength in patients with respiratory muscle weakness. The traditional method of strengthening skeletal muscle groups is to alternate periods of exercise and periods of rest (similar to the T-piece trials) and not to continually use the fatigued muscles (which is what IMV does). This concept is simplified, particularly because the diaphragm is continually in use in either method of weaning. However, the concept of rest for a fatiguing muscle is valid, and at least the accessory muscle will rest periodically using the T-piece method of weaning.

The choice of weaning method is not the important issue in the ability to wean from mechanical ventilation because weaning is not a therapy for the removal of mechanical ventilation. Remember:

> The ability to wean depends on the severity of the underlying problem and not on the method of weaning. When the underlying problem is corrected, the patient should wean regardless of the method used.

COMMON PROBLEMS

The following problems often arise during a difficult wean and require a decision about continuing the wean or resuming mechanical ventilation.

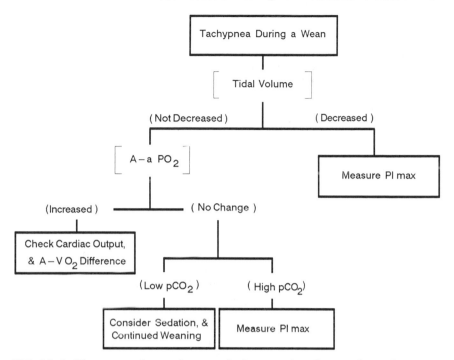

FIG. 30–4. The approach to tachypnea during weaning. See text for explanation.

TACHYPNEA

The most common scenario in a difficult wean is the appearance of agitation and tachypnea. The immediate concern is to distinguish anxiety from muscle weakness or a cardiopulmonary problem.

Spontaneous Tidal Volume. The exhaled tidal volume can be monitored when the patient is kept connected to the ventilator during the wean. Failure to wean is often associated with a decreasing tidal volume,[14] but not invariably.[15] The interpretation of the tidal volume in the setting of tachypnea is shown in Figure 30–4. An increase in the tidal volume suggests hyperventilation from anxiety, while a drop in tidal volume suggests muscle weakness.

The A-a PO_2 Gradient. The alveolar-arterial PO_2 (A-a PO_2) gradient might help to differentiate anxiety from a cardiopulmonary problem.

> An increase in the A-a PO_2 gradient indicates a ventilation-perfusion imbalance or a reduced mixed venous PO_2, while a normal or unchanged A-a PO_2 gradient indicates anxiety or muscle weakness.

Unfortunately, an increase in the A-a PO_2 gradient might not always rule out anxiety as a cause of hypoxemia. There are two mechanisms whereby anxiety could elevate the A-a PO_2 gradient. First, the anxiety-induced tachypnea could produce auto-PEEP and thereby create a ventilation-perfusion mismatch (see Chapter 29). Second, increased work of breathing from anxiety could increase oxygen consumption and reduce mixed venous P_{O_2}. Both processes would increase the A-a P_{O_2} gradient.

Recommendations. If the tidal volume is maintained in the setting of tachypnea, obtain an arterial blood sample and check the A-a P_{O_2} gradient. Continue the wean only if the patient is not in extremis. Otherwise, resume mechanical ventilation until the problem is uncovered. If the A-a P_{O_2} gradient is unchanged, consider sedating the patient and continuing the wean. If the A-a P_{O_2} gradient is increased, then search for an underlying cardiac or pulmonary problem. The workup of an elevated A-a P_{O_2} gradient is outlined in the next section.

HYPOXEMIA

The approach to hypoxemia or an increase in A-a P_{O_2} gradient is presented in Chapter 3 and outlined in Figure 3–5. This approach considers two sources for an increase in A-a P_{O_2} gradient:

Mixed Venous Oxygen. A decrease in mixed venous P_{O_2} can increase the A-a P_{O_2} gradient if there is an underlying intrapulmonary shunt (which is usually the case in ventilator-dependent patients). The causes of a low $P\bar{v}_{O_2}$ during a wean include:

1. Oxygen cost of spontaneous breathing
2. Low cardiac output from negative pressure breathing[18]

The first step in the approach to hypoxemia should be to measure the $P\bar{v}_{O_2}$ or $S\bar{v}_{O_2}$ to determine if the problem is in the thorax (normal $S\bar{v}_{O_2}$) or in the peripheral oxygen extraction (low $S\bar{v}_{O_2}$).

Intrapulmonary Shunt. The shunt fraction should increase when mechanical ventilation is discontinued in most patients because the tidal volume will decrease from 10 to 15 ml/kg (during mechanical ventilation) to 5 ml/kg (during spontaneous breathing). Further increases in shunt fraction during the wean might result from the following:

1. Atelectasis
2. Secretions
3. Airflow obstruction from forced expirations

HYPERCAPNIA

The appearance of hypercapnia during a wean is an ominous sign and usually indicates immediate return to mechanical ventilation. The bedside approach to hypercapnia is presented in Chapter 3 and outlined in Figure 3–7. The end-tidal P_{CO_2} (ET_{CO_2}) should be monitored during a difficult wean because the gradient between ET_{CO_2} and arterial P_{CO_2} (Pa_{CO_2}) can help to identify the problem.

An increase in the Pa_{CO_2}-ET_{CO_2} gradient indicates an increase in dead space ventilation while a constant gradient suggests respiratory muscle weakness or enhanced CO_2 production.

Extrapulmonary Causes. The two extrapulmonary causes of hypercapnia in the weaning patient are:[17]

1. Respiratory muscle weakness
2. Increased CO_2 production from spontaneous breathing.

Both processes are likely to play a role in the weaning patient. The strength of the inspiratory muscles can be monitored during the wean by measuring the PImax at regular intervals. A decrease in PImax to below 25 to 30 cm H_2O is taken as evidence for muscle weakness. Hypercapnia alone can depress the contractile strength of the diaphragm,[3] and this will confuse the interpretation of a decrease in PImax during a wean.

Dead Space Ventilation. The causes of dead space ventilation during a wean are:

1. Low cardiac output from negative pressure breathing
2. Auto-PEEP from high respiratory rates

The cardiac output can be monitored at regular intervals during a difficult wean but auto-PEEP can be monitored only during mechanical ventilation. However, the combination of tachypnea and an increase in dead space ventilation suggests auto-PEEP. In this situation, the judicious use of sedation is not unreasonable if the CO_2 retention is acute and the degree of elevation is mild.

SPECIAL CONSIDERATIONS

SEDATION

There are clear benefits to sedation during a wean. First, reducing anxiety might reduce O_2 consumption and CO_2 production and this can itself improve the arterial blood gases (see Chapter 3). Second, limiting respiratory rate will reduce (or limit the risk for) auto-PEEP. Because auto-PEEP can produce ventilation-perfusion abnormalities (see Chapter 29), sedation might improve gas exchange if auto-PEEP is present.

Several agents are available for sedation and these are presented in some detail in Chapter 26. Two of the more popular agents are listed in Table 30–3.

Haloperidol is becoming the preferred agent for sedation in the ICU because of its lack of cardiovascular or pulmonary side effects.[19] This agent will reduce the level of anxiety and the sense of dyspnea, but might not reduce the respiratory rate. The **benzodiazepines** can produce unwanted levels of sedation leading to CO_2 retention and can reduce the respiratory rate but can also produce unwanted levels of sedation leading to CO_2 retention, particularly in the elderly. One of the popular methods of sedation is to combine haloperidol and lorazepam and reduce the recommended dose of each by 50%. This allows for adequate sedation with a reduction in respiratory rate but reduces the risk for CO_2 retention.

	TABLE 30–3. PARENTERAL THERAPY OF AGITATION	
Drug	IV Dose* (Agitation Level)	Comments
Haloperidol[1] (Haldol)	0.5–2 mg (mild) 5–10 mg (moderate) >10 mg (severe)	1. Can be given IV push 2. Allow 15–20 min for full effect, then double the dose if needed 3. No respiratory depression 4. No hypotension unless given with beta-blockers or hypovolemia 5. Dose interval must be individualized 6. Not FDA approved for IV use, but is proven effective and safe[1]
Lorazepam[2] (Ativan)	0.04 mg/kg (mild) 0.05 mg/kg (severe) DO NOT exceed 2 mg/min	1. Allow 15–20 min for full effect 2. Produces an amnesic effect that may be desirable 3. Can produce hypotension and respiratory depression, particularly in the elderly 4. Dose interval must be individualized

[1]From Tesar GE, Stern TA. J Intensive Care Med 1986; 1:137–148.
[2]From Drug facts and comparisons. St. Louis: J.B. Lippincott, 1985.
*Dose based on 70 kg adult.

AMINOPHYLLINE

The observation that aminophylline increases the contractility of the diaphragm has led to the recommendation that aminophylline be used to facilitate a difficult wean.[20] There are several problems associated with this recommendation. First, the effects of theophylline on diaphragm contractility does not mean it will augment the power output of the diaphragm (the transdiaphragmatic pressure). Recent studies show that maximum inspiratory pressure is unchanged during theophylline therapy.[21] Second, the use of aminophylline assumes that the diaphragm is the major reason for the inability to wean. This has not been verified.[22] Finally, if a skeletal muscle is fatigued, the traditional approach is to rest the muscle rather than stimulate the muscle continuously (with aminophylline). Constant stimulation of a tired or weak muscle will further deplete high energy phosphate stores and add to the problem.

Summary. At the present time, there is no evidence to support the routine use of aminophylline to facilitate weaning from mechanical ventilation.

REFERENCES

REVIEWS

1. Karpel JP, Aldrich TK. Respiratory failure and mechanical ventilation: Pathophysiology and methods to promote weaning. Lung 1986; 164:309–324.

2. Sporn PHS, Morganroth ML. Discontinuation of mechanical ventilation. Clin Chest Med 1988; 9:113–126.
3. Rochester DF, Arora NS. Respiratory muscle failure. Med Clin North Am 1983; 67:573–598.

WEANING CRITERIA

4. Benedixen HH, et al. Respiratory care. St. Louis: C.V. Mosby Co. 1965; 137–156.
5. Stetson JB. Introductory essay in prolonged tracheal intubation. Int Anesthesiol Clin 1970; 8:774–775.
6. Pontoppidan H, Laver MA, Geffin B. Acute respiratory failure in the surgical patient. Adv Surg 1970; 4:163–254.
7. Sahn SA, Lakshminarayan S. Bedside criteria for discontinuation of mechanical ventilation. Chest 1973; 63:1002–1005.
8. Morganroth ML, et al. Criteria for weaning from prolonged mechanical ventilation. Arch Intern Med 1984; 144:1012–1016.

OXYGEN COST OF BREATHING

9. Harpin RP, Baker JP, Downer JP, et al. Correlation of the oxygen cost of breathing and length of weaning from mechanical ventilation. Crit Care Med 1987; 15:807–812.
10. Nashimura M, Taenaka N, Takezawa J, et al. Oxygen cost of breathing and inspiratory work of ventilator as weaning monitor in critically ill. Crit Care Med 1984; 12:258.

METHODS OF WEANING

11. Venus B, Smith RA, Mathru M. National survey of methods and criteria used for weaning from mechanical ventilation. Crit Care Med 1987; 15:530–533.
12. Ashutosh K. Gradual vs abrupt weaning from respiratory support in acute respiratory failure and advanced chronic obstructive lung disease. South Med J 1983; 76:1244–1248.
13. Prakash O, Meij MS, Van Der Borden B. Spontaneous ventilation test vs. intermittent mandatory ventilation. Chest 1982; 81:403–405.

COMMON PROBLEMS DURING WEANING

14. Tobin MJ, Perez W, Guenther SM, et al. The pattern of breathing during successful and unsuccessful trials of weaning from mechanical ventilation. Am Rev Respir Dis 1986; 134:1111–1118.
15. Pourriat JL, Lamberto C, Hoang PH, et al. Diaphragmatic fatigue and breathing pattern during weaning from mechanical ventilation in COPD patients. Chest 1986; 90:703–707.
16. Wolff G, Gradel E. Hemodynamic performance and weaning from mechanical ventilation following open heart surgery. Eur J Intensive Care Med 1975; 1:99–104.
17. Weinberger SE, Schwartzstein RM, Weiss JW. Hypercapnia. N Engl J Med 1989; 321:1223–1230.
18. Pinsky M. The influence of positive pressure ventilation on cardiovascular function in the critically ill. Crit Care Clin 1985; 1:699–717.

SPECIAL CONSIDERATIONS

19. Tesar GE, Stern TA. Evaluation and treatment of agitation in the intensive care unit. J Intensive Care Med 1986; 1:137–148.
20. Aubier M, DeTroyer A, Sampson M, et al. Aminophylline improves diaphragm contractility. N Engl J Med 1981; 305:249–252.
21. Brophy C, Miler A, Moxham J, Green M. The effect of aminophylline on respiratory and limb muscle contractility in man. Eur Respir J 1989; 2:652–655.
22. Swartz M, Marino PL. Diaphragm strength during weaning from mechanical ventilation. Chest 1985; 88:736–739.

section IX
ACID-BASE DISORDERS

It is not enough that our premises should be true, they must also be known.
Bertrand Russell

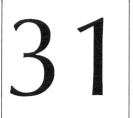

ALGORITHMS FOR ACID-BASE INTERPRETATIONS

The approach to acid-base disorders is a good example of a "rule-oriented" system because a set of well-defined rules is used to make the interpretations.[1-6] These rules are a series of IF:THEN statements called algorithms. The algorithm is the dominant stucture in clinical problem solving and is particularly dominant in the interpretation of acid-base disorders. It also resembles the binary ON:OFF logic used by computers. In fact, the algorithms used in this chapter are taken from a computer program we developed that interprets blood gases.[4]

PHYSICIAN PERFORMANCE

Acid-base interpretation is an area that Alexander Pope was describing when he wrote "A little learning is a dangerous thing." At one university teaching hospital, one-third of blood gases were interpreted incorrectly by senior residents and many of these interpretations led to inappropriate therapy.[7] At another university medical center, 70% of the non-pulmonary staff physicians claimed a mastery of blood gas analysis and did not want any further instruction in the subject. However, those same physicians could correctly interpret only 40% of the blood gases presented to them.[8]

BASIC CONCEPTS

The hydrogen ion (H^+) concentration in blood is determined by the balance between carbon dioxide (PCO_2) and the serum bicarbonate (HCO_3). This relationship can be expressed as follows:[8]

$$H^+ \ (mEq/L) = 24 \times [PCO_2/HCO_3^-]$$

TABLE 31-1.   PRIMARY AND SECONDARY ACID-BASE DISORDERS

$$\text{Goal: } \frac{P_{CO_2}}{HCO_3^-} = K$$

Primary Disorder	Compensatory Response
↑ P_{CO_2} (Respiratory Acidosis)	↑ HCO_3^- (Metabolic Alkalosis)
↓ P_{CO_2} (Respiratory Alkalosis)	↓ HCO_3^- (Metabolic Acidosis)
↓ HCO_3^- (Metabolic Acidosis)	↓ P_{CO_2} (Respiratory Alkalosis)
↑ HCO_3^- (Metabolic Alkalosis)	↑ P_{CO_2} (Respiratory Acidosis)

A change in H^+ of 1 mEq/L corresponds to a change in pH of 0.01 units. This relationship predicts that the serum H^+ will change in the same direction as the P_{CO_2} and in the opposite direction from the serum HCO_3. This relationship forms the basis of the four primary and compensatory acid-base disorders, which are shown in Table 31–1.

The goal of compensation is to keep the P_{CO_2}/HCO_3 ratio constant. When one of the two components becomes abnormal, adjustments are made to change the other component in the same direction. It is important to emphasize that compensation will limit the change in serum pH but will not entirely prevent a change, that is, compensation is not synonymous with correction.

COMPENSATORY RESPONSES

The respiratory system provides the compensation for metabolic disorders (see Table 31–1) and the response occurs immediately. Metabolic acidosis stimulates ventilation and the resultant decrease in P_{CO_2} helps to counteract the primary decrease in serum HCO_3. Metabolic alkalosis inhibits ventilation and the increase in P_{CO_2} will balance the increase in HCO_3.

The kidneys provide the compensation for respiratory disorders by adjusting HCO_3 reabsorption in the proximal tubules. Respiratory acidosis stimulates HCO_3 reabsorption and the resultant increase in serum HCO_3 will counteract the increase in P_{CO_2}. Respiratory alkalosis inhibits HCO_3 reabsorption and the decrease in serum HCO_3 will balance the decrease in P_{CO_2}. The renal response is not immediate (unlike the respiratory response), but begins to develop at 6 to 12 hours and requires a few days to reach maximum. The respiratory disorder will be "partially compensated" during this time period.

TABLE 31–2. EXPECTED COMPENSATORY RESPONSES	
Primary Disorder	**Expected Response**
Metabolic Acidosis	Expected P_{CO_2} = 1.5 × HCO_3^- + 8 (±2)
Metabolic Alkalosis	Expected P_{CO_2} = 0.7 × HCO_3^- + 20 (±1.5)
Respiratory Acidosis	$\dfrac{\Delta pH}{\Delta P_{CO_2}} = \dfrac{0.008 \text{ (Acute)}}{0.003 \text{ (Chronic)}}$
Respiratory Alkalosis	$\dfrac{\Delta pH}{\Delta P_{CO_2}} = \dfrac{0.008 \text{ (Acute)}}{0.017 \text{ (Chronic)}}$

THE RULES OF ACID-BASE INTERPRETATION

The compensatory responses can be quantified and the observed response can be compared to the expected response. The expected or normal responses are shown in Table 31–2. These equations will be used to formulate the rules that are followed in acid-base interpretation. The normal ranges for arterial blood gas variables are shown below:

pH: 7.36 to 7.44

P_{CO_2}: 36 to 44 mm Hg

HCO_3: 22 to 26 mEq/L

PRIMARY METABOLIC DISORDERS

Rule 1: A primary metabolic disorder is present if:
A. The pH and P_{CO_2} change in the same direction, or
B. The pH is abnormal but the P_{CO_2} is normal.
The algorithm format would state:
   IF: The pH and P_{CO_2} change in the same direction,
   AND: The pH is not normal,
THEN: The primary disorder is metabolic.
Rule 2: The following equations will identify an associated respiratory disorder:
A. For metabolic acidosis
   Expected P_{CO_2} = 1.5 (HCO_3) + 8 (+/−2)
B. For metabolic alkalosis
   Expected P_{CO_2} = 0.7 (HCO_3) + 20 (+/−1.5)

That is, if the P_{CO_2} is higher than expected, then there is an associated respiratory acidosis, and if the P_{CO_2} is lower than expected, there is an associated respiratory alkalosis.

Unlike the highly predictable respiratory stimulation that occurs in metabolic acidosis, the respiratory depression in metabolic alkalosis is variable. As a result, several equations have been proposed to define the relationship between Pco_2 and HCO_3 in metabolic alkaloses.[9] The one presented here seems to be the most accepted equation, at least up to a serum HCO_3 of 40 mEq/L.

PRIMARY RESPIRATORY DISORDERS

Rule 3: A primary respiratory disorder is present if the pH and the Pco_2 change in opposite directions.

Rule 4: The relationship between the change in Pco_2 and the change in pH can be used to identify an associated metabolic disorder or an incomplete compensatory response.[8]

A. For Respiratory Acidosis

Acute uncompensated acidosis—The pH changes 0.008 units for every 1 mm Hg change in Pco_2.

Chronic compensated acidosis—The pH changes 0.003 units for every 1 mm Hg change in Pco_2. Therefore:

Change in pH/Pco_2	Disorder
above 0.008	Associated metabolic acidosis
0.003 to 0.008	Partially compensated respiratory acidosis
below 0.003	Associated metabolic alkalosis

B. For Respiratory Alkalosis

Acute uncompensated alkalosis—The pH/Pco_2 change is the same as for acute respiratory acidosis (0.008).

Chronic compensated alkalosis—The serum pH changes 0.017 units for every 1 mm Hg change in Pco_2. Therefore:

Change in pH/Pco_2	Disorder
above 0.008	Associated metabolic alkalosis
0.002 to 0.008	Partially compensated respiratory acidosis
below 0.002	Associated metabolic acidosis

MIXED METABOLIC–RESPIRATORY DISORDERS

Rule 5: A mixed metabolic–respiratory disorder is present if the pH is normal and the Pco_2 is abnormal.

RULE-ORIENTED BLOOD GAS INTERPRETATION

The rules just stated can now be used to interpret arterial blood gases for any patient. The following system requires only recognition of the

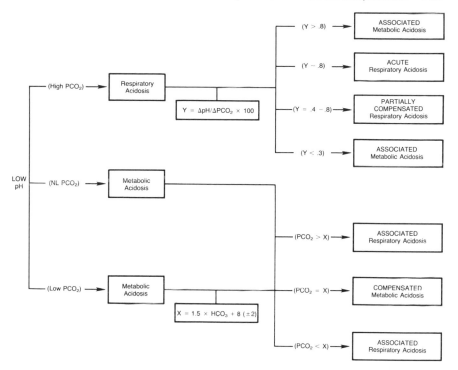

FIG. 31–1. Flow diagram for blood gas interpretation when the serum pH is low.

arterial pH and PCO_2 to start with. Figures 31–1 and 31–2 are flow diagrams that illustrate this process starting with the arterial pH.

WHEN THE pH IS LOW:

A. A low or normal PCO_2 indicates a primary metabolic acidosis (Rules 1A and 1B).
   1. The equation [$PCO_2 = 1.5(HCO_3) + 8 (+/-2)$] in Rule 2A is then used to identify an associated respiratory disorder.

B. A high PCO_2 indicates a primary respiratory acidosis (Rule 3).
   1. The change in pH/PCO_2 ratio is then used to determine the degree of compensation and to identify an associated metabolic disorder (Rule 4).

WHEN THE pH IS HIGH:

A. A high or normal PCO_2 indicates a primary metabolic acidosis (Rules 1A and 1B).
   1. The equation [$PCO_2 = 0.7(HCO_3) + 20(\pm1.5)$] in Rule 2B is then used to identify an associated respiratory disorder.

B. A low PCO_2 indicates a primary respiratory alkalosis (Rule 3).
   1. The pH/PCO_2 ratio is then used to determine the degree of com-

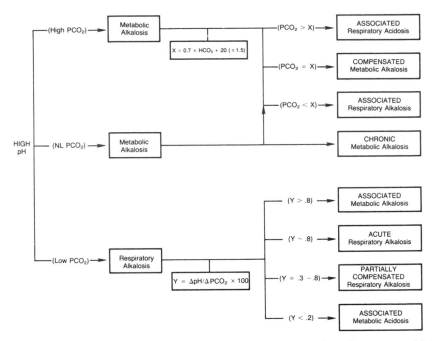

FIG. 31–2. Flow diagram for blood gas interpretation when the serum pH is high.

pensation and to identify an associated metabolic disorder (Rule 4B).

WHEN THE pH IS NORMAL:
A. A high Pco_2 indicates a mixed respiratory acidosis-metabolic alkalosis (Rule 5).
B. A low Pco_2 indicates a mixed respiratory alkalosis-metabolic acidosis (Rule 5).
C. A normal Pco_2 may indicate normal acid-base status but does not rule out a combined metabolic acidosis-metabolic alkalosis. In this situation, the anion gap can prove to be valuable.

METABOLIC ACIDOSES

The metabolic acidosis are separated into two groups by the anion gap. The high anion gap acidoses are characterized by the addition of a fixed acid (e.g., lactic acid), and the nonanion gap acidoses are characterized by loss of bicarbonate buffer (e.g., diarrhea). In the latter condition, chloride replaces the lost bicarbonate for electrical neutrality and the increase in serum chloride produces a "hyperchloremic metabolic acidosis." The common metabolic acidoses are shown in Figure 31–3, grouped according to the anion gap.

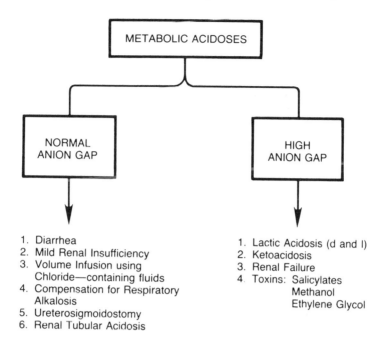

FIG. 31–3. Classification of metabolic acidoses according to the anion gap.

THE ANION GAP

The basis of the anion gap is the assumption that the negatively-charged anions and positively-charged cations in the serum must be equal for electrical neutrality.[10] If so, then the unmeasured anions and unmeasured cations can be determined using the serum chloride (Cl), bicarbonate (HCO_3), and sodium (Na). This is shown in Table 31–3. The difference between the unmeasured anions and cations in the serum is the "anion gap" or AG. As shown in Table 31–3, the normal AG is 12 mEq/L.[10,11] When a fixed acid like lactic acid donates a proton (H^+) to the serum, the bicarbonate decreases 1 mEq/L for every 1 mEq/L of H^+ added and the anion gap will, therefore, increase by the same amount. When bicarbonate is lost in the urine or stool, the compensatory increase in chloride maintains the negative equivalency of bicarbonate and the anion gap is unchanged.

OTHER INFLUENCES ON THE ANION GAP

As shown in Table 31–3, most of the unmeasured anion pool in the serum represents serum proteins; therefore, a low serum albumin can

TABLE 31–3. THE SERUM ANION GAP				
Unmeasured Anions (UA)			**Unmeasured Cations (UC)**	
Protein	15 mEq/L		K	4.5 mEq/L
PO$_4$	2		Ca	5.0
SO$_4$	1		Mg	1.5
Organic Acids	5			
Total	23		Total	11

$$\text{Anion Gap: UA} - \text{UC} = 12 \text{ mEq/L}$$
$$\text{UA} + (\text{Cl}^- + \text{HCO}_3^-) = \text{Na}^+ + \text{UC}$$

$$\boxed{\text{UA} - \text{UC} = \text{Na}^+ - (\text{Cl}^- + \text{HCO}_3^-)}$$

decrease the anion gap. Other causes of a reduced anion gap are abnormal paraproteins (which have a net positive charge), an increase in unmeasured cations (K, Mg, and Ca), and hyponatremia.

Hypoalbuminemia. This is probably the most common cause of a reduced anion gap in critically ill patients. Serum albumin contributes about half (11 mEq/L) of the total anionic equivalency of the unmeasured anion pool, which is 23 mEq/L.[11] Therefore, a 50% decrease in serum albumin will cause a 25% decrease in the total anion equivalency. Assuming normal serum electrolytes,

A 50% reduction in serum albumin will decrease the anion gap by 5 to 6 mEq/L.[11]

Therefore, an anion gap of 12 mmHg should be corrected to 17 to 18 mmHg when the serum albumin is half normal. This is an important correction factor because of the prevalence of hypoalbuminemia in the ICU patient population and because it could make a difference in uncovering an elevated anion gap acidosis.

Hyponatremia. This is another common cause of a reduced anion gap but the mechanism is not clear.[5,10] Because most causes of hyponatremia involve water overload, the extra free water should decrease the serum chloride as much as the serum sodium leaving the anion gap unchanged. However, the chloride does not show an equivalent reduction in most cases of hyponatremia. One possible mechanism is that other unmeasured cations (Mg and Ca) increase in the serum during hyponatremia and the chloride is needed to match electrical neutrality.[10]

URINARY ANION GAP

The urine anion gap is used to identify a defect in renal tubular acidification (renal tubular acidosis) in patients with a hyperchloremic (normal anion gap) metabolic acidosis.[15] The principle is the same as that

TABLE 31–4. THE URINE ANION GAP		

Anion Gap:

$$Total\ Anions = Total\ Cations$$
$$UA + Cl^- = Na^+ + K^+ + UC$$
$$UA - UC = (Na^+ + K^+) - Cl^-$$

Urine Anion Gap	Urine pH	Diagnosis
Negative	<5.5	Normal
Positive	>5.5	RTA
Negative	>5.5	Diarrhea

for the serum anion gap and is shown in Table 31–4. The usual electrolytes measured in urine are sodium, potassium, and chloride. The major unmeasured cation in the urine is ammonium and ammonium is the excretion form for titratable acid (H^+ binds to ammonia to form ammonium). When urine ammonium normally increases in response to an acid load, the urine anion gap decreases and becomes negative. However, when urine acidification is deranged, the urine ammonium is reduced and the anion gap will increase (become more positive). Table 31–4 shows how the urine anion gap can be used to differentiate GI bicarbonate losses from defective renal tubular acidification.

MIXED METABOLIC DISORDERS

Mixed metabolic disorders may be common in the ICU. For example, a patient with diabetic ketoacidosis may also have a hyperchloremic acidosis from diarrhea or early renal insufficiency. Mixed metabolic disorders can be identified using the relationship between the increase in anion gap and the decrease in serum bicarbonate. This ratio of anion gap excess to bicarbonate deficit is sometimes called the "gap–gap."

$$AG\ Excess/HCO_3\ Deficit = [AG - 12/24 - HCO_3]$$

The ratio associated with different metabolic disorders is shown in Figure 31–4.

MIXED METABOLIC ACIDOSES

When an acid like lactic acid is added to blood, the decrease in serum HCO_3 is equivalent to the increase in anion gap, so the [AG-excess/HCO_3-deficit] ratio will be unity. When a hyperchloremic acidosis is present, the ratio will approach zero. When a mixed acidosis is present (combined high AG and hyperchloremic acidoses), the [AG-excess/HCO_3-deficit] ratio will indicate the relative contribution of each to the

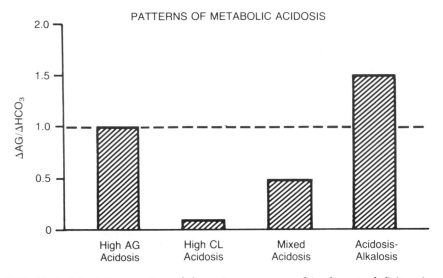

FIG. 31–4. The interpretation of the anion gap excess/bicarbonate deficit ratio. See text for explanation.

acidosis. For example, a ratio of 0.5 would indicate an equivalent contribution from each type of acidosis.

DIABETIC KETOACIDOSIS

The therapy of diabetic ketoacidosis changes the [AG-excess/HCO_3-deficit] ratio and this should be monitored instead of the serum bicarbonate. During therapy with insulin and intravenous fluids, the high anion gap will begin to decrease (as will the delta-delta ratio) but the serum HCO_3 will remain low because of the dilutional effect of the intravenous fluids. Therefore, if you follow the serum HCO_3, you will be misled into thinking that the therapy is inadequate. However, a decreasing delta-delta ratio indicates that the acidosis is changing from a high gap to a low gap and that the ketones are being cleared.

MIXED ACIDOSIS-ALKALOSIS

When alkali is added in the presence of a high anion gap acidosis, the decrease in serum bicarbonate will be less than the decrease in anion gap and the [AG-Excess/HCO_3-deficit] ratio will be greater than 1. Metabolic alkalosis is common in the ICU, primarily because of the common use of nasogastric suction and diuretics. Therefore, this type of combined metabolic disorder may also be common.

ARTERIAL OR VENOUS BLOOD?

The traditional practice is to use arterial blood for the P_{CO_2} and the pH measurements and to use venous blood for the electrolytes and bicarbonate determinations. These two sources of blood can differ considerably in patients who are hemodynamically unstable or who are receiving vasoconstrictor agents.[16] In fact, the venous blood should be a closer approximation of the acid-base status at the tissue level under normal circumstances, while the arterial blood depicts pulmonary gas exchange. However, in critically ill and septic patients, the normal venous blood may not mirror the tissues because of microcirculatory shunts that divert blood away from metabolizing tissues. Therefore, the value of venous blood will depend on the clinical condition of the patient.

When cardiac output falls, the arterial pH and lactate may look normal but the venous blood reveals a lactic acidosis. Venous P_{CO_2} may also increase in low-flow states because of the increase in lactic acid in the venous effluent. Therefore,

> When a patient is hemodynamically unstable, never assume that the arterial blood is an accurate measure of tissue acid-base status.

In this situation, a mixed venous blood sample (or any venous sample) should be checked periodically while monitoring the arterial blood gases.

REFERENCES

GENERAL

1. Cohen JJ, Kassirer JP eds. Acid-base. Boston: Little Brown & Co. 1982.
2. Arieff AI, DeFronzo RA eds. Fluid electrolyte and acid-base disorders. New York: Churchill Livingstone, 1985.
3. Kurtzman NA, Battle DC eds. Acid-base disorders. Med Clin North Am 1983; 67:751–929.

SOFTWARE

4. Krasner J, Marino PL. Respiratory expert. Philadelphia: W.B. Saunders, 1987.

REVIEWS

5. Narins RG, Emmett M. Simple and mixed acid-base disorders: A practical approach. Medicine 1980; 59:161–187.
6. Fencl V, Rossing TH. Acid-base disorders in critical care medicine. Ann Rev Med 1989; 40:17–29.

PHYSICIAN PERFORMANCE

7. Broughton JO, Kennedy TC. Interpretation of arterial blood gases by computer. Chest 1984; *85*:148–149.
8. Hingston DM. A computerized interpretation of arterial pH and blood gas data: Do physicians need it? Respir Care 1982; *27*:809–815.

METABOLIC ALKALOSIS

9. Javaheri S, Kazemi H. Metabolic alkalosis and hypoventilation in humans. Am Rev Respir Dis 1987; *136*:1011–1016.

THE ANION GAP

10. Emmet M, Narins RG. Clinical use of the anion gap. Medicine 1977; *56*:38–54.
11. Oh MS, Carroll HS. The anion gap. N Engl J Med 1977; *297*:814–817.
12. Goodkin DA, Krishna GG, Narins RG. The role of the anion gap in detecting and managing mixed metabolic acid-base disorders. Clin Endocrinol Metab 1984; *13*:333–349.
13. Gabow PA, Kaehny WD, Fennessey PV, et al. Diagnostic importance of an increased serum anion gap. N Engl J Med 1980; *303*:854–858.
14. Paulson WD. Anion gap-bicarbonate relationship in diabetic ketoacidosis. Am J Med 1986; *81*:995–1000.

URINE ANION GAP

15. Battle DC, Hizon M, Cohen E, et al. The use of the urinary anion gap in the diagnosis of hyperchloremic metabolic acidosis. N Engl J Med 1988; *318*:594–599.

ARTERIAL VERSUS VENOUS BLOOD

16. Griffith KK, McKenzie MB, Peterson WE, Keyes JL. Mixed venous blood-gas composition in experimentally induced acid-base disturbances. Heart Lung 1983; *12*:581–586.

c h a p t e r

LACTIC ACID, KETOACIDS, AND ALKALI THERAPY

The accumulation of organic acids is a marker for a metabolic abnormality and is not a primary illness. The important dictum here is not to focus on the acid because the problem is the underlying metabolic abnormality. This will help to place bicarbonate therapy in the proper perspective when it surfaces later in the chapter.

LACTIC ACIDOSIS

Lactic acid is an end-product of glucose metabolism and is produced at an average rate of 1 mEq/kg/hr.[1,2] Normal serum lactate levels are 2 mEq/L or less but severe exercise can raise the serum lactate to 4 mEq/L.[2] Most of the lactate is cleared by the liver and used either for gluconeogenesis or for energy production. The liver has a large capacity for clearing lactate and can clear 10 times the normal rate of lactate production. Disorders associated with lactic acidosis are listed in Table 32–1. I have classified them as being common, overemphasized, or overlooked. This list is far from complete, but it includes the clinical disorders that you should be aware of in the ICU. For a more complete list, see reference 2.

CLINICAL SHOCK

The predominant cause of lactic acidosis is clinical shock, which is defined in Chapter 12 as a state of inadequate tissue oxygenation. Of the three major shock syndromes, cardiogenic shock and septic shock are the predominant causes of lactic acidosis. Sepsis can produce lactic

427

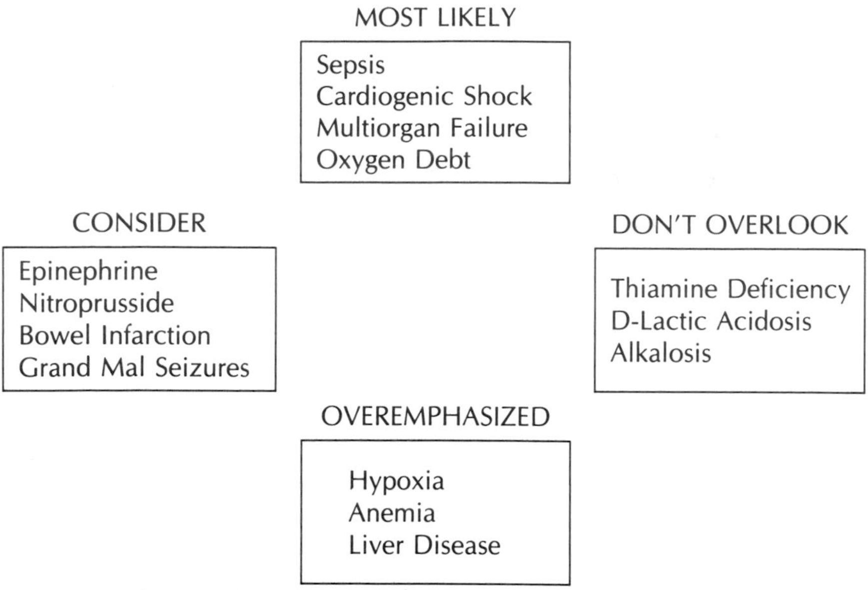

MOST LIKELY

Sepsis
Cardiogenic Shock
Multiorgan Failure
Oxygen Debt

CONSIDER

Epinephrine
Nitroprusside
Bowel Infarction
Grand Mal Seizures

DON'T OVERLOOK

Thiamine Deficiency
D-Lactic Acidosis
Alkalosis

OVEREMPHASIZED

Hypoxia
Anemia
Liver Disease

FIG. 32–1. Causes of lactic acidosis in the ICU.

acidosis in the absence of hypotension or other outward clinical signs of shock, but this condition still represents shock at the tissue level. The rise in serum lactate in clinical shock is the result of a combination of increased lactate production and decreased lactate clearance by the liver. The reduced clearance is a result of diminished blood flow to the liver as a part of the global hypoperfusion. The appearance of lactate in any clinical shock syndrome carries a poor prognosis,[3] regardless of the etiology of the shock.

DOES ANEMIC SHOCK EXIST?

Hypoxemia, anemia, and liver disease are routinely listed as causes of lactic acidosis,[2] yet there is little or no experimental evidence to confirm the association. Patients with respiratory insufficiency have been shown to tolerate an arterial PO_2 as low as 22 mmHg without developing lactic acidosis.[4] More severe hypoxemia is almost never encountered in clinical practice, therefore, it is unlikely that hypoxemic respiratory failure causes lactic acidosis. When lactate appears in a patient with respiratory insufficiency, the problem is usually a low cardiac output,[4] although respiratory alkalosis can contribute (see later in this chapter).

Severe anemia is listed as a cause of lactic acidosis,[2] yet there is no evidence for an illness called "anemic shock." Most of the information in this area has come from experience with Jehovah's Witnesses (who will not accept blood products for religious reasons) where postoperative hemoglobin levels as low as 3.0 mg/dl have been tolerated without the appearance of lactic acidosis.[5] The important factor in the ability to tol-

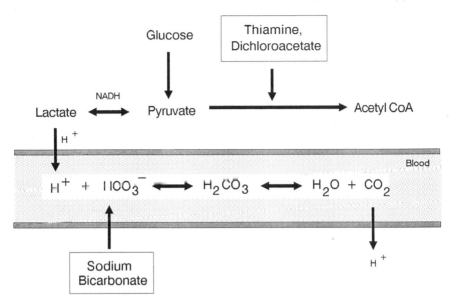

FIG. 32–2. The mechanisms behind the treatment of lactic acidosis with bicarbonate, thiamine, and dichloroacetate. See text for explanation.

erate anemia is the ability to increase cardiac output to maintain oxygen delivery in the face of a reduced hemoglobin. The less the cardiac response to anemia, the more the likelihood for lactate production in anemia.

Liver disease is listed as a cause of lactic acidosis primarily because of the role played by the liver in clearing venous lactate. However, patients with severe liver disease alone will not develop lactic acidosis unless there is hypotension or some other sign of clinical shock.[6] A defect in hepatic clearance is likely to play a role in the lactic acidosis that appears in clinical shock syndromes, but the mechanism is reduced hepatic blood flow rather than hepatocellular disease.

THIAMINE DEFICIENCY

Thiamine deficiency can cause lactic acidosis by reducing the mitochondrial oxidation of pyruvate.[7] Thiamine is a cofactor for the conversion of pyruvate to acetyl coenzyme A, as indicated in Figure 32–2. Thiamine deficiency will block this conversion and divert pyruvate to the production of lactate. The hallmark of lactic acidosis in thiamine deficiency is its appearance in the absence of severe cardiovascular derangements and its response to thiamine injection.[7] Thiamine deficiency may be common in critically ill patients,[4] therefore, it must be considered in every case of lactic acidosis that appears in patients who are hemodynamically stable or when the serum lactate levels are out of proportion to the degree of cardiovascular compromise.

LACTIC ALKALOSIS

Increased serum lactate levels have been associated with severe metabolic and respiratory alkalosis.[4,8] The proposed mechanism is an increase in lactate production caused by enhanced activity of pH-dependent enzymes in the glycolytic pathway. The liver is usually able to handle any increase in lactate production caused by alkalosis, so that severe alkalosis (serum pH over 7.6) is usually necessary to produce a significant rise in serum lactate levels.[8] However, when hepatic clearance is reduced in low-flow states, alkalosis-associated lactate production may become important during alkali therapy. This is discussed again in the section on alkali therapy.

D-LACTIC ACIDOSIS

The lactic acid produced by mammalian tissues is the levo-isomer (bends light to the left), while the dextro-isomer (bends light to the right) is produced by bacterial fermentation of glucose in the colon. Several species of bacteria are capable of producing d-lactic acid, including *Bacteroides fragilis* and the aerobic gram-negative enteric pathogens like *Escherichia coli*.[9] D-lactic acidosis has been reported mostly in patients with extensive small bowel resection and jejunoilial bypass for morbid obesity.[10,11] However, several of the common bowel inhabitants can produce d-lactic acid,[9] so it is possible that this illness is more common than suspected.

D-lactic acidosis should be suspected in any patient with a poorly explained metabolic acidosis and a high anion gap. The presence of diarrhea or a history of bowel surgery should heighten the suspicion. The standard assays for serum lactate will measure only the levo form of lactate and you will have to request a special assay for d-lactate. This assay should be available in most large clinical laboratories.

DRUGS AND LACTIC ACID

The drugs most likely to cause lactic acidosis in the ICU are epinephrine and nitroprusside.

Epinephrine stimulates glycogen breakdown in skeletal muscle and increases the rate of lactate production. Vasoconstriction in small arterioles from epinephrine may also play a role. There is little use for epinephrine as a cardiovascular drug unless the problem is anaphylaxis or electromechanical dissociation.

Nitroprusside releases cyanide when it is metabolized and the cyanide can uncouple oxidative phosphorylation. As mentioned in Chapter 20, lactic acidosis is a late finding in cyanide toxicity and significant increases in cyanide can occur with no increase in serum lactate levels.

DIAGNOSIS

Lactic acidosis should be suspected as the cause of any metabolic acidosis associated with an elevated anion gap.

The Anion Gap. The anion gap is virtually never normal in lactic acidosis but the degree of elevation can vary. In the absence of factors that can falsely lower the anion gap, an organic acidosis is almost always present when the anion gap is greater than 30 mEq/L, even in the presence of renal insufficiency.[12] Therefore, in the absence of ketoacidosis or toxin ingestion, an anion gap above 30 mEq/L indicates probable lactic acidosis. An anion gap from 20 to 30 may not represent lactic acidosis or ketoacidosis.

The Blood Sample. Venous blood reflects lactate production and arterial blood reflects the net effect of production and hepatic clearance. I prefer to use a sample obtained from the superior vena cava or the pulmonary artery because the correlation between the lactate from these sites and arterial lactate is excellent in some reports.[13] The blood sample should be immediately placed on ice to limit lactate production by red cells in the sample. Remember that the standard assay for lactate measures l-lactate only and you must specifically request a d-lactate assay.

THERAPY FOR LACTIC ACIDOSIS

The primary goal of therapy is to correct the underlying problem and this usually involves some type of hemodynamic manipulation to improve oxygen delivery to the tissues. The hemodynamic management of clinical shock syndromes has been covered in Chapters 12–15 and will not be repeated here. The following are some specific aspects of therapy that have not been mentioned. This therapy is aimed at the acid load and its adverse effects.

BICARBONATE THERAPY

Sodium bicarbonate therapy for lactic acidosis has received much attention in the past few years because of its questionable efficacy and its potential for adverse effects. The controversy centers on a few questions and each is addressed briefly.

Is Acidemia Harmful? Systemic acidosis will decrease myocardial contractility but cardiac output usually increases because acidosis also stimulates catecholamine release and reduces systemic vascular resistance.[14,15] Patients with cardiac disease may respond differently to an acid load but this has not been studied.

One of the best arguments for the lack of adverse effects from acidemia is the evidence that patients with diabetic ketoacidosis can tolerate a serum pH below 7.0 without suffering a life-threatening cardiovascular collapse (see later in this chapter).

Is Bicarbonate Harmful? Bicarbonate therapy can produce a number of undesirable effects including hyperosmolarity, hypotension, a reduced cardiac output, and an increase in serum lactate levels.[15,16] The hypotension and reduced cardiac output may be the result of calcium binding by the bicarbonate.[15] The increase in serum lactate levels may be caused by enhanced production of lactate by red blood cells, which is known to occur under alkalotic conditions.[18]

Is Bicarbonate Effective? Bicarbonate therapy is often ineffective in reducing the serum pH despite massive infusion of alkali in some cases. This is because of the ability of bicarbonate to produce CO_2, as shown in Figure 32–2. The CO_2 is usually eliminated by the lungs but it may also diffuse into cells and combine with water to produce hydrogen ions. This aggravates the underlying acidosis and favors the formation of additional lactate. This is considered one of the major drawbacks of bicarbonate therapy and has led to the development of alkaline solutions that do not increase CO_2 production.

Recommendations. The standard recommendation for alkali therapy in lactic acidosis has been to keep the arterial pH above 7.2. This is not to be applied strictly, however, because patients with diabetic ketoacidosis often tolerate a pH below 7.2 without serious consequences (see later).

One indication for alkali therapy is hypotension refractory to volume and catecholamine infusion. The response to bicarbonate infusion will help to predict the need for further alkali therapy. The normal response to an intravenous bolus of bicarbonate is a decrease in blood pressure, possibly because of the binding of calcium by the administered bicarbonate. Therefore, if the blood pressure increases after a bolus injection of bicarbonate, with no response to an equivalent volume of normal saline, this can be taken as evidence that the acid should be treated.

The amount of bicarbonate (HCO_3) needed to correct the pH can be estimated as follows:

$$HCO_3 \text{ deficit} = 0.5 \times \text{wt (kg)} \times (\text{desired } HCO_3 - \text{serum } HCO_3)$$

The serum HCO_3 that will keep the pH above 7.20 will depend on the arterial P_{CO_2}. In the absence of a superimposed respiratory acidosis or alkalosis, a serum HCO_3 of 15 mEq/L should be sufficient. Respiratory acidosis should always be corrected before considering bicarbonate therapy because bicarbonate infusion will increase CO_2 production.

The usual recommendation is to give one-half of the HCO_3 deficit as an intravenous bolus and to replace the remaining deficit over the next 4 to 6 hours. This will underestimate bicarbonate requirements when acid production continues, so periodic determinations of the HCO_3 deficit are necessary.

ALTERNATIVES

The disadvantages of bicarbonate therapy have created some interest in the following alternative therapies.

TABLE 32–1. ALKALI SOLUTIONS		
	Carbicarb	NAHCO$_3$
Na$^+$	1000	1000 (mmol/L)
HCO$_3$	333	1000
CO$_3^{2-}$	333	0
P$_{CO_2}$	3	over 200 (mmHg)
pH 25°C	9.6	8.0
Osmolality	1667	2000 (mOsm/kg)

From Sun JH, Filley GF, Hord K, Kindig NB, Bartle EJ, Carbicarb: An effective substitute for NAHCO$_3$ for the treatment of acidosis. Surgery 1987; 102:835–839.

Carbicarb. Carbicarb is a buffer solution with less bicarbonate than sodium bicarbonate, as shown in Table 32–1. The substitution of carbonate for bicarbonate reduces the tendency to produce CO$_2$. As a result, Carbicarb has proven superior to bicarbonate for increasing the serum pH while not increasing serum lactate levels.[18] The clinical experience with Carbicarb is limited at present but the preliminary results are encouraging.

Dichloroacetate. Sodium dichloroacetate (DCA) can reduce the formation of lactate by stimulating pyruvate dehydrogenase and diverting pyruvate toward mitochondrial oxidation (Fig. 32–2). The result will be a decrease in serum lactate levels, which has been confirmed in clinical trials.[19] There is also a positive inotropic effect from DCA that will help to counteract the myocardial depression from acidosis. The concept behind DCA is appealing, however, there has been no improvement in clinical outcome with DCA.[19]

KETOACIDOSIS

Ketoacids are the products of fatty acid metabolism in the liver and are used as energy sources when oral intake is low. Each gram of ketoacid yields 4 kcal compared to 3.4 kcal/gm for carbohydrate. The major ketoacids are acetoacetate (AcAc) and beta-hydroxybutyrate (BOHB), both existing in equilibrium with the other. The balance favors the formation of beta-hydroxybutyrate from acetoacetate and this is exaggerated in a reduced redox state.

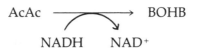

THE ANION GAP

Unlike the high anion gap in lactic acidosis (often over 30 mEq/L), the anion gap in ketoacidosis may only be mildly elevated (15 to 20 mEq/L) and can even be normal.[22,23] The anion gap is much lower in patients with normal renal function because the ketoacids are excreted in the urine and chloride is reabsorbed for electrical neutrality.[23] At present, the character of the acid-base abnormality at the outset has little predictive value.

THE NITROPRUSSIDE TEST

The nitroprusside test is a colorimetric method for detecting ketoacids in blood and urine. The test is available using tablets (Acetest) or strips (Ketostix) and measures only the serum **acetoacetate** and acetone levels.[20] The test is positive when acetoacetate levels rise above 3 mEq/L, as illustrated in Figure 32–3. The problem with the nitroprusside test is the distribution of the ketoacids because the unmeasurable beta-hydroxybutyrate predominates in all types of ketoacidosis. The ratio of ketoacids in diabetic and alcoholic ketoacidosis is shown in Figure 32–3. As illustrated, the levels of acetoacetate are barely above threshold for detection using the Acetest tablets. This indicates that the severity of the standard tests for ketoacids will not correlate with the severity of the acid-base problem in ketoacidosis.

DIABETIC KETOACIDOSIS

Diabetic ketoacidosis represents an exaggerated form of the normal response to starvation. The precipitating event is often inappropriate insulin dosing although concurrent illness can be responsible in 60% of cases.[21] The mortality can exceed 50% in select patient groups such as the elderly.

DIAGNOSIS

The typical clinical presentation is difficult to miss with the presence of hyperglycemia, a high anion gap metabolic acidosis, and ketones in urine and blood.[21] However, the diagnosis is not always this straightforward.

Diabetic ketoacidosis can present with a serum glucose below 350 mg/dl,[22] a normal anion gap,[23] or an alkaline serum pH.[24]

The most common of the "atypical" presentations is the normal or mildly elevated anion gap. This illness has always been described as a high anion gap acidosis but it is common to have an anion gap below 20 mEq/L on presentation. This is because of a hyperchloremic metabolic acidosis produced by enhanced chloride reabsorption in the renal tubules to

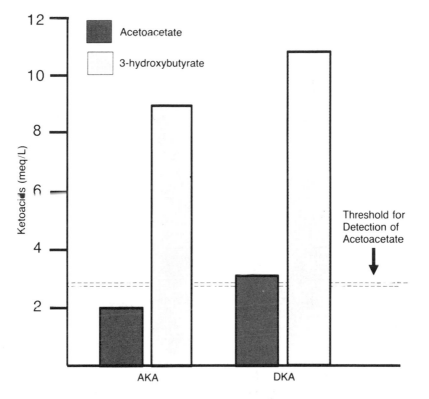

FIG. 32–3. The serum level of ketoacids in alcoholic and diabetic ketoacidosis. Height of bars indicates means. AKA: alcoholic ketoacidosis, DKA: diabetic ketoacidosis.

counteract the renal excretion of ketoacids.[25] The anion gap is highest in patients who are dehydrated because the ketoacids are not readily excreted.

TREATMENT

The standard recommendations for the therapy of DKA are presented in Table 32–2. A few points deserve mention.

1. Volume losses average 10 to 15% of the body weight,[21] and normal saline has been the standard fluid for the initial resuscitation. However, the risk of cerebral edema and pulmonary edema is significant and has dampened the enthusiasm for crystalloid fluids.[21] Colloid fluids such as 5% albumin may prove to be superior because of their greater tendency to remain in the vascular space (see Chapter 17). It may not be wise to use hydroxyethyl starch in this setting because of the increase in serum amylase that is associated with hydroxyethyl starch (see Chapter 17).

2. Potassium depletion is almost universal and averages 3 to 5 mEq/kg. However, the serum K^+ can be normal or high at presentation.

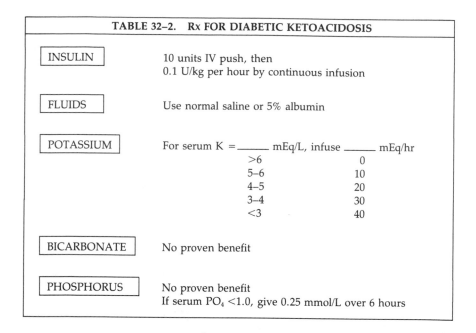

TABLE 32–2. Rx FOR DIABETIC KETOACIDOSIS	
INSULIN	10 units IV push, then 0.1 U/kg per hour by continuous infusion
FLUIDS	Use normal saline or 5% albumin
POTASSIUM	For serum K =_____ mEq/L, infuse _____ mEq/hr

<table>
<tr><td></td><td>>6</td><td>0</td></tr>
<tr><td></td><td>5–6</td><td>10</td></tr>
<tr><td></td><td>4–5</td><td>20</td></tr>
<tr><td></td><td>3–4</td><td>30</td></tr>
<tr><td></td><td><3</td><td>40</td></tr>
</table>

BICARBONATE	No proven benefit
PHOSPHORUS	No proven benefit If serum PO_4 <1.0, give 0.25 mmol/L over 6 hours

Potassium should be replaced as soon as possible and the recommended schedules are shown in Table 32–2.

3. Phosphorus depletion is also common and averages 1 to 1.5 mmol/kg. However, phosphorus supplementation has not improved outcome in DKA and it is not recommended as a routine practice. Therapy is reserved for patients with severe hypophosphatemia (below 1 mEq/dL) because of the risk for adverse effects at this level. See Chapter 38 for more on hypophosphatemia.

4. Bicarbonate infusion is no longer recommended as a routine practice. Not only does bicarbonate not improve outcome,[26] it stimulates the formation of ketoacids. The only situation where you might consider bicarbonate is the patient with refractory hypotension.

The End-Point of Therapy. The end-point of therapy is neither the serum glucose nor the serum bicarbonate. The glucose should decline within 6 hours,[21] while the acidemia can take twice as long to correct. When the serum glucose reaches 250 mg/dl, dextrose is added to the intravenous fluids and the insulin infusion is continued until the serum bicarbonate increases to 15 mmHg. The value of the serum HCO_3 as an endpoint is explained below.

The most appropriate end-point is the pattern of acidosis. Volume therapy will produce hyperchloremia by increasing the renal clearance of ketoacids (which increases chloride reabsorption) and simply by infusion of chloride in the solutions. This hyperchloremia will decrease the anion gap but will maintain the metabolic acidosis. Therefore, it is important not to follow the serum bicarbonate or pH alone during therapy because these may not change immediately, despite the fact that the ketoacidosis is resolving. The ratio of anion gap excess to bicarbonate deficit (discussed in Chapter 30) should be monitored during therapy. This ratio approaches 1.0 with a pure organic acidosis and will be zero in a pure hyperchloremic metabolic acidosis. Therefore, this ratio will decrease during therapy of DKA as the hyperchloremic metabolic acidosis develops.

ALCOHOLIC KETOACIDOSIS

Alcoholic ketoacidosis is probably the result of several factors.[27] Food intake is usually poor, resulting in starvation ketosis. In addition, the oxidation of ethanol to acetaldehyde in the liver generates NADH, which also promotes the formation of ketoacids. Finally, dehydration will result in decreased renal clearance of ketoacids.

DIAGNOSIS

In contrast to ethanol-induced lactic acidosis (which occurs during a period of heavy consumption), alcoholic ketoacidosis (AKA) usually develops 1 to 3 days after a period of heavy consumption. The acidosis can be severe and serum ethanol levels may be negligible. Like DKA, the anion gap can vary.

The NADH generated by the oxidation of ethanol in the liver promotes the conversion of acetoacetate to hydroxybutyrate. Because the nitroprusside assay for serum ketones (Acetest) detects only acetoacetate, **serum ketone levels in AKA may be negligible** (see Fig. 32–3). The clinical setting is, therefore, important in the diagnosis of AKA. Although mild hyperglycemia can occur in AKA, the absence of significant hyperglycemia (over 300 mg/dL) will differentiate AKA from DKA.

TREATMENT

AKA usually resolves within 24 hours when saline and glucose are infused (5% Dextrose in 0.9% sodium chloride). The glucose infusion will decrease ketoacid formation in the liver and the saline infusion will promote the renal clearance of ketoacids. Potassium replacement is necessary only when the serum potassium is low. Bicarbonate therapy should not be necessary.

REFERENCES

LACTIC ACIDOSIS

1. Kruse JA, Carlson RW. Lactate metabolism. Crit Care Clin 1987; 3:725–746.
2. Mizock BA. Lactic acidosis. Disease-A-Month 1989; 35:237–300.
3. Weil MH, Afifi AA. Experimental and clinical studies on lactate and pyruvate as

indicators of the severity of acute circulatory failure (shock). Circulation 1970; *16*:989–1001.

4. Eldridge F. Blood lactate and pyruvate in pulmonary insufficiency. N Engl J Med 1966; *274*:878–882.
5. Ott DD, Cooley DA. Cardiovascular surgery in Jehovah's Witnesses. Report of 542 operations without blood transfusions. JAMA 1977; *238*:1256–1263.
6. Kruse JA, Zaidi SAJ, Carlson RW. Significance of blood lactate levels in critically ill patients with liver disease. Am J Med 1987; *83*:77–82.
7. Campbell CH. The severe lactic acidosis of thiamine deficiency: Acute pernicious or fulminating beriberi. Lancet 1984; *1*:446–449.
8. Bersin RM, Arieff AI. Primary lactic alkalosis. Am J Med 1988; *85*:867–871.

D-LACTIC ACIDOSIS

9. Smith SM, Eng RHK, Buccini F. Use of D-lactic acid measurements in the diagnosis of bacterial infections. J Infect Dis 1986; *154*:658–664.
10. Stolberg L, Rolfe R, Giflin N, et al. D-lactic-acidosis due to abnormal gut flora. N Engl J Med 1982; *306*:1344–1348.
11. Dahlquist NR, Perrault J, Callaway CW, Jones JD. D-lactic acidosis and encephalopathy after jejunoileostomy: Response to overfeeding and to fasting in humans. Mayo Clin Proc 1984; *59*:141–145.

DIAGNOSIS

12. Gabow PA, Kaehny WD, Fennessey PV, et al. Diagnostic importance of an increased serum anion gap. N Engl J Med 1980; *303*:854–858.
13. Weil MH, Michaels S, Rackow EC. Comparison of blood lactate concentrations in central venous, pulmonary artery and arterial blood. Crit Care Med 1987; *15*:489–490.

ALKALI THERAPY

14. Mehta PM, Kloner RA. Effects of acid-base disturbance, septic shock, and calcium and phosphorous abnormalities on cardiovascular function. Crit Care Clin 1987; *3*:747–758.
15. Graf H, Arieff AI. The use of sodium bicarbonate in the therapy of organic acidosis. Intensive Care Med 1986; *12*:286–288.
16. Stacpoole PW. Lactic Acidosis. The case against bicarbonate therapy. Ann Intern Med 1986; *105*:276–279.
17. Narins RG, Cohen JJ. Bicarbonate therapy for organic acidosis: The case for its continued use. Ann Intern Med 1987; *106*:615–618.
18. Sun JH, Filley GF, Hord K, Kindig NB, Bartle EJ. Carbicarb: An effective substitute for $NAHCO_3$ for the treatment of acidosis. Surgery 1987; *102*:835–839.

DICHLOROACETATE

19. Stacpoole PW, Lorenz AC, Thomas RG, Harman EM. Dichloroacetate in the treatment of lactic acidosis. Ann Intern Med 1988; *108*:58–63.

KETOACIDOSIS

20. Owen OE, Caprio S, Reichard G, et al. Ketosis of starvation: A revisit and new perspectives. Clin Endocrin Metab 1983; *12*:359–379.
21. Kriesberg RA. Diabetic ketoacidosis: An update. Crit Care Clin 1987: *3*:817–834.
22. Brandt KR, Miles JM. Relationship between severity of hyperglycemia and metabolic acidosis in diabetic ketoacidosis. Mayo Clin Proc 1988; *63*:1071–1074.
23. Gamblin GT, Ashburn RW, Kemp DG, Beuttel SC. Diabetic ketoacidosis presenting with a normal anion gap. Am J Med 1986; *80*:758–760.
24. Zonszein J, Baylor P. Diabetic ketoacidosis with alkalemia: A review. West J Med 1988; *149*:217–219.
25. Androgue HJ, Wilson H, Boyd AE, et al. Plasma acid-base patterns in diabetic ketoacidosis. N Engl J Med 1982; *307*:1603–1610.
26. Morris LR, Murphy MB, Kitabchi AE. Bicarbonate therapy in severe diabetic ketoacidosis. Ann Intern Med 1986; *105*:836–840.
27. Kriesberg RA. Acid-base and electrolyte disturbances in the alcoholic. In: Problems in Critical Care: The Substance Abuser. Dellinger RP (ed), Philadelphia, J.B. Lippincott, Vol. 1, pp. 66–77, 1987.
28. Kriesberg RA. Acid-base and electrolyte disturbances in the alcoholic. In: Dellinger RP ed. The substance abuser. Philadelphia: J.B. Lippincott, 1987; 66–77.

33

METABOLIC ALKALOSIS

Metabolic alkalosis is the most common acid-base disorder in hospitalized patients,[1,2] probably because of the widespread and often indiscriminant use of diuretics. Although this condition is considered a nuisance illness, the associated mortality is 40% when the serum pH rises above 7.55.[3]

The signal for a metabolic alkalosis is not a pH above 7.44 but a serum bicarbonate that is higher than expected for the arterial P_{CO_2} (see Chapter 31). The problem with metabolic alkalosis is not the initial event that created the alkalosis but the ability of the alkalosis to sustain itself despite correction of the inciting process. This is attributed to chloride depletion, which limits bicarbonate excretion in the urine by promoting reabsorption and reducing secretion into the renal tubules.

COMMON ETIOLOGIES

The common sources of metabolic alkalosis are loss of gastric acid and renal retention of bicarbonate. The latter phenomenon is often due to chloride depletion.

GASTRIC ACID LOSS

The hydrogen ion concentration in gastric juice averages 50 to 100 mEq/L so large volumes of gastric secretions must be lost to produce significant hydrogen ion loss. Continuous nasogastric suction produces alkalosis through several mechanisms including loss of sodium, potassium, chloride, and hydrogen ion as well as volume depletion. The alkalosis can often be corrected by replacing sodium and chloride losses without replenishing hydrogen ion losses. However, severe losses of hydrogen ion will require specific replacement therapy. The hydrogen ion loss can be estimated by subtracting the chloride concentration in the gastric juice from the sum of sodium and potassium concentrations.

DIURETICS

Diuretics promote alkalosis through electrolyte losses and volume contraction. The following electrolytes are involved:

1. **Chloride** excretion increases with diuresis because the chloride follows the sodium that is lost in the urine. The chloride that is not reabsorbed is replaced by bicarbonate, to maintain electrical neutrality. The enhanced bicarbonate reabsorption maintains the alkalosis.

2. **Potassium** is lost in the urine because more sodium is delivered to the distal tubule where the sodium-potassium exchange pump is located. Potassium depletion promotes an alkalosis by allowing more hydrogen ion to be secreted in the distal tubule.[3] However, the actual mechanism involved is not clear.

3. **Magnesium** is also lost in the urine during diuresis. This promotes potassium loss through unclear mechanisms. Magnesium depletion is underappreciated during diuresis, and must be corrected before potassium deficits can be corrected. See Chapter 37 for more details on magnesium.

These electrolyte deficits will maintain the metabolic alkalosis once it is established, because they do not allow the kidneys to excrete bicarbonate.

VOLUME CONTRACTION

A decrease in extracellular volume can promote a metabolic alkalosis in two ways. First, the free water loss will concentrate the bicarbonate and increase serum bicarbonate concentration. Second, the decrease in circulating blood volume will stimulate aldosterone release and promote loss of potassium and hydrogen ions in the distal tubule. The value of hypovolemia as a factor in alkalosis is not proven, because electrolyte losses are also present in this situation. In fact, a decrease in renal blood flow should cause an acidosis, not an alkalosis.

ALKALI ADMINISTRATION

Alkali infusion will not cause a metabolic alkalosis normally, because the infused alkali is rapidly excreted in the urine. However, when there are electrolyte abnormalities that interfere with renal bicarbonate excretion (e.g., chloride depletion), alkali administration can produce a sustained metabolic alkalosis. The common sources of exogenous alkali are lactate (Ringer's lactate), acetate (parenteral nutrition), and citrate (whole

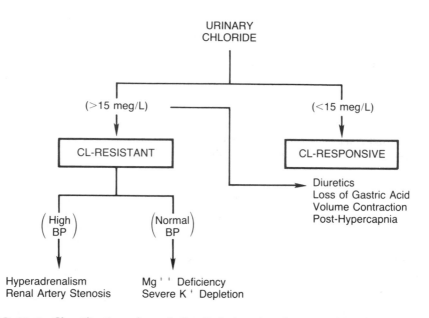

FIG. 33–1. Classification of metabolic alkalosis using the urine chloride concentration (random urine sample).

blood). Of these, massive blood transfusion is the only one reported to cause a significant metabolic alkalosis.[4]

CLASSIFICATION

Metabolic alkalosis can be classified as chloride-responsive or chloride-resistant according to the urinary chloride. This is shown in Figure 33–1, along with a list of the disorders in each category. A chloride concentration of 10–15 mEq/L in a random (spot) urine sample is used to separate the two types; i.e., a concentration less than 10–15 mEq/L identifies a chloride-responsive alkalosis, while a higher concentration identifies a chloride-resistant alkalosis. The exception to this rule is diuretic therapy, which will cause a chloride-sensitive alkalosis that is associated with a high urine chloride (indicated by the arrow in Figure 33–1).

CHLORIDE-RESPONSIVE ALKALOSIS

Cl-responsive alkalosis is characterized by chloride depletion and volume depletion. This is the most common type of alkalosis encountered in the ICU, and usually results from gastrointestinal loss of hydrochloric acid (e.g., vomiting or nasogastric suction) and aggressive diuretic therapy. The loop diuretics (e.g., furosemide) and the thiazides cause alkalosis by several mechanisms, including chloride and potassium loss in the urine, and volume contraction.

CHLORIDE-RESISTANT ALKALOSIS

Chloride-resistant alkalosis is characterized by volume expansion and potassium depletion and is caused by mineralocorticoid excess. The clinical disorders responsible for this form of alkalosis are rarely encountered in the ICU, with the possible exception of aggressive steroid therapy, and magnesium depletion.

COMPLICATIONS

There are several potential adverse effects of metabolic alkalosis but the significance of these is not clear. Moderate degrees of alkalosis seem to be well tolerated. Severe alkalosis (serum HCO_3 over 50 mEq/L) and alkalemia (serum pH over 7.6) rarely occur but could cause seizures and cardiac arrhythmias. Respiratory alkalosis seems to have a greater potential for adverse effects than metabolic alkalosis, probably because of the greater propensity for respiratory alkalosis to influence intracellular pH.

The most frequently quoted complications of metabolic alkalosis are hypoventilation, generalized seizures, and cardiac arrhythmias. The latter two have been explained by the decrease in ionized calcium caused by alkalosis, but this is being questioned.[1] In fact, few of the stated complications of alkalosis seem to be a problem in the ICU. The effects of alkalosis on ventilation and peripheral oxygen balance deserve mention.

DOES METABOLIC ALKALOSIS CAUSE HYPOVENTILATION?

There is no doubt that a metabolic acidosis will stimulate ventilation, but the opposite cannot be said of a metabolic alkalosis. The ventilatory response to metabolic alkalosis is variable and can be absent. An example of this is patients who receive diuretics because most of these patients have a metabolic alkalosis yet few of them show any CO_2 retention. There are several formulas that predict the PCO_2 expected in the face of a metabolic alkalosis, and the one that is popular at present is:[5]

$$\text{Expected } PCO_2 = 0.7 \times HCO_3 + 20 \, (\pm 1.5)$$

The PCO_2 at different levels of metabolic alkalosis is shown in Table 33–1, using this equation to determine the expected PCO_2. As is evident, the serum HCO_3 must increase substantially before significant CO_2 retention

TABLE 33–1. THE ESTIMATED EFFECT OF METABOLIC ALKALOSIS ON THE ARTERIAL P_{CO_2}*	
Serum HCO₃	**Arterial P_{CO_2} (Range)**
30 mEq/L	42 mmHg (40.5–43.5)
35	46 (44.5–47.5)
40	49 (47.5–50.5)
45	52.5 (51.0–54.0)
50	56 (54.5–57.5)

*Expected P_{CO_2} = 0.7 × [HCO₃] + 20 (±1.5)
Equation from Javeheri S, Kazemi H. Metabolic alkalosis and hypoventilation in humans. Am Rev Respir Dis 1987; 136:1011–1016.

occurs. This illustrates the lack of ventilatory response to metabolic alkalosis.

The explanation for the lack of hypoventilation during a metabolic alkalosis may be related to the baseline activity of peripheral chemoreceptors, where metabolic acid-base disorders exert most of their effects on ventilation. That is, the peripheral chemoreceptors are not active under normal conditions so there is little input from these receptors to the brainstem respiratory centers. This means there is little activity for the alkalosis to inhibit, while acidosis can increase the firing in these receptors and produce hyperventilation. Whatever the case, the important thing to remember is that there is little risk of hypoventilation until profound alkalosis is present.

PERIPHERAL OXYGEN BALANCE

The adverse effects of alkalosis are easiest to organize using the principles of tissue oxygenation (see Chapter 2). The levels of tissue oxygen are determined by the balance between oxygen supply (rate of oxygen delivery) and oxygen demand (oxygen consumption). As shown in Figure 33–2, alkalosis will depress oxygen delivery by decreasing cardiac output and shifting the oxyhemoglobin dissociation curve to the left (Bohr effect). In addition, oxygen consumption can increase because of the ability of alkalosis to stimulate glycolysis.[6] Therefore, alkalosis will reduce oxygen supply while increasing oxygen demand and this might promote inadequate tissue oxygenation. The significance of these effects is not known at present but it is a reasonable way to view the potential complications of alkalosis.

MANAGEMENT STRATEGIES

Therapy is aimed at repleting electrolyte losses to allow the kidneys to excrete bicarbonate. The following options are available.

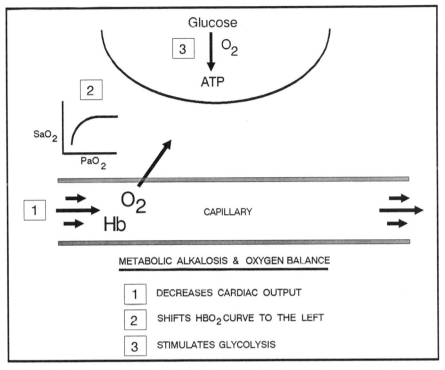

FIG. 33-2. Effects of metabolic alkalosis on the factors that determine tissue oxygen balance.

CHLORIDE REPLACEMENT

Most of the metabolic alkaloses in the ICU are chloride-responsive alkaloses, therefore, the mainstay of treatment for most alkaloses will be chloride replacement. The chloride can be replaced as a sodium salt (saline), a potassium salt (KCl), or as a chloride-containing acid (hydrochloric acid).

Sodium Chloride. Sodium chloride is indicated for patients with a low extracellular volume. The volume of 0.9% saline can be estimated by calculating the chloride deficit, as shown in Table 33-2. For example, if the serum Cl is 80 mEq/L in a 70 kg (154 lb) adult and the desired serum Cl is 100 mEq/L, the chloride deficit will be 378 mEq ($0.27 \times 70 \times 20$). Because 0.9% NaCl (normal saline) contains 154 mEq of chloride per L, this deficit would be corrected by infusion of 2.3 L of the saline solution.

TABLE 33-2. CORRECTING METABOLIC ALKALOSIS WITH SALINE
Cl Deficit (mEq) = 0.27 × WT (kg) × (100 − Present [Cl])
Volume of Saline (L) = Cl Deficit / 154*
*154 = Chloride (mEq) in 1 L of 0.9% saline

TABLE 33–3. CORRECTING METABOLIC ALKALOSIS WITH HCl INFUSION
H$^+$ Deficit (mEq) = 0.5 × WT (kg) × (Present HCO$_3$ − Desired [HCO$_3$])
Volume (L) of 0.1N HCl = H$^+$ Deficit / 100*
0.25N HCl = H$^+$ Deficit / 250*
Infusion Rate = 0.2 mEq/kg per hour
*The mEq of H$^+$ per L of solution

Potassium Chloride. Potassium replacement must be guided by several factors and this is presented in more detail in Chapter 36. Magnesium must be repleted before it will be possible to replete potassium (see Chapter 37). Potassium chloride replacement will not be sufficient by itself to correct chloride deficits because the amount of chloride that can be given is small. However, hypokalemia must be corrected because hypokalemia will sustain a metabolic alkalosis when the chloride deficits are replaced. Therefore, potassium chloride therapy is essential in the therapy of metabolic alkalosis.

Hydrochloric Acid. Infusion of hydrochloric acid is usually reserved for severe alkalemia (pH over 7.5), when saline and potassium replacement are ineffective. Various concentrations of HCl can be used but the 0.1 N HCl solution (100 mEq H$^+$ per L) is popular because it is close to the normal acid content of the stomach (50 to 150 mEq H$^+$ per L). The amount of HCl required to correct the alkalosis can be determined by estimating the hydrogen ion (H$^+$) deficit, as shown in Table 33–3 below.

With a pure metabolic alkalosis, a serum HCO$_3$ less than 35 mEq/L is a safe end-point.[1] If the serum [HCO$_3$] is 45 mEq/L in a 70 kg (154 lb) adult, the H$^+$ deficit is then 350 mEq (0.5 × 70 × 10). Using a standard 0.1 N HCl solution (100 mEq H$^+$ per L), infusion of 3.5 L should correct the problem (in the absence of ongoing losses). When volume is a concern, a more concentrated HCl solution (0.25 N HCl) can be used safely.[8] In the present example, 1.4 L of 0.25 N HCl (250 mEq H$^+$ per L) will correct the estimated H$^+$ deficit. The infusion rate can be adjusted for body size, as shown in the table, or an infusion rate of 100 to 125 ml/hr can be used for most patients.[8,9]

Infusion of HCl solutions has proven to be safe and effective in correcting severe metabolic alkalosis.[7–9] The major drawback is the need for central venous access because of the sclerosing properties of the solutions. These solutions have been given via peripheral vein in combination with fat emulsions,[9] but this needs to be studied further before any conclusions can be drawn.

Other chloride-containing acids such as ammonium chloride (NH$_4$Cl) and arginine hydrochloride (HCl) have been used to correct metabolic alkalosis. However, these solutions have drawbacks in selected patients. Arginine HCl can produce severe hyperkalemia in patients with renal insufficiency. Ammonium chloride is not recommended in patients with liver disease because it will increase circulating ammonia levels (which are believed by some to participate in the manifestations of hepatic encephalopathy).

DRUG THERAPY

Acetazolamide. Acetazolamide (250 to 500 mg) inhibits bicarbonate reabsorption in the proximal tubule and can be used to treat metabolic alkalosis when extracellular volume is high. The problem with this approach is that it does not correct the underlying problem (e.g., chloride depletion). Furthermore, acetazolamide can cause potassium depletion and volume depletion, both of which will negate the effects of the drug on the alkalosis. This approach is used for temporary control only, because the underlying problem must still be corrected.

Histamine H2-Blockers. In the presence of nasogastric suction that drains gastric acid, intravenous H2 blockers (e.g., ranitidine) can limit H^+ loss by limiting gastric acid secretion.[1] However, you must first check gastric pH to determine if the stomach is actively secreting acid. Try to avoid H2-blockers whenever possible because of their side effects. If forced to use an H2-blocker, monitor the gastric pH frequently and maintain the pH above 5.

CONTINUOUS HEMOFILTRATION

Continuous arteriovenous hemofiltration (CAVH) can be valuable for severe metabolic alkalosis associated with a high extracellular volume, particularly when diuresis with acetazolamide is ineffective. CAVH alone will not decrease serum HCO_3 but must be combined with infusion of chloride-containing solutions. When fluid overload is present, the fluids should be infused at a slower rate than the ultrafiltration removal rate.

CORRECTING CHLORIDE-RESISTANT ALKALOSIS

Because extracellular volume is high in chloride-resistant alkalosis, saline infusion will not correct the alkalosis. The alkalosis from mineralocorticoid excess is maintained by potassium depletion, therefore, potassium replacement or mineralocorticoid antagonists such as aldactone may be effective.

REFERENCES

REVIEWS

1. Rimmer JM, Gennari FJ. Metabolic alkalosis. J Intensive Care Med 1987; 2:137–150.
2. Riley LJ, Ilson BE, Narins RG. Acute Metabolic Acid-Base Disturbances. Crit Care Clin 1987; 3:699–724.
3. Galla JH, Luke RG. Pathophysiology of metabolic alkalosis. Hosp Pract 1987; (Oct): 95–118.

SELECTED TOPICS

4. Driscoll DF, Bistrian BR, Jenkins RL. Development of metabolic alkalosis after massive transfusion during orthotopic liver transplantation. Crit Care Med 1987; 15:905–908.
5. Javeheri S, Kazemi H. Metabolic alkalosis and hypoventilation in humans. Am Rev Respir Dis 1987; 136:1011–1016.
6. Rastegar HR, Woods M, Harken AH. Respiratory alkalosis increases tissue oxygen demand. J Surg Res 1979; 26:687–692.
7. Williams DB, Lyons JH. Treatment of severe metabolic alkalosis with intravenous infusion of hydrochloric acid. Surg Gynecol Obstet 1980; 150:315–321.
8. Brimioulle S, Vincent JL, Dufaye P, et al. Hydrochloric acid infusion for treatment of metabolic alkalosis: Effects on acid-base balance and oxygenation. Crit Care Med 1985; 13:738–742.
9. Duncan DA. Use of intravenous hydrochloric acid for the treatment of metabolic acidosis in renal or hepatic failure. Int Med Spec 1984; 5:56–63.

section X
FLUID AND ELECTROLYTE DISORDERS

A slight instability is the necessary condition for the true stability of the organism.
Charles Richet

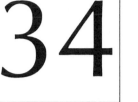

BEDSIDE STRATEGIES
FOR OLIGURIA

Oliguria (less than 400 ml/24h) can be an ominous sign because acute oliguric renal failure carries a mortality as high as 90%.[1] This chapter presents a simple approach to oliguria using invasive hemodynamic monitoring. Although not applicable to the general wards, the principles in the approach are the important message.

PRIMER

The sources of oliguria are traditionally separated into three categories, as shown in Figure 34 1. Each category is placed in series starting at the renal arteries, continuing through the renal parenchyma, and ending in the urinary collecting system.

PRERENAL CONDITIONS

The first class of disorders is characterized by a decrease in renal blood flow. This "prerenal" condition can be the result of a low cardiac output or an inadequate renal perfusion pressure. The common clinical disorders in this category are hypovolemia, vasodilatation, and acute heart failure.

RENAL DISORDERS

Two intrinsic renal disorders are responsible for most cases of acute oliguric renal failure (AORF); acute tubular necrosis, and acute interstitial

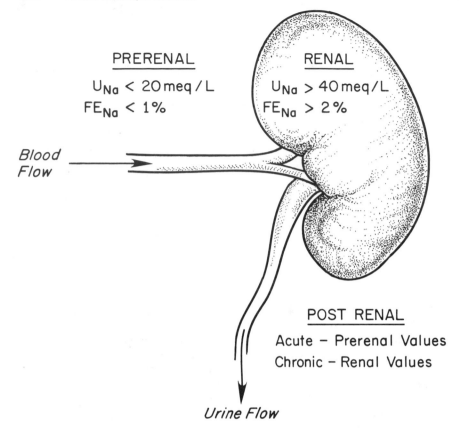

PRERENAL

$U_{Na} < 20\,meq/L$
$FE_{Na} < 1\%$

RENAL

$U_{Na} > 40\,meq/L$
$FE_{Na} > 2\%$

Blood
Flow

POST RENAL

Acute – Prerenal Values
Chronic – Renal Values

Urine Flow

FIG. 34–1. The classification system for the causes of oliguria. See text for explanation.

nephritis. Acute glomerulonephritis is not a common culprit in the adult ICU population.

Acute tubular necrosis (ATN) is a poorly understood disorder produced by a variety of insults including sepsis, toxins, drugs, and pigments (e.g., myoglobin). **Acute interstitial nephritis** (AIN) is an immunogenic disorder produced by at least 40 different drugs, most commonly the penicillins and nonsteroidal anti-inflammatory agents.[5] The clinical presentation often does not differentiate AIN from ATN. Although AIN classically presents with fever, rash, and arthralgias,[5] the rash may be fleeting and fever can be absent in 40% of cases.[5]

Unified View. Acute oliguric renal failure (AORF) in the ICU setting is usually a sign of another problem. That problem is usually a systemic illness like sepsis or multiorgan failure or a toxic manifestation of a drug, dye, or pigment. The association of AORF with multiorgan failure means the renal dysfunction is merely part of the larger syndrome. Therefore, when AORF appears, it should prompt a search for another process. The role of drugs is becoming more prominent and the aminoglycosides are primary offenders. Recent estimates are that **1 of every 4 courses of**

aminoglycoside therapy is complicated by acute renal failure.[3] If this is a valid estimate, aminoglycosides may be the most common cause of acute renal failure in the ICU.

POSTRENAL CONDITIONS

The final category includes obstructive processes in the renal outflow tracts. This "postrenal" category includes obstruction in the collecting system (papillary necrosis), the ureters (retroperitoneal tumours), and the bladder outlet (e.g., strictures and prostatism). Obstruction is an uncommon cause of oliguria, but must be considered in certain high-risk conditions (e.g., solitary kidney).

URINE EVALUATION

Urine indices identify two categories: prerenal and renal disorders.[7] The prerenal category also includes acute glomerulonephritis and acute postrenal obstruction, while the renal category also includes chronic postrenal obstruction (Fig. 34–1).

URINE SODIUM

When renal perfusion is diminished, there is an increase in sodium reabsorption and a decrease in urinary sodium excretion. Conversely, acute renal failure is associated with impaired sodium reabsorption and an increase in urinary sodium excretion. The sodium concentration in a random urine sample proves valuable for discriminating between prerenal and renal causes of oliguria.

> In the setting of oliguria, a urine sodium below 20 mEq/L usually indicates a prerenal condition. However, a urine sodium above 40 mEq/L might not indicate acute renal failure.[3]

A urine sodium above 40 mEq/L can occur in prerenal conditions when there is prior renal dysfunction, or it may indicate ongoing diuretic therapy. Elderly patients often have an obligatory sodium loss in the urine and they can have an inappropriately high urine sodium in the face of diminished renal blood flow. Therefore, a urine sodium in the range of 40 mEq/L should not be used in isolation to make the diagnosis of acute renal failure.[3]

FRACTIONAL EXCRETION OF SODIUM

The fractional excretion of sodium (FE_{Na}) represents the fraction of sodium filtered at the glomerulus that is excreted in the urine.[5] The FE_{Na}

is determined by comparing the urine sodium clearance to the urine creatinine clearance (U: urine concentration; P: plasma concentration):

$$FE_{Na} = \frac{(U/P)\ Na}{(U/P)\ Cr} \times 100$$

$$FE_{Na} < 1\% = \text{prerenal azotemia}$$

$$FE_{Na} > 2\% = \text{acute renal failure}$$

The FE_{Na} is considered one of the most reliable urinary tests for identifying renal failure. However, an FE_{Na} less than 1% has been reported in cases of AORF from myoglobinuria and contrast agents.[5] The problem here is, when the FE_{Na} is below 1, how is the diagnosis of ATN possible? In other words, if the FE_{Na} is below 1 in the face of oliguria, then the renal tubules are functioning and this is against the diagnosis of ATN. At present, the FE_{Na} remains the single best urine laboratory test for differentiating prerenal conditions from AORF.[5,6]

URINE MICROSCOPIC EXAM

The urine sediment should be examined in every case of suspected acute renal failure.

1. In prerenal conditions, the urine contains nonspecific elements such as hyaline casts or finely granular casts.

2. In ATN, the characteristic sediment contains an abundance of epithelial cells and epithelial cell casts along with coarsely granular casts.

3. In AIN, the sediment may contain white cells and white cell casts. Red cell casts are characteristic of acute glomerulonephritis, but are occasionally seen in other forms of acute renal failure.

URINE SEDIMENT VERSUS FE_{Na}

The urine microscopic exam is taken as the gold standard for the diagnosis of ATN if the sediment contains epithelial cell casts or other highly characteristic findings. However, the FE_{Na} is a measure of the reabsorptive function of the tubules, which seems to be the more important test. For example, if the urine sediment shows epithelial cell casts but the FE_{na} is below 1, the diagnosis is ATN (based on the sediment) but the tubules are functional because they can reabsorb sodium. The FE_{Na}, therefore, seems to be the test that provides the most information concerning the functional status of the kidneys.

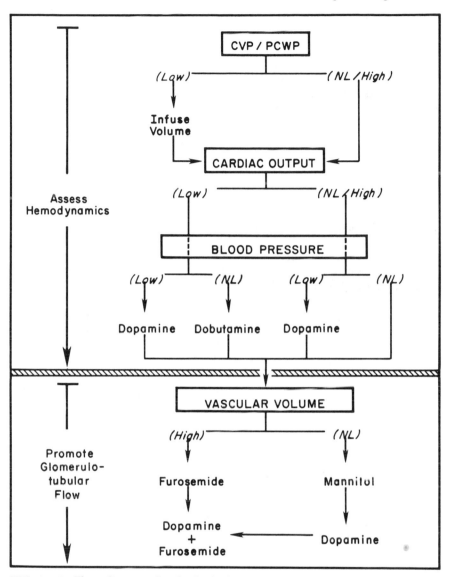

FIG. 34–2. Flow diagram for the bedside approach to oliguria.

STEPWISE APPROACH TO OLIGURIA

The first concern with acute onset of oliguria or anuria is to make sure that the bladder drainage catheters are functional. This is particularly important when the urine flow is less than 100 ml per 24 hours (anuria), because renal disorders do not usually cause anuria.

Oliguria can be approached systematically in three stages, as outlined in Figure 34–2. This approach requires invasive hemodynamic monitoring with pulmonary artery catheters.

STAGE 1: ASSESS HEMODYNAMIC STATUS

The initial goal is to optimize the hemodynamic forces that govern renal blood flow. This is done in the following two steps:

Ventricular Filling Pressures. The first step is to determine the adequacy of the ventricular filling pressures; the central venous pressure (CVP) or the pulmonary capillary wedge pressure (PCWP). A decrease of 4 mmHg or greater in either of these is taken as a significant change.[8] If these pressures have not been monitored previously, a CVP of 10 to 12 mmHg or a PCWP of 15 to 20 mmHg can be used, in most instances, as evidence for an adequate intravascular volume.

If the filling pressures are inadequate, infuse volume until the PCWP is 15 mmHg. If the oliguria persists, measure the cardiac output.

Cardiac Output. The cardiac output is measured only after the filling pressures have been optimized. If the cardiac output is low, immediate steps should be taken to determine the cause (e.g., acute MI or tamponade). Therapy is determined by the blood pressure. If the blood pressure is normal, inotropic therapy with dobutamine (10 to 20 mcg/kg/min) can be started. If the blood pressure is low, dopamine (5 to 15 mcg/kg/min) may be more appropriate.

If the cardiac output is normal or high and the patient is hypotensive (e.g., sepsis), immediate drug therapy will be geared to increasing vascular resistance without compromising renal blood flow. Dopamine (5 to 15 mcg/kg/min) may be preferred here because of its potential for stimulating dopaminergic receptors in the renal circulation and promoting renal perfusion. Potent vasoconstrictors, such as neosynephrine, should be avoided at all costs.

STAGE 2: OBTAIN URINE FOR DIAGNOSTIC TESTS

When oliguria persists after the hemodynamics are satisfactory, a blood and urine sample should be obtained to determine the FE_{Na} and a portion of the urine sample should be saved for microscopic analysis, if needed. A urine sample should always be obtained before giving diuretics to preserve the diagnostic value of a high urine sodium. While waiting for the laboratory tests to be performed, the following steps can be performed to help improve urine flow.

STAGE 3: IMPROVING GLOMERULOTUBULAR FLOW

The persistence of oliguria in the face of normal hemodynamics suggests acute renal failure. In this situation, low-dose dopamine (1 mcg/kg/min) is given to counteract the vasoconstriction that accompanies acute renal failure and intravenous furosemide is given to promote renal tubular flow and reduce back pressure (which reduces net filtration pressure across the glomerulus). Unfortunately, these maneuvers do not improve renal function even when they increase urine output. One observation seems consistent:

Patients who show an increase in urine flow with dopamine and furosemide have received therapy within 48 hours after the onset of oliguria.[2,9-11]

Unnecessary delay can be the difference between oliguric and nonoliguric renal failure. Although renal function is not improved in the latter situation, the improved urine flow makes it easier to manage the patient.

Colloid Infusion. Infusion of mannitol has been shown to improve GFR if given very soon after the onset of acute renal failure.[9] The response to infusion of 50 to 100 ml of a 25% solution should appear within 2 hours. Other colloids have had similar success,[10] and it is possible that a decrease in blood viscosity is the important factor for supporting renal perfusion.[10] Whatever the mechanism, the observations with colloid infusion suggest that the plasma volume should be kept as high as possible to promote renal perfusion in patients with early renal failure.

Furosemide. The practice of using intravenous furosemide in early acute renal failure is confusing. Intravenous furosemide causes vasoconstriction and a reduced cardiac output when given intravenously in high doses.[11] This observation hardly justifies its use to improve renal flow, but an occasional patient will show an improvement in urine output.[1-3]

> To prevent any further hemodynamic embarrassment, the cardiac output and circulating blood volume must be optimal before intravenous furosemide is given.

The optimal dose of furosemide is not known and intravenous doses as high as 600 mg have been recommended.[12] A starting dose of 100 mg (given slowly) seems reasonable and the response should be evident within an hour.

Dopamine. Low-dose dopamine infusion (1 to 2 mcg/kg/min) can selectively stimulate dopaminergic receptors in the renal circulation.[13] Urine output has improved with this regimen in persistent oliguria,[13] and the effect of furosemide is enhanced if the drug is given in combination with dopamine.[14] When there is a response to dopamine in early renal failure, the infusion should be continued for 24 to 72 hours and then tapered.[11]

PERSISTENT OLIGURIA

Persistent oliguria or azotemia after the above maneuvers are evidence for acute oliguric renal failure. At this point, the drugs and medications shown in Table 34-1 should be withheld or changed.

NEPHROTOXIC DRUGS

Aminoglycosides should be stopped in all patients unless the organism is resistant to all other antibiotics or the patient is neutropenic and has a *Pseudomonas* infection. Aztreonam is proving to be an effective alternative to aminoglycosides and has no renal toxicity. **Amphotericin**

TABLE 34–1. DRUGS THAT SHOULD BE DISCONTINUED IN ACUTE RENAL FAILURE	
Nephrotoxic Drugs	**Alternatives**
Aminoglycosides	Aztreonam (?)
Amphotericin	None (Continue at ½ dose)
Pentamidine	Trimethoprim-Sulfamethoxazole (?)
Allergic Nephritis	
All Penicillins	Erythromycin, Vancomycin
Cephalothin	Vancomycin
TMP—SMX	Pentamidine
Furosemide	Bumetanide
Thiazides	Bumetanide
Cimetidine	Sucralfate, Antacids
Non-steroidals	Acetaminophen

B has no suitable alternative but can be stopped for 24 hours and re-started at half the dose (see Appendix). **Pentamidine and Trimethoprim-Sulfamethoxazole (TMP–SMX)** are both common causes of renal insufficiency in AIDS victims and can sometimes be exchanged for each other if renal toxicity develops.

INTERSTITIAL NEPHRITIS

Drug-induced interstitial nephritis may be difficult to identify clinically because the fever is nonspecific and the rash and eosinophilia can be fleeting.[4,5] In fact, fewer than one-third of the patients will exhibit the classic triad of fever, rash, and eosinophilia.[4] Therefore, it is wise to stop all possible offending drugs. The **penicillins** and **nonsteroidals** are at the top of the list. **Furosemide** is on everyone's list and can be substituted with bumetanide (Bumex) at a 1:40 ratio of bumetanide to furosemide (if the patient was receiving 40 mg furosemide, the dose of bumetanide is 1 mg). **Cimetidine** should not be overlooked as a possible offender and should be discontinued in favor of sucralfate or antacids.

RENAL ELIMINATION OF DRUGS

Common ICU drugs and medications that are eliminated by the kidneys are shown in Table 34–2. **Magnesium-containing antacids** must be stopped or alternated with other antacids. **Digoxin** should also be stopped, if possible, because the creatinine clearance will be changing and the dose will have to be continually adjusted. **Nitroprusside** should not be continued for more than 3 days in the face of renal failure because of the risk for thiocyanate toxicity (see Chapter 20). If aminoglycosides are continued in acute renal failure, the dose must be adjusted. The

TABLE 34–2. ADJUSTMENTS IN DRUG THERAPY IN ACUTE RENAL FAILURE

Medication	Recommendation
Magnesium-containing antacids	Switch to aluminum hydroxide antacids or sucralfate
Digoxin	Reduce daily dose to 25% normal or Switch to Verapamil or Esmolol for Rx SVT Switch to Dobutamine for inotropy
Nitroprusside	Can infuse up to 3 mcg/kg/min for 72 hours, but would: Switch to Trimethaphan for high BP Switch to Amrinone for normotensive heart failure
Procainamide	Use ½ maintenance dose Follow NAPA levels
Aminoglycosides	Adjusted dose: 3–5 mg/kg/day ÷ serum creatinine Adjusted interval: q8h × serum creatinine

methods used to adjust aminoglycoside doses are shown in Table 34–2. The adjustment can either involve the total daily dose of the drug (with a dosing interval of 8 hours), or the dosing interval can be adjusted while the daily recommended dose remains the same. There is no evidence that one method is superior to the other in influencing the clinical outcome.

RHABDOMYOLYSIS

Acute myonecrosis with myoglobinuric renal failure is usually a self-limited condition if renal tubular flow is maintained with aggressive volume infusion. One of the signs of possible myonecrosis is the daily rate of rise in the serum creatinine and the other variables shown in Table 34–3. The creatinine should not increase more than 1 mg/dl in a 24-hour period and the blood urea nitrogen should not rise more than 30 mg/dl.[12] When the criteria in Table 34–3 are present, an immediate

TABLE 34–3. MARKERS OF HYPERCATABOLISM OR MYONECROSIS IN ACUTE RENAL FAILURE*

Serum Chemistry	Daily Increment	Final Level
BUN	> 30 mg/100 ml	
Creatinine	> 1 mg/100 ml	
Potassium	> 1 mEq/L	
Uric Acid		> 15 mg/100 ml
Phosphorous		> 10 mg/100 ml

*From Schrier RW. Acute renal failure. Kidney Int 1979; 15:205–216.

search for rhabdomyolysis is indicated. The serum CPK is a good screening test because a normal level virtually excludes the diagnosis. However, an elevated serum CPK does not secure the diagnosis unless the rise in CPK is precipitous. Severe myonecrosis can release enough creatinine to elevate the CPK MB bands in circulating blood. When the CPK level is elevated and MB bands are present, a serum aldolase level will help to determine if the source of the problem is cardiac or skeletal muscle. Aldolase is an enzyme confined to skeletal muscle, so that an elevated serum aldolase level will identify skeletal muscle as the site of the myonecrosis. Volume infusion should begin immediately when the problem is uncovered because early aggressive management should ensure a favorable prognosis.

The routine management of acute oliguric renal failure involves fluid and electrolyte adjustments and many of these are covered in the next few chapters. The intricacies of acute hemodialysis and hemofiltration will not be covered because you will not be performing these procedures.

REFERENCES

REVIEWS

1. Corwin HL, Bonventre JV. Acute renal failure in the intensive care unit. Parts 1 and 2. Intensive Care Med 1988; 14:10–16; 86–96.
2. Hou SH, Cohen JJ. Diagnosis and management of acute renal failure. Acute Care 1985; 11:59–84.
3. Sillix DH, McDonald FD. Acute renal failure. Crit Care Clin 1987; 5:909–925.

DRUGS AND RENAL FAILURE

4. Sonheimer JH, Migdal SD. Toxic nephropathies. Crit Care Clin 1987; 5:883–907.
5. Linton AL, Clark WF, Driedger AA, et al. Acute interstitial nephritis due to drugs. Ann Intern Med 1980; 93:735–741.

URINE EVALUATION

6. Steiner RW. Interpreting the fractional excretion of sodium. Am J Med 1984; 77:699–702.
7. Miller TR, Anderson RJ, Linas SL, et al. Urinary diagnostic indices in acute renal failure. Ann Intern Med 1978; 89:47–50.

BEDSIDE MANEUVERS

8. Niemens EJ, Woods SL. Normal fluctuations in pulmonary artery and pulmonary capillary wedge pressures in acutely ill patients. Heart Lung 1982; 11:393–398.
9. Luke RG, Briggs JD, Allison MEM, Kennedy AC. Factors determining response to mannitol in acute renal failure. Am J Med Sci 1970; 259:168–172.
10. Rajagopalan PR, Reines HD, Pulliam C, et al. Reversal of acute renal failure using hemodilution with hydroxyethyl starch. J Trauma 1983; 23:795–800.

11. Francis GS, Siegel RM, Goldsmith SR, et al. Acute vasoconstrictor response to intravenous furosemide in patients with chronic congestive heart failure. Ann Intern Med 1985; *103*:1–6.
12. Schrier RW. Acute renal failure. Kidney Int 1979; *15*:205–216.
13. Schwartz LB, Gewertz B. The renal response to low dose dopamine. J Surg Res 1988; *45*:574–588.
14. Lindner A. Synergism of dopamine and furosemide in diuretic-resistant oliguric renal failure. Nephron 1983; *33*:121–126.

chapter

HYPERTONIC AND HYPOTONIC SYNDROMES

The clinical disorders described in this chapter are caused primarily by disturbances in total body water (TBW). The abnormal water balance is reflected in the serum sodium concentration because the serum (extracellular) sodium is determined more by TBW than by total body sodium stores. Therefore, the serum sodium is used as a marker for disturbances in free-water balance. The focus of this chapter is on the general features of sodium and water imbalance and not on the specific clinical features of each hypertonic and hypotonic syndrome.

BASIC CONCEPTS

The following definitions and equations will be valuable for identifying the specific problem in salt and water balance and selecting appropriate therapy.

OSMOTIC ACTIVITY

The osmotic activity of a solute is an expression of the concentration of solute or density of solute particles in a fluid. This activity is expressed in milliosmoles (mOsm), which is equivalent to milliequivalents (mEq) for monovalent ions. The osmotic activity of a fluid is the sum of the individual osmotic activities of each solute in the fluid. This is shown below for isotonic saline:

$$0.9\% \text{ NaCl} = 154 \text{ mEq Na} + 154 \text{ mEq Cl}$$

$$= 154 \text{ mOsm Na} + 154 \text{ mOsm Cl}$$

$$= 308 \text{ mOsm/L}$$

Salts like sodium chloride will dissociate completely in water and yield a final osmolality that is twice the concentration of each electrolyte.

Osmolarity is the term for expressing osmotic activity per volume of solution (solutes plus solvent). **Osmolality** is the term for expressing osmotic activity per volume of solvent (water). Because osmotic activity is expressed in relation to water, osmolality is the more accurate term for describing the osmotic activity of a fluid. For biologic fluids, the volume of water far exceeds the number of electrolyte particles and there is little difference between osmolality and osmolarity. Therefore, the two terms can be used interchangeably in clinical medicine.

OSMOLALITY VERSUS TONICITY

Tonicity or "effective osmolality" describes the difference in osmotic activity between two fluid compartments. This difference provides a gradient for water to move from one compartment to the other. A solute that equilibrates fully between two fluid compartments will increase the osmolality of both compartments but will not increase the tonicity of either compartment. Examples of solutes that produce hyperosmolality without hypertonicity are urea and the alcohols (ethanol, methanol, and ethylene glycol).

PLASMA OSMOLALITY

The osmolality of the plasma (extracellular fluid) can be measured in the clinical laboratory using the freezing point of water. A plasma sample is placed in a refrigerated bath and the temperature at which the water in the sample freezes is converted directly to osmolality (A one osmolal solution freezes at $-1.86°C$). This is called the "freezing point depression" method.

The plasma osmolality can also be calculated using the concentrations of sodium, chloride, glucose, and urea (the major solutes in the extracellular fluid). The calculation below uses a plasma sodium of 140 mEq/

L, a blood glucose of 90 mg/dL, and a blood urea nitrogen (BUN) of 14 mg/dL.

$$\text{Plasma Osmolality} = 2 \times [\text{Na}] + \frac{[\text{Glucose}]}{18} + \frac{[\text{Urea}]}{2.8}$$

$$= 2 \times (140) + \frac{90}{18} + \frac{14}{2.8}$$

$$= 290 \text{ mOsm/kg } H_2O$$

The sodium concentration is doubled to include the osmotic contribution of chloride. The serum glucose and urea are measured in mg/dL and the factors 18 and 2.8 (the atomic weights divided by 10) are used to convert mg/dL to mOsm/kg H_2O.

PLASMA TONICITY

The "effective osmolality" or tonicity of plasma is calculated by eliminating urea from the equation because urea passes freely across cell membranes and does not create an osmotic gradient between intracellular and extracellular fluid compartments.

$$\text{Plasma Tonicity} = 2 \times [\text{Na}] + \frac{[\text{glucose}]}{18} \quad (\text{mOsm/kg } H_2O)$$

$$= 2 \times (140) + \frac{90}{18}$$

$$= 285 \text{ mOsm/kg } H_2O$$

The difference between osmolality and tonicity of plasma is negligible in healthy subjects because the urea contributes little to the total extracellular solute pool. In the setting of azotemia, the difference between osmolality and tonicity is increased. However, pure hyperosmolar syndromes without hypertonicity produce no water shifts across cell membranes and are of little consequence.

THE OSMOLAL GAP

The difference between the measured and calculated plasma osmolality is proportional to the concentration of osmotically active solutes other than those included in the osmolality equation (e.g., magnesium, calcium, proteins, etc.). This difference is called the "osmolal gap" and is normally 10 mEq/L or less.[4]

An osmolal gap above 10 mEq/L must be interpreted in light of the

TABLE 35–1. RELATIVE CHANGES IN SODIUM AND WATER IN HYPERNATREMIA AND HYPONATREMIA			
Serum Sodium	Extracellular Volume	Total Body	
		Sodium	Free Water
High	Low	↓	↓ ↓
	Normal	→	↓
	High	↑ ↑	↑
Low	High	↑	↑ ↑
	Normal	→	↑
	Low	↓ ↓	↓

calculated serum osmolality. If the calculated osmolality is low, the problem is a decrease in the aqueous phase of plasma caused by hyperproteinemia or hyperlipidemia. If the calculated osmolality is in the normal range, an elevated osmolal gap indicates the presence of toxins like ethanol, methanol, and ethylene glycol or some other osmotically active substances like mannitol or those elusive "middle molecules" that accumulate in renal failure. The osmolal gap has been recommended as a reliable test for distinguishing acute from chronic renal failure because the gap should be normal in acute renal failure and elevated in chronic renal failure.[1]

HYPERNATREMIA

Hypernatremia, defined as a serum Na over 145 mEq/L, is the result of either one of two conditions; loss of fluid with a sodium concentration less than the plasma sodium concentration or gain of a fluid with a sodium concentration greater than the plasma sodium concentration. Loss of hypotonic fluids is the most common cause of hypernatremia. Infusion of hypertonic fluids occurs only with hypertonic saline or bicarbonate infusions.

THE EXTRACELLULAR VOLUME

The problem in sodium and water balance can be determined for any case of hypernatremia by assessing the state of the extracellular volume (ECV). This is illustrated in Table 35–1. The clinical assessment of ECV includes an evaluation of intravascular volume like the one presented in Chapter 13. Unfortunately, the clinical evaluation of ECV can be deceiving. If invasive hemodynamic monitoring is available, the ventricular filling pressures and cardiac output can provide valuable information (see Chapters 12 and 13). The sodium concentration in a random urine sample might also help. A urine sodium less than 10 mEq/L suggests a low ECV while a higher urine sodium is against a low ECV (in the absence of diuretics or renal failure). The following strategies are applied to each state of the ECV.

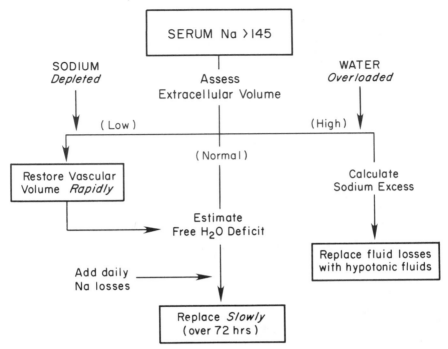

FIG. 35–1. The approach to hypernatremia based on the extracellular volume (ECV). The calculations for free H_2O deficit and sodium excess are in the text. From Marino PL, Krasner J, O'Moore P. Fluid and Electrolyte Expert. Philadelphia: W.B. Saunders, 1987. (Software.)

Low ECV—Indicates loss of sodium and water with water losses exceeding sodium losses. Common causes are diuresis, vomiting, and diarrhea. The management strategy is to correct sodium (volume) deficits first and then to correct free-water deficits slowly over a few days.

Normal ECV—Indicates net loss of free-water. The management here involves calculating and replacing free-water deficits slowly while replacing ongoing sodium and water losses.

High ECV—Indicates an excess of sodium and water with sodium gain more than water gain. This is uncommon and is usually seen only with excessive infusion of hypertonic saline or bicarbonate solutions.

The management strategies based on the ECV are shown in the flow diagram in Figure 35–1. Each strategy is described in the sections that follow.

HYPOVOLEMIC HYPERNATREMIA

The sodium concentration in some commonly lost body fluids is shown in Table 35–2. With the exception of small bowel and pancreatic secretions, loss of any body fluid should result in hypernatremia. Note that all of the fluids contain some sodium. This means that fluid losses

TABLE 35–2.	THE SODIUM CONCENTRATION IN FLUIDS COMMONLY LOST	
Fluid	**Sodium (mEq/L)**
Gastric	55
Pancreatic	145
Ileostomy	145
Perspiration	80
Diarrhea	40
*Urine	<10
Furosemide Diuresis	70–80
*Urine sodium will vary according to sodium intake	

will be accompanied by sodium (volume) deficits as well as free-water deficits.

HYPOVOLEMIA VERSUS HYPERTONICITY

The two consequences of hypotonic fluid loss are hypovolemia (from sodium loss) and hypertonicity (from free-water loss).

Hypovolemia is the more life-threatening of the two consequences because of the risk for hypovolemic shock. However, hypovolemia is usually not prominent in hypertonic conditions because the increase in plasma colloid osmotic pressure from the hypertonicity will draw fluid into the vascular space and protect the intravascular volume.

Hypertonicity leads to cellular dehydration. The clinical manifestations are most prominent in the central nervous system and usually involve an altered sensorium. The degree of mental status change is proportional to the magnitude of the hyperosmolality and the acuity of the change. Serum osmolalities in excess of 350 mOsm/kg H_2O are often accompanied by frank coma.[4] Seizures and focal neurologic deficits are also observed in hypertonic syndromes and focal deficits can disappear when the hypertonicity is corrected.[4]

FLUID THERAPY

The general approach to hypovolemic hypernatremia can be summarized as follows.

Volume (sodium) deficits are replaced rapidly to prevent hypovolemic shock and free-water deficits are replaced slowly to prevent unwanted edema.

Remember that the hypovolemia can be life-threatening and should be corrected as soon as possible. The replacement therapy for volume deficits can be estimated using the methods presented in Chapter 13 (see Figure 13–6). When solute losses produce significant volume deficits and hemodynamic instability, colloid fluids (5% albumin or 6% hetastarch) are much more effective for rapid expansion of the vascular space than crystalloid fluids (see Chapter 17). Restoration of blood pressure should not be the sole end-point of acute volume therapy, as discussed in Chapter 12. When using crystalloid fluids for acute volume replacement, always infuse isotonic saline and avoid less concentrated fluids like half-normal saline. Remember that hypovolemia indicates profound sodium deficits even in the face of hypernatremia, and sodium must be replaced if the vascular volume is to be restored. Infusion of less concentrated saline solutions like half-normal saline are indicated only for replacing free-water deficits and these fluids must be avoided in the setting of significant hypovolemia.

FREE-WATER DEFICIT

Once volume deficits are replaced, the free-water deficit can be calculated. The assumption behind the calculation is that the deficit in total body water (TBW) is proportional to the increase in plasma sodium (P_{Na}). The normal TBW is 60% of lean body weight and the normal plasma sodium is assumed to be 140 mEq/L.

$$\text{Current (TBW} \times P_{Na}) = \text{Normal (TBW} \times P_{Na})$$

$$\text{Current TBW} = 0.6 \times \text{wt (kg)} \times (140/\text{Current } P_{Na})$$

The water deficit in L is then taken as the difference between the current TBW and the normal TBW (or 60% of the ideal body weight).

$$\text{TBW Deficit (L)} = 0.6 \times \text{wt (kg)} \times [(\text{Current } P_{Na}/140) - 1]$$

The free-water deficit for a 70 kg adult (premorbid weight) with a plasma sodium of 160 mEq/L would be [0.6 × 70 × (160/140 − 1)] or 6 L.

REPLACEMENT FLUID VOLUME

The volume of replacement therapy needed to deliver the free-water deficit will depend on the concentration of sodium in the fluid. For example, 1 L of half-normal saline (0.45% NaCl) represents 500 ml of free water and 500 ml of normal saline, so twice the volume of half-normal saline is needed to replace the calculated free-water deficit. This relationship can be expressed as follows:

$$\text{Fluid Replacement (L)} = \text{TBW Deficit} \times (1/1 - K)$$

where K = replacement fluid (Na)/154. If the water deficit of 6 L is replaced with half-normal saline (K = 0.5), the volume of replacement fluid is 12 L [6 L × (1/0.5)].

COMPLICATIONS OF REPLACEMENT THERAPY

The major complication of replacement therapy is edema, particularly pulmonary and cerebral edema. The brain initially shrinks in response to the hypertonic state but this is a transient phenomenon. The volume quickly returns to baseline and this can take place in just a few hours in hypertonic states caused by hyperglycemia.[4] The mechanism is the appearance of osmotically active substances that pull water back from the vascular compartment. These "idiogenic osmoles" help the brain to control its volume in hypertonic states but increase the risk for cerebral edema during replacement therapy.

DIABETES INSIPIDUS

Diabetes insipidus (DI) is a general term for conditions that impair renal water conservation. This condition results in excessive loss of urine that is almost pure water (devoid of solute). The underlying problem is with antidiuretic hormone (ADH), a hormone secreted by the posterior pituitary gland that promotes water reabsorbtion in the distal renal tubules. This hormone is released in response to an increase in extracellular fluid osmolality and it serves to increase water retention and limit the rise in osmolality. There are two defects in ADH that can occur and this creates two categories of DI.

MECHANISMS

Central DI is caused by inhibition of ADH release from the posterior pituitary. Common causes of central DI in the critically ill patient population include closed head injury, anoxic encephalopathy, and meningitis.[4] The onset is heralded by polyuria that is usually evident within 24 hours of the inciting event.

Nephrogenic DI is the second form and is the result of end-organ unresponsiveness to ADH. Common associated conditions in the critically ill are aminoglycosides, amphotericin, radiocontrast dyes, and the polyuric phase of ATN. The defect in urine concentrating ability is not as severe in nephrogenic DI as it is in central DI.

DIAGNOSIS

The hallmark of DI is a dilute urine in the face of hypertonic plasma (plasma osmolality can exceed 350 mOsm/L).

In central DI, the urine osmolality is often below 200 mOsm/L while in nephrogenic DI urine osmolality can range from 200 to 500 mOsm/L.[4]

The diagnosis of DI is confirmed by noting the urinary response to fluid restriction. Failure of the urine osmolality to increase more than 30 mOsm/L in the first hours of complete fluid restriction is diagnostic of DI. The fluid losses can be excessive during fluid restriction in DI (particularly central DI) and this must be done carefully. Once the diagnosis of DI is confirmed, the response to aqueous vasopressin (5 units IV) will differentiate central from nephrogenic DI. In central DI, the urine osmolality will increase abruptly by at least 50% of baseline while in nephrogenic DI, the urine osmolality remains unchanged after the intravenous vasopressin.

MANAGEMENT

The fluid loss in DI is almost pure water so the replacement strategy is aimed at replacing free-water deficits only. Once again, free water is given slowly to limit the risk for edema formation. Ongoing sodium and water losses must also be replaced during the free-water replacement period. **In severe cases of central DI**, vasopressin administration may be necessary. The usual dose is **5 to 10 units of aqueous vasopressin subcutaneously every 4 to 6 hours**.[4] The serum sodium must be monitored carefully during vasopressin therapy because there is a risk for water intoxication and hyponatremia if the central DI begins to resolve.

HYPERGLYCEMIC NONKETOTIC SYNDROME

The syndrome of severe hyperglycemia and hypertonicity without ketosis is a disorder of adults with mild diabetes (or no history of diabetes) who have enough endogenous insulin to prevent ketosis.[8–10] The blood glucose is often above 900 mg/dL,[10] (in contrast to diabetic ketoacidosis, where the blood glucose is often below 600 mg/dL). The persistent loss of glucose in the urine produces an osmotic diuresis that can lead to profound volume (solute) depletion. Predisposing factors include infection, parenteral nutrition, beta-blockers, diuretics, and steroid therapy.

GLUCOSE CORRECTIONS

An increase in the glucose concentration in plasma will draw water from the intracellular space if the glucose is not transported into cells. This will expand the aqueous phase of plasma and create a dilutional decrease in the measured Na of plasma. The dilutional effect of hyperglycemia is corrected as follows.

Each increase in serum glucose of 100 mg/dL will decrease the serum Na^+ by 1.6 mEq/L in euvolemic subjects,[4] and by 2 mEq/L in hypovolemic patients.[5]

Most patients with hyperglycemia are hypovolemic, so the 2 mEq/L correction factor is appropriate in most cases. A patient who presents with a blood glucose of 500 mg/dL and a serum Na of 145 mEq/L will have a corrected sodium of 153 mEq/L. This correction not only brings out the hypertonic state, it identifies the correct Na for designing fluid therapy (see later).

CLINICAL MANIFESTATIONS

The patients usually have altered mental status and signs of hypovolemia. Hypovolemic shock can be present initially but is often easy to correct. Despite the common term of "hyperosmolar nonketotic coma," coma is present in less than half the patients on admission.[8] Furthermore, there is no correlation between the severity of the hyperosmolality and the severity of the mental status changes in individual patients.[10] Generalized seizures and focal neurologic deficits can be part of this syndrome. Prerenal azotemia can be severe but renal failure is uncommon.

MANAGEMENT

The primary goal is to correct volume deficits as soon as possible (as done for any case of hypovolemic hypernatremia). Volume loss tends to be severe because of the osmotic diuresis associated with glycosuria. Insulin must be used cautiously because insulin requirements will diminish as the hypertonic state is corrected. **The usual insulin dose is 2 to 5 units per hour by continuous intravenous infusion.** Potassium abnormalities are common and often appear during volume therapy.

Once volume is restored, free-water deficits can be estimated as shown previously. The plasma Na must be corrected for the hyperglycemia before calculating free-water deficits. Water replacement should be done cautiously here because the risk for cerebral edema is particularly high in hyperglycemia, as explained previously. Half-normal saline is the most common fluid used for replacement therapy.

HYPERVOLEMIC HYPERNATREMIA

Hypernatremia from hypertonic fluid gain is uncommon, and is usually the result of sodium bicarbonate infusion to relieve metabolic acidosis. The sodium bicarbonate solutions used at many hospitals contain 1 mEq sodium per ml, which means the solution has a sodium concentration of 1000 mEq/L! The amount of excess sodium gained from sodium bicarbonate infusion can be calculated as follows.

$$\text{Sodium Excess (mEq)} = 0.6 \times \text{wt (kg)} \times (\text{Current } P_{Na} - 140)$$

The sodium excess is eliminated by diuresis, so that the sodium concentration in the urine during diuresis can be used to determine the volume of diuresis needed to eliminate the excess sodium.

$$\text{Urine Volume (L)} = \text{Na Excess/Urine}_{Na}$$

So, a sodium excess of 300 mEq with a urine sodium of 100 mEq/L would mean that 3 L of urine would have to be lost to excrete all the excess sodium:

$$\text{Urine Volume} = 300 \text{ mEq}/100 \text{ mEq/L} = 3 \text{ L}$$

Urine losses must be replaced partly with D_5W to prevent further increases in serum sodium from the loss of hypotonic urine.

HYPONATREMIA

Hyponatremia (serum sodium less than 135 mEq/L) is found in 1% of the general hospital population,[11] and in 4 to 5% of postoperative patients.[12] The high prevalence of this disorder in hospitalized patients is probably a result of nonosmotic release of vasopressin that occurs during periods of stress. The approach to hyponatremia can proceed in a logical fashion, but first be sure that the hyponatremia is associated with hypotonicity (water excess).

PSEUDOHYPONATREMIA

Extreme elevations in serum lipids or proteins will increase the plasma volume and reduce the serum sodium concentration. However, the increase in volume is in the nonaqueous phase, while the sodium is contained in the aqueous portion of plasma. Therefore, the hyponatremia will not be associated with excess water; that is, this condition is not hypotonic hyponatremia. The correction factors for hyperlipidemia and hyperproteinemia are as follows:

1. Plasma triglycerides (g/L) $\times$ 0.002 = mEq/L decrease in P_{Na}
2. Plasma [protein] above 8 g/dL $\times$ 0.025 = mEq/L decrease in P_{Na}

Significant elevations in plasma lipids and protein are necessary to reduce the serum sodium concentration, because the nonaqueous phase normally represents only 7% of the total plasma volume.

The conventional method for measuring serum sodium concentration

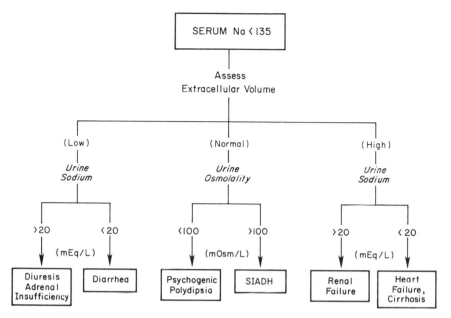

FIG. 35–2. Flow diagram for the approach to hyponatremia.

(flame emission spectrophotometry) measures the total volume (aqueous and nonaqueous), however the newer technique using ion-specific sodium electrodes will measure only the aqueous phase of plasma, and will not produce a spurious decrease in serum sodium.[13] Your hospital laboratory will tell you what method is being used.

HYPOTONIC HYPONATREMIA

True (hypotonic) hyponatremia represents an excess of free water relative to sodium in the extracellular space. It does *not* represent an excess volume in this space; that is, the extracellular volume can be low, normal, or high. Table 35–1 shows the disturbances in sodium and water expected at each level of ECV in hyponatremic states. The approach to hyponatremia begins with the assessment of ECV, as was done for the approach to hypernatremia. The diagnostic approach is outlined in Figure 35–2.

HYPOVOLEMIC HYPONATREMIA

This condition is characterized by loss of fluid that is isotonic to plasma (e.g., a secretory diarrhea) combined with volume replacement using a hypotonic fluid. This creates a net sodium loss, which will decrease the extracellular volume and decrease the extracellular sodium concentration.

Common Cause	Urine Sodium
1. Diuretics	> 20 mEq/L
2. Adrenal Insufficiency	> 20 mEq/L
3. Secretory Diarrhea	< 10 mEq/L

The urine sodium concentration (spot sample) can help to identify the site of the sodium loss (renal or extrarenal). However there may be some overlap for a variety of reasons, and the clinical history is often helpful in selected cases. Remember that adrenal insufficiency can be an occult process that becomes evident only during an intercurrent illness.

"ISOVOLEMIC" HYPONATREMIA

This condition is characterized by a small gain in free water, but not enough to be clinically detected (about 5 L of excess water is necessary to produce visible edema in the average-sized adult).

Clinical Disorder	Urine Sodium	Urine Osmolality
Inappropriate ADH	> 20 mEq/L	> 100 mOsm/Kg H_2O
Acute Water Intoxication	< 10 mEq/L	< 100 mOsm/kg H_2O

The syndrome of inappropriate ADH (SIADH) is a condition produced by sustained (nonosmotic) release of vasopressin in the face of a hypotonic extracellular fluid. This condition is associated with a variety of tumors and chronic infections, and can produce severe hyponatremia (serum sodium less than 120 mEq/L). The hallmark of SIADH is an inappropriately concentrated urine (urine osmolality above 100 mOsm/L) in the face of a hypotonic plasma (plasma osmolality below 290 mOsm/L).[14] The concentrated urine is the result of sustained release of vasopressin, which is not inhibited by the usual osmotic influences. This nonosmotic release of vasopressin is also seen in certain groups of "stressed" patients in the hospital, such as postoperative patients.[10]

HYPERVOLEMIC HYPONATREMIA

This condition represents an excess of sodium and water, with water gain being greater than sodium gain.

Common Causes	Urine Sodium
1. Heart Failure	< 20 mEq/L
2. Renal Failure	> 20 mEq/L
3. Cirrhosis	< 20 mEq/L

The urine sodium can help to identify the cause if necessary, but can be misleading if the patient is receiving diuretics. The clinical picture is usually helpful, although these three conditions often coexist.

SEVERE HYPONATREMIA

Severe hyponatremia (less than 120 mEq/L) is a serious condition with a mortality than can exceed 50%.[10] However, rapid correction of the serum sodium can itself produce a serious illness called **central pontine myelinolysis,** a demyelinating brainstem lesion that causes permanent neurological deficits and can be fatal.[14] The available evidence suggests that this lesion is produced by rapid correction of hyponatremia only when the serum sodium is corrected to normal or supranormal levels.[14,15] The issue then is not so much the rate of the correction, but the final goal of correction. The following recommendations are generally accepted.

RAPID CORRECTION

The rate of correction of the hyponatremia is determined by the clinical condition of the patient. The presence of neurologic abnormalities is evidence for aggressive management, because symptomatic hyponatremia can carry a mortality over 50%.[10] The neurologic manifestations can vary from mild lethargy to coma, generalized seizures, and respiratory arrest.

In symptomatic patients, increase serum sodium at a rate of 1 to 2 mEq/ L per hour until the level reaches 125 to 130 mEq/L.[10,14] For alcoholic or malnourished patients, the end-point of rapid correction should be a serum sodium of 125 mEq/L. NEVER correct sodium to normal levels when using rapid correction methods.

The important aspect of rapid correction is to avoid returning the serum sodium to normal levels, to minimize the risk of central pontine myelinolysis. Alcoholics and malnourished patients may be at particular risk for this brainstem lesion,[14] and therefore it seems wise to select a lower end-point for these patients.

MANAGEMENT PROTOCOLS

The use of hypertonic saline and diuresis is determined by the state of the extracellular volume (ECV). In symptomatic patients, hypertonic saline is preferred to isotonic saline for rapid correction.
1. **Low ECV**—Use 3% saline until the serum sodium increases to 125 to 130 mEq/L.
2. **Normal ECV**—Start with furosemide diuresis, then begin infusion of 3% saline (severe symptoms) or isotonic saline (mild or absent symptoms).
3. **High ECV**—Use furosemide-induced diuresis only, until serum sodium rises to 125 to 130 mEq/L.

USEFUL CALCULATIONS

When the ECV is normal or reduced, the therapy involves the infusion of sodium in the form of hypertonic saline (3% NaCl). The amount of sodium that is needed can be determined by estimating the sodium deficit.

$$\text{Sodium Deficit (mEq)} = \text{TBW} \times (125 - \text{Current } P_{Na})$$

The desired plasma sodium is 125 mEq/L, because the sodium is not to be corrected to normal or even near-normal levels. The volume of hypertonic saline needed for the correction can then be determined easily if 3% saline is used (3% NaCl contains 513 mEq sodium per 500 ml container or about 1 mEq/ml).

$$\text{Volume 3\% NaCl (ml)} = \text{Sodium Deficit (mEq)}$$

Once the volume of saline is determined, the rate of infusion can be calculated according to the infusion rate that is appropriate. If the problem is a high extracellular volume, prompt diuresis is warranted if possible. Although not necessary, you can get some idea of the volume of diuresis needed using the following equation:

$$\text{Water Excess} = \text{TBW} \times (125/\text{Current } P_{Na}) - 1$$

If you know the sodium concentration in the urine, you can determine the volume of urine needed to eliminate the water excess using the following equation:

$$\text{Urine Volume (ml)} = \text{Water Excess} \times (1/1 - \text{Urine Na}/154)$$

For example, if the water excess is 2 L and the urine sodium is 75 mEq/L (or one-half normal saline), then the urine volume needed would be 4 L (2 L $\times$ 1/0.5).

REFERENCES

REVIEWS

1. Rose BD. New approach to disturbances in the plasma sodium concentration. Am J Med 1986; *81*:1033–1040.
2. Alvis R, Geheb M, Cox M. Hypo- and hyperosmolar states: Diagnostic approaches. In: Arieff AI, DeFronzo R eds. Fluid, electrolyte and acid-base disorders. New York: Churchill Livingstone, 1985; 185–221.
3. Narins RG, Jones ER, Stom MC, et al. Diagnostic strategies in disorders of fluid, electrolyte and acid-base homeostasis. Am J Med 1982; *72*:496–520.

HYPERTONIC SYNDROMES

4. Geheb M. Clinical approach to the hyperosmolar patient. Crit Care Clin 1987; 5:797–815.
5. Katz MA. Hyperglycemia-induced hyponatremia—calculation of expected serum sodium depression. N Engl J Med 1973; 289:843–844.
6. Moran SM, Jamison RL. The variable hyponatremic response to hyperglycemia. West J Med 1985; 142:49–53.
7. Feig PU. Hypernatremia and hypertonic syndromes. Med Clin North Am 1981; 65:271–290.
8. Khadori R, Soler NG. Hyperosmolar hyperglycemic nonketotic syndrome. Am J Med 1984; 77:899–903.
9. Daugirdas JT, Kronfol NO, Tzamaloukas AH, Ing TS. Hyperosmolar coma: Cellular dehydration and the serum sodium concentration. Ann Intern Med 1989; 10:855–857.

HYPONATREMIA

10. Arieff AI. Osmotic failure: Physiology and strategies for treatment. Hosp Pract 1988; 22:131–152.
11. Anderson RJ, Chung HM, Kluge R, Schrier RW. Hyponatremia: A prospective analysis of its epidemiology and the pathogenic role of vasopressin. Ann Intern Med 1985; 102:164–168.
12. Chung HM, Kluge R, Schrier RW, Anderson RA. Postoperative hyponatremia. A prospective study. Arch Intern Med 1985; 146:333–336.
13. Weisberg LS. Pseudohyponatremia: A reappraisal. Am J Med 1988; 86:315–318.
14. Ayus JC, Krothapalli RK, Arieff AI. Changing concepts in treatment of severe symptomatic hyponatremia. Am J Med 1985; 78:897–902.
15. Dubois GD, Arieff AI: Symptomatic hyponatremia: The case for rapid correction. In: Narins RG ed. Controversies in Nephrology and Hypertension. New York: Churchill Livingstone, 1984; 393–407.

c h a p t e r

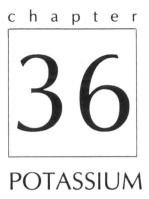

POTASSIUM

The average 70 kg (154 lb) adult contains about 3500 mEq of potassium (50 mEq/kg body weight), but less than 70 mEq (<2%) is located in the extracellular space.[1,2] This is the result of the sodium-potassium membrane pump that pumps potassium into cells and maintains a 30:1 gradient across the cell membrane. The intracellular predominance limits the value of serum potassium as a marker of total body potassium stores.

LIMITATIONS OF SERUM POTASSIUM

The uneven distribution of potassium between the intracellular and extracellular space creates a nonlinear relationship between whole body potassium and serum potassium.[1] This is shown in Figure 36–1.

The slope of the line decreases sharply on the "deficit" side of the graph, indicating that potassium depletion causes less of a change in serum potassium than does potassium excess. The insensitivity of extracellular potassium to potassium depletion is explained by the ability of the intracellular potassium pool to replenish extracellular deficits. The serum potassium is also a poor marker of potassium excess but the correlation between serum potassium and potassium excess is far better than the correlation between serum potassium and potassium deficits.

HYPOKALEMIA

Hypokalemia is defined here as a serum potassium concentration below 3.5 mEq/L.[1,2] The causes of hypokalemia are classified according to whether there is an intracellular shift of potassium (transcellular shift) or whether there is a net loss of potassium (potassium depletion). The

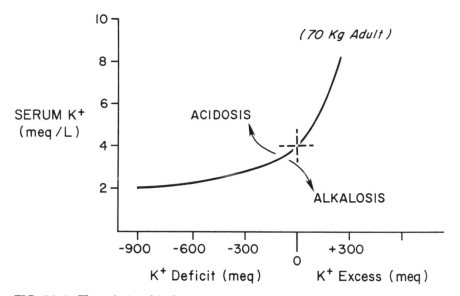

FIG. 36–1. The relationship between serum potassium and whole body potassium at different levels of potassium deficit and excess.

following are some clinical disorders that cause hypokalemia and are likely to be encountered in the ICU. (See Reference 3 for a more complete list of disorders that cause hypokalemia.)

TRANSCELLULAR SHIFT

Potassium movement into muscle cells is facilitated by **beta receptor agonists** like epinephrine and dobutamine.[4a] The latter agent can diminish serum potassium by 0.5 mEq/L at a dose of 10 mcg/kg/min.[4b] However, the clinical impact of this is not clear at present. The other factor promoting transcellular shift is alkalosis, particularly **metabolic alkalosis.**[1,2] The mechanism is a potassium-hydrogen exchange across the cell membrane. Alkalosis also increases potassium secretion in the distal tubules of the kidneys, presumably because of competition between potassium and hydrogen ions for receptor sites.

POTASSIUM DEPLETION

The clinical disorders associated with potassium depletion can be separated into renal and extrarenal losses using the urine potassium. This approach is outlined in Figure 36–2.

Renal Potassium Loss (Urine K above 30 mEq/L). The most common cause of renal potassium wasting is **diuretic therapy.** Other causes in the ICU include nasogastric suction, vomiting, hyperventilation, cirrhosis, and steroid therapy.

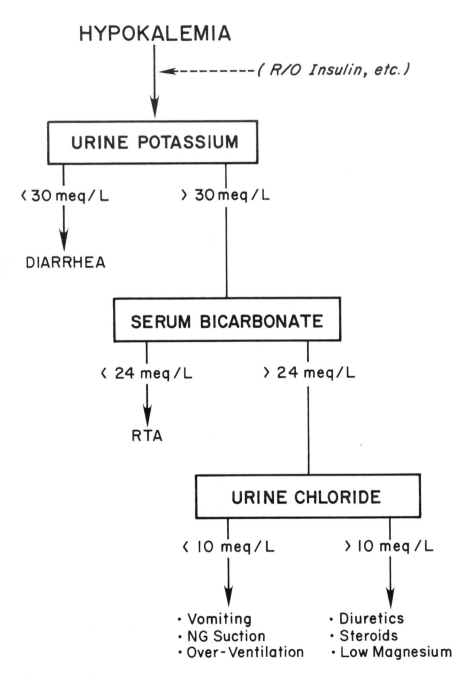

FIG. 36–2. Flow diagram for the approach to hypokalemia.

When hypokalemia is associated with metabolic alkalosis, the urine chloride will help to identify the cause.[4b]

The urine chloride will be low (below 10 mEq/L) when nasogastric suction or vomiting is the cause, but will be high (above 10 mEq/L) when diuretics are responsible.

Extrarenal Loss (Urine K below 30 mEq/L). The major cause of extrarenal potassium depletion is **diarrhea.** The potassium concentration in stool is 75 mEq/L in normal subjects[2] but the stool volume is only 100 to 150 ml/day. The increased volume from diarrhea (which can reach over 10 L a day!) can result in significant potassium depletion. Villous adenoma is often singled out for its high potassium secretion,[5] but the diarrheal fluid from villous adenoma is no richer in potassium than any other diarrheal fluid.[2]

CLINICAL PRESENTATION

Muscle weakness and mental status changes can accompany severe hypokalemia (below 2.5 mEq/L) but milder cases are often asymptomatic. The ECG will be abnormal in over 50% of cases,[6] showing prominent U waves and a decrease in T wave amplitude. Neither change is specific for hypokalemia as they can also be seen with digitalis or left ventricular hypertrophy.

There is a misconception about the ability of hypokalemia to cause arrhythmias.

Hypokalemia alone does not usually produce serious arrhythmias but it can potentiate digitalis-toxic arrhythmias.[6]

Hypokalemia increases the binding of digitalis to the sodium-potassium membrane pump and potentiates the arrhythmias caused by digitalis toxicity.[7] The presence of arrhythmias (usually ventricular ectopics), in association with the combination of digitalis therapy and hypokalemia, should prompt aggressive measures to correct the serum potassium.

MANAGEMENT

Remember that a decrease in serum potassium is a late finding in potassium depletion. When the serum potassium falls below 3.5 mEq/L there is already a 200 mEq deficit in potassium that must be corrected.[1] Therefore, **any decrease in serum potassium is significant, regardless of the magnitude.**

The first concern in hypokalemia is to eliminate agents that promote intracellular potassium accumulation (i.e., bronchodilators). If the problem is potassium depletion, estimate the potassium deficit.

Each 1 mEq/L decrease in serum potassium from 4.0 to 2.0 mEq/L represents a 10% decrease in total body potassium.[8]

This does not apply to serum potassium less than 2.0 mEq/L because

TABLE 36–1. ESTIMATED POTASSIUM DEFICITS FOR A 70 KG ADULT*		
Serum K+	**K+ Deficit**	
(mEq/L)	**Total (%)**	**mEq**
3.0	10	350
2.5	15	470
2.0	20	700
*Based on a total body K+ of 50 mEq/kg lean body weight		

the relationship between serum and whole body potassium is no longer linear in this range.[2]

The estimated potassium deficits for a 70 kg (154 lb) adult is shown in Table 36–1. These estimates are based on a total body potassium of 50 mEq/kg lean body weight.[10]

The estimated potassium deficit can vary widely, partly because it does not account for any contribution from transcellular shifts. However, it may give you an idea of the magnitude of the problem and this should help to reduce any tendency to underestimate the potassium deficit.

Dose Recommendations

1. Use KCl when there is a metabolic alkalosis, and $KHCO_3$ when treating renal tubular acidosis.

2. Recommended IV dose is 0.7 mEq/kg lean body weight over 1 to 2 hours.[2] For obese subjects, give 30 mEq/M^2 body surface area.

The chloride salt is necessary for correcting the metabolic alkalosis, because most of the administered potassium will be lost in the urine if the alkalosis persists. When a metabolic acidosis is present, potassium replacement is not advised (because of the risk of severe hyperkalemia) unless the diagnosis is renal tubular acidosis.

The dose recommendations given above are for the intravenous route, which is the recommended route if the serum K is 2.5 mEq/L or less or if there are ECG changes or muscle weakness. The dose should not increase serum K by more than 1 to 1.5 mEq/L unless there is an acidosis (in which case the need for any therapy must be assessed). This regimen, therefore, should not produce hyperkalemia, even when you start at a serum K of 3 to 3.5 mEq/L.

When the hypokalemia is severe (below 2.0 mEq/L) or there is troublesome ventricular ectopy, the recommended dose is up to 80 to 100 mEq potassium over 1 hour.[2]

> If potassium infusion exceeds 40 mEq/hr, do not use a central vein for the infusion. Instead, split the dose into two equal portions and administer each portion via a separate peripheral vein.

Infusion of high-dose potassium into the superior vena cava or right atrium can produce life-threatening cardiotoxicity and is never recommended. When infusing high-dose potassium peripherally, the use of two separate veins will minimize sclerosis from the infusion.

Response Time. The increase in serum potassium may be gradual, particularly at the outset, because of the gradual slope of the curve as shown in Figure 36–1. Replacement usually takes a few days, particularly if potassium losses are ongoing.

> When the serum potassium is resistant to aggressive replacement therapy, consider magnesium depletion.[9]

Magnesium depletion promotes potassium loss in the urine and impairs the movement of potassium into the extracellular space. The mechanism is not clear but magnesium is needed for the membrane pump that determines potassium movement. The problem with magnesium depletion is that it may not be accompanied by a decrease in serum magnesium. The diagnosis and therapy of magnesium is presented in the next chapter.

HYPERKALEMIA

Hyperkalemia is defined as a serum potassium above 5.5 mEq/L. This can be a life-threatening condition and should be managed much more aggressively than hypokalemia.

PSEUDOHYPERKALEMIA

Hemolysis during the venipuncture can produce a spurious elevation in serum potassium. This is not uncommon and has been reported in 20% of blood samples showing an elevated serum potassium.[10] Hemolysis is usually noted by the pink color of the serum (from hemoglobin) and is reported as a hemolyzed specimen when noted. However, this may be missed. Unexpected hyperkalemia should always be reinvestigated immediately, with careful attention paid to avoid cell trauma during the collection of the blood sample.

Excessive leukocytosis (over 50,000) and thrombocytosis (1 million/mm³) can also produce pseudohyperkalemia from potassium release during clot formation in the collection tube. When this is suspected, obtain a simultaneous serum potassium from a clotted and unclotted blood specimen. Pseudohyperkalemia will produce an increase in the potassium from the clotted sample, which will be at least 0.3 mEq/L higher than in the unclotted specimen.

If the hyperkalemia is real, the problem is either transcellular shift of potassium into the extracellular space or reduced renal excretion of potassium, or both. The problem is usually evident but the urine potassium can be used to identify the problem if needed. A high urine potassium (above 30 mEq/L) suggests a transcellular shift and a low urine potassium indicates reduced renal excretion.

TRANSCELLULAR SHIFT

The following can cause release of potassium into the extracellular fluid.[11]

1. **Myonecrosis**—Direct release of potassium from disruption of cell membranes.

2. **Insulin Lack**—Insulin promotes potassium uptake into the muscles and liver.

3. **Acidosis**—Enhanced potassium-hydrogen shift across cell membranes plus reduced renal excretion. Respiratory acidosis produces little or no effect but metabolic acidosis can increase serum potassium by 1.0 mEq/L.[2] Lactic acidosis and ketoacidosis have much less effect on transcellular shift than the mineral acidoses.

4. **Digitalis toxicity**—Damage to the membrane sodium-potassium pump that normally keeps potassium intracellular.

With the exception of acidosis, all of these should be associated with a high urine potassium (above 30 mEq/L) unless there is also some degree of renal insufficiency.

REDUCED RENAL EXCRETION

Renal insufficiency alone will not cause hyperkalemia until the glomerular filtration rate (GFR) is below 10 ml/min or the urine output falls to 1 L/day or less.[11] Exceptions are interstitial nephritis and hyporenin hypoaldosteronism.[11] The latter condition is seen in elderly diabetic patients who have defective renin release in response to reduced renal blood flow.

Adrenal insufficiency is a well-known cause of hyperkalemia from reduced renal excretion but this is probably not common in the ICU.

Drugs may be common offenders.[10] The drugs most commonly implicated are angiotensin-converting enzyme (ACE) inhibitors, potassium-sparing diuretics, and nonsteroidal anti-inflammatory agents.[10,12] The hyperkalemia usually appears when potassium supplements are continued along with drug therapy. Therefore, it is imperative to eliminate potassium supplements during therapy with these drugs. Heparin has been associated with hyperkalemia, even in small doses used to prevent thromboembolism.[13] This is because of inhibition of aldosterone synthesis and is reversible.

CLINICAL PRESENTATION

The predominant clinical features of hyperkalemia are skeletal muscle weakness and cardiac conduction abnormalities. In some cases, the ECG begins to change at a serum potassium of 6.0 mEq/L and is always abnormal when the serum level reaches 8.0 mEq/L.[11] Figure 36–3 illustrates the ECG changes associated with progressive hyperkalemia.

The earliest change is a tall narrow T wave most evident on precordial leads V2–V4. The "tented" T wave of hyperkalemia is characterized more

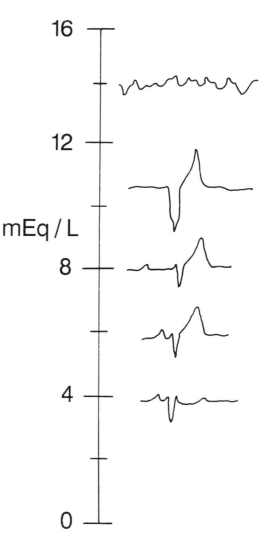

16

12

mEq / L

8

4

0

FIG. 36–3. The ECG manifestations of hyperkalemia. Adapted from Burch GE, Winsor T. A primer of electrocardiography. Lea & Febiger: Philadelphia, 1966; 143.

by its narrow base than by its height.[14] Tall T waves can be a normal variant, which makes the narrow, tapered shape of the T wave in hyperkalemia an important discriminative feature. As the hyperkalemia progresses, the P wave amplitude decreases and the PR interval increases until eventually the P waves disappear. The QRS duration then becomes prolonged and the final event is ventricular asystole.

Neuromuscular weakness is always mentioned as a clinical feature of hyperkalemia[2] and there is a severe flaccid quadriplegia occasionally reported.[15] However, the prevalence of muscle weakness with hyperkalemia is unknown.

TABLE 36–2. ACUTE THERAPY OF HYPERKALEMIA		
Condition	Therapy	Comment
ECG changes	Calcium gluconate (10%) 10 ml IV over 3 minutes. Repeat in 5 minutes if needed	Lasts only 30 to 60 minutes. No bicarbonate after calcium
AV block with no response to calcium	Transvenous pacemaker and 10 U regular insulin in 500 ml D_{20} over 1 hour	Should drop serum K^+ by 1 mEq/L over 1 to 2 hours
Digitalis toxicity	Digitalis antibodies $MgSO_4$—2 gm IV bolus	Avoid calcium. Insulin may be ineffective
After acute phase or if no ECG changes	Kayexalate: Oral dose of 30 gm in 50 ml sorbitol (20%). Rectal dose of 50 gm in 200 ml sorbitol (20%) as retention (30 to 45 min) enema	Oral dose preferred. Enemas not tolerated by patients or nurses
If renal failure	Hemodialysis as soon as possible	

MANAGEMENT

Therapy is guided by the serum potassium levels and the ECG. The serum potassium has priority in dictating the need for therapy.

Therapy is always advised when serum K exceeds 6.0 mEq/L, regardless of the ECG findings, because ventricular tachycardia can appear without premonitory signs on the ECG.[2]

Several approaches are available and these are listed in Table 36–2.
Direct Membrane Antagonists. Calcium gluconate is indicated when the ECG shows advanced changes such as loss of P waves and prolonged QRS duration. Some recommend calcium also when the serum K exceeds 7.0 mEq/L.
Dose:
1. 10 to 20 ml of a 10% solution IV over 3 minutes. Repeat in 5 minutes if no response.
2. If the patient is on digitalis, add 10 ml of 10% solution to 100 ml normal saline and infuse over 20 to 30 minutes.

Calcium increases the membrane threshold and directly antagonizes the action of potassium. The effects last only 20 to 30 minutes, and the problem will return unless another therapy is instituted in the intervening time period. The response to calcium should be evident within a few minutes and a second dose can be given if there is no response by 5 minutes. A third dose will not be effective if there is no response to the second dose. Calcium must be given cautiously to patients on digitalis because hypercalcemia can potentiate digitalis cardiotoxicity.

Transcellular Shift. An **insulin-glucose** infusion will cause a prompt shift of potassium into cells, particularly in skeletal muscle.

> Dose: Add 10U regular insulin to 500 ml of 20% dextrose and infuse over 1 hour.

This regimen should decrease serum potassium 1 mEq/L after 1 to 2 hours. The glucose is given to prevent hypoglycemia. **Sodium bicarbonate** can shift potassium into cells but may be ineffective in some patients.[16]

> Dose: 1 to 2 amps (44 to 88 mEq) over 5 to 10 minutes.

Bicarbonate infusion can aggravate intracellular acidosis and promote lactic acid accumulation (see Chapter 32). Bicarbonate can also bind calcium and should not be used after calcium infusion. The risks of bicarbonate therapy always seem to outweigh the benefits.

Promote Potassium Clearance. Furosemide or ethacrynic acid can be used to promote renal excretion of potassium but will be ineffective in oliguric renal failure.

> Dose: 40 mg IV.

A response should be seen in 20 to 30 minutes. A repeat dose of up to 200 mg IV (over 2 to 3 minutes) can be tried while other measures for potassium elimination are being instituted.

Polystyrene sulfonate resin (Kayexalate) is a cation exchange resin that can be given orally or by retention enema. Each mEq potassium removed will add 2 to 3 mEq of sodium.

> Oral Dose: 30 g Kayexalate in 50 ml of 20% sorbitol.
> Rectal Dose: 50 g Kayexalate in 200 ml 20% sorbitol as an enema.
> Retain solution for 30 to 45 minutes if possible.

Dialysis is the most effective means of removing potassium (particularly hemodialysis) and may be necessary if diuretics and exchange resins are not effective.

BIBLIOGRAPHY

Tannen RL ed. Potassium metabolism. Semin Nephrol. 1987; 7(Sep):171–273.

REFERENCES

REVIEWS

1. Brown RS. Extrarenal potassium homeostasis. Kidney Int 1986; 30:116–127.
2. Smith JD, Bia MJ, DeFronzo RA. Clinical disorders of potassium metabolism. In: Arieff

AI, DeFronzo RA. Fluid, electrolyte and acid-base disorders. New York: Churchill Livingstone, 1985; 413–509.
3. Narins RG, Jones ER, Stom MC, et al. Diagnostic strategies in disorders of fluid, electrolyte and acid-base balance. Am J Med 1982; 72:496–520.

HYPOKALEMIA

4. Parker MS, Oster JR, Perez GO, Taylor AL. Chronic hypokalemia and alkalosis. Arch Intern Med 1980; 140:1336–1337.
5. Knochel JP. Etiologies and management of potassium deficiency. Hosp Pract 1987; 22(Jan):153–162.
6. Flakeb G, Villarread D, Chapman D. Is hypokalemia a cause of ventricular arrhythmias? J Crit Illness 1986; 1:66–74.
7. Surawicz B. Factors affecting tolerance to digitalis. J Am Coll Cardiol 1985; 5(Suppl):69A–81A.
8. Stanaszek WF, Romankiewicz JA. Current approaches to management of potassium deficiency. Drug Intell Clin Pharm 1985; 19:176–184.
9. Solomon R. The relationship between disorders of potassium and magnesium homeostasis. Semin Nephrol 1987; 7:253–262.

HYPERKALEMIA

10. Rimmer JM, Horn JF, Gennari FJ. Hyperkalemia as a complication of drug therapy. Arch Intern Med 1987; 147:867–869.
11. Williams ME, Rosa RM. Hyperkalemia: Disorders of internal and external potassium balance. J Intensive Care Med 1988; 3:52–64.
12. Ponce SP, Jennings AE, Manias NE, Harrington JT. Drug-induced hyperkalemia. Medicine 1985; 64:357–370.
13. Edes TE, Sunderrajan EF. Heparin-induced hyperkalemia. Arch Intern Med 1985; 145:1070–1072.
14. Fisch C. Electrocardiography and vectorcardiography. In: Braunwald E ed. Heart disease. A textbook of cardiovascular medicine. Philadelphia: W.B. Saunders, 1988; 180–222.
15. Villabona C, Rodriguez P, Joven J. Potassium disturbances as a cause of metabolic neuromyopathy. Intensive Care Med 1987; 13:208–210.
16. Blumberg A, Weidmann P, Shaw S, Gradinger M. Effect of various therapeutic approaches on plasma potassium and major regulating factors in terminal renal failure. Am J Med 1988; 85:507–512.

c h a p t e r

MAGNESIUM: THE HIDDEN ION

Magnesium has been the forgotten cousin of potassium and calcium despite the fact that it is the second most abundant intracellular cation (next to potassium) in the body. Magnesium is a cofactor for all enzyme reactions that involve ATP and it is part of the membrane pump that maintains electrical excitability in muscle and nerve cells.[1] The real problem with magnesium is the lack of a reliable measure of total body magnesium status. This will be stressed repeatedly in the chapter that follows.

MAGNESIUM BALANCE

One of the important features of magnesium (Mg) balance is the non-uniform distribution of the ion in the body fluid compartments. The distribution of magnesium in the normal adult is shown in Table 37–1. Over half of the total body stores are located in bone and less than 1% is in plasma. The lack of representation in the circulating blood creates a problem in diagnosing alterations in magnesium balance.

TABLE 37–1. MAGNESIUM DISTRIBUTION IN ADULTS		
Tissue	Content	Total Body Mg (%)
Serum	2.6 mmoles	0.3 ←
RBC	5.0	0.5
Soft Tissue	193	19.3
Muscle	270	27
Bone	530	53
From Elin RJ. Magnesium metabolism in health and disease. Disease-A-Month 1988(Apr); 34:173.		

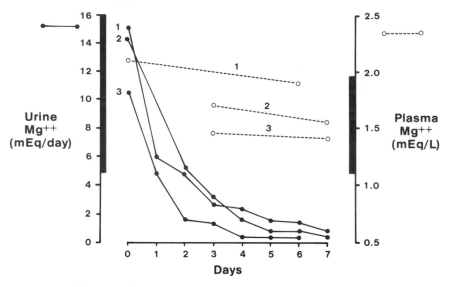

FIG. 37–1. Plasma and urine magnesium levels in three healthy volunteers in the first week after eliminating magnesium from the diet. Individual numbers identify the values obtained in each subject. Solid vertical bars indicate the normal ranges for urine and plasma magnesium. From Shils ME. Experimental human magnesium deficiency. Medicine 1969; 48:61–82.

The serum magnesium is not a reliable measure of total body magnesium balance and serum levels can be normal in the face of magnesium depletion or excess.[2]

This means that alterations in magnesium balance are difficult to detect without clinical markers. These markers will be presented later in the chapter.

The recommended daily intake for magnesium (Mg) is 6 to 10 mg/kg/day.[2] Elimination of Mg intake can lead to clinically significant Mg depletion in just a few days, as shown in Figure 37–1. The urine magnesium in the figure begins to drop off precipitously in the first few days while the plasma magnesium declines much more gradually. The urine magnesium is, therefore, the more sensitive indicator of magnesium balance. The ability to reduce urinary magnesium excretion is the major defense against magnesium depletion when intake is poor. The regular use of diuretics and other agents that promote urinary magnesium excretion will eliminate the renal adjustment to reduce intake and can produce profound magnesium depletion in just a few days.

MAGNESIUM DEPLETION

Magnesium depletion may be the most common electrolyte abnormality in hospitalized patients.[3] This is because of the lack of daily intake of magnesium in intravenous fluids combined with the use of diuretics, aminoglycosides, and other agents that enhance urinary magnesium excretion and blunt the renal conservation response.

PREVALENCE

The true prevalence of magnesium depletion is unknown because most studies have used serum Mg levels as an index of total-body stores. The incidence of hypomagnesemia in ICU patients is summarized below.

Situation	Number of Patients	Patients with Low Serum Mg (%)	Reference
Admission to MICU	102	20	5
Admission to MICU	94	65	6
*Residing in CCU	104	7	7
Admission to SICU	193	61	8
*53% of the patients in this study had low levels of Mg in lymphocytes			

These figures will underestimate the actual frequency of this disorder in the hospital because serum levels show little or no correlation with intracellular magnesium levels. At our hospital some 4 years ago, Dr. William Novick measured erythrocyte magnesium levels in 20 consecutive patients immediately after cardiopulmonary bypass and found diminished red cell magnesium levels in all but one patient. Serum magnesium levels showed no correlation with red cell magnesium levels (Novick W. Personal communication). Analysis of intracellular Mg levels (erythrocytes or lymphocytes) are needed to document the true prevalence of magnesium depletion in ICU patients.

> Magnesium depletion may be almost universal in ICU patients because of the lack of daily supplements and the enthusiastic use of diuretics.

Remember that a normal serum magnesium concentration (1.5 to 2.0 mEq/L) should not sway you from considering hypomagnesemia when the clinical presentation is suggestive of magnesium depletion.

COMMON CAUSES

Table 37–2 lists the causes of magnesium depletion. The most prevalent cause is enhanced renal losses from diuretics and aminoglycosides.

Diuretics that inhibit sodium reabsorption in the loop of Henle (e.g., furosemide and ethacrynic acid) also block magnesium absorption at this site (where most of the magnesium is reabsorbed) and cause urine magnesium wasting.[9]

Aminoglycosides are also common offenders because approximately 30% of patients receiving these antibiotics will develop hypomagnesemia.[1] The mechanism is reduced magnesium reabsorption in the loop of Henle, much like the effect of diuretics.

Alcoholism may be the most common cause of magnesium depletion in general hospital populations. Alcohol has several actions that reduce

TABLE 37–2. COMMON CAUSES OF MAGNESIUM DEPLETION
IN THE ICU

Intravenous fluids with no Mg
Diarrhea
Osmotic Diuresis
Cisplatin

ANTIBIOTICS
Aminoglycosides
Amphotericin
Ticarcillin

DIURETICS
Furosemide
Ethacrynic Acid
Thiazides

serum magnesium but urine magnesium losses are probably the pre-dominant cause. Severe hypomagnesemia can develop in the first few days of hospitalization for ethanol withdrawal and should be watched for carefully in these patients.[1]

Diarrhea is also likely to be a common contributing factor because this condition is present in almost 50% of patients who reside in an ICU (see Chapter 6). Lower GI tract secretions are rich in magnesium (10 to 14 mEq/L) but upper tract secretions are not (1 to 2 mEq/L). Therefore, vomiting is not a likely cause of hypomagnesemia.

Reduced intake of magnesium is unlikely as a sole cause of magnesium depletion because 2 months of fasting has been shown to cause only a 20% deficit in total-body magnesium stores.[1] However, in ICU patients who are likely to have abnormal losses, daily magnesium (4.0 mmoles per day) is recommended. Intravenous administration is the most ef-fective route because changes in gastric pH can alter absorption of certain oral magnesium preparations (see later).

CLINICAL MARKERS

Because the serum levels of magnesium can be misleading, the di-agnosis of magnesium depletion often must be made on clinical grounds. The physiologic effects of magnesium depletion can be used as "clinical markers" that should heighten your suspicion for a problem in mag-nesium balance. Remember to not let a normal serum level influence your diagnosis when the clinical situation suggests magnesium defi-ciency.

The "Hypo's." Magnesium depletion is commonly associated with other electrolyte abnormalities, as shown in the following report.[10]

Abnormality	% with Hypomagnesemia
Hypokalemia	40
Hypophosphatemia	30
Hyponatremia	27
Hypocalcemia	22

Refractory hypokalemia is a prominent feature of hypomagnesemia and the magnesium deficit must be corrected before it will be possible to correct the potassium deficit. The mechanism behind the association may be the inhibition of the membrane pump that keeps potassium intracellular, but this remains unproven.[1] What is known is that Mg depletion is associated with a decrease in intracellular potassium and repletion of Mg stores will return these levels to normal.[3,10] The link between hypocalcemia and hypomagnesemia is reduced parathyroid hormone secretion reported in magnesium-depleted patients.[1]

Arrhythmias in Acute MI. Magnesium depletion is considered to be a risk factor for arrhythmias in acute myocardial infarction because magnesium infusion reduces the incidence of arrhythmias in this patient population.[11-13] Hypomagnesemia can also precipitate coronary vasospasm because it enhances calcium entry into vascular smooth muscle.[14,15] However, the role of coronary vasospasm in the arrhythmias of hypomagnesemia is not clear. Furthermore, magnesium might have a nonspecific antiarrhythmic effect that is unrelated to body magnesium stores.[16] The fact that low intracellular Mg levels have been found in patients in a coronary care unit should increase your suspicion for Mg depletion in patients with acute MI.[7]

Digitalis Cardiotoxicity. Magnesium depletion plays an important role in potentiating digitalis-induced arrhythmias and may be more important than hypokalemia in increasing the risk for digitalis cardiotoxicity.[16-18] Because digitalis works by inhibiting the Mg-dependent membrane pump that allows calcium to move into cardiac muscle fibers,[16] it is no surprise that hypomagnesemia exaggerates the digitalis effect. For this reason, Mg deficiency should be considered in any case of suspected digitalis toxicity.

Magnesium can be effective in abolishing digitalis-induced tachyarrhythmias even when serum Mg levels are not depressed.[16-18]

Intractable Arrhythmias. Difficult arrhythmias can sometimes respond to intravenous Mg when conventional antiarrhythmic therapy fails.[14] It is not clear if this is a nonspecific antiarrhythmic action of Mg or if the arrhythmias are caused by Mg depletion that is not being detected by the serum Mg levels. Regardless of the mechanism, Mg infusion should be seriously considered in any patient with intractable tachyarrhythmias (except sinus tachycardia), even when the serum Mg levels are in the normal range.

Muscle Strength. There are isolated reports of muscle weakness associated with hypomagnesemia, including respiratory muscle weakness.[19] However, the clinical significance of this is yet to be determined. It seems unlikely that hypomagnesemia has a profound influence on respiratory muscle strength because Mg depletion is common in hospitalized patients and clinically evident respiratory muscle weakness (i.e., causing hypoventilation) is not. Nevertheless, the possibility for respiratory muscle weakness is just another reason for trying to maintain adequate Mg stores in the critically ill.

Miscellaneous. The following effects are either uncommon or are of questionable clinical significance:

1. Neuromuscular excitability (positive Chvostek's and Trousseau's signs)
2. Seizures
3. Psychiatric disturbances
4. Prolonged QT interval on ECG
5. Tremors

MAGNESIUM REPLACEMENT PROTOCOLS

Magnesium can be given via the oral, intramuscular, or intravenous routes. In symptomatic cases, intravenous therapy is recommended. Remember that it is almost impossible to produce hypermagnesemia for prolonged periods of time if renal function is normal because of the capacity of the kidneys to eliminate excess magnesium. The following protocols are recommended only for patients with normal renal function. These recommendations are taken from an excellent review listed at the end of the chapter.[20]

GENERAL GUIDELINES

The following guidelines can be adopted for most patients with symptomatic magnesium depletion and normal renal function.[20]

1. Estimated deficit: 1 to 2 mEq/kg
2. Replacement fluid: Magnesium sulfate, available as 10% or 50% solution. Each ml of the 50% solution provides ½ gram of magnesium, or 4 mEq of elemental magnesium. Five ml of the 10% solution will provide ½ gram magnesium.
3. Replacement Protocol: 1 mEq/kg for the first 24 hours and 0.5 mEq/kg/day for the next 3 to 5 days

About twice the estimated magnesium deficit is replaced because 50% of the administered parenteral dose will be lost in the urine even in the face of significant magnesium depletion.[20] Magnesium chloride is preferred to magnesium sulfate in hypocalcemic patients because sulfate can bind calcium and aggravate the hypocalcemia. The 50% solution of $MgSO_4$ must be diluted when using the intravenous route.[20]

LIFE-THREATENING HYPOMAGNESEMIA

If serious cardiac arrhythmias or seizures are present:
1. Infuse 2 g magnesium (4 ml of 50% $MgSO_4$) intravenously over 1 to 2 minutes.
2. Follow with 5 g magnesium (10 ml of 50% $MgSO_4$ in 500 ml saline) over the next 6 hours.
3. Continue 5 g $MgSO_4$ every 12 hours (as continuous infusion) for the next 5 days.

The initial bolus dose of magnesium will acutely increase serum levels but levels begin to decline at 15 minutes.[11] Therefore, it is important to follow with a continuous infusion of magnesium. It will usually take several days to replete body magnesium stores even though serum levels may normalize within 1 day of replacement therapy. Make sure not to use Ringer's lactate as the diluent solution because it contains calcium.

MODERATE DEPLETION

This situation usually arises when serum magnesium levels are depressed but there are no signs of serious clinical sequelae of magnesium depletion. Refractory electrolyte abnormalities (e.g., hypokalemia and hypocalcemia) can be included in this category unless the hypokalemia is severe (below 3.0 mEq/L).
1. Infuse 6 g $MgSO_4$ (12 ml of 50% $MgSO_4$ in 500 ml saline) over 3 hours.
2. Follow with 5 g $MgSO_4$ in 500 ml saline infused continuously over the next 6 hours.
3. Continue with 5 g $MgSO_4$ infused every 12 hours for the next 5 days.

RENAL INSUFFICIENCY

Severe magnesium deficiency is not at all common in patients with renal failure but can occur when renal insufficiency is mild and creatinine clearance is greater than 30 ml/min.[1] Careful magnesium replacement can be given in mild renal insufficiency by reducing the recommended replacement amounts by 50%.[1,20] Aggressive intravenous magnesium replacement is never recommended in patients with established renal failure, unless serious, life-threatening arrhythmias must be treated.

For renal insufficiency and serious arrhythmias:
1. Infuse 2 g $MgSO_4$ intravenously over 5 minutes and check the serum magnesium level in 15 minutes.
2. Repeat 2 g $MgSO_4$ over 5 minutes if the serum level is not elevated and if serious arrhythmias persist.

TABLE 37–3. MAGNESIUM-CONTAINING MEDICATIONS	
Medication	Dose (per 5 ml)
Antacids	
Mylanta	7 mEq
Riopan	10
Gelusil	8
Magnesium Citrate	7
Laxatives	
Milk of Magnesia	13–15
Magnesium sulfate	8

MONITORING REPLACEMENT THERAPY

The replacement therapy is empiric because serum levels are misleading. The serum magnesium levels will normalize within 24 hours of initiating therapy yet it often requires days to replete tissue magnesium stores. Therefore, serum levels serve only to monitor for unwanted hypermagnesemia from overly aggressive therapy. Urine magnesium excretion has been recommended by some but the value of this is unproven at present.[20]

MAGNESIUM EXCESS

Magnesium excess is (like Mg depletion) difficult to detect because of the unreliability of serum Mg levels. However, hypermagnesemia is less prevalent than hypomagnesemia, occurring in 10% of hospitalized patients.[1]

CAUSES

Virtually all cases of hypermagnesemia are associated with renal failure, usually in combination with excess Mg ingestion. The most common source of excess Mg ingestion is the aggressive use of Mg-containing antacids or cathartics. Some magnesium-containing oral preparations are listed in Table 37–3. Magnesium containing antacids and cathartics should be avoided whenever possible in patients with acute or chronic renal failure. There is little justification for using Mg-containing antacids in the ICU. The aggressive use of antacids to prevent stress ulceration is falling out of favor because of the colonization of gastric contents that occurs with increased gastric pH (see Chapter 5). If antacids are used in patients with renal failure, aluminum-containing antacids are favored (for short-term use) because the aluminum binds phosphorous and helps limit the risk for hyperphosphatemia in renal failure. Long-term use of aluminum-containing antacids in chronic renal failure is being questioned because of the risk for aluminum toxicity but this should not be an issue with short-term antacid administration in the ICU. If the constipating effects of aluminum are not desirable, magnesium-containing antacids can be alternated with its aluminum-containing counterparts.

Other causes of hypermagnesemia in renal failure are disease processes that cause magnesium transport out of cells. The most common ICU illness that can produce this effect is **diabetic ketoacidosis.** Pheochromocytoma can also produce hypermagnesemia through this mechanism but this is not encountered commonly in the general ICU patient population.

CONSEQUENCES

The most feared complication is **hypotension,** which can be seen at serum Mg levels of 3.0 to 5.0 mEq/L and is common at higher levels.[2] The hypotension is classically refractory to the usual therapeutic maneuvers. Complete heart block can be seen at serum levels of 7.5 mEq/L and respiratory depression and coma can occur at serum levels of 10 mEq/L.[2]

TREATMENT

Hemodialysis is the therapy recommended in many texts. However, intravenous calcium (two 10 ml ampules of calcium gluconate or 0.47 mEq calcium per ml) can be effective in reversing hypotension without hemodialysis.[21] If fluid therapy will be tolerated in patients with renal insufficiency, aggressive volume infusion combined with loop diuretics (e.g., furosemide) may be effective by enhancing renal Mg losses.

REFERENCES

1. Elin RJ. Magnesium metabolism in health and disease. Disease-A-Month 1988; Apr 34:173.
2. Reinhart RA. Magnesium metabolism. A review with special reference to the relationship between intracellular content and serum levels. Arch Intern Med 1988; 148:2415–2420.
3. Whang R. Magnesium deficiency: Pathogenesis, prevalence, and clinical implications. Am J Med 1987; 82(3A):24–29.
4. Whang R, Oci TO, Watawabe A. Frequency of hypomagnesemia in hospitalized patients receiving digitalis. Arch Intern Med 1985; 145:655–656.
5. Reinhart RA, Desbiens NA. Hypomagnesemia in patients entering the ICU. Crit Care Med 1985; 13:506–507.
6. Ryzen E, Wagers PW, Singer FR, Rude RK. Magnesium deficiency in a medical ICU population. Crit Care Med 1985; 13:19–21.
7. Ryzen E, Elkayam U, Rude RK. Low blood mononuclear cell magnesium in intensive cardiac care unit patients. Am Heart J 1986; 111:475–480.
8. Chernow B, Bamberger S, Stoiko M, et al. Hypomagnesemia in patients in postoperative intensive care. Chest 1989; 95:391–397.
9. Ryan MP. Diuretics and potassium/magnesium depletion. Am J Med 1987; 82(3A):38–47.

10. Whang R, Oei TO, Aikawa JK, et al. Predictors of clinical hypomagnesemia. Arch Intern Med 1984; *144*:1794–1796.
11. Iseri LT, Freed J, Bures AR. Magnesium deficiency and cardiac disorders. Am J Med 1975; *58*:837–846.
12. Abraham AS, Rosenmann D, Kramer M, et al. Magnesium in the prevention of lethal arrhythmias in acute myocardial infarction. Arch Intern Med 1987; *147*:753–755.
13. Rasmussen HS, Suenson M, McNair P, Nooregard P, Balsev S. Magnesium infusion reduces the incidence of arrhythmias in acute myocardial infarction. A double-blind placebo-controlled study. Clin Cardiol 1987; *10*:351–356.
14. Iseri LT. Magnesium in coronary artery disease. Drugs 1984; *28*(Suppl 1):151–160.
15. Iseri LT, French JH. Magnesium: Nature's physiologic calcium blocker. Am Heart J 1984; *108*:188–193.
16. Laban E, Charbon GA. Magnesium and cardiac arrhythmias: Nutrient or drug? J Am Coll Nutr 1986; *5*:521–532.
17. Cohen L, Kitzes R. Magnesium sulfate and digitalis-toxic arrhythmias. JAMA 1983; *249*:2808–2810.
18. French JH, Thomas RG, Siskind AP, Brodsky M, Iseri LT. Magnesium therapy in massive digoxin intoxication. Ann Emerg Med 1984; *13*:562–566.
19. Molloy DW, Dhingra S, Solven F, Wilson A, McCarthy DS. Hypomagnesemia and respiratory muscle power. Am Rev Respir Dis 1984; *129*:497–498.
20. Oster JR, Epstein M. Management of magnesium depletion. Am J Nephrol 1988; *8*:349–354.
21. Fassler CA, Rodriguez RM, Badesch DB, Stone WJ, Marini JJ. Magnesium toxicity as a cause of hypotension and hypoventilation. Arch Intern Med 1985; *145*:1604–1606.

38

CALCIUM AND PHOSPHORUS

The focus on calcium and phosphorus imbalance is not so much on the prevalence of the abnormalities but rather on their relevance. Hypocalcemia and hypophosphatemia seem to be well tolerated in most patients despite their potential for adverse effects. In fact, it seems that abnormal serum levels of calcium and phosphorus serve as markers of illness severity more than primary disorders requiring immediate attention and aggressive management.

CALCIUM

The diagram in Figure 30–1 illustrates the three fractions of calcium in blood. About 50% of the calcium is bound to serum proteins, with albumin accounting for 80% of the protein binding. An additional 5 to 10% is complexed with anions like bicarbonate and the remainder is present as the free or ionized form. The ionized fraction contains the physiologically active form of the ion but the clinical laboratory measures all three fractions as the "total" serum calcium. The normal values for total and ionized calcium in serum are shown below. The total calcium is reported in milligrams per deciliter (mg/dL) and the ionized calcium is usually reported in millimoles per L (mM/L). The normal range for ionized calcium may vary slightly at each hospital.

Normal Range

Total calcium = 8.5 to 10.2 mg/dL

or 2.1 to 2.5 mM/L

Ionized calcium = 4.8 to 7.2 mg/dL

or 1.1 to 1.3 mM/L

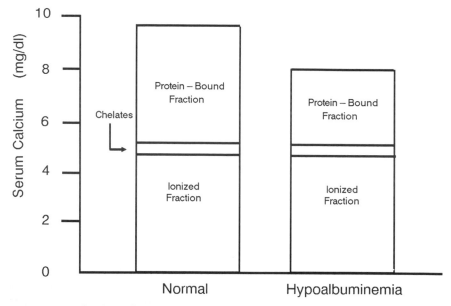

FIG. 38–1. The three fractions of calcium in the blood. Left: Normal distribution. Right: Hypoalbuminemia.

TOTAL SERUM CALCIUM

The total serum calcium is unreliable as a measure of the active (ionized) fraction in certain situations, as illustrated in Figure 38–1. The height of the columns in this figure indicate the total serum calcium and the column on the right illustrates how a decrease in the protein-bound fraction can reduce the total serum calcium while the ionized fraction remains unchanged. This shows how the total serum calcium can be misinterpreted without a simultaneous measure of serum albumin.

Correction Factor. The total serum calcium can be adjusted for changes in serum albumin using a correction factor that increases the total calcium by 0.8 mg/dL for each 1 mg/dL decrease in serum albumin.[1] For example, if the total calcium is 8.0 mg/dL and the serum albumin is 3.0 mg/dL, the adjusted calcium is 8.8 mg/dL which is in the normal range. This adjustment is used widely but has not proven reliable when compared to the ionized calcium measurement.[4] Therefore, a direct measurement of ionized calcium is recommended to insure accuracy.

IONIZED CALCIUM

Ion specific electrodes are available for measuring the ionized calcium in blood and many clinical laboratories now have the ability to perform this measurement.

TABLE 38–1. THE FACTORS THAT ALTER THE ACCURACY OF IONIZED CALCIUM	
Condition	Change in Ionized Calcium
Acid pH	Increases
Alkaline pH	Decreases
Heparin	Decreases
Serum Na <120 mEq/L	Decreases
Serum Na >155 mEq/L	Increases
Room Temperature	Increases
Blood Cell Metabolism	Increases

Blood Collection. The blood sample used for the ionized calcium determination must be collected properly to insure accuracy. The factors that alter accuracy are listed in Table 38–1. Acid pH decreases the binding of calcium to serum proteins and increases ionized calcium, while alkalosis has the opposite effect.[1, 2] This means that a blood sample allowed to sit in the collection tube can generate CO_2 and falsely elevate the ionized calcium. To minimize metabolic CO_2 production in the blood sample, collect the blood anaerobically and separate the cells as soon as possible. Anticoagulants like heparin and citrate can bind calcium in the sample and reduce the ionized fraction,[2] so these must be avoided. Other factors that influence the ionized calcium is the sodium concentration and temperature of the sample. Hyponatremia increases calcium binding to serum proteins and reduces ionized calcium, while hypernatremia has the opposite effect.[2] Ionized calcium will increase if the sample falls to room temperature, so ionized calcium should be measured at body temperature.

IONIZED HYPOCALCEMIA

As many as two-thirds of the patients entering a medical ICU will have a low serum calcium on admission.[5,6] The common disorders associated with "ionized hypocalcemia" are listed in Table 38–2, along with their prevalence in a medical ICU.[6] **The most common causes are sepsis and magnesium depletion.** Hypoparathyroidism is a leading cause of hypocalcemia in outpatients but is not a consideration in the ICU unless the patient has had recent neck surgery. The following is a brief description of the more common causes of hypocalcemia in the ICU patient population.

TABLE 38–2. COMMON CAUSES OF IONIZED HYPOCALCEMIA IN A MICU*	
Condition	% Total
Sepsis	50
Hypomagnesemia	28
Renal Insufficiency	8
Alkalosis	6
Acute Pancreatitis	3

*From Desai TK, et al. Prevalence and clinical implications of hypocalcemia in acutely ill patients in a medical intensive care setting. Am J Med 1988; 84:209–214.

COMMON CAUSES

Magnesium Depletion. Magnesium deficiency can reduce serum calcium by inhibiting parathormone secretion and reducing the end-organ response to parathormone. The hallmark of hypocalcemia from magnesium depletion is the inability to raise the serum calcium because the infused calcium is excreted in the urine as a result of the diminished parathormone action.

Hypocalcemia should always trigger a search for magnesium depletion because it is a common cause for hypocalcemia and because the serum calcium will not correct until the magnesium deficit is corrected.

The problem is that the serum magnesium can be normal in the face of significant magnesium depletion (see Chapter 37). When this occurs, empiric magnesium loading is advisable unless the patient has renal insufficiency. The method of magnesium loading is described in Chapter 37.

Alkalosis. An increase in serum pH promotes the binding of calcium to albumin and reduces ionized calcium. Both metabolic and respiratory alkalosis are common in the ICU. Metabolic alkalosis is usually produced by diuretics and nasogastric suction and respiratory alkalosis is produced by sepsis, anxiety, and mechanical ventilation. The albumin correction factor will be misleading in the setting of alkalosis and the ionized calcium must be measured.

Sepsis. Sepsis is often associated with hypocalcemia,[7] presumably as a result of calcium efflux across a disrupted microcirculation. However, respiratory alkalosis may also play a role. It is also possible that hypocalcemia and sepsis are just common disorders and are not causally linked. The appearance of hypocalcemia in sepsis carries a poor prognosis,[7] possibly because these patients are more prone to hypotension and circulatory instability.

Renal Failure. The hypocalcemia of renal failure is attributed to phosphorus retention and to defective conversion of vitamin D to its active metabolite. The hyperphosphatemia promotes the formation of insoluble calcium phosphate crystals that can accumulate in soft tissues. The treatment of hypocalcemia in renal failure is aimed at lowering serum phosphate levels with antacids that block intestinal absorption of phosphorus. The hypocalcemia itself is usually asymptomatic because the tendency for acidosis in renal failure reduces protein binding and maintains the ionized calcium within normal limits.

Miscellaneous. The other causes of hypocalcemia include pancreatitis, burns, fat embolism syndrome, massive blood transfusion, cardiopulmonary bypass, burns, and drugs. Pancreatitis and burns may cause a decrease in parathormone secretion, while fat embolism syndrome is associated with elevated circulating free fatty acids that can bind calcium. In massive blood transfusion, the citrate preservative in bank blood can bind calcium directly.

CLINICAL MANIFESTATIONS

Hypocalcemia is often a laboratory diagnosis because the clinical manifestations are minimal or absent. The manifestations that do surface are caused by neuromuscular excitability and decreased cardiac contractility.

Neuromuscular Excitability. Virtually every text on the subject lists hyperreflexia, tetany, and seizures as consequences of hypocalcemia, yet there is little evidence that these complications actually occur in the clinical setting. The hyperreflexia is undocumented and the characteristic Chvostek and Trousseau signs are far from reliable.

Chvostek's sign is present in 25% of the general population and is absent in 30% of patients with hypocalcemia.[2]

Trousseau's sign is even less sensitive and specific than Chvostek's sign. Although neither of these signs is a reliable marker of hypocalcemia, their presence should prompt immediate steps to correct the serum calcium.

Cardiovascular Effects. The list of cardiovascular complications in most texts includes peripheral vasodilatation, hypotension, a prolonged QT interval, and left ventricular failure. Once again, the significance of these complications is in question. There are occasional reports of heart failure that improve with calcium infusion, but this is not a common phenomenon.

CALCIUM INFUSION THERAPY

The infusion of calcium can promote vasoconstriction and this may be beneficial or harmful in selected patients. Calcium infusion has been recommended for cardiogenic shock following cardiopulmonary bypass surgery.[8] However, low cardiac output syndromes are characterized by peripheral vasoconstriction, and calcium infusion can aggravate the vasoconstriction and further reduce blood flow. The role of calcium in heart failure seems limited to the few patients who have hypocalcemia and systolic heart failure that is refractory to therapy with inotropes and vasodilators. Remember that calcium can reduce ventricular compliance

TABLE 38–3. INTRAVENOUS CALCIUM THERAPY*		
Salt	**Contents Per 10 ml Vial**	**Maximum Rate**
Calcium Chloride (10%)	272 mg (13.6 mEq) Ca^{++}	1.0 ml/min
Calcium Gluconate (10%)	90 mg (4.5 mEq) Ca^{++}	0.5 ml/min
Preparation: For IV Use Only Dilute 10 ml vial in 100 ml D5W (To prevent vein irritation) Warm to body temperature (To prevent precipitation)		
Dose Recommendations: For Acute Symptoms Initial Dose: 100–200 mg Ca^{++} over 10 minutes		
Maintenance: 1–2 mg/kg/hr		
*From Drug Facts and Comparisons, St. Louis, Lippincott, 1985, p. 111–112.		

and this will aggravate any pre-existing diastolic heart failure (see Chapter 14).

The ability of calcium to promote vasoconstriction has been used as an explanation for the "no-reflow" phenomenon that describes the persistent hypoperfusion that follows periods of hypotension or cardiac arrest (see Chapter 12). This is one of the reasons that calcium infusion has been restricted in cardiopulmonary resuscitation and it should also be a reason to restrict unwarranted calcium infusions for asymptomatic hypocalcemia.

Calcium Infusion Protocols. Some recommendations for calcium infusion are shown in Table 38–3. Calcium can be very irritating to veins and should be infused through the large central veins if possible. Neither calcium chloride nor calcium gluconate should be given by the intramuscular route.

HYPERCALCEMIA

Hypercalcemia can appear in 4% of hospitalized patients[9] and is often asymptomatic. The most common cause in the general population is hyperparathyroidism, while malignancy is the predominant cause in the ICU.

MANAGEMENT OF SEVERE HYPERCALCEMIA

The indications for treating hypercalcemia are the presence of symptoms or a serum calcium of 13 mg/dL or higher. The symptoms of hypercalcemia include altered mental status, ileus, hypotension and renal failure. Mental status changes can be mild or can progress rapidly to obtundation and coma. The appearance of these symptoms is considered a medical emergency that warrants immediate therapy.

TABLE 38–4. THERAPY FOR SEVERE HYPERCALCEMIA		
Agent	Dose	Interval
Furosemide	40–80 mg IV	q2 hr
Saline	Infusion rate = Urine flowrate	
Calcitonin	4 U/kg IM or SubQ	q12 hr
Mithramycin	25 mcg/kg IV	q2–3 days

THERAPEUTIC STRATEGIES

The therapeutic approach to severe hypercalcemia is summarized in Table 38–4.[9–12] The goal of acute therapy is to promote calcium excretion in the urine.

Saline and Loop Diuretics. Hypercalcemia is usually accompanied by increased calcium excretion in the urine and the hypercalciuria causes an osmotic diuresis that can lead to profound volume depletion. The decrease in intravascular volume produces a concentration effect that can cause the serum calcium concentration to increase even further. The hallmark of the therapy here is aggressive volume infusion. Saline is preferred as the resuscitation fluid because the natriuresis itself promotes calcium excretion in the urine.

Aggressive volume infusion is often successful in reducing the serum calcium to acceptable levels with no other interventions.[11,12] However, loop diuretics are commonly added to further promote calcium excretion. Furosemide is given intravenously in doses of 40 to 100 mg every 2 hours. The urine output is monitored every hour and the output from the previous hour is replaced with a saline infusion. Failure to replace urine losses will be counterproductive and the saline infusion should be adjusted every hour to match the urine output.

Calcitonin. Thyrocalcitonin reduces serum calcium by inhibiting bone resorption. Synthetic salmon calcitonin has the greatest potency, and can return the serum calcium to normal levels in 2 to 3 hours.[9] The usual dose is 4 units/kg IM or subcutaneously every 12 hours for two doses. If this is ineffective, the dose can be doubled after 2 days have elapsed. Calcitonin is well tolerated, but can cause nausea and vomiting.

Mithramycin. Mithramycin is an antineoplastic agent that inhibits bone resorption. It is more effective than calcitonin, but the response takes 24 to 36 hours to appear.[9] The usual dose is 25 mcg/kg given intravenously, either as a bolus or as a 6-hour infusion. The dose can be repeated after two days if needed. This dose of mithramycin for hypercalcemia is lower than the antineoplastic dose, and bone marrow depression should not develop. The drug is well tolerated if a time period of 2 to 3 days is allowed between doses.

Dialysis. Hemodialysis is effective for removing calcium from the blood, but is not practical for routine therapy. Dialysis is indicated only when the other measures are ineffective. Hemodialysis is much more effective than peritoneal dialysis.[9]

TABLE 38–5. COMMON CAUSES OF SEVERE HYPOPHOSPHATEMIA*	
Condition	% Total
Dextrose Infusion	73
Refeeding	50
Phosphate-Binding Antacids	50
Etoh Withdrawal	32
Respiratory Alkalosis	10
Recovery from Diabetic Ketoacidosis	9
Parenteral Nutrition	5

*From King AL, et al. Severe hypophosphatemia in a general hospital population. South Med J 1987; *80*:831–834.

PHOSPHORUS

Phosphorus is predominantly an intracellular ion (like magnesium and potassium) and less than 1% is located in the extracellular fluid. The serum phosphorus levels show a diurnal variation of up to 1.5 mg/dL.[13] Levels are lowest in the morning (8 AM to noon) and highest at night (2 AM to 6 AM). This change may be due to food intake or to diurnal patterns for parathormone secretion.

Normal range = 3.0 to 4.5 mg/dL

Low Normal: 8 AM to 12 NOON

High Normal: 2 AM to 6 AM

HYPOPHOSPHATEMIA

Hypophosphatemia is not common in hospitalized patients. One study of over 1,000 consecutive hospitalized patients reported an incidence of only 0.24%.[14] The conditions associated with severe hypophosphatemia (serum PO_4 below 0.5 mg/dL) in this report are shown in Table 38–5. Note that many of the patients in this study had more than one predisposing condition. Most of these conditions promote the movement of phosphorus into cells where it is used as a co-factor for the metabolism of glucose.

PREDISPOSING FACTORS

Dextrose Infusion. Glucose infusions are the leading cause of hypophosphatemia in hospitalized patients.[13–16] The patients are usually alcoholic or otherwise debilitated and the nadir in the serum phosphorus

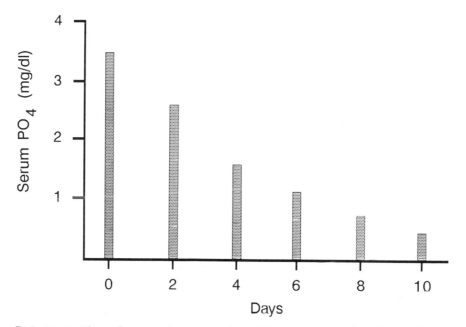

FIG. 38–2. The influence of parenteral nutrition on serum phosphorus. From Knochel JP. The pathophysiology and clinical characteristics of severe hypo-phosphatemia. Arch Intern Med 1977; *137*:203–220.

appears in the first few days after admission to the hospital. Figure 38–2 shows the change in serum phosphorus during the first 10 days after intravenous nutrition is started. The serum phosphorus levels gradually fall during the first week and can reach extremely low levels. This reduction in serum phosphate is one of the reasons that intravenous feedings are usually not started at full strength but are gradually increased to full strength over 5 to 7 days.

The hypophosphatemia associated with dextrose infusion is due to insulin-supported transport of glucose and phosphorus into skeletal muscle and liver. Once in the cells, the phosphorus is used as a cofactor for glycolysis. In patients who are adequately nourished, dextrose infusion will not produce hypophosphatemia. In malnourished patients, glucose infusion can reduce serum phosphate levels to below 0.5 mg/dL in just a few days. This can be seen with the standard 5% dextrose solutions used for maintenance intravenous fluid therapy.

The Nutritional Recovery Syndrome. Aggressive feeding of repatriated prisoners of war in World War II produced an illness characterized by lethargy, diarrhea, weakness, and multiple electrolyte abnormalities. This illness proved fatal in some cases and was called the "nutritional recovery syndrome." One of the features of this illness was hypophosphatemia, produced by overzealous carbohydrate feeding. This is one of the reasons that feedings are gradually increased in malnourished or otherwise ill patients.

Respiratory Alkalosis. Respiratory alkalosis is a common cause of hypophosphatemia.[13] The increase in intracellular pH accelerates glycolysis, and the enhanced glucose phosphorylation promotes transcellular phosphate influx. This may be an important cause of hypophosphatemia in patients receiving mechanical ventilation, because respiratory alkalosis is common in these patients.

Sepsis. Septicemia from either gram-positive or gram-negative organisms is a common cause of hypophosphatemia in some studies.[15] The mechanism is not clear but may be related to an increased demand for phosphorus to support the hypermetabolism of sepsis. Hypophosphatemia can appear early in the course of sepsis,[18] and an unexplained drop in serum phosphorus levels should always prompt a search for infection.

Diabetic Ketoacidosis. Glycosuria increases urinary phosphate excretion and patients who present with diabetic ketoacidosis are usually phosphate depleted despite a normal or even high serum phosphorus level. Insulin therapy drives the remaining phosphorus into the cells and quickly uncovers the hypophosphatemia. Although this is a common scenario, aggressive phosphorus supplementation does not alter the outcome in diabetic ketoacidosis.[3] However, any patient who presents with hypophosphatemia in combination with ketoacidosis is severely phosphate depleted and will benefit from early aggressive phosphorus replacement.

Antacids. Antacid preparations that contain aluminum hydroxide will bind phosphorus in the bowel lumen and can produce a state of phosphate depletion. Commercially available antacids with aluminum include Amphogel, Alternagel, and Basalgel. Sucralfate is an aluminum-containing gel that is used to maintain the integrity of the upper GI tract mucosa and this agent can also bind phosphorus. Sucralfate is becoming popular for stress ulcer prophylaxis (see Chapter 5) but there is no study of its ability to produce hypophosphatemia in the ICU setting. All preparations capable of binding phosphorus in the bowel (including sucralfate) should be discontinued in patients who are hypophosphatemic.

CLINICAL FEATURES

The clinical consequences of hypophosphatemia may not be prominent, even at serum phosphate levels considered to be dangerously low. In one study of hospitalized patients who developed severe hypophosphatemia (serum PO_4 below 1.0 mg/dL), not one patient showed evidence of a complication from the hypophosphatemia.[14] This creates some doubt about the ability of hypophosphatemia to produce adverse reactions. The following consequences are reported occasionally, but their relationship to phosphate depletion remains to be shown conclusively.

Oxygen Transport. Hypophosphatemia can be detrimental to oxygen delivery for a number of reasons. This can be demonstrated using the determinants of oxygen delivery, as illustrated in Figure 38–3. Hypo-

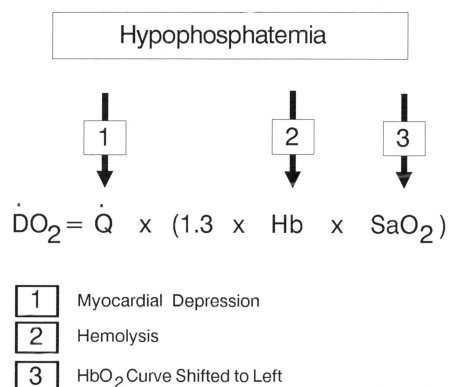

FIG. 38–3. The influence of hypophosphatemia on the components of oxygen delivery ($\dot{D}o_2$). Q: cardiac output, Hb: hemoglobin concentration, Sao_2: arterial O_2 saturation.

phosphatemia has an adverse influence on each of the components of the oxygen delivery equation:

1. **Cardiac Output**—Phosphate deficiency reduces cardiac contractility, and chronic phosphate deficiency has been implicated as a cause of cardiomyopathy.[16]

2. **Hemoglobin**—Hemolysis can occur at very low phosphorus levels, but is uncommon.[14]

3. **Oxygen Saturation**—Phosphate depletion is associated with depletion of 2,3 diphosphoglycerate, and this causes a leftward shift of the oxyhemoglobin dissociation curve.[13] As a result, the oxygen bound to hemoglobin is less readily released to the tissues.

Skeletal Muscle. Hypophosphatemia can impair ATP generation needed for skeletal muscle to perform work, and muscle weakness can result. Respiratory muscle weakness has been reported that is severe enough to impair weaning from mechanical ventilation.[17] Respiratory muscle weakness is common when serum phosphorus levels are below 2.5 mg/dL, but the weakness is not clinically significant in most patients.[19] At present, it seems that more than just hypophosphatemia is needed to produce clinically relevant muscle weakness.

TABLE 38–6. PARENTERAL PHOSPHORUS THERAPY		
	Contents	
Preparation	Phosphorus*	Other
Sodium Phosphate	3 mM (93 mg) per ml	Na^+ = 4 mEq/ml
Potassium Phosphate	3 mM (93 mg) per ml	K^+ = 4.3 mEq/ml
Neutral Sodium Phosphate	0.09 mM (2.8 mg) per ml (1 mMole = 31 mg)	Na^+ = 0.16 mEq/ml
Dose Recommendations†		
Serum PO_4	Dose	
<0.5 mg/dl	15 mg/kg (0.5 mM/kg) over 4 hours	
0.5–1.0 mg/dl	7.7 mg/kg (0.25 mM/kg) over 4 hours	

*From Lentz RD, et al. Treatment of severe hypophosphatemia. Ann Intern Med 1978; 89:941–944.
†From Kingston M, Badawi Al-Siba'i M. Treatment of severe hypophosphatemia. Crit Care Med 1985; 13:16–18.

MANAGEMENT

Intravenous replacement is recommended for all patients with a serum phosphorus below 1.0 mg/dL, even if there are no clinical sequelae. The recommended intravenous replacement therapies are shown in Table 38–6.[21,22] Rapid infusion is usually well tolerated but can be associated with hypotension.[22] When replacing phosphorus, remember to monitor serum calcium, magnesium, and potassium, because these electrolytes are commonly depleted in patients with hypophosphatemia. Serum levels should return to normal in 90% of patients within 3 days.[14]

HYPERPHOSPHATEMIA

The most common causes of hyperphosphatemia are renal failure and widespread cell necrosis. **Renal failure** causes phosphorus retention when the glomerular filtration rate (GFR) drops to less than 25 ml/min.[13] **Rhabdomyolysis and tumor lysis syndromes** produce hyperphosphatemia by releasing phosphorus from damaged cells. Diabetic ketoacidosis can present with elevated serum phosphate levels, but the patients are usually phosphate deficient and the serum levels decrease rapidly when insulin therapy is started. This is an example of transcellular shift as a cause of hyperphosphatemia.

The management of hyperphosphatemia is usually aimed at correcting the underlying problem. In renal failure, a common practice is to administer aluminum-containing antacids (Amphogel, Basalgel) to bind phosphorus in the bowel. This is not usually a concern in the ICU, and is more a therapy for chronic renal failure in outpatients.

REFERENCES

CALCIUM

1. Kassirer JP, Hricik DE, Cohen JJ. Repairing body fluids. Philadelphia: W.B. Saunders, 1989; 73–99.
2. Zaloga GP, Chernow B. Calcium metabolism. In: Geelhoed GW, Chernow B eds. Endocrine aspects of acute illness. Clinics in critical care medicine. Vol. 5. New York: Churchill Livingstone, 1985.

Hypocalcemia

3. Desai TK, Carlson RW, Geheb MA. Hypocalcemia and hypophosphatemia in acutely ill patients. Crit Care Clin 1987; 5:927–941.
4. Ladenson JH, Levius JW, Boyd JC. Failure of total calcium corrected for protein, albumin and pH to correctly assess free calcium status. J Clin Endocrinol Metab 1978; 46:986–991.
5. Chernon B, Zaloga G, McFadden E, et al. Hypocalcemia in critically ill patients. Crit Care Med 1982; 10:848–851.
6. Desai TK, Carlson RW, Geheb MA. Prevalence and clinical implications of hypocalcemia in acutely ill patients in a medical intensive care unit setting. Am J Med 1988; 84:209–214.
7. Zaloga GP, Chernow B. The multifactorial basis for hypocalcemia during sepsis. Studies of the parathyroid hormone–Vitamin D axis. Ann Intern Med 1987; 107:36–41.
8. Neville WE. Intensive care of the surgical cardiopulmonary patient. 2nd ed. Chicago: Year Book Medical Publishers, 1983; 77.

Hypercalcemia

9. Roswell RH. Severe hypercalcemia: Causes and specific therapy. J Crit Illness 1987; 2:14–21.
10. Green L, Ringenberg QS. Current concepts in the management of hypercalcemia of malignancy. Hosp Form 1988; 23:268–287.
11. Baker JK, Wray HL. Early management of hypercalcemic crisis: Case report and literature review. Milit Med 1982; 147:756–760.
12. Hosking DJ, Cowley A, Bucknall CA. Rehydration in the treatment of severe hypercalcemia. QJ Med 1981; 22:473–481.

PHOSPHORUS

13. Yu GC, Lee DB. Clinical disorders of phosphorus metabolism. West J Med 1987; 147:564–576.

Hypophosphatemia

14. King AL, Sica DA, Miller G, Pierpaoli S. Severe hypophosphatemia in a general hospital population. South Med J 1987; 80:831–835.
15. Halevy J, Bulvik S. Severe hypophosphatemia in hospitalized patients. Arch Intern Med 1988; 148:153–155.
16. Janson C, Birnbaum G, Baker FJ. Hypophosphatemia. Ann Emerg Med 1983; 12:107–116.

17. Agusti AGN, Torres A, Estopa R, Agusti-Vidal A. Hypophosphatemia as a cause of failed weaning: The importance of metabolic factors. Crit Care Med 1984; 12:142–143.
18. Shoenfeld Y, Hager S, Berliner S, et al. Hypophosphatemia as a diagnostic aid in sepsis. NY State Med J 1982; 82:163–165.
19. Gravelyn TR, Brophy N, Siegert C, Peters-Golden M. Hypophosphatemia-associated respiratory muscle weakness in a general inpatient population. Am J Med 1988; 84:870–875.
20. Youssef HAE. Hypophosphatemic respiratory failure complicating total parenteral nutrition. An iatrogenic potentially lethal hazard. Anesthesiology 1982; 57:246.
21. Lentz RD, Brown DM, Kjellstrand CM. Treatment of severe hypophosphatemia. Ann Intern Med 1978; 89:941–944.
22. Kingston M, Al-Siba MB. Treatment of severe hypophosphatemia. Crit Care Med 1985; 13:16–18.

NUTRITION AND METABOLISM

Energy expenditure is the most representative parameter of the life process.
Max Kleiber

c h a p t e r

39

NUTRITIONAL REQUIREMENTS

The goal of nutritional support is to design a regimen that is tailored to the needs of the individual patient. This chapter will highlight the more important nutritional needs of hospitalized patients, with emphasis on hypermetabolic patients in the ICU.

ENERGY AND METABOLISM

The process of metabolism involves the oxidation of basic nutrients to produce thermal energy or heat. As illustrated in Figure 39–1, this process converts oxygen into carbon dioxide, water, and heat. The heat is dissipated through the skin and is measured as kilocalories. The quantities of oxygen, carbon dioxide, and heat involved in nutrient combustion are shown in Table 39–1. The information in this table can be rearranged as follows:

1 g GLUCOSE + 0.74 L of O_2 yields 0.74 L of CO_2 + 3.75 kilocalories

The summed metabolism of all three substrates will determine the overall O_2 consumption ($\dot{V}O_2$), CO_2 production ($\dot{V}CO_2$), and energy expenditure (EE) in any individual patient. Because heat production is not easy to measure, the $\dot{V}O_2$ and $\dot{V}CO_2$ can be used as indirect measures of the

TABLE 39–1. METABOLIC PROFILES			
Item	Lipid	Protein	Glucose
O_2 Consumption (L/g)	2.0	0.96	0.74
CO_2 Production (L/g)	1.4	0.78	0.74
Respiratory Quotient	0.7	0.80	1.00
Energy (kcal/g)	9.1	4.0	3.75

From Bursztein S, et al. Energy metabolism, indirect calorimetry, and nutrition. Baltimore: Williams & Wilkins, 1989:55.

metabolic energy expenditure in individual subjects. This is the principle behind "indirect calorimetry," which is the standard method for measuring energy expenditure in the clinical setting.

ENERGY REQUIREMENTS

The daily caloric needs of each patient can be estimated or measured.[1-6] The usual practice is to estimate the caloric needs and to measure the requirements only in selected patients who need careful adjustments in nutrient intake.

PREDICTIVE EQUATIONS

The Harris-Benedict Equations shown below are used to predict the basal energy expenditure (BEE), which is the basal metabolic rate in the resting and fasting state.
BEE (kcal/day):

$$\text{Males: } 66 + (13.7 \times \text{Wt}) + (5 \times \text{Ht}) - (6.7 \times \text{A})$$

$$\text{Females: } 655 + (9.6 \times \text{Wt}) + (1.8 \times \text{Ht}) - (4.7 \times \text{A})$$

where Wt: weight in kg, Ht: height in cm, A: age in years. The actual body weight is used for patients who are well-nourished and the ideal body weight is used for patients who are malnourished, obese, or edematous.
The following rule is also used to estimate daily calories:[7]

$$\text{BEE (kcal/day): } 25 \times \text{Wt (in Kg)}$$

This simple estimate has proven to be as accurate as the complicated Harris-Benedict Equations but it has not been tested rigorously.[7] This is the rule we use on our daily rounds to estimate daily energy needs.

Adjustments in BEE. A common practice is to adjust the estimated BEE for daily activity and for the hypermetabolism that characterizes critically ill patients. The common correction factors are shown below:

Minimal Activity: BEE × 1.2
Fever: BEE × 1.1 (for each degree C)
Mild Stress: BEE × 1.2
Moderate Stress: BEE × 1.4
Severe Stress: BEE × 1.6

The actual adjustment for severe illness can vary widely in individual patients.[5] The difference between estimated and measured energy expenditure in ICU patients has ranged from as little as 2 to 3%,[3] to as great as 50%.[3-5] The predictive equations are least reliable in patients who are hypermetabolic, and direct measurements of energy needs may be necessary in these patients.

INDIRECT CALORIMETRY

As mentioned earlier, indirect calorimetry measures the daily energy expenditure as the oxygen consumption ($\dot{V}O_2$) and the carbon dioxide production ($\dot{V}CO_2$). This is illustrated in Figure 39–1. The $\dot{V}O_2$ and $\dot{V}CO_2$ are determined by measuring the concentration of O_2 and CO_2 in inhaled and exhaled gas with an apparatus called a "metabolic cart." These devices can be wheeled to the bedside and placed in series with the ventilator tubing to measure the gas exchange across the lungs. The resting energy expenditure (REE) is then calculated as follows:[1,2]

$$REE \text{ (kcal/min): } 3.94 \ (\dot{V}O_2) + 1.1 \ (\dot{V}CO_2)$$

$$REE \text{ (kcal/day): } REE \times 1440$$

The gas exchange measurements are usually obtained over a 15 to 30 minute period and the REE is extrapolated to 24 hours. For patients who are not active, the REE measured over a limited time period is only 15 to 20% less than the 24-hour energy expenditure.[6] The REE is, therefore, increased by 20% to account for daily activity. The REE is similar to the BEE but also includes the thermal effect of food (because ICU patients are frequently receiving enteral tube feedings or intravenous nutrition). However, these two measurements are considered essentially the same for clinical purposes.

Indirect calorimetry is the most accurate means of determining the daily caloric needs in the clinical setting. However, the method is expensive, time consuming, and not universally available. In addition, the oxygen sensor in the metabolic carts is not reliable at inspired oxygen levels above 50%, so the methodology is only applicable to selected patients.

NONPROTEIN CALORIES

Carbohydrates and lipids are used to provide the calories and protein is used to maintain or replete protein stores. The proportion of calories provided by lipids and carbohydrates is a matter of some debate, although there is no clear evidence that one substrate is superior to the other as a source of calories.

CARBOHYDRATES

Carbohydrates supply 60 to 90% of the total calories in the average American diet. Much of it is used by the central nervous system, which

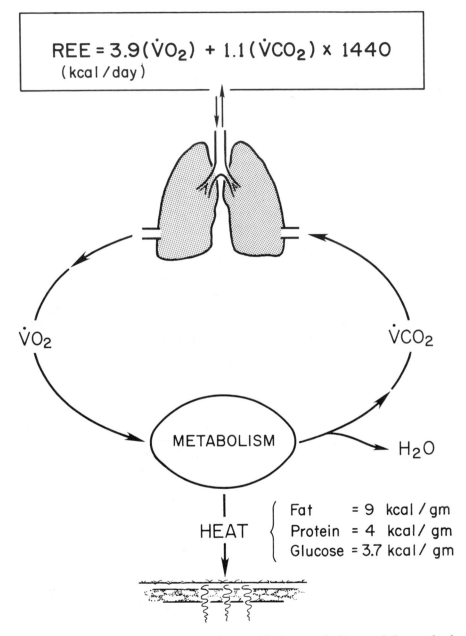

$$REE = 3.9(\dot{V}O_2) + 1.1(\dot{V}CO_2) \times 1440$$
(kcal/day)

$\dot{V}O_2$

$\dot{V}CO_2$

METABOLISM

H_2O

HEAT

Fat = 9 kcal/gm
Protein = 4 kcal/gm
Glucose = 3.7 kcal/gm

FIG. 39–1. The energy conversion from oxidative metabolism and the method of measuring resting energy expenditure (REE) from pulmonary gas exchange.

TABLE 39–2. FUEL COMPOSITION OF NORMAL MAN		
Fuel	Amount (kg)	Calories (kcal)
Fat	15	141,000
Muscle Protein	6	24,000
Glycogen (muscle)	0.015	600
Glycogen (liver)	0.075	300
Total		165,900
From Cahill GF Jr. N Engl J Med 1970; 282:668–675.		

relies heavily on glucose as its principal fuel. Otherwise, glucose has some disadvantages as a major fuel source.

1. Carbohydrate utilization may be impaired in sepsis and other "stress states" and this can promote hyperglycemia in diabetic patients.[8]

2. Carbohydrates stimulate insulin release and insulin inhibits the mobilization of free fatty acids from adipose tissue. This impairs the ability of the body to rely on endogenous fat stores during periods of inadequate nutrition (see Table 39–2).

3. Excess carbohydrates are used for fatty acid synthesis in adipose tissue and liver and this can lead to fatty infiltration of the liver.

4. Carbohydrate metabolism produces an abundance of CO_2, which can be detrimental for patients with compromised lung function.[9]

The Respiratory Quotient. The RQ is the ratio of CO_2 production to O_2 consumption ($RQ = \dot{V}CO_2/\dot{V}O_2$). Table 39–1 lists the RQ for each of the basic substrates. Glucose has the highest RQ (1.0) and fat has the lowest (0.7). The RQ from indirect calorimetry will measure the average contribution from all three substrates and will provide an index of the major fuel source in the individual patient. This may be valuable in detecting excess carbohydrate ingestion.

Because the RQ of carbohydrates is 1.0, **an overall RQ above 0.9 indicates excess carbohydrate calories in the diet.**[9] In this situation, the fraction of carbohydrate calories can be reduced 40% or even lower. This may be particularly valuable in patients with respiratory failure, to limit the tendency for CO_2 retention. The goal of nutrition in these patients is to deliver the desired calories while maintaining the RQ below 0.9.

LIPIDS

Lipids have the highest caloric value of the three basic substrates (9 kcal/gm) and it is no surprise that the body relies on fat stores during periods of starvation. The supply of energy in stored fat is shown in Table 39–2. Note that the calories supplied as glycogen are miniscule compared to the energy supplied from fat. The glycogen stores are barely capable of supplying one day's worth of calories.

Lipids usually provide 30 to 50% of the ingested calories in hospitalized patients and they may be the preferred fuel in sepsis.[8] Linoleic acid is the only essential fatty acid that must be provided in the diet, and should provide 4% of the total calorie intake to prevent essential fatty acid deficiency.[10]

Essential fatty acid deficiency is produced by a deficiency in linoleic acid intake and is usually seen after a few weeks of fat-free intravenous nutrition. The clinical manifestations include an eczema-like rash with neutropenia and thrombocytopenia.[10] The syndrome is quickly reversed with intravenous lipid preparations or oral ingestion of safflower oil (10 to 15 ml/day). Topical application of safflower oil (10 to 15 ml TID) is also effective.

PROTEIN REQUIREMENTS

The daily protein requirements are usually estimated at first and measured later, if necessary. The recommended intake of protein is as follows:[11]

Minimum Intake: 0.54 gm/kg/day

Recommended Intake: 0.8 gm/kg/day

Catabolic States: 1.2–1.6 gm/kg/day

These estimates are limited because of the variability in protein breakdown in individual patients in the ICU. The protein catabolism can be measured in each patient as the urinary nitrogen excretion per 24 hours. The goal then is to deliver more protein than is broken down. This is accomplished by performing a nitrogen balance.

NITROGEN BALANCE

The urine is the major route of nitrogen elimination, containing two-thirds of all the nitrogen derived from protein breakdown.[11] Because protein is 16% nitrogen, each gram of urinary nitrogen (UN) represents 6.25 grams of degraded protein. The nitrogen (N) balance can be expressed as:

$$\text{N Balance (gm)} = (\text{Protein Intake}/6.25) - (\text{UN} + 4)$$

where UN is the nitrogen in a 24-hour urine collection, and the factor 4 represents the nonurinary nitrogen loss in grams. The urine collection must be obtained during steady-state conditions, when renal function is not changing.

The goal of the nitrogen balance is to keep the intake higher than the losses. The extrarenal nitrogen losses are likely to be underestimated in critically ill patients because these patients frequently have enhanced

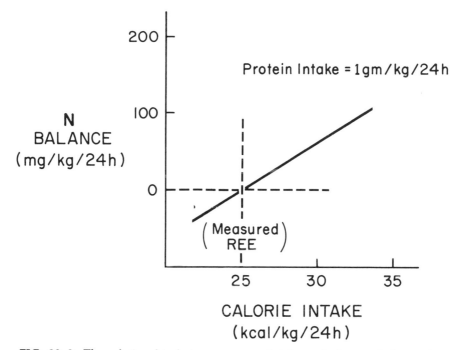

FIG. 39–2. The relationship between energy intake and nitrogen balance. Protein intake is constant.

fecal nitrogen loss from diarrhea, blood loss, or accelerated rates of mucosal sloughing. In these patients, the nonurinary nitrogen loss should be assumed to represent 6 g per day.

NITROGEN BALANCE AND ENERGY INTAKE

The graph in Figure 39–2 shows the relationship between the intake of nonprotein calories and the nitrogen balance. At a given protein intake, the nitrogen balance will become positive only when the caloric intake exceeds 25 kcal/kg/day. This graph illustrates the fact that protein will be used for calories when nonprotein calories are insufficient. When the nonprotein calories are adequate, exogenous protein can then be added to the protein pool.

ESSENTIAL VITAMINS

There are 12 essential vitamins that should be supplied each day. Table 39–3 shows the recommendations for daily supplementation in normal subjects and hospitalized patients. The daily requirements may be much higher than this in seriously ill or hypermetabolic patients. In fact, one study revealed that 25% of adult males on a general surgical service had laboratory evidence of deficiencies in at least one of the essential vita-

TABLE 39–3.	RECOMMENDED DAILY DOSES OF VITAMINS	
Vitamin	IV Dose*	RDA
A	3300	4000 IU
D	200	400 IU
E	10	15 IU
C	100	45 mg
Thiamine	3	1.5 mg
Riboflavin	3.6	1.8 mg
Niacin	40	19 mg
Pantothenate	15	10 mg
Pyridoxine	4	2 mg
B_{12}	5	3 mcg
Folate	400	400 mcg
Biotin	60	200 mcg

*Multivitamin preparations for parenteral use. A statement by the Nutrition Advisory Group. JPEN 1979; 3:258–262.

mins.[12] More disturbing was the finding that intravenous replacement therapy failed to correct the abnormal laboratory values in 40% of the patients, even when higher than normal doses were given.[12]

The vitamin deficiencies are most prevalent with vitamins A, C, E, and folate,[12] and thiamine deficiency may be more common than suspected.[13] The assays and normal reference levels for many of the vitamins are listed in the Appendix.

FOLATE

The recommended folate requirement is 400 mcg/day in normal subjects but there are no published recommendations for critically ill patients. Folate requirements may be increased in sepsis and following surgery.[14] Folate deficiency can develop within a few days of admission to the ICU,[14] and the first sign is usually a decrease in platelets. Serum folate levels may be normal and the diagnosis may require a bone marrow biopsy to look for megaloblastic changes.[14] Daily replacement of folate in the usual recommended doses may not be sufficient to prevent the depletion.[13]

THIAMINE

Thiamine is a component of the enzyme thiamine pyrophosphate (TPP), which is involved in glucose metabolism. The usual daily requirement in adults is up to 1.5 mg,[12] but the requirement in ICU patients is not known. There may be enhanced thiamine requirements in patients with sepsis and other states of hypermetabolism.[15] Little is stored in the

TABLE 39–4. DAILY ALLOWANCE FOR TRACE ELEMENTS IN THE ICU*	
Trace Element	**Intravenous Dose**
Chromium	10–15 mcg
Copper	0.5–1.5 mg
Iodine	1–2 mcg/kg
Iron	1–2.5 mg
Manganese	0.15–0.8 mg
Molybdenum	20 mcg
Selenium	30–200 mcg
Zinc	2.5–4 mg

*From Shenkin A. Trace elements in intensive care. Intensive Crit Care Digest 1988; 7:20–23.

body, so supplementation must begin soon after admission to the ICU. Thiamine deficiency is not restricted to alcoholics and can develop in poorly nourished patients who are suddenly presented with a glucose load after admission. The enhanced rate of glycolysis will exhaust the stores of thiamine to generate TPP.

There are three clinical manifestations of thiamine deficiency: (1) beriberi heart disease, (2) Wernicke's encephalopathy, and (3) lactic acidosis. The encephalopathy is the most common presentation of thiamine deficiency. It is often associated with ocular findings, particularly nystagmus and lateral gaze paralysis.[16] Other signs of encephalopathy, such as confusion, are present but non-specific.

The transketolase activity in red blood cells is the diagnostic test for thiamine deficiency. This enzyme requires TPP as a co-factor and the activity is quickly restored after thiamine replacement begins, so it should be checked as soon as the diagnosis is considered (see Appendix for the normal levels). The ocular findings may resolve within a few hours of receiving small doses (1 to 3 mg) of thiamine, but the mental status may never fully recover.[16]

ESSENTIAL TRACE ELEMENTS

Trace elements are gaining more attention because of the potential for deficiencies in the ICU patient population. There are nine trace elements that are considered essential (i.e., associated with a deficiency syndrome) and these are listed in Table 39–4. The intravenous maintenance doses in Table 39–4 are meant as general guidelines only because the daily maintenance doses for the ICU population is unknown. A few of the substances that you should be aware of are mentioned next.[17–18]

CHROMIUM

Chromium is a cofactor for the action of insulin.[18] A deficiency of chromium can produce insulin resistance and progressive hyperglycemia. Chromium is commonly added to enteral feeding solutions and is included in mineral packs used in parenteral nutrition regimens. Serum chromium levels are normally 0.04 to 0.35 mcg/ml.[17]

The incidence of chromium deficiency in the ICU is not known but insulin resistance is not uncommon in patients who remain in the hospital for prolonged periods of time. We have recently discovered two patients with low serum chromium levels in the surgical ICU. Both developed increasing insulin requirements while receiving intravenous nutrition with daily chromium supplements. Neither patient was septic and both were receiving human insulin to minimize the risk for insulin antibodies. I mention this to highlight the fact that chromium deficiency is a real phenomenon in patients with insulin resistance. The next few years might uncover the true incidence of this mineral deficiency in hospitalized patients.

SELENIUM

Selenium is a cofactor for glutathione peroxidase, an enzyme that converts hydrogen peroxide to water and thereby limits formation of the highly reactive hydroxyl ion that produces lipid peroxidation and promotes cell damage (see Chapter 25, Figure 25–4). Selenium deficiency should theoretically increase the risk for oxygen toxicity but the only documented manifestations of selenium deficiency are a cardiomyopathy and a skeletal muscle myopathy.[19]

The selenium content of many enteral feeding formulas is below the recommended daily requirement.[20] The recommended daily dose of selenium is 50 mcg/day,[20] which can be given intravenously as sodium selenite.

ZINC

Zinc deficiency may be common in the ICU because of the prevalence of predisposing factors such as diarrhea, diuresis, malnutrition, alcoholism, chronic renal failure, burns, and chronic debilitating diseases.[21] Zinc is involved in nucleic acid synthesis and lymphocyte transformation, and the deficiency syndrome increases susceptibility to infection. The diagnosis requires a decrease in plasma zinc levels, although the magnitude of decrease required to produce the deficiency syndrome may vary.[22] Effective replacement to correct deficits may require a daily dose of 4 mg elemental zinc.

COPPER

Copper deficiency has been reported as a result of intravenous nutrition without copper replacement. Because copper is excreted in the bile, continuous nasogastric suction predisposes to deficiency states.[18] The major clinical feature of copper deficiency is a pancytopenia. The anemia is hypochromic and microcytic and is a late finding. Replacement is recommended with a daily dose of 0.5 to 1.5 mg elemental copper.[18]

BIBLIOGRAPHY

GENERAL

Burzstein S, Elwyn DH, Askanazi J, Kinney JM eds. Energy metabolism, indirect calorimetry, and nutrition. Baltimore: Williams & Wilkins, 1989.

Proceedings of the First International Workshop on Nutrition and Metabolism in Hospital Nutrition. JPEN 1987; 11(Suppl) (Sep–Oct).

Weissman C ed. Nutritional support in the critically ill patient. Critical Care Clinics. Philadelphia: W.B. Saunders, (Jan) 1987.

REFERENCES

ENERGY AND PROTEIN REQUIREMENTS

1. Jequier E. Measurement of energy expenditure in clinical nutritional assessment. JPEN, 1987; 11(Suppl):86S–89S.
2. Westenskow DR, Schipke CA, Raymond JL, et al. Calculation of metabolic expenditure and substrate utilization from gas exchange measurements. JPEN 1988; 12:20–24.
3. Long CL, Schaffel N, Geiger JW, et al. Metabolic response to injury and illness: Estimation of energy and protein needs from indirect calorimetry and nitrogen balance. JPEN 1979; 3:452–456.
4. Weissman C, Kemper M, Askanazi J, Hyman AI, Kinney JM. Resting metabolic rate of the critically ill patient: Measured versus predicted. Anesthesiology 1986; 64:673–679.
5. Mann S, Westenskow DR, Houtchens BA. Measured and predicted caloric expenditure in the acutely ill. Crit Care Med 1985; 13:173–177.
6. Swanimar DL, Phang PT, Jones RL, et al. Twenty-four hour energy expenditure in critically ill patients. Crit Care Med 1987; 15:637–643.
7. Paauw, JD, McCamish MA, Dean RE, Ouellette TR. Assessment of caloric needs in stressed patients. J Am Coll Nutr 1984; 3:51–59.
8. Askanazi J, Carpentier YA, Elwyn DH, et al. Influence of total parenteral nutrition on fuel utilization in injury and sepsis. Ann Surg 1980; 191:40–46.
9. Stein TP. Why measure the respiratory quotient of patients on total parenteral nutrition? J Am Coll Nutr 1985; 4:501–513.
10. Linscheer WG, Vergroesen AJ. Lipids. In: Shils ME, Young VR eds. Modern nutrition in health and disease. 7th ed. Philadelphia: Lea & Febiger, 1988; 72–107.
11. Munro HN, Crim MC. The proteins and amino acids. In: Shils ME, Young VR eds. Modern nutrition in health and disease. 7th ed. Philadelphia: Lea & Febiger, 1988; 1–37.

VITAMINS AND TRACE ELEMENTS

12. Dempsey DT, Mullen JL, Rombeau JL, et al. Treatment effects of parenteral vitamins in total parenteral nutrition patients. JPEN 1987; *11*:229–237.
13. Campillo B, Zittoun J, de Gialluly E. Prophylaxis of folate deficiency in acutely ill patients: Results of a randomized clinical trial. Intensive Care Med 1988; *14*:640–645.
14. Beard M, Hatipov C, Hamer J. Acute onset of folate deficiency in patients under intensive care. Crit Care Med 1980; *8*:500–503.
15. McConachie I, Haskew A. Thiamine status after major trauma. Intensive Care Med 1988; *14*:628–631.
16. Reuler JB, Girard DE, Cooney TG. Wernicke's encephalopathy. NEJM 1985; *312*:1035–1038.
17. Shenkin A. Trace elements in intensive care. Intensive Care Digest 1988; *7*:20–23.
18. Aggett PJ. Physiology and metabolism of essential trace elements: An outline. Clin Endocrinol Metab 1985; *14*:513–543.
19. Neve J, Vertongen F, Molle L. Selenium deficiency. Clin Endocrinol Metab 1985; *14*:629–656.
20. Martin RF, Young VR, Janghorbani M. Selenium content of enteral formulas. JPEN 1986; *10*:213–215.
21. Prasad AS. Clinical, endocrinological and biochemical effects of zinc deficiency. Clin Endocrinol Metab 1985; *14*:567–589.
22. Takagi Y, Okada A, Itakura T, Kawashama Y. Clinical studies on zinc metabolism during total parenteral nutrition as related to zinc deficiency. JPEN 1986; *10*:195–201.

40

ENTERAL NUTRITION

When oral feeding is not possible, liquid feeding formulas can be placed in the stomach or small bowel whenever possible, to allow nutrient substrates to be processed in the normal fashion.[1] The presence of nutrients in the bowel lumen has several benefits in addition to nutrient absorption. One of these is the trophic effects of enteral feeding on the mucosal barrier that isolates luminal organisms from the bloodstream. This is receiving much attention because the bowel is now being recognized as a common source of sepsis in critically ill patients. This chapter will begin with an introduction to trophism before tackling the more practical issues in enteral nutrition.

TROPHISM AND SEPSIS

One of the more convincing arguments in support of enteral feedings over intravenous nutrition is the fact that complete bowel rest produces atrophy of the intestinal mucosa.[1,2] The degenerative changes in the bowel wall appear after just a few days of bowel rest and the atrophic changes progress despite the administration of full intravenous nutrition.[2] The influence of luminal nutrients on the structure of the bowel mucosa is shown in Figure 40–1. The photomicrographs in this figure are taken from an animal study examining the influence of protein-calorie malnutrition on the small bowel mucosa.[3] Panel A shows the normal mucosa of the small bowel with numerous fingerlike projections extending out into the bowel lumen. These projections are called microvilli and they increase the surface area for nutrient absorption. Panel B shows the mucosal changes that appear after one week of a diet deficient in protein and calories. The degenerative changes range from

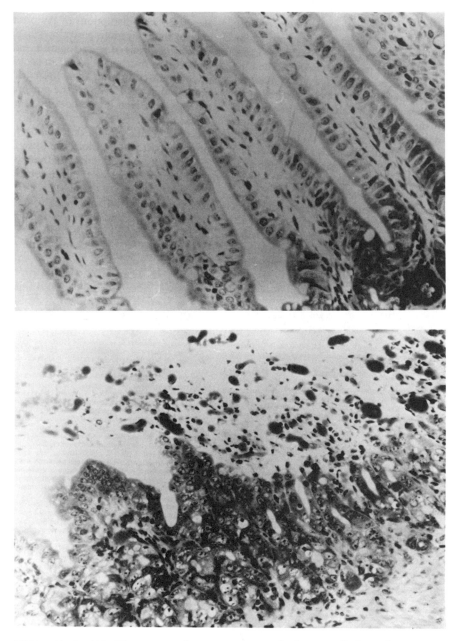

FIG. 40–1. (A) The normal appearance of the small bowel mucosa. (B) The mucosal changes after 1 week of a protein-deficient diet. From Deitch EA, et al. Ann Surg 1986; *205*:681–690.

shortening and atrophy of the microvilli to total disruption of the surface architecture. This kind of disruption is not desirable in any circumstance.

The degenerative changes in the bowel mucosa are presumably caused by the absence of nutrients in the bowel lumen that are normally taken up by mucosal cells and used for energy. Proteins may play an important part in this process and glutamine has been identified as a primary fuel for the surface epithelium.[4] Enteral feedings also may stimulate the release of trophic substances (biliary IgA, etc.) and indirectly promote mucosal growth.[2]

The mucosal disruption that develops when luminal nutrients are removed will result in malabsorption when feeding resumes. This explains the phenomenon of "refeeding diarrhea" seen after prolonged periods of bowel rest, and emphasizes the need to continue enteral feedings in any volume possible to limit the refeeding syndrome.

TRANSLOCATION

The bowel mucosa also serves as a protective barrier to isolate the pathogens in the bowel lumen from the systemic circulation.[2] When this barrier is disrupted (like it is in Figure 40–1B), enteric pathogens can invade the mucosa and gain access to the bloodstream. This process is called translocation and it may be the most important source of occult sepsis in seriously ill patients.[2-5] Translocation is considered to be the initial step that leads to a syndrome called the "multi-organ failure syndrome."[5] This syndrome has a high mortality considered by some to be the leading cause of death in critically ill patients.[5]

The role played by luminal nutrients maintaining the mucosal barrier and preventing translocation is not known at present. However, this area points to a "non-nutritive" function of enteral feedings as part of an antibacterial defense system that helps limit sepsis in the seriously ill. To summarize the observations in this area:

> Enteral feedings can maintain the absorptive function of the intestinal mucosa and may help to maintain the mucosal barrier that isolates enteric pathogens from the systemic circulation. These non-nutritive effects may be as important as the nutritional benefits of enteral feedings.

GUIDELINES FOR TUBE FEEDINGS

The following recommendations for tube feedings are taken from an official statement of the American Society of Parenteral and Enteral Nutrition.[1]

INDICATIONS

In the absence of contraindications, full enteral support is recommended in the following situations.

1. Malnourished patients with inadequate oral intake for 5 days.
2. Well nourished patients with inadequate oral intake for 7 to 10 days.
3. Patients with full-thickness burns.
4. Following massive (up to 90%) small bowel resection.
5. Enterocutaneous fistulas with a low output (less than 500 ml/day).

After small bowel resection, enteral nutrients are important to help the small bowel mucosa regenerate. The specific benefit from enteral feedings in burns is not clear at present but there is some evidence that early and aggressive enteral feeding limits sepsis and massive protein loss from the bowel in burn patients.[1]

CONTRAINDICATIONS

Enteral feeding in any amount is contraindicated in the following conditions.
1. Clinical shock
2. Complete bowel obstruction
3. Intestinal ischemia
4. Ileus
5. When the patient or legal guardian does not desire nutritional support and this action is in accordance with hospital policy and existing laws

The following conditions are contraindications to full enteral support but not necessarily to partial enteral support.
1. Partial bowel obstruction
2. Severe, unrelenting diarrhea
3. Enterocutaneous fistulas with an output over 500 ml/day
4. Severe pancreatitis or pseudocyst

The conditions listed here can be given low volume enteral feeding in selected cases. The goal of low volume enteral feeding is not necessarily to provide calories but to help maintain the integrity of the bowel mucosa.

NASOENTERAL TUBE FEEDING

Tube feedings are usually administered via specialized tubes inserted through the nose and advanced into the stomach or duodenum. The original feeding tubes were large-bore (14 to 16-French) rigid tubes placed in the stomach. The newer feeding tubes are narrower (8 French), more flexible, and are available in longer lengths for intubation of the small bowel.[6] The newer feeding tubes are designed to improve patient comfort and reduce the risk for reflux and aspiration pneumonia.[7] The major drawback of the small-bore tubes is the risk for silent tracheal intubation and pneumothorax.[8,9]

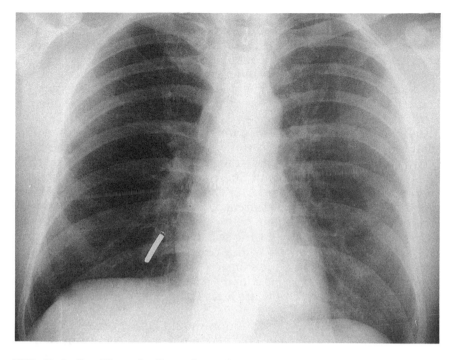

FIG. 40–2. Small bore feeding tube in the lower lobe of the right lung. Courtesy of Dr. Wallace Miller, M.D.

TUBE PLACEMENT

The length needed to reach the stomach from the entrance to the nares can be estimated by measuring the distance from the tip of the nose to the earlobe and then from the ear to the xiphoid process.[10] A rigid stylet is required to insert the flexible small-bore feeding tubes and this stylet facilitates passage of the tubes through the larynx and into the upper airways. The narrow tubes can pass easily around the inflated cuffs on tracheal tubes. Patients who require enteral feedings often have a depressed mental status and will not cough or develop other signs of tracheal intubation. Therefore, tubes can be advanced deep into the lungs without warning and can be advanced into the pleural space.

CHECKING TUBE POSITION

The tendency for intubation of the lungs is demonstrated in the chest film shown in Figure 40–2. The opaque end of a small-bore feeding tube is evident in the right lung. This film was obtained as a routine practice after tube insertion in an asymptomatic patient. The lack of symptoms from tracheal placement is not uncommon in ICU patients and this highlights the need to perform some test to verify tube position after each insertion and before feeding commences.

Chest Films. The standard practice is to obtain chest films after each insertion. Although this can verify thoracic placement of feeding tubes (like the film in Figure 40–2), the converse is not true. That is, a feeding tube that is situated below the dome of the diaphragm shadow can still be in the chest because the posterior costophrenic sulcus runs down as far as the fourth lumbar vertebral body.[9] A lateral view is necessary for accurate localization of tube placement. However, lateral views are not obtained easily at the bedside.

Auscultation. A popular method for evaluating tube position is to auscultate the left upper quadrant while insufflating air through the tube. A gurgling sound in the subcostal region is taken as evidence that the tube is in the stomach. However, this can be misleading because sounds emanating from a tube in the lower chest can be transmitted to the left upper quadrant.[9] At present, auscultation is not considered reliable for documenting gastric placement.[9]

Gastric pH. Aspiration of gastric secretions can help if the secretions have an acid pH. Secretions with a pH of 3 or below can be used as evidence that the tube is in the stomach.[8] However, aspiration of gastric secretions is often not possible with the small-bore feeding tubes because they collapse when suction is applied. This limits the value of the aspiration test.

Summary. Some test of tube position should be performed after each insertion. If an aspirate can be obtained, a pH of 3 or below can be used as evidence for gastric placement. Otherwise, a chest x-ray should be obtained after each insertion. Single views are acceptable in most cases. At the present time, the risk for placing tubes in the posterior costophrenic gutter is considered too small to justify routine lateral chest films after each insertion.

THE FEEDING SITE

The liquid feeding formulas can be delivered directly into the stomach or duodenum. The choice of feeding site is a matter of personal preference because there is little evidence to support one site over the other.

Gastric Feeding. Intragastric feeding takes advantage of the reservoir capacity of the stomach and the dilutional effect of gastric secretions. Gastric secretions can mix with the feeding solutions and reduce osmolality and the risk for diarrhea. In addition, the buffering properties of the feeding formulas are considered effective for prophylaxis against stress ulcer bleeding (see Chapter 5). Finally, gastric distention from feedings will stimulate the release of trophic hormones like biliary IgA that promote the integrity of the bowel mucosa.

The major disadvantage of gastric feeding is the risk for regurgitation and pulmonary aspiration. This is reported in 1 to 38% of patients,[7] although the true incidence is hard to document. The risk varies in different patient populations, being the highest in patients who are comatose or paralysed.

Duodenal Feeding. The proposed advantage of duodenal placement is reduced risk for reflux and aspiration pneumonia. However, there is no evidence to support this theory at the present time. The drawbacks of duodenal placement include difficulty advancing the tubes through the pylorus and increased risk for diarrhea. If duodenal placement is desired, the following steps may help to facilitate transpyloric passage of the tubes.

1. Insert the tube a length of at least 85 cm from the nares (so the tube will coil in the stomach), and wait for 24 hours. One-third of tubes may pass into the duodenum at this time.[11]
2. If the tube does not pass spontaneously after 24 hours, place the patient in the right lateral decubitus position for a few hours and check tube position with a chest x-ray.
3. For patients with gastric atony (particularly from diabetes), metoclopramide (10 mg given 15 minutes prior to tube placement) may facilitate transpyloric migration.[12]
4. If all fails, fluoroscopy will be necessary.

Recommendation. I prefer gastric feedings for the many advantages (particularly trophic effects) and because there is little evidence to support the reduced risk of aspiration with duodenal placement. We often add food coloring to the tube feedings in intubated patients and monitor the color of the upper airway secretions for evidence of aspiration.

STARTING TUBE FEEDINGS

The first concern is to determine if tube feeding will be safe at the desired volume and rate. The next step involves the pattern of feeding and the use of starter regimens.

GASTRIC RETENTION

A test infusion is always indicated prior to feeding to determine the safety of gastric feedings. A volume of water or saline equivalent to the desired hourly feeding volume is selected and infused over one hour. The feeding tube is then clamped for 30 minutes and the residual volume is aspirated. If the volume is less than 50% of the infused volume, gastric feeding is considered appropriate.[10] However, it may be wise to start at small volumes when the residual volume is significant. When performing this test, do not give the test volume as a bolus because this produces acute gastric distension that can delay gastric emptying and produce a residual volume that is greater than would be seen after slow infusion.

FEEDING PATTERN

The popular method for delivery is continuous infusion over 16 hours each day. Intermittent infusions more closely mimic the normal process of eating but the volumes required to meet daily requirements are large and this increases the risk for aspiration and diarrhea. Continuous infusion is better tolerated and also produces more weight gain and positive nitrogen balance.[13]

STARTER REGIMENS

The traditional approach to tube feeding begins with "starter regimens" that use a dilute formula and slow infusion rate at first and gradually advance the volume and infusion rate over the following few days until the desired intake is achieved. The rationale here is to allow the GI tract time to regenerate after a period of bowel rest. The drawback to starter regimens is the time required to reach full nutritional support, particularly if the patient is malnourished at the outset.

The value of starter regimens as a routine practice for all patients has been questioned by two clinical studies, one performed in normal subjects[14] and the other in patients with inflammatory bowel disease.[15] Both studies report that full nasogastric feeding could be delivered immediately (without a starter regimen) with no apparent ill effects.

Recommendations. Starter regimens should not be necessary for gastric feedings because the gastric secretions should dilute the feeding formula and improve tolerance. Starter regimens are reserved for patients with significant gastric residual, prolonged bowel rest, or depressed mental status. If a starter regimen is used for gastric feedings, it should be possible to advance to full feeding in 24 hours. Starter regimens are to be used for all small bowel feedings.

GASTROSTOMY

A gastrostomy is a fistulous tract between the stomach and the abdominal wall. These tracts are used for chronic enteral feeding, particularly in patients who repeatedly extubate themselves. Gastrostomies were also believed to reduce the risk of aspiration compared to nasogastric feedings, but this does not seem to be the case.[17] Gastrostomies can be created surgically, or with the aid of an endoscope.[18] Both methods have an associated morbidity, and the choice of procedure may be dictated by the experience at each hospital.

PERCUTANEOUS ENDOSCOPIC GASTROSTOMY (PEG)

The percutaneous method was introduced in 1979 as a less expensive alternative to surgical gastrostomy. Figure 40–3 illustrates a recently developed PEG technique using a Foley catheter.[19] An endoscope is passed into the stomach and the stomach is distended with air to bring the anterior wall close to the abdominal wall. The light beam from the endoscope can be seen on the abdomen and used to mark the point where the stomach is close to the surface. A 9-French introducer catheter and sheath is inserted percutaneously using the Seldinger technique

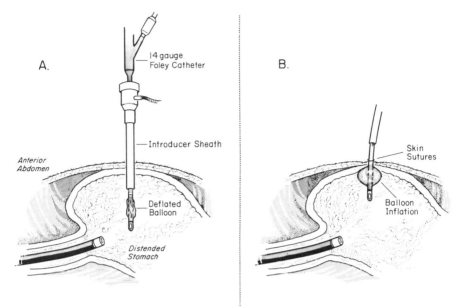

FIG. 40–3. Percutaneous endoscopic gastrostomy (PEG) using an introducer sheath and a Foley catheter.

(see Chapter 4) and a Foley catheter is introduced through the sheath into the stomach. The balloon on the Foley catheter is inflated, and the catheter is pulled back until taut and then sutured to the abdominal wall.

The PEG technique is reported as safe if done by experienced personnel.[19] The reported incidence of complications from PEGs varies from 2 to 75%.[10] The most feared complication is spillage of bowel contents into the peritoneum, because this can be fatal.[18] Because of the potential for complications, gastrostomy should only be considered if there is an obstruction in the esophagus, or if feedings will be necessary for prolonged periods of time.[18]

JEJUNOSTOMY

The jejunostomy takes advantage of the fact that small bowel motility is restored immediately after abdominal surgery. The jejunum can be used for immediate postoperative nutrition after surgery on the esophagus, stomach, biliary tree, liver, spleen, and pancreas. There may be little risk for aspiration, although this has not been studied. The only contraindications are regional enteritis, radiation enteritis, ileus, and bowel obstruction distal to the feeding tube.

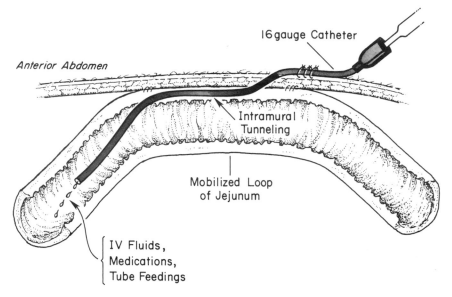

FIG. 40–4. Needle catheter jejunostomy.

NEEDLE CATHETER JEJUNOSTOMY

The jejunostomy is performed as a "complimentary" procedure at the end of the laparotomy and only takes 5 to 10 minutes.[20] Figure 40–4 illustrates the course of a jejunostomy catheter. A loop of jejunum is mobilized to the anterior abdominal wall. A 14-gauge needle is used to create a tunnel in the small bowel mucosa, and a 16-gauge jejunostomy catheter is inserted through the tunnel and advanced 30 to 45 cm within the bowel lumen. The catheter is passed out to the skin surface and sutured in place, while the intraperitoneal portion is secured to the underside of the abdominal wall.

Feeding Method. The small bowel does not have the reservoir capacity of the stomach and diarrhea is common unless starter regimens are used. An isotonic feeding formula is usually diluted to one-quarter the original strength, and feeding is started at 25 ml/hr.[21] The infusion rate is advanced 25 ml/hr every 12 hours until the target infusion rate is reached.[20] At this point, the concentration of the feeding solution is gradually increased over the next few days. Using this method, full nutrition can be achieved after 4 days.[21] Each feeding is given over a 6-hour period.

Complications. The potential for serious complications is high, with one study reporting an 8% mortality rate from the procedure![22] The most common complications are diarrhea and occluded feeding tubes. The present recommendation is to use jejunostomies as a temporary measure only.

ENTERAL DIET FORMULATIONS

The list of enteral feeding formulas is growing each year. The following characteristics will help select an appropriate formula for each individual patient.[23]

CALORIC DENSITY

The caloric density of each formula is determined primarily by the carbohydrate content of the formula. Some examples are listed below.

1. 1.0 kcal/ml   (Osmolite, Isocal, and Ensure)
2. 1.5 kcal/ml   (Ensure Plus)
3. 2.0 kcal/ml   (Isocal HCN and Osmolite HN)

The formulas that provide 1 kcal/ml are isotonic to plasma and are preferred for small bowel feedings. The higher density formulas are favored when fluid intake must be limited. The high density formulas should be placed in the stomach, whenever possible, to dilute them with gastric secretions and reduce the risk for diarrhea.

OSMOLALITY

The osmolality of feeding formulas varies from 300 to 1100 mOsm/kg H_2O and is determined by the caloric density. Although there is no clear relationship between osmolality and diarrhea,[6] it may be wise to limit osmolality in patients with diarrhea by placing the feeding in the stomach or using isotonic formulas.

PROTEIN CONTENT

The average American diet provides about 10% of the calories as protein. Most enteral formulas provide up to 20% of the total calories as protein. High protein formulas provide 22 to 24% of the total calories as protein and are popular for trauma and burn victims. There is no evidence that the high protein feeding formulas improve outcome.

1. Protein < 20% of calories (most formulas)
2. Protein > 20% of calories (Sustacal, Traumacal)

PROTEIN COMPLEXITY

Intact protein is more difficult to absorb than hydrolysed protein and therefore the latter is popular in malabsorption and rapid transit disorders (e.g., short bowel syndrome). There is some evidence that peptide-based formulas can reduce diarrhea from tube feeding[16] but this needs further verification.

1. Intact protein (Isocal, Osmolite, Ensure)
2. Hydrolysed protein (Vital, Reabolan)

FAT COMPLEXITY

Fat is provided as long chain triglycerides (LCTs) or medium chain triglycerides (MCTs). MCTs are easier to absorb than LCTs and are favored in patients with malabsorption. Most enteral solutions contain LCTs, but some have a mix of both (e.g., Isocal and Osmolite).

PLANT FIBER

Plant fiber is not a single substance but a variety of polysaccharides that resist common routes of carbohydrate metabolism. There are two classes of fiber.[24]

1. **Fermentable fiber.** These substances (cellulose and pectin) are metabolized by intestinal bacteria to produce short-chain fatty acids (acetate, proprionate, and butyrate) which can be used as an energy source by the bowel mucosa.[24] This type of fiber delays gastric emptying and can be beneficial in treating diarrhea.

2. **Nonfermentable fiber.** These substances (lignins) are not degraded by intestinal bacteria and they can exert an osmotic force that draws water into the bowel lumen. This type of fiber increases stool bulk and may help to treat constipation.

There are two commercial tube feeding products with added fiber at present, and these are listed below. Each has equivalent amounts of both fiber types and neither is useful, in theory, for constipation or diarrhea.

1. Enrich—12.5 gm fiber/L
2. Jevity—13.5 gm fiber/L

Fiber-containing solutions are recommended for chronic tube feedings although the benefit is not documented. Fiber is not recommended for patients with liver failure because fermentable fiber promotes the proliferation of bacteria in the colon. Fiber can be added to feedings in the form of Metamucil (nonfermentable fiber) or Kaopectate (fermentable fiber).

CLASSIFICATIONS

Liquid feeding formulas are classified according to the complexity of the nutrients,[23] or ease of absorption. The more salient features of enteral tube feedings are listed below:

Blenderized Formulas. These are liquid forms of table food and they cause diarrhea in lactose intolerant adults.

Indications: Popular for elderly patients with normal GI tracts who cannot eat or feed themselves.
Examples: Compleat B (1 kcal/ml)

Lactose-Free Formulas. These are the standard feeding formulas used in hospitalized patients and are better tolerated by adults than the blenderized formulas.

Indications: Patients with a normal GI tract who will not tolerate lactose.
Examples: 1 kcal/ml . . . Isocal, Ensure, Sustacal, and Osmolite
1.5 kcal/ml . . . Sustacal HC and Ensure Plus
2 kcal/ml . . . Magnacal and Isocal HCN

Chemically-Defined Formulas. These formulas contain hydrolysed protein instead of intact protein to facilitate absorption.

Indications: Patients with impaired ability to absorb nutrients.
Examples: Criticare HN, Vital HN, Citrotein, Isotein, Travasorb HN, and Precision HN

Elemental Formulas. The elemental formulas contain crystalline amino acids. Most of the nutrients are easily ingested, and are completely absorbed in the first part of the small bowel.

Indications: Patients with limited absorptive capacity. Popular for jejunostomy feedings.
Examples: Vivonex and Vivonex T.E.N. (1 kcal/ml)

SPECIAL FORMULATIONS

The following conditions have specialized feeding formulas to satisfy the specific requirements of each.
1. **Hepatic Encephalopathy.** The feeding formulas for this disorder are rich in branched chain amino acids (BCAA). The rationale here is that hepatic encephalopathy is the result of the accumulation of aromatic amino acids in the brain. BCAAs inhibit aromatic uptake across the blood-brain barrier.
Examples: Hepaticaid and Travenol Hepatic.
2. **Trauma/Stress.** These formulas are also rich in BCAA (50% of total amino acids compared to the normal 25 to 30%). The rationale here is that the hormonal response to stress promotes hydrolysis of branched chain amino acids in skeletal muscle and this prevents degradation of other proteins for energy. These formulas have a caloric density of 1 kcal/ml and are very hyperosmolar (up to 900 mOsm/kg H_2O).
Examples: Trauma-Aid HBC.
3. **Renal Failure.** The renal failure formulas are rich in essential amino acids and have no added electrolytes. The rationale here is that degradation of essential amino aids will limit the increase in blood urea nitrogen because the nitrogen is recycled to the synthesis of nonessential amino acids.
Examples: 1. Travasorb Renal, 2. Amino Aid

4. **Respiratory Failure.** Low carbohydrate, high fat enteral formulas are used to limit CO_2 production in patients with severe lung disease. These formulas should provide at least 50% of the total calories as fat. The main drawback of this diet is the malabsorption of fat and steatorrhea.

Examples: Pulmocare

COMPLICATIONS

The common complications of tube feedings are diarrhea and reflux of gastric contents into the upper airways.[25] Diarrhea is presented in detail in Chapter 6 and is summarized only briefly here.

DIARRHEA

Diarrhea occurs in 10 to 20% of patients receiving enteral tube feedings. The diarrhea is partly caused by osmotic forces and partly caused by malabsorption. Tube feeding diarrhea is not bloody and is not accompanied by signs of sepsis. When the diagnosis is uncertain, the following measures might help:
1. Avoid using agents that decrease bowel motility (e.g., paregoric and lomotil). This is unlikely to remedy the situation, and it can produce problems by promoting ileus.
2. Use isotonic solutions and gastric installation if possible. Eliminate any hypertonic medications added to the feeding formulas.
3. Discontinue any magnesium-containing antacids or other medications that can promote diarrhea (e.g., theophylline).
4. Consider using a fermentable fiber like pectin. This fiber delays gastric emptying, and thus may help by allowing the stomach to more effectively decrease the osmolality of the feeding solutions. Pectin can be added to feeding solutions as Kaopectate (30 ml BID or TID) or as unprocessed apple juice (100 ml per feeding bag).
5. If small bowel feedings are being used, decrease the infusion rate by 50%, and slowly increase over the next 3 to 4 days. Try not to dilute the formula because this will increase the water content of the stool.
6. Start peripheral (protein sparing) nutrition to prevent negative nitrogen balance while the enteral feeding is being adjusted.
7. DO NOT STOP THE TUBE FEEDING, as this will further aggravate the diarrhea when you wish to start the enteral feeding at a future time.

See Chapter 6 for more information on the approach to nosocomial diarrhea.

ASPIRATION

The risk for reflux of gastric contents into the upper airways is over-emphasized. The reported incidence of documented aspiration varies from 1 to 44%.[16] Although aspiration is felt to be reduced when feeding tubes are placed in the small bowel, this has not been confirmed. For patients at risk for aspiration (eg., comatose patients), the addition of food coloring to the tube feedings can be valuable for detecting aspiration by the change in color of the respiratory secretions.

MECHANICAL PROBLEMS

The narrow feeding tubes can become obstructed in about 10% of patients.[25] The usual cause is a feeding formula that has coalesced to form an occlusive plug. This problem is reduced by flushing the tubes with 10 ml of warm water before and after each infusion period.[10] When formula is not infusing, the tubes are filled with water and plugged. If a tube becomes obstructed, there are several methods that have proven useful. The fluids used with some success include such scientific solutions as Coke Classic, Mountain Dew, and Adolf's Meat Tenderizer (papain). Viokase seems to be particularly effective when given in the following mixture: Crush one tablet of Viokase and one tablet bicarbonate (324 mg) and add 5 ml tap water.[25] Inject this mixture into the tube and clamp the tube for 5 minutes. If this is unsuccessful, the feeding tube will have to be replaced.

BIBLIOGRAPHY

Rombeau JL, Caldwell MD eds. Enteral and tube feeding. 1st ed., Philadelphia: W.B. Saunders, Co., 1984.

REFERENCES

REVIEWS

1. A.S.P.E.N. Board of Directors. Guidelines for the use of enteral nutrition in the adult patient. JPEN 1987; *11*:435–439.

TROPHIC INFLUENCES

2. Wilmore DW, Smith RJ, O'Dweyer ST, et al. The gut: A central organ after surgical stress. Surgery 1988; *104*:917–923.
3. Deitch EA, Wintertron J, Li MA, Berg R. The gut is a portal of entry or bacteremia. Ann Surg 1987; *205*:681–690.
4. Fox AD, Kripke SA, Berman JR, Settle RG, Rombeau JL. Reduction of severity of enterocolitis by glutamine-supplemented enteral diets. Surg Forum 987; *38*:43–44.

5. Cerra FB. Metabolic manifestations of multiple systems organ failure. Crit Care Clin 1989; 5:119–132.

NASOENTERAL FEEDING

6. Ramos SM, Lindine P. Inexpensive, safe and simple nasoenteral intubation—an alternative for the cost conscious. JPEN 1986; 10:78–81.
7. Metheny NA, Eisenberg P, Spies M. Aspiration pneumonia in patients fed through nasoenteral tubes. Heart Lung 1986; 15:256–261.
8. Raff MH, Cho S, Dale R. A technique for positioning nasoenteral feeding tubes. JPEN 1987; 11:210–213.
9. Valentine RJ, Turner WW, Jr. Pleural complications of naso-enteric feeding tubes. JPEN 1985; 9:605–607.
10. Rombeau JL, Caldwell MD, Forlaw L, Geunter PA eds. Atlas of nutritional support techniques. Boston: Little, Brown & Co., 1989; 77–106.
11. Rees, RGP, Payne-James JJ, King C, Silk DBA. Spontaneous transpyloric passage and performance of 'fine-bore' polyurethane feeding tubes: a controlled clinical trial. JPEN 1988; 12:469–472.
12. Whatley K, Turner WW, Dey M, Leonard J, Guthrie M. When does metoclo600promide facilitate transpyloric intubations? JPEN 1984; 8:679–681.

DELIVERY METHODS

13. Jones BMJ. Enteral feeding: Techniques and administration. Gut 1986; 27(Suppl):47–50.
14. Zarlin EJ, Parmar JR, Mobarhan S, Clapper M. Effect of enteral formula infusion rate, osmolality, and chemical composition upon clinical tolerance and carbohydrate absorption in normal subjects. JPEN 1986; 10:588–590.
15. Rees RGP, Keohane PP, Grimble GK, Forst PG, Attrill H, Silk DBA. Elemental diet administered nasogastrically without starter regimens to patients with inflammatory bowel disease. JPEN 1986; 10:258–262.
16. Koruda M, Geunther P, Rombeau J. Enteral nutrition in the critically ill. Crit Care Clin 1987; 3:133–153.

TUBE ENTEROSTOMIES

17. Hassett JM, Sunby C, Flint LM. No elimination of aspiration pneumonia in neurologically disabled patients with feeding gastrostomy. Surg Gynecol Obstet 1988; 167:383–388.
18. Gauderer MWL, Stellato TA. Gastrostomies: Evolution, techniques, indications, and complications. Current Probl Surg 1986; 23:660–719.
19. Ponsky JL, Gauderer MWL. Percutaneous endoscopic gastrostomy: Indications, limitations, techniques, and results. World J Surg 1989; 13:165–170.
20. Ryan JA, Page CP. Intrajejunal feeding: Development and current status. JPEN 1984; 8:187–198.
21. Sarr MG. Needle catheter jejunostomy: An unappreciated and misunderstood advance in the care of patients after major abdominal operations. Mayo Clin Proc 1988; 63:565–572.
22. Adams MB, Seabrook GR, Quebbemen EA, Condon RE. Jejunostomy. Arch Surg 1986; 121:236–238.

FORMULAS AND COMPLICATIONS

23. Heimburger DC, Weinsier RL. Guidelines for evaluating and categorizing enteral feeding formulas according to therapeutic equivalence. JPEN 1985; *9*:61–67.
24. Jenkins DJA. Dietary fiber. In: Shils ME, Young VR eds. Modern nutrition in health and disease. 7th ed. Philadelphia: Lea & Febiger, 1988; 52–71.
25. Marcuard CP, Segall KL, Trogdon S. Clearing obstructed feeding tubes. JPEN 1989; *13*:81–83.

chapter

41

PARENTERAL NUTRITION

The enthusiasm for total parenteral nutrition (TPN) is now being tempered by the risks of intravenous route and the benefits of the enteral route for nutrition support. This chapter will introduce you to the basic features of TPN including how to create a TPN regimen and some complications to be aware of during TPN.

INDICATIONS

The indications for TPN include any condition in which the bowel will not tolerate or process bulk nutrients. This situation most commonly occurs with bowel obstruction and bowel ischemia. The point to emphasize here is that TPN should never be used as the sole means of nutrition when the bowel is functional. This means that TPN may be inappropriate in conditions like anorexia nervosa and cancer cachexia.

BOWEL SOUNDS

Auscultation of the abdomen for bowel sounds can be misleading because the absence of bowel sounds does not mean the absence of bowel function. Bowel sounds are produced by air being propelled along the bowel and most bowel sounds originate in the stomach and colon. The small bowel, which is the site of nutrient absorption, does not contribute much to the bowel sounds because the small bowel is usually devoid of air. This means that there should be no correlation between bowel sounds and the absorptive function of the bowel. In fact, the small bowel remains functional after most operative procedures (except aortic surgery and certain types of resectional surgery) despite the absence of

TABLE 41–1. DEXTROSE SOLUTIONS			
Concentration (mg/dl)	Dextrose (gm/L)	Energy (kcal/L)	Osmolarity (mOsm/L)
10%	100	340	505
20%	200	680	1010
50%	500	1700	2525
70%	700	2380	3535

bowel sounds in the first few postoperative days. This indicates that bowel sounds should not be used to decide about TPN.

TPN SOLUTIONS

There are three elemental nutrients in TPN: (1) dextrose, (2) triglycerides, and (3) amino acids. These are available in a variety of solutions and the TPN regimen combines these solutions to meet the energy and protein needs of the patient.

DEXTROSE SOLUTIONS

Dextrose (glucose) is available in concentrations ranging from 10 to 70% (gm/L), as shown in Table 41–1. Since dextrose is not a potent energy source (3.4 kcal/gm for dextrose versus 9 kcal/gm for fat), concentrated solutions must be used to provide the needed calories. As a result, the dextrose solutions used for TPN are hyperosmolar and must be infused through large central veins.

AMINO ACID SOLUTIONS

Protein is supplied as solutions of crystalline amino acids that contain equivalent proportions of essential and non-essential amino acids. The amino acid concentration (mg/dl) varies from 3 to 10%, with the higher concentrations favored in adults who need full TPN via central veins. All are hypertonic to plasma, although the 3% amino acid mixture can be given safely via peripheral veins.

Modified amino acid formulas are available for specific clinical situations. Table 41–2 shows a special formula recommended for patients with hepatic encephalopathy, compared to a standard 7% amino acid solution. The liver failure formula is rich in branched-chain amino acids (leucine, isoleucine, and valine) and deficient in aromatic amino acids (methionine, phenylalanine, tyrosine, and tryptophan). The basis for this formula is a theory that hepatic encephalopathy is caused by an excess of aromatic amino acids and a deficit in circulating branched-chain amino acids. The other specialized formula is for patients with

TABLE 41–2. STANDARD AND SPECIALIZED AMINO ACID MIXTURE		
	7% Aminosyn	8% Hepatamine
Protein (gm/L)	70	80
Osmolality (mOsm/L)	700	785
Branched-Chain Amino Acids		
Leucine	660	1100
Isoleucine	510	900
Valine	560	840
Aromatic Amino Acids		
Phenylalanine	280	100
Tryptophan	120	66
Methionine	280	100
Tyrosine	44	—

renal failure. These latter solutions are rich in essential amino acids, which might limit azotemia because they produce less urea than the nonessential amino acids.

DEXTROSE-AMINO ACID MIXTURES

The dextrose and amino acid solutions are mixed together in equal volumes (usually 500 ml of each). These mixtures are named according to the premixed concentration of each substrate rather than the final concentration. Therefore,

> When 500 ml of 50% dextrose (D50) is added to 500 ml of 10% amino acids (A10), the final mixture is called A10–D50 even though the final concentration is A5–D25.

This is a confusing practice but it is necessary to realize this if you are to accurately define the characteristics of each TPN formula. For example, 1 L of A10–D50 contains 250 grams of dextrose and provides 850 nonprotein calories (3.4 kcal × 250 gm) whereas 1 L of D50 provides 1700 calories (twice the amount).

FAT EMULSIONS

Fat is provided as chylomicron suspensions or emulsions derived from safflower or soybean oils. These emulsions are rich in linoleic acid, the essential fatty acid that the body is unable to produce. Commercial fat emulsions are available in 10% and 20% concentrations (gm fat/100 ml) and these provide 1 kcal/ml and 2 kcal/ml, respectively. The composition of a few of the available fat emulsions is shown in Table 41–3. Note that the osmolarity of each solution is similar to that of plasma. This permits fat emulsion to be infused via peripheral veins, eliminating the risks associated with central venous cannulation.

TABLE 41–3. COMMERCIAL FAT EMULSIONS			
Emulsion	**Liposyn 10%**	**Intralipid 10%**	**Intralipid 20%**
Fat Source	Safflower Oil	Soybean Oil	Soybean Oil
Fatty Acids (%)			
Linoleic	66	50	50
Oleic	18	26	26
Linolenic	4	9	9
Palmitic	9	10	10
Kcal/ml	1.1	1.1	2.0
Osmolarity	320	260	268

Fat is infused in 250 to 500 ml aliquots, at a rate of 50 ml per hour. The chylomicrons introduced into the bloodstream are not cleared for 8 to 10 hours, so no more than one fat infusion is recommended each day. Fat cannot be combined with the dextrose-amino acid mixtures because it is insoluble in these solutions. The fat emulsions can, however, be infused along with the dextrose-amino acid solutions if Y-shaped tubing is used and each solution is introduced in a separate arm of the tubing.

Despite the value of fat emulsions as a concentrated source of calories that does not require central venous cannulation, fat is used primarily to prevent essential fatty acid deficiency. This can be accomplished by infusing 500 ml of the 10% fat emulsion twice a week. This regimen provides only 5 to 10% of the total energy needs in most adults.[2] However, when carbohydrate calories are not tolerated (as in diabetes), fat can be used to provide up to 60% of the non-protein calories in TPN.

ADDITIVES

Commercial preparations are available for electrolytes, vitamins, and trace elements, and these are added directly to the dextrose-amino acid mixtures. Table 41–4 shows one commercial additive for electrolytes and one for trace elements.

TABLE 41–4. ELECTROLYTE AND TRACE ELEMENT ADDITIVES			
Electrolytes (per 20 ml)		**Trace Elements (per ml)**	
Sodium*	45 mEq	Zinc	1.0 mg
Potassium	43 mEq	Copper	0.4 mg
Phosphate	6 mM	Manganese	0.1 mg
Magnesium	8 mEq	Chromium	4.0 mcg
Calcium	5 mEq		

*as acetate

ELECTROLYTES

Commercial electrolyte mixtures contain sodium, potassium, magnesium, calcium, and phosphorous in about half the amount recommended as the normal daily requirement. One unit volume of the electrolyte solution is added to each L of dextrose-amino acid mixture so that daily infusion of 2 L of TPN will replace normal daily electrolyte losses. Excess electrolyte losses are common in ICU patients and these must be replaced by adding additional amounts of each electrolyte to the TPN solution. Some of the crystalline amino acid solutions contain electrolytes that have been added by the manufacturer and this must be considered when ordering electrolyte additives.

VITAMINS AND TRACE ELEMENTS

A standard multivitamin preparation is added to one of the dextrose-amino acid bottles each day. These preparations are devoid of vitamin K, therefore, vitamin K must be added separately (5 mg/day). Remember that the daily requirement for vitamins has not been determined for critically ill patients so provision of daily vitamins does not eliminate the possibility of vitamin deficiencies.

Trace element mixtures usually contain zinc, copper, manganese, and chromium, like the preparation shown in Table 41–4. As with vitamin requirements, the daily requirements for trace elements in seriously ill patients is not known and routine infusion of these elements does not necessarily prevent deficiencies.

CREATING A TPN FORMULATION

The following sequence is one method for creating a TPN regimen. The steps involved in this approach are outlined in Table 41–5. The patient in this example will be a 70 kg (154 lb) adult who is not nutritionally depleted.

STEP 1. DAILY REQUIREMENTS

The first task is to estimate the daily protein and calorie needs. The methods available for this were presented in Chapter 39. For this patient, the estimated daily requirements will be 25 kcal/kg for calories and 1.4 gm/kg for protein.

Daily calories (70 kg × 25) = 1750 kcal

Protein (70 kg × 1.4) = 98 grams

TABLE 41–5.   CREATING A TPN FORMULA

Determine Daily Requirements
Calories   = 25 kcal/kg/day
Protein   = 1.4 gm/kg/day

Calculate Volume Needed for Protein Needs
A10–D50   = 50 gm protein/L
L/Day   = Daily protein needs/50 gm

Dextrose Calories Provided by A10–D50 Per Day
A10–D50   = 250 gm dextrose/L
= 3.4 kcal/gm × 250 gm/L
= 850 kcal/L from dextrose
Dextrose kcal   = 850 × daily volume of A10–D50

Lipid Volume for Remaining Caloric Needs
10% Emulsion   = 1 kcal/ml
Lipid volume   = Daily kcal needs − dextrose kcal
= mls/day

STEP 2. VOLUME OF A10–D50 TO SUPPLY PROTEIN

A standard 50% dextrose—10% amino acid mixture is used, which has 50 grams of protein per L. Therefore, the total volume needed to deliver 98 grams of protein is:

$$\text{Volume} = (98 \text{ gm}/50 \text{ gm/L})$$

$$= 1.9 \text{ L}$$

If the TPN is infused over 24 hours, the infusion rate will be:

$$\text{Infusion rate} = 1900 \text{ ml}/24 \text{ hrs}$$

$$= 81 \text{ ml/h or } 81 \text{ } \mu \text{ drops/min}$$

STEP 3: DEXTROSE CALORIES PROVIDED

The number of nonprotein calories provided by the infusion in Step 2 is then determined by multiplying the volume (1.9 L) and the amount of dextrose in 1 L of 50% dextrose (250 gm). This is the total amount of dextrose infused each day, which, when multiplied by the caloric value of dextrose (3.4 kcal/gm), yields the dextrose calories provided each day.

$$\text{Amount of dextrose infused: } 250 \text{ gm/L} \times 1.9 \text{ L}$$

$$= 475 \text{ gm}$$

$$\text{Daily calories from dextrose: } 475 \text{ gm} \times 34 \text{ kcal/gm}$$

$$= 1615 \text{ kcal}$$

$$\text{Estimated daily need: } = 1750 \text{ kcal}$$

Therefore, all but 135 calories per day will be provided by dextrose. The rest will be provided by a lipid emulsion.

STEP 4. VOLUME OF LIPID EMULSION

$$\text{Daily calories from lipid: } 135 \text{ kcal/day}$$

$$\text{Weekly lipid calories: } 135 \text{ kcal/day} \times 7 \text{ days}$$

$$= 945 \text{ kcal/week}$$

$$\text{Volume of } 10\% \text{ emulsion} = 945 \text{ ml/week}$$

Since fat emulsions are available in 500 ml aliquots, the remaining calories will be provided by infusing one 500 ml aliquot on 2 days of the week.

FORMULA: The TPN orders can be written as follows:
1. Standard TPM wth A10–D50 to infuse at 80 gtts/min
2. Add standard lytes to each L.
3. Daily multivitamins and mineral pack.
4. 10% intralipid (500 ml) on Tuesday and Thursday to run at 50 gtts/min.

STARTING TPN

It is common to see glucose intolerance when TPN is started and this can be minimized by starting the infusion at 2 mg dextrose/kg/min. This is continued for 12 to 24 hours and a step increase is made to an infusion rate of 4 to 5 mg/kg/min. This step increase is well-tolerated and it eliminates the tedium involved in gradually increasing the infusion in several small steps.

TABLE 41–6. ESTIMATING INSULIN ADDITIVE FOR TPN	
Serum Glucose During Infusion of 5% Dextrose	Amount of Insulin Per 250 gm Glucose
130 mg/dL	6 U (Regular insulin)
150	10 U
200	18 U
250	25 U

INSULIN

If the serum glucose is consistently above 200 mg/dl after TPN is started, insulin can be added directly to the dextrose-amino acid mixture. Insulin adsorbs to glass and plastic surfaces and as much as 50% of the insulin added to the TPN will be lost to the walls of the tubing and containers.[2] Albumin has been added to TPN to reduce this insulin binding, but this practice is unproven and is not recommended as a routine practice.[2]

Insulin has undesirable effects of its own and should be avoided whenever possible. Insulin inhibits lipoprotein lipase, which limits the ability to mobilize fat from adipose tissue. This prevents the body from using endogenous fuels and propagates the cycle where glucose is needed for nonprotein energy because triglycerides are unavailable. The logical solution to adding insulin to a TPN regimen is to reduce the glucose load and use fat to provide more nonprotein calories.

If insulin must be added, Table 41–6 shows one scheme that can be used to determine the amount of insulin needed. The insulin is added to each 250 grams of dextrose, which is equivalent to 500 ml of 50% dextrose. The estimated insulin amount is then added to each L of amino acid-dextrose mixture when the dextrose solution is D50.

PROTEIN-SPARING NUTRITION

The immediate response to fasting involves the breakdown of muscle protein into amino acids that are converted to glucose for cerebral energy needs. The conversion of amino acids into glucose takes place in the liver and is called gluconeogenesis. The principle of protein-sparing nutrition is to prevent muscle breakdown during a fast by providing enough glucose to satisfy the nonprotein calorie needs of metabolism. This form of nutrition will not build up protein stores and will not create a positive nitrogen balance.

> Protein-sparing nutrition is indicated only for short-term maintenance therapy in patients who have adequate protein stores.

When patients are malnourished or protein-depleted, full nutrition should be delivered either intravenously or enterally.

Protein-sparing nutrition is given via peripheral veins, which means that the amino acid and dextrose solutions must be dilute. Admixture of 3% amino acids and 20% dextrose is the most common solution used for peripheral nutrition. The final concentration is 1.5% amino acid, 10% dextrose. The dextrose will provide 340 kcal per L and the amino acids will provide 15 grams of protein per L.

The daily glucose requirement for cerebral metabolism is 150 gm/day. This corresponds to 510 kcal from carbohydrates. Because the 10% dextrose provides 340 kcal/L, 1.5 L will be needed to provide the necessary number of nonprotein calories.

One problem with protein-sparing nutrition is the volumes that are necessary to deliver the needed calories. When volume restriction is required, fat emulsions can be substituted using a 20% solution. This supplies 2 kcal/ml, so 250 ml will deliver the 500 kcal needed each day.

COMPLICATIONS

Complications can develop in over 50% of patients receiving TPN.[5] These complications are either related to the catheters placed in the large central veins or they are related to the biochemical effects of the TPN solutions.

Mechanical Complications

The hypertonic TPN solutions require infusion into a large central vein (see Chapter 4 for the techniques of catheter insertion). The catheter tips should rest in the superior vena cava but this is not always possible. Figure 41–1 shows a catheter that has been advanced into the internal jugular vein. This kind of problem can go undetected unless a chest film is obtained soon after each insertion. When the tip is malpositioned like the one in Figure 41–1, a guidewire can be used to reposition the catheter tip in the superior vena cava.[7] The other problems with catheter insertion (e.g., pneumothorax and infection) are presented in Chapters 4, 29, and 45.

Metabolic Complications

There are a variety of metabolic complications from TPN and the most prevalent are indicated on the body map in Figure 41–2. Each of the three nutrient substrates has its own specific complications

Carbohydrate Complications

Aggressive infusion of dextrose can create a variety of problems and the more common ones are discussed below.

Hyperglycemia is the most common complication of TPN and is particularly prevalent at the outset.[5] The hyperglycemia can be severe enough to precipitate hyperosmolar nonketotic coma, but this is uncommon. The preferred method of reducing the risk for hyperglycemia is to provide fewer nonprotein calories as glucose and more as lipids. This eliminates the need for insulin and its adverse effects on endogenous

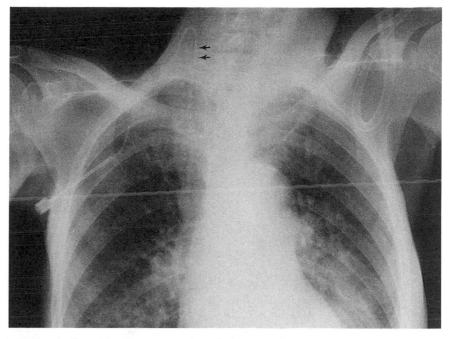

FIG. 41–1. Portable chest x-ray of a subclavian catheter that has been advanced into the ipsilateral internal jugular vein.

fat mobilization. Another factor that may promote glucose intolerance during TPN is chromium deficiency, which is discussed in Chapter 39.

Hypophosphatemia is reported in 30% of patients receiving TPN.[5] The mechanism is enhanced phosphate uptake into cells associated with enhanced glucose uptake. The consequences of hypophosphatemia include respiratory muscle weakness, hemolysis, and impaired O_2 release from hemoglobin. These may be particularly prominent when serum PO_4 falls below 1.0 mg/dl. The therapy for hypophosphatemia is presented in Chapter 38.

Fatty liver can be seen when glucose infusion exceeds the daily caloric requirements.[6] This is because the production of fatty acids from excess glucose and impaired ability to mobilize the fat for energy needs. Fat accumulation eventually leads to abnormal liver enzyme elevations in the serum, particularly alkaline phosphatase. The long-term consequences of fatty liver are not clear but at present there seem to be no serious residua.

Carbon dioxide retention can develop when excess glucose is given to patients with severe lung disease.[10] As discussed in Chapter 39, glucose metabolism produces a larger quantity of CO_2 for each L of O_2 consumed than the other two nutrient substrates. When the ability to eliminate CO_2 via alveolar ventilation is impaired, this enhanced CO_2 production can produce hypercapnia and impaired ability to wean from mechanical ventilation.[10]

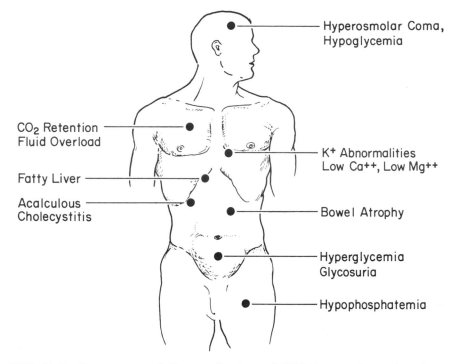

Hyperosmolar Coma, Hypoglycemia

CO₂ Retention
Fluid Overload

K⁺ Abnormalities
Low Ca⁺⁺, Low Mg⁺⁺

Fatty Liver

Acalculous
Cholecystitis

Bowel Atrophy

Hyperglycemia
Glycosuria

Hypophosphatemia

FIG. 41–2. Common metabolic complications of TPN. See text for explanation.

Monitoring Glucose Excess

The consequences of excess glucose infusion (i.e., fatty liver and CO_2 retention) can be prevented or minimized by periodic measurements of the respiratory quotient ($RQ = \dot{V}CO_2/\dot{V}O_2$) using indirect calorimetry.

The RQ associated with glucose breakdown is 1.0 versus the RQs of 0.8 for protein breakdown and 0.7 for fat metabolism. Therefore, an RQ that approaches 1.0 indicates a predominance of glucose metabolism for energy needs.

> An RQ greater than 0.95 is evidence for excess carbohydrate calories and an RQ greater than 1.0 indicates extensive lipogenesis in the liver.

The general rule of thumb is to keep the RQ below 0.95 during TPN to reduce the risks of excess carbohydrate infusion.

Complications of Lipid Infusion

Impaired oxygenation has been demonstrated in association with lipid infusion.[4] Free fatty acids are well-known for their ability to damage the pulmonary capillaries (e.g., fat embolism syndrome) and oleic acid infusion is the standard method for producing experimental ARDS. However, the risk for pulmonary injury from fat emulsions seems to be minimal in the clinical setting.[4]

Hyperlipemia has been observed as a result of impaired clearance of triglycerides from the blood but this is uncommon. Fat deposition in reticuloendothelial cells and macrophages has been reported;[12] however, there is no evidence that lipid accumulation impairs immunity in hospitalized patients.

ELECTROLYTE ABNORMALITIES

Several electrolyte abnormalities can appear during TPN, including hyponatremia, hypokalemia, hypomagnesemia, hypocalcemia, and hypophosphatemia.[5] The most noted electrolyte abnormality is hyponatremia, which is produced by excessive infusion of free water in the TPN solutions. The hyponatremia can be prevented by matching the sodium concentration in the dextrose-amino acid mixtures to the sodium concentration in the urine and other lost fluids. The hypophosphatemia from TPN is due to excessive glucose infusion (see earlier); the hypomagnesemia is the result of failure to replete daily magnesium losses in the urine. Magnesium depletion might also be responsible for the hypokalemia and hypocalcemia reported during TPN. The approach to these electrolyte abnormalities is presented in Section X of the book and will not be repeated here.

GI COMPLICATIONS

Two complications of TPN are related to the absence of nutrients in the bowel lumen.

Bowel Atrophy

As presented in Chapter 40, bowel rest leads to degenerative changes in the small bowel mucosa after only a few days (see Figure 40-1), and TPN does not prevent these atrophic changes. Bowel atrophy during TPN is now considered a major risk because disruption of the normal mucosal barrier might allow intestinal microbes to enter the systemic circulation.

Acalculous Cholecystitis

The absence of lipids in the proximal small bowel prevents cholecystokinin-mediated contraction of the gallbladder and the bile stasis that results may promote acalculous cholecystitis. This clinical disorder is presented in Chapter 43.

BIBLIOGRAPHY

Rombeau JL, Caldwell MD eds. Parenteral nutrition. Philadelphia: Lea & Febiger, 1986.
Weissman C ed. Nutritional support. Crit Care Clin 1987; 3(1)(Jan):97.
Askanazi, J ed. Nutrition and respiratory disease. Clin Chest Med 1986; 7:141.

REVIEWS

1. Gilder H. Parenteral nourishment of patients undergoing surgical or traumatic stress. J Parenter Enter Nutr 1986; 10:88–99.
2. Louie N, Niemiec PW. Parenteral nutrition solutions. In: Rombeau JL, Caldwell MD eds. Parenteral nutrition. Philadelphia: W.B. Saunders, 1986.
3. Rodriguez JL, Askanazi J, Weissman C, et al. Ventilatory and metabolic effects of glucose infusions. Chest 1985; 88:512–518.
4. Skeie B, Askanazi J, Rothkopf M, et al. Intravenous fat emulsions and lung function. A review. Crit Care Med 1988; 16:183–193.

COMPLICATIONS

5. Weinsier RL, Bacon PHJ, Butterworth CE. Central venous alimentation: A prospective study of the frequency of metabolic abnormalities among medical and surgical patients. J Parenter Enter Nutr 1982; 6:421–425.
6. Baker AL, Rosenberg IH. Hepatic complications of total parenteral nutrition. Am J Med 1987; 82:489–497.
7. Bernotti PN, Bistrian BR. Practical aspects and complications of total parenteral nutrition. Crit Care Clin 1987; 3:115–131.
8. Stein TP. Why measure the respiratory quotient of patients on total parenteral nutrition? J Am Coll Nutr 1985; 4:501–503.
9. Weinsier R, Krumdieck C. Death resulting from overzealous total parenteral nutrition: The refeeding syndrome revisited. Am J Clin Nutr 1981; 34:393–399.
10. Amene PC, Sladen RN, Feeley TW, Fisher R. Hypercapnia during total parenteral nutrition with hypertonic dextrose. Crit Care Med 1988; 15:171–172.
11. Askanazi J, Matthews D, Rothkopf M. Patterns of fuel utilization during parenteral nutrition. Surg Clin North Am 1986; 66:1091–1103.
12. Jensen GL, Seidner DL, Mascioli EA, et al. Fat emulsion infusion and reticuloendothelial system function in man. J Parenter Enter Nutr 1988; 12:4551.

c h a p t e r

42

ADRENAL AND THYROID
DISORDERS IN THE ICU

The adrenal and thyroid glands are capable of causing serious problems while escaping notice themselves. These endocrine disorders can be clinically silent until a serious illness occurs and they then serve as a catalyst to enhance the severity of the underlying disease. The adrenal and thyroid disorders in this chapter differ in severity from the ones you learned about in outpatients. Adrenal insufficiency with hyperpigmentation now becomes adrenal crisis with hypotension and refractory shock. Hypo- and hyperthyroidism now become myxedema coma and thyroid storm, respectively.

ADRENAL INSUFFICIENCY

The adrenal insufficiency in this chapter is limited to primary adrenal failure, because hypopituitarism is rare in ICUs.

NORMAL ADRENAL RESPONSE

The adrenal gland plays a major role in the adaptive response to stress. In the ICU, stress means hypotension, trauma, sepsis, and major surgery. The adrenals release glucocorticoids, mineralocorticoids, and catecholamines in these situations, and these substances help to maintain (1) cardiac output, (2) vascular tone, (3) plasma volume, and (4) blood glucose for cerebral energy needs. Plasma cortisol levels rise to 2 to 3 times normal following the conditions cited above, and the levels can reach 5 to 6 times normal in moribund patients.[1,2]

RISK FACTORS

Specific conditions that can damage the adrenal glands are hypotension, hypovolemia, sepsis, severe coagulopathy, and low cardiac output.[1,2,5,6] More than 90% of the adrenal tissue must be destroyed before adrenal insufficiency becomes clinically evident,[7] and this surely protects many of the patients at risk in the ICU. The group at particular risk are the patients who had occult adrenal insufficiency prior to the onset of the acute illness. However, this group is impossible to identify after the acute illness begins.

INCIDENCE

Despite the prevalence of risk factors in ICU patients, there are few studies of the incidence of adrenal insufficiency in the ICU patient population. One study performed in a medical ICU showed that primary adrenal insufficiency was uncommon;[4] however, this was far from an exhaustive study of the problem. At present, the illness should be considered in any patient with refractory shock or a catastrophic deterioration in clinical status.

CLINICAL PRESENTATION

As mentioned, mild illness is clinically silent or associated with nonspecific complaints. Anorexia, lethargy, and weight loss are the most common early manifestations. Skin hyperpigmentation is a characteristic sign of primary (not secondary) adrenal failure, but is not always present.[8] Orthostasis and certain electrolyte abnormalities (hyponatremia and hyperkalemia) can develop as the illness progresses and these usually increase suspicion for the illness. In acute or profound adrenal failure, the following manifestations are prominent.

Hypotension. This is the most common and most life-threatening feature of acute adrenal failure. The hypotension results from several factors, including hypovolemia and a reduced arterial resistance. **Orthostatic or labile hypotension** can be the expression of hypovolemia but is more often the result of an inability to adjust vascular tone in response to a decrease in cardiac output. **Refractory hypotension** is also common and may be caused by the "permissive effect" of glucocorticoids on the vascular response to catecholamines. Adrenal insufficiency should be considered in any case of refractory hypotension, regardless of the inciting event.

Hemodynamic Profiles. Invasive hemodynamic measurements with a pulmonary artery catheter can help in suspected cases of adrenal failure. The following profiles are possible (see Chapter 9 for an explanation of hemodynamic profiles and the abbreviations that are used).
1. Low PCWP/Low CI/Low SVRI
   This profile occurs in cardiovascular collapse, which is the expected finding in adrenal crisis.

2. Low PCWP/Low CI/Normal SVRI

   This profile results from the combination of hypovolemia and the inability to vasoconstrict in response to low cardiac output. This is the expected profile in milder forms of adrenal insufficiency.

3. Low or normal PCWP/High CI/Low SVRI

   High cardiac output is not an expected finding in acute adrenal failure, although this profile has been observed in human subjects with adrenal failure.[9] This profile is common in septic shock, which predisposes to adrenal necrosis,[6] so it is possible that hyperdynamic profiles reflect the predisposing condition and not the adrenal failure itself.

Electrolyte Abnormalities. Aldosterone deficiency causes a decrease in both sodium reabsorption and potassium secretion in the distal renal tubules. The expected result is hyponatremia and hyperkalemia. The prevalence of these findings in acutely ill patients is not clear. In one autopsy series, hyponatremia was present in 60% of those autopsied and hyperkalemia was present in 20%.[5] Because acute adrenal failure is frequently accompanied by hypotension and shock, the resultant decrease in renal perfusion may prevent the development of these electrolyte abnormalities.

Any patient who develops hyponatremia or hyperkalemia should have a urine sodium and potassium measured. If the urine sodium is high or the urine potassium is low, adrenal failure is a possibility.

Hypoglycemia. Although hypoglycemia is theoretically possible in adrenal failure, this seems to be a rare finding.[5] Probably the most common cause of hypoglycemia in the ICU is sepsis, liver failure, and malnutrition.

THE CORTROSYN TEST

The diagnostic test of choice for primary adrenal insufficiency is the rapid ACTH-stimulation test, also named after the synthetic ACTH (Cortrosyn) that is used in the test.

The Method. A baseline serum cortisol is obtained and 250 mcg of Cortrosyn is injected intravenously. A repeat serum cortisol is obtained one hour later. This test can be performed at any time of the day or night because diurnal variations in cortisol secretion are lost in critical illness.

The Results. An example of the adrenal response to synthetic ACTH is shown in Figure 42–1. In the stressed state (which most ICU patients experience), the baseline cortisol level is elevated, and the response to ACTH is blunted compared to the normal response. In adrenal insufficiency, the baseline cortisol is low and the ACTH response is blunted.

The rules for interpretation of the Cortrosyn test are outlined in Figure 42–2 and are listed below.

1. A baseline serum cortisol above 22 mcg/dl is evidence for normal adrenal responsiveness. In unstressed patients, a serum level greater than 14 mcg/dl is considered normal. A baseline cortisol would suffice in some cases but it is usually more expeditious to

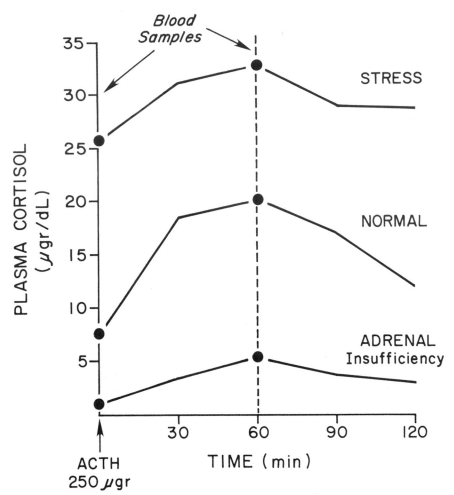

FIG. 42–1. The rapid ACTH stimulation test. Redrawn from Chernow B. Hormonal and metabolic considerations in critical care medicine. In: Thompson WL, Shoemaker W. Critical care: State of the art, Vol. 3. Fullerton: Society of Critical Care Medicine, 1982.

perform the entire test because of the lag time that is usually involved in performing the serum cortisol assays.

2. When the serum cortisol is below 22 mcg/ml, the increment in cortisol produced by the ACTH injection is the critical measure, that is, **an increase in serum cortisol less than 7 mcg/dl one hour after ACTH stimulation is evidence of primary adrenal failure.**

The Cortrosyn test is simple and should be performed at the slightest hint of adrenal dysfunction. We perform this test on most patients with refractory hypotension. Steroid treatment can be started before performing the Cortrosyn test, as described in the next section.

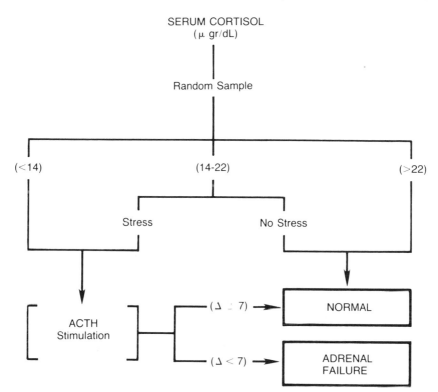

FIG. 42–2. The interpretation of the ACTH stimulation test.

Starting Steroids. When hypotension is severe or difficult to control, steroids can be started immediately, even before the test is performed. The following recommendations are made:

1. Dexamethasone does not interfere with serum cortisol measurements and can be given immediately.[7] The recommended dose is 10 mg IV as a bolus.
2. Methylprednisolone can be given if the cortisol assay is a radioimmunoassay (RIA) but not if the protein displacement method is used.[7] The initial dose is 60 mg IV.
3. Aggressive volume replacement is also indicated when adrenal failure is suspected, unless there is a specific indication for fluid overload by hemodynamic measurements.
4. After the test is performed, start intravenous hydrocortisone therapy at 250 mg as an intravenous bolus, followed by 100 mg every 6 hours.[7] Continue until test results are available.

If the ACTH stimulation test is normal, the hydrocortisone is discontinued (no taper needed). If the test confirms adrenal insufficiency, the drug is continued in a dose of 100 mg IV every 6 hours until the patient is no longer in a stress state. When this occurs, decrease the dose of hydrocortisone to a daily dose of 20 to 30 mg, which is the normal daily amount of cortisol released by the nonstressed adrenal gland.[7]

THYROID DYSFUNCTION

Thyroid dysfunction is present in up to 5% of hospitalized patients,[10] which is why thyroid function tests are performed so frequently in hospitalized patients. The following tests are available to evaluate thyroid function.

THYROID FUNCTION TESTS[3,11]

Serum T3 and T4. Thyroxine (T4) is the major hormone secreted by the thyroid, but triiodothyronine (T3) is the active form and is produced by conversion of T4 in extrathyroidal tissues. Both T4 and T3 are readily bound to carrier proteins, like thyroid binding globulin. The assay is a radioimmunoassay (RIA) that measures total T4 and T3, that is, it measures both the bound (inactive) forms and the free (active) forms. This means that abnormal results for "total" T4 and T3 may not represent thyroid illness but may be a reflection of abnormal carrier proteins.

T3 Resin Uptake. The T3 resin uptake (T3RU) has a misleading name because it is not a measure of serum T3. Rather, this test measures the ability of carrier proteins to bind radiolabelled T3 that is added to the blood sample. The remaining unbound fraction of T3 is then absorbed by a resin. Therefore, an increase in T3 resin uptake indicates a decrease in protein binding and vice-versa.

An increase in T3RU can occur (1) when there is more T4 bound to carrier proteins (hyperthyroidism), (2) when other substances are bound to the proteins (e.g., fatty acids), or (3) when there is a decrease in the amount of carrier proteins (e.g., severe illness or malnutrition). Conversely, a decrease in T3RU occurs when there is less T4 to bind to the proteins (hypothyroidism) or when the amount of carrier protein increases (e.g., during acute illness).

Free Thyroxine Index (FTI). The free thyroxine index (FTI) is the product of the serum T4 and T3RU. This test is used to determine if abnormal serum T4 levels are caused by thyroid illness or by changes in the binding of T4 by carrier proteins.

> When the T4 and T3RU change in the same direction (FTI changing), the problem is thyroidal illness. When the T4 and T3RU change in opposite directions (FTI unchanged), the problem is binding to carrier proteins.

Both T4 and T3RU are increased in hyperthyroidism and decreased in hypothyroidism.

Free T3 and T4. The free or unbound fraction of T3 and T4 is more reliable as a measure of thyroid function. The technique involves measuring the amount of hormone that crosses a semipermeable membrane. The test is complex and expensive and may not be available in all hospitals.

Thyroid Stimulating Hormone (TSH). TSH is released by the anterior pituitary gland and is under negative feedback control from the thyroid hormones. Serum levels of TSH are normally low (1 to 5 microunits/ml) and the levels typically rise above 20 microunits/ml in primary hypothyroidism.[11] This is the hallmark of primary hypothyroidism. Increases in serum TSH to less than 20 microunits/ml can occur without thyroid illness. Remember that serum TSH can be low in secondary hypothyroidism from pituitary insufficiency; therefore, the absence of an elevated serum TSH does not rule out hypothyroidism. TSH has little value for diagnosing hyperthyroidism because the normal serum levels are low to begin with.

Reverse T3. T4 is converted to T3 (the active metabolite) and reverse T3 (an inactive form). The reverse T3 in serum is elevated in hyperthyroidism and in acute illness. The reverse T3 is used to interpret a low total T4 because the reverse T3 will be low in hypothyroidism and will be normal or high in non-thyroidal illness.

RATIONAL USE OF THYROID FUNCTION TESTS

The total T4 is used as a screening test and the blood can be held in the laboratory for further tests if necessary. A normal serum T4 level excludes the diagnosis of hypo- or hyperthyroidism. If the serum T4 is abnormal, a T3RU should be performed on the remaining blood sample. The following schemes can then be used to interpret the problem.

High Serum T4. The approach to a high serum T4 level is outlined in Figure 42–3. An increase in the FTI (serum T4 × T3RU) indicates hyperthyroidism although a normal FTI does not rule it out. If the FTI is normal but hyperthyroidism is clinically suspected, a serum T3 can be obtained. A free T3 index (serum T3 × T3RU) that is elevated indicates hyperthyroidism. If the free T3 index is normal but hyperthyroidism is still suspected, a radioiodine uptake test should be performed.

Low Serum T4. Low serum T4 levels can be seen in close to half of the critically ill patient population,[12] and the approach to this problem is shown in Figure 42–4. The most common cause is not hypothyroidism but a decrease in serum binding proteins. A low serum T4 that results from diminished protein binding is called the "euthyroid sick" syndrome. A normal FTI indicates a decrease in protein binding (euthyroid sick). However, a low FTI can occur in both hypothyroid and euthyroid sick patients.[13] Therefore, when the FTI is low a serum TSH should be obtained. **A serum TSH >20 μU/cc is evidence of primary hypothyroidism.** A slightly elevated TSH (5 to 19 μU/cc can be seen in the euthyroid sick patients or mild hypothyroidism. If a hypothyroid state is suspected, a free T4 or reverse T3 level can be obtained. If these levels are low, primary hypothyroidism is possible. A normal serum TSH is evidence of a euthyroid state. If the TSH is low, a free T4 or reverse T3 should be obtained to rule out hypothyroidism from pituitary failure (secondary hypothyroidism).

HYPERTHYROIDISM

CLINICAL PRESENTATION

The clinical manifestations that may alert you to the possibility of hyperthyroidism are listed in Table 42–1. Persistent unexplained sinus

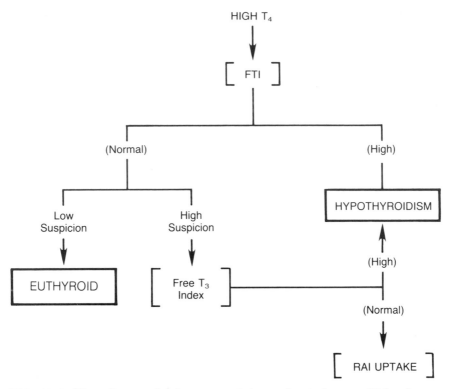

FIG. 42–3. Flow diagram for the approach to an elevated serum T4 level.

tachycardia should always raise the possibility of a hyperthyroid state. Elderly patients with lethargy and atrial fibrillation (apathetic thyrotoxicosis) should also be tested for hyperthyroidism. Thyroid storm can be precipitated by acute illness or by surgery, and is characterized by fever, severe agitation, high-output heart failure, and progression to hypotension and coma.

DIAGNOSIS

As mentioned in the preceeding section, the serum T4 can be used as a screening test. A normal value virtually excludes significant thyrotoxicosis. If the serum T4 is elevated, the flow diagram in Figure 42–3 can be used to determine if hyperthyroidism is present.

TREATMENT[12,14]

Propylthiouracil (PTU) is the most effective agent for treating hyperthyroidism. This drug not only inhibits thyroid hormone synthesis but also inhibits peripheral conversion of T4 to T3. The drug is only available in oral form. A loading dose of 600 to 1,000 mg is given at the start of

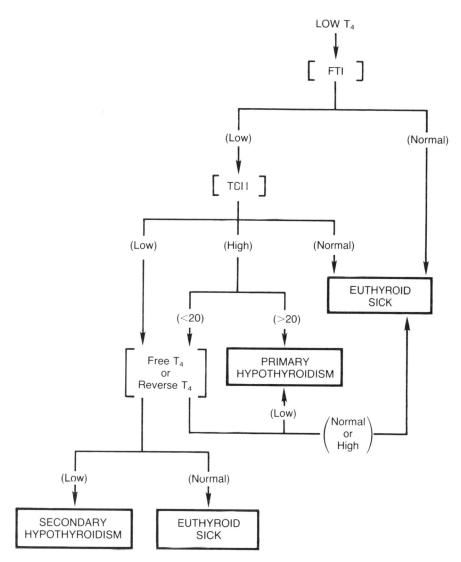

FIG. 42–4. Flow diagram for evaluating a low serum T4 level. Serum TSH expressed in microunits/mL

therapy and is followed by a maintenance dose of 150 to 200 mg TID. Skin rash can occur in 5 to 10% of patients. More serious reactions (hepatotoxicity and agranulocystosis) occur in less than 1% of patients.

In severe cases, **iodide** (which blocks release of performed thyroid hormone) can be given 1 to 2 hours after the loading dose of PTU. Because the inhibition of T4 release by iodide can be overcome, hormone synthesis should be blocked first with PTU. Iodide can be given orally (Lugol's solution, 4 drops q 12 hrs) or intravenously (sodium iodide, 500 to 1,000 mg q 12 hrs). If iodide allergy exists, lithium (300 mg po q

TABLE 42–1. CLUES TO THYROID ILLNESS IN THE ICU

Hyperthyroidism
1. Persistent sinus tachycardia
2. Atrial fibrillation in the elderly
3. High output heart failure
4. Persistent agitation
5. Unexplained fever and hypotension (thyroid storm)
 	
Hypothyroidism
1. Bradycardia
2. Unexplained cardiac dysfunction
3. Depressed mental status and coma
4. The "hypos":
    Hypoventilation
    Hypothermia
    Hyponatremia
    Hypotension

8 hrs) can be used.

Propranolol can be given for severe tachyarrhythmias or for tachycardia in patients with coronary artery disease. If immediate control is necessary, intravenous propranolol (1 mg given over 3 to 5 min and repeated every 5 to 10 min until desired effect is reached) can be used. Oral maintenance therapy can vary from 20 to 120 mg every 6 hrs.

Thyroid storm can accelerate glucocorticoid metabolism and cause a relative adrenal insufficiency. For this reason, **hydrocortisone** (300 mg IV loading dose, followed by 100 mg q 8 hrs) can be given in severe cases and continued until the hypermetabolism is controlled.

The remaining therapy in thyroid storm consists of general supportive measures and treatment of the precipitating event (e.g., infection). Hypovolemia is common as a result of increased insensible fluid losses, vomiting, and diarrhea. Aggressive volume replacement is often necessary.

HYPOTHYROIDISM

CLINICAL PRESENTATION

The early manifestations of hypothyroidism can be nonspecific. However, the onset of acute illness can precipitate severe thyroid failure. The clinical manifestations that should alert you to the possibility of hypothyroidism in the ICU are shown in Table 42–1. Myxedema coma has a high mortality and early recognition of this disorder is important.[12]

DIAGNOSIS

As mentioned in the preceding section, a serum T4 should be obtained as a screening test. A normal serum T4 should virtually exclude the

TABLE 42–2. TREATMENT OPTIONS FOR MYXEDEMA COMA	
Agent	**Dose**
Thyroxine (T4)	300–500 mcg IV (initial dose)
	75–100 mcg IV (daily dose)
Triiodothyronine (T3)	12.5–25 mcg IV q6h
Combination Rx	
T4	250 mcg IV (initial dose)
	100 mcg IV (day 2)
	50 mcg IV (daily dose)
T3	12.5 mcg PO q6h

possibility of significant hypothyroidism. If the serum T4 is low, the flow diagram in Figure 42–4 can be used to differentiate hypothyroidism from nonthyroidal illness.

TREATMENT

The treatment of mild hypothyroidism is oral thyroxine (T4) in a single daily dose of 50 to 200 mcg. The optimal treatment for severe hypothyroidism and myxedema coma is not clear. Although oral therapy can be effective,[15] it may be wise to use intravenous replacement (at least initially) because of the risk for impaired GI motility in severe hypothyroidism. Table 42–2 shows the regimens recommended for myxedema coma.[14] Replacement therapy using T3 instead of T4 seems logical because T3 is the active form of thyroid hormone and conversion of T4 to T3 is depressed in serious illness. An intravenous form of T3 is not available but can be prepared by dissolving 100 mcg of T3 in 2 ml of 0.1 N NaOH and then adding this solution to 2 ml of 2% albumin solution.[14] The final concentration of T3 in this solution will be 25 mcg/ml.

BIBLIOGRAPHY

Geelhoed GW, Chernow B eds. Endocrine aspects of acute illness. Clinics in critical care medicine. New York: Churchill Livingstone, 1985.

REFERENCES

REVIEWS

1. Felicetta JV, Sowers JR. Endocrine changes with critical illness. Crit Care Clin 1987; 3:855–870.
2. Knowlton AI. Adrenal insufficiency in the intensive care setting. Intensive Care Med 1989; 4:35–45.
3. Zaloga GP, Smallridge RC. Thyroid alterations in acute illness. Semin Respir Med 1985; 7:95–107.

ADRENAL INSUFFICIENCY

4. Drucker D, Shandling M. Variable adrenocortical function in acute medical illness. Crit Care Med 1985; 13:477–479.
5. Xarli VP, Steele A, Davis PJ, et al. Adrenal hemorrhage in the adult. Medicine 1978; 57:211–221.
6. Sibbald WJ, Short A, Cohen MP, Wilson RF. Variations in adrenocortical responsiveness during severe bacterial infections. Ann Surg 1977; 186:29–33.
7. Passmore JM, Jr. Adrenal cortex. In: Geelhoed SW, Chernow B eds. Endocrine aspects of acute illness. Clinics in critical care medicine. Vol 5. New York: Churchill Livingstone, 1985; 97–134.
8. Barnett AH, Espiner EA, Donald RA. Patients presenting with Addison's disease need not be pigmented. Postgrad Med J 1982; 58:690–692.
9. Dorin RI, Kearns PJ. High output circulatory failure in acute adrenal insufficiency. Crit Care Med 1988; 16:296–297.

THYROID DISORDERS

10. Morley JE, Slag MF, Elson MK, Shafer RB. The interpretation of thyroid function tests in hospitalized patients. JAMA 1983; 249:2377–2379.
11. Koenig RJ, Larsen PR, Enrique Silva J. Current approach to the euthyroid patient with abnormal thyroid function tests. Resident & Staff Physician 1987; 33:49–62.
12. Zaloga GP, Chernow B. Thyroid function in acute illness. In: Geelhoed GW, Chernow B eds. Endocrine aspects of acute illness. Clinics in critical care medicine. Vol 5. New York: Churchill Livingstone, 1985:67–96.
13. Chopra IJ, Solomon DH, Hepner GW, Morgenstein AA. Misleading low free thyroxine index and usefulness of reverse triiodothyronine measurement in nonthyroidal illnesses. Ann Intern Med 1979; 90:905–912.
14. Ehrmann DA, Sarne DH. Early identification of thyroid storm and myxedema coma. J Crit Illness 1988; 3:111–118.
15. McCulloch W, Price P, Hinds CJ, Wass JAH. Effects of low dose triiodothyronine in myxedema coma. Intensive Care Med 1985; 11:259–262.

section XII
INFECTIOUS DISEASE

The advances . . . over the past three decades do not appear to have had a significant impact on mortality due to gram-negative bacillary bacteremia. While it is difficult for most of us today to accept such a conclusion, it is not unique in infectious diseases.

Jay P. Sanford, MD

chapter

APPROACHES TO NOSOCOMIAL FEVER

Humanity has but three great enemies:
Fever, famine and war.
Of these, by far the greatest,
By far the most terrible, is fever.
                Sir William Osler

Nosocomial fever (one that appears 24 hours after admission) occurs in as many as 30% of hospitalized patients.[1] One of every three patients who develops a fever after admission will not survive the hospitalization, representing a fourfold increase in mortality when compared to their afebrile neighbors.[1] This lends some credence to Osler's harsh statements about fever and emphasizes the importance of approaching fever as a life-threatening problem.

OVERVIEW

This chapter is organized in four sections. The first presents the salient features of the febrile response and the methods available for monitoring body temperature. The second section outlines a bedside approach to fever according to the clinical setting in which the fever appears. The third section contains a variety of illnesses that can cause fever in an adult ICU. The chapter ends with a section on the early therapeutic strategies for febrile patients. This chapter does not focus on fever in the immunocompromised host.

THE FEBRILE RESPONSE

Body temperature normally varies from 36°C (AM) to 38°C (PM) over 24 hours, with a mean temperature of 37°C (98.6°F). Fever is traditionally defined as a rectal temperature that rises above the upper limit of normal, or 38°C (100.4°F) in the normal adult.[1,3,4] In certain patient groups (the elderly, the malnourished, etc.), the mean temperature may be below the norm of 37°C, so that a fever may be present at a temperature below 38°C. The important point here is to know the usual temperature range for each of your patients.

SEVERITY

There is a tendency to assume that the height of the fever is proportional to the severity of the underlying illness. However, **neither the height of the fever nor the clinical appearance of the patient will correlate with the presence or severity of infection.**[1,3] High fevers and rigors can be associated with benign processes (drug fever), and minor temperature elevations can be associated with life-threatening sepsis. Therefore, the clinical presentation should not influence the workup of fever, or the decision to start antibiotics.

MONITORING TECHNIQUES

The traditional mercury glass thermometers used to measure rectal or oral temperatures are being replaced by rapid-response thermistors equipped with digital displays. The electronic thermistors achieve steady state readings in 30 seconds whereas the mercury thermometers require up to 9 minutes to reach steady-state recordings.[2]

Oral and axillary temperatures are 0.5 and 1°C below core temperature, respectively.[2,3] Rectal temperatures are close approximations of the core, and rectal measurements are the standard in many ICUs. Alternative methods of monitoring core temperature are now available using thermistors placed on bladder catheters, pulmonary artery catheters, and ear probes. However, the rectum remains the most popular site for monitoring body temperature.

THE CLINICAL SETTING

The common sources of nosocomial fever are indicated on the body map in Figure 43–1.[1,3,4]

When first learning of a fever in an individual patient, the clinical setting will dictate the initial evaluation of fever at the bedside. The following settings are relevant.

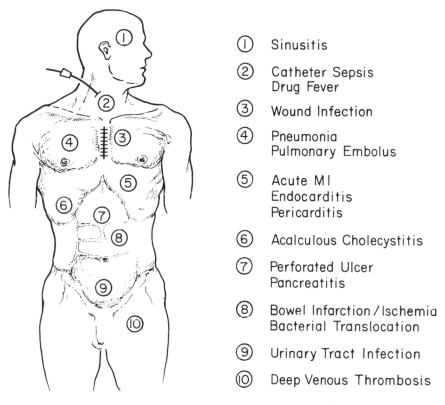

①	Sinusitis
②	Catheter Sepsis Drug Fever
③	Wound Infection
④	Pneumonia Pulmonary Embolus
⑤	Acute MI Endocarditis Pericarditis
⑥	Acalculous Cholecystitis
⑦	Perforated Ulcer Pancreatitis
⑧	Bowel Infarction/Ischemia Bacterial Translocation
⑨	Urinary Tract Infection
⑩	Deep Venous Thrombosis

FIG. 43–1. Common causes of nosocomial fever in the ICU.

POSTOPERATIVE FEVER

Approximately 15% of patients will develop a fever in the first week following general surgery but infection is absent in two-thirds of patients.[6] Most of the noninfectious fevers occur as a single episode and are not recurrent or persistent.[7] For the first episode of fever, a thorough physical exam should be sufficient to identify an underlying infection.[6] If the physical exam is unrevealing, no clinical tests need be obtained unless the patient is immune deficient or the fever recurs.

Malignant Hyperthermia

This is a rare disorder (1:50,000 to 1:100,000 adults) caused by an abnormal release of calcium in skeletal muscle in response to general anesthetics and muscle relaxants.[8] The clinical features and therapy are outlined in Table 43–1. The onset is characterized by tachycardia, ventricular arrythmias, labile blood pressure, and muscle rigidity, the latter the result of abnormal release of calcium from the sarcoplasmic reticulum of skeletal muscle. Fever is a late finding and occurs in less than 50% of patients.[8] Aggressive treatment with dantrolene is imperative to reduce mortality and prevent myoglobinuric renal failure. The average

TABLE 43–1. MALIGNANT HYPERTHERMIA	
1. CLINICAL FEATURES:	Tachycardia (96%)
	Muscle Rigidity (84%)
	Labile Blood Pressure (86%)
	Cyanosis (71%)
	Fever (31%)
2. TREATMENT	Dantrolene Sodium
Acute:	1 to 2 mg/kg IV Bolus. Repeat q
	15 min to maximum of 10 mg/kg
Maintenance:	1 to 2 mg/kg PO qid × 3 days

Henschel, EO ed. Malignant Hyperthermia: Current Concepts. Atlanta: Appleton-Century-Crofts, 1983.

dose needed for acute control is 2.5 mg/kg. All patients should be given a bracelet to wear to prevent further episodes and the family should be informed of the possibility that they may have a predeliction for this disorder.

Wound Infections

Surgical wounds are classified as clean (abdomen and chest unopened), contaminated (abdomen or chest opened), and dirty (direct contact with pus or bowel contents), and the infection rates are reported at 2%, 20%, and 40%, respectively.[9] Most infections are "uncomplicated," meaning that the skin and subcutaneous tissues alone are involved. The treatment is debridement and local drainage, while vancomycin is used to eradicate skin organisms.

Necrotizing wound infections are produced by clostridia or beta-hemolytic streptococci. Unlike the other wound infections (which appear 5 to 7 days after surgery), the necrotizing infections are evident in the first few postoperative days. There is marked edema around the incision, and the surrounding skin may have fluid-filled bullae. Crepitance and deep spread to muscle occurs often, and rhabdomyolysis with myoglobinuric renal failure can become a problem. The treatment is intravenous penicillin and extensive debridement. Mortality is high (60 to 80%) if diagnosis is delayed.

Atelectasis

Atelectasis is commonly regarded as a cause of fever in the postoperative period despite little experimental support. Atelectasis is a radiographic diagnosis that can be a nonspecific finding in supine patients. This is shown in Figure 43–2. The chest film on the left (arrow pointing down) shows loss of lung volume with coalescence of markings at the lung bases. This film could be interpreted as atelectasis, however, it was taken only minutes after the chest film on the right, using the same subject. The difference between the two x-rays is the body position; the film on the right is in the upright position (arrow up), while the one on

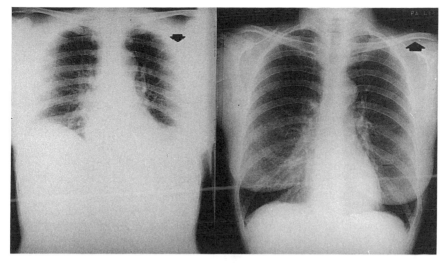

FIG. 43–2. The influence of body position on the chest film. Both films obtained from the same subject. Arrow up indicates upright position. Arrow down indicates supine position.

the left is in the supine position (arrow down). The radiographic appearance of basilar atelectasis can therefore be a nonspecific finding in the supine position.

Atelectasis is a decrease in functional residual capacity (FRC), which is the volume of air in the lungs at end-expiration. The FRC decreases 40% to 70% after upper abdominal surgery, and remains diminished for 1 week.[10] If atelectasis causes fever, then significant fever should also be common after major abdominal surgery. Yet fever is reported in only 15% of postoperative patients in one large series.[6] Other evidence against a causal link between atelectasis and fever is the lack of fever from atelectasis in chronic conditions like pulmonary fibrosis, or neuromuscular disease.

> The lack of proof for a causal relationship between atelectasis and fever means that problems can arise when a fever is attributed to an x-ray finding while the actual cause of fever is overlooked.

Thromboembolism

Thromboembolism can produce fever to 39°C or higher for as long as 1 week.[23] The risk for thromboembolism is highest in postoperative patients, particularly following orthopedic procedures on the hip and knee. Other high-risk conditions are acute MI, acute cerebrovascular accidents, and neoplasm. Acute pulmonary embolism can be associated with a normal leg exam in over half the patients, so the absence of leg swelling, tenderness, or erythema in the face of a fever does not rule out acute embolism. See Chapter 7 for more information on thromboembolic disease.

Adrenal Insufficiency

Adrenal insufficiency can be an obscure illness in outpatients because the early manifestations are either absent or nonspecific. The full clinical syndrome can surface after the stress of surgery. The diagnosis and therapy of adrenal failure is presented in Chapter 42.

PROCEDURES

The following procedures are associated with fever in the absence of infection.

Hemodialysis

Febrile reactions during hemodialysis are attributed to endotoxin contamination of the dialysis equipment, but bacteremia occurs on occasion.[11] If the patient appears toxic, the dialysis is stopped, blood cultures are obtained, and antibiotics are started immediately. The dialysis need not be stopped if the patient is doing well otherwise, but blood cultures should always be obtained. When empiric antibiotic therapy is started, the antibiotics should cover both gram-positive and gram-negative organisms. Vancomycin is used for gram-positive coverage, particularly because of the risk for *Staphylococcus epidermidis.*

Bronchoscopy

Fever can appear after 15% of bronchoscopies,[12] and usually becomes evident in the first few hours after the procedure. Pneumonia has been reported following 6% of bronchoscopies,[12] but bacteremia is rare.

Iatrogenic Fever

Iatrogenic fever from a faulty heating element in mattresses and ventilators can cause fever by transference. The lung has a surface area the size of a tennis court, and the temperature of inspired air can have a profound effect on core temperature. It only takes a minute to check the thermometers on mattresses and ventilators, but it can take far longer to explain why you missed a simple and easily corrected problem.

Blood Transfusion

Febrile reactions appear in 1 to 4% of patients receiving blood products. The fever appears within 6 hours of receiving the transfusion and is caused by antileukocyte antibodies and not by hemolysis. See Chapter 18 for a discussion of febrile transfusion reactions.

INFECTIOUS FEVERS

In one report of nosocomial fevers in internal medicine patients, 70% of the fevers resulted from an infectious process.[1] The proportion of fevers due to infectious processes is not reported for an ICU patient population. However, there are several infections that must be considered in any case of nosocomial fever in an ICU, and the following are some of the infections to consider.

COMMON INFECTIONS

The predominant infections in the ICU are pneumonia (37%) and urinary tract infections (23%), accounting for half of the total number of infections. The other common infections are catheter sepsis and wound infection. The first three disorders are presented separately in the next three chapters, and are mentioned here only briefly. The fourth has already been mentioned in this chapter.

Pneumonia

Look for sputum production or change in sputum quality. All sputum samples should be examined microscopically to determine if the specimen is from the lower airways. Only deep specimens are to be cultured. The gram stain is used to decide about antibiotic therapy. See the next chapter for more on this topic.

Urosepsis

This is the most common nosocomial infection, occurring predominantly in patients with indwelling bladder catheters. Diagnosis is often difficult without culture results. Urine gram stain often has limited value, as discussed in Chapter 45.

Catheter Sepsis

Vascular catheters (arterial or venous) are suspects in any unexplained fever when they have been in place for longer than 2 days (or less if they were placed in an emergency situation). Table 43–2 lists some guidelines for vascular catheters. Catheter sepsis is presented in Chapter 46.

UNCOMMON INFECTIONS

When the more common infections are not evident, look for the infections in the following paragraphs.

TABLE 43–2.   GUIDELINES FOR INTRAVASCULAR CATHETERS
1. If purulent material can be expressed from the insertion site, remove the catheter immediately. A new skin site must be used for continued venous access
2. Otherwise, change the catheter over a guidewire in the following situations: a. Catheter in place longer than 48 hours b. Catheter placed in emergency situation, regardless of the duration of cannulation
3. All catheter tips should be cultured by the semiquantitative method. Do not request broth cultures

Sinusitis

Nasal tubes can block the sinus ostia and lead to accumulation of infected secretions in the paranasal sinuses. The incidence of sinusitis from nasal intubation ranges from less than 5% to as high as 25%.[13,14] Unlike community-acquired sinusitis, this infection is serious and even life-threatening.

Diagnosis is often possible with bedside films like the one shown in Figure 43–3. The opacification of the left maxillary and frontal sinuses in this film is typical of the distribution of sinusitis from nasal tubes, which is usually a pansinusitis but almost always involves the maxillary sinuses.[13] (Note the nasal tubes in the x-ray.) Air-fluid levels may also be seen if the sinuses are not completely filled. If bedside sinus films are not available or are suboptimal, a CT scan of the paranasal area is the best method for visualizing the sinuses.

Opacification of a sinus does not always indicate infection, and bedside aspiration of the sinuses (usually maxillary) is necessary to make the diagnosis and to identify the responsible pathogens. Once the diagnosis is confirmed, remove all nasal tubes, and start broad-spectrum antibiotic therapy to cover gram-positive cocci (including methicillin-resistant staphylococci) and gram-negative enteric organisms. If the response to antibiotics is not prompt, surgical drainage should be seriously considered.

Acalculous Cholecystitis

This disorder is being recognized more often, and is prevalent in patients receiving intravenous nutrition.[15,16] The proposed mechanism is edema of the cystic duct with stasis, infection, and perforation of the gallbladder. The salient features are listed below.

1. The cardinal sign is right upper quadrant tenderness, but this can be absent in 30% of cases,[15] particularly in comatose or obtunded patients.
2. Liver enzymes and serum bilirubin levels are neither sensitive nor specific markers of the disease,[16] and should not be used to make diagnostic decisions.
3. Bedside ultrasound of the right upper quadrant can be misleading,

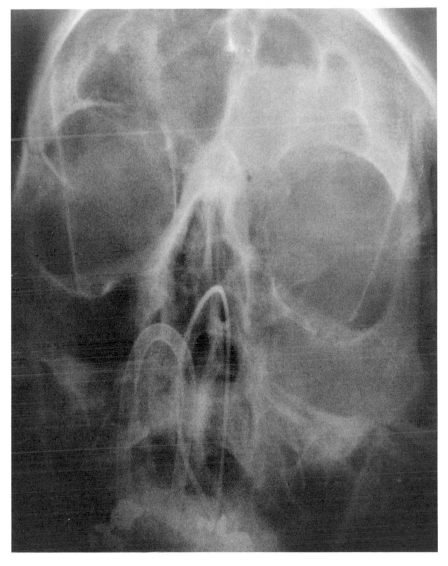

FIG. 43-3. Bedside anteroposterior film of the paranasal sinuses. Note opacification of the left maxillary and frontal sinuses with a fluid level in the frontal sinus. Nasal tubes represent a nasotracheal tube and a nasogastric feeding tube.

because abnormal findings (sludge, dilatation, thickened walls) can be seen with prolonged bowel rest.[16]

4. Hepato-biliary scans that visualize the gallbladder in 2 hours can exclude the illness, but reduced hepatic uptake of tracer is common in critically ill patients, reducing the accuracy of this test.[16]

The diagnosis is usually based on the combination of physical findings, ultrasound, and radionuclide scans. Non-specific findings should not discourage definitive therapy because this illness can be fatal.[16] Therapy involves cholecystectomy or tube cholecystostomy with local anesthesia, combined with antibiotics.

Abdominal Abscess

Localized collections in the abdomen are usually seen after trauma or abdominal surgery. Blood cultures can be positive in 50% of cases,[17] so these collections may be a source of unexplained bacteremia. The best diagnostic test is the computed tomographic scan, which can be positive in 96% of cases.[17] Treatment includes antibiotic coverage for anaerobes (particularly *Bacillus fragilis*) and gram-negative enteric pathogens, combined with drainage (percutaneous if possible).

Bowel Flora

The flora of the large and small bowel can produce fever in a number of ways. The toxin-producing *Clostridium difficile* can be responsible in patients with prior antibiotic exposure (see Chapter 5). Bowel flora can gain access to the systemic circulation by "translocation" across a damaged mucosal barrier. An expression of translocation in cirrhotics with ascites is "spontaneous bacterial peritonitis." This disorder can present with fever only and can be associated with growth of organisms in the ascites without evidence for bacteremia. Diagnosis requires a peritoneal tap. Cultures of peritoneal fluid are positive in about 90% of cases, and a leukocyte count over 250/mm^3 in the fluid is considered an indication for early antibiotic therapy.[18]

Meningitis

Purulent meningitis is a concern only in selected patients (e.g., neurosurgical patients, trauma victims, pneumococcal bacteremia, and disseminated candidiasis). Meningeal involvement from septicemia is uncommon and lumbar puncture should not be considered a routine part of the nosocomial fever workup unless the patient falls into one of the high-risk categories. The diagnosis of meningitis is covered in detail in reference 19 at the end of the chapter.

NON-INFECTIOUS SOURCES

If the infections mentioned above are not evident, consider the following noninfectious sources.

Pancreatitis

Pancreatitis is reported following cardiac surgery,[20] or as part of the multiple organ failure syndrome. Elevated amylase levels are relatively nonspecific, and serum lipase elevation is required for the diagnosis.[21] The lipase levels can be normal in the first few days of the illness. When the diagnosis is uncertain, a computed tomographic scan of the abdomen can be revealing.

Bowel Infarction

Mesenteric ischemia and infarction are often accompanied by abdominal pain and tenderness, but these may be masked in patients with altered mental status. Unfortunately, the diagnosis is often difficult, because physical findings and laboratory tests are neither sensitive nor specific.[22] Plain radiographs of the abdomen are often unrevealing, but can be diagnostic if there is gas in the bowel wall or portal venous gas, like the film in Figure 43–4. Unfortunately, these radiographic findings are far from common, but you should be aware of what they look like. The diagnosis often requires laparotomy.

Drug Fever

The diagnosis of drug fever is often suggested by excluding other causes of fever. The features of drug fever are shown in Table 43–3. The important points in the table are the uncommon appearance of rash and eosinophilia and the common appearance of rigors and tachycardia.

> Contrary to prior teaching, the patient with drug fever can appear as ill as the patient with a serious infection.[24]

The only characteristics that may separate drug fever from infection are an urticarial rash and eosinophilia, but these are uncommon findings in drug fever, as shown in Table 43–3. Virtually any drug can cause fever, and Table 43–4 lists the common and uncommon offenders.

When drug fever is a possibility, discontinue as many drugs as possible, or switch to alternative agents. The fever should disappear in 2 to 3 days if the drug is responsible.

Tumor Fever

A variety of neoplasms can produce a fever, particularly during chemotherapy. Naproxen (250 mg BID) is a nonsteroidal anti-inflammatory agent that can reduce fever of neoplastic origin within 24 hours, but may not reduce fever from infections.[25]

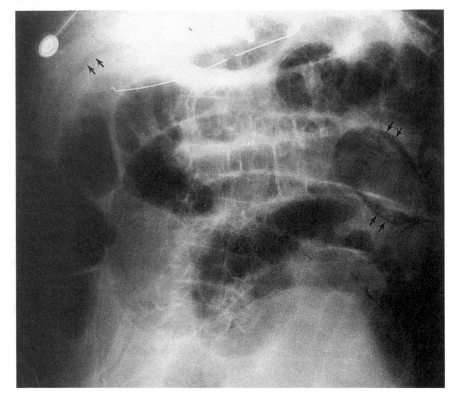

FIG. 43–4. Supine film of the abdomen showing air in wall of the small bowel (outlined by arrows) and air in the hepatic veins (arrows in upper left). Patient expired only a few hours after this film was obtained.

TABLE 43–3. FEATURES OF DRUG FEVER	
Feature	**Sensitivity (%)**
Rigors	41
Tachycardia	89
Hypotension	18
Rash	18
Urticaria	7
Eosinophilia	22
Deaths	4

From Mackowiak PA, LeMaistre CF. Drug fever: A critical appraisal of conventional concepts. Ann Intern Med 1987; *106*:728–733.

TABLE 43–4. CAUSES OF DRUG FEVER IN THE ICU		
Common	Occasional	Almost Never
Amphotericin B	Cimetidine	Digitalis
Penicillins	Dextrans	Insulin
Phenytoin	Folate	
Procainamide	Hydralazine	
Quinidine	Streptokinase	
Sulfas	Vancomycin	

Dressler's Syndrome

Fever that appears 2 to 3 weeks (range of 1 to 12 weeks) after acute myocardial infarction or cardiac surgery may represent a pleuropericarditis that is autoimmune in origin.[26] Chest pain is prominent, and can be pleuritic. There may be pericardial and pleural rubs, along with effusions. Treatment consists of aspirin or nonsteroidal anti-inflammatory agents, and steroids if needed.

Miscellaneous

The other noninfectious causes of fever include drug withdrawal (e.g., ethanol withdrawal), thyroid storm, adrenal insufficiency, thromboembolism, and the whole-body inflammation of multiorgan failure.

BLOOD CULTURES

Blood cultures should be obtained in all cases of nosocomial fever except: 1) The first episode of fever in the postoperative period; 2) Strong suspicion for drug fever; 3) Clinical evidence for deep vein thrombosis in the legs. The published guidelines for obtaining blood cultures for nosocomial fever are shown in Table 43–5. The number of venipunctures (one venipuncture is called one "set" of blood cultures) is dictated by the likelihood of bacteremia from the suspected infection. A low or moderate probability of bacteremia, like that expected from a pneumonia or urinary tract infection, merits two sets of cultures. A high-probability

TABLE 43–5. GUIDELINES FOR THE USE OF BLOOD CULTURES TO DIAGNOSE BACTEREMIA	
Likelihood of a Positive Culture	Number of Blood Culture Sets to Obtain*
Low or Moderate	2
High	3
High + Antibiotics	4 or more
*1 set = 1 venipuncture site	
From Aronson MD, Bor DH. Blood cultures. Ann Intern Med 1987; 106:246–253.	

TABLE 43–6. BLOOD CULTURE METHODS
1. DO NOT obtain blood from an indwelling catheter
2. Skin Preparation: Alcohol first, then 2% iodine or iodophor. Let stand 1 minute
3. Gloves: To be worn while palpating venipuncture site
4. Volume: 10 ml per set minimum 20–30 ml preferred

bacteremic disorder like endocarditis requires at least three sets of blood cultures.

The technique for obtaining blood cultures is shown in Table 43–6.[27] The specimen should never be drawn through an indwelling catheter.[27] The volume of blood in the specimen is one of the most important factors for determining the yield from blood cultures. Up to 20 or 30 ml per set is now recommended as the optimal volume,[27] but the volume of blood placed in each bottle of broth should not exceed 5 ml.

EARLY ANTIBIOTIC THERAPY

The decision to start antibiotics is usually dictated by the results of gram stains or other tests aimed at documenting infection. In the absence of an identifiable source of fever, empiric antibiotic therapy is usually given to seriously ill patients (e.g., fever with hypotension) or neutropenic patients.

THE NEUTROPENIC PATIENT

Empiric antibiotics are indicated in every patient with fever and neutropenia (neutrophil count below 500 per mm^3). The rationale for this practice is the observation that bacteremia in neutropenic patients (particularly gram-negative bacteremia) can be rapidly fatal.[28] Common antibiotic regimens for neutropenic patients is shown in Table 43–7. The basic ingredient is an aminoglycoside because the most common pathogens are gram-negative enteric pathogens, including *Klebsiella pneumoniae* and *Pseudomonas aeruginosa.* Added to this is an antipseudomonal

TABLE 43–7. EMPIRIC COVERAGE FOR FEVER AND NEUTROPENIA		
Double Coverage for Pseudomonas	**+**	**Added Gram-Positive Coverage**
Aminoglycoside + Antipseudomonal Penicillin or Ceftazidime	+	Vancomycin
[1]Aminoglycoside + Aztreonam	+	Vancomycin
[1]If there is a history of anaphylaxis from penicillin		

penicillin (e.g., ticarcillin) or a cephalosporin with antipseudomonal activity (ceftazidime). Gram-positive coverage with an antistaphylococcal agent is added if there is suspicion for gram-positive infection or if methicillin-resistant staphylococci are prominent in your hospital.[28] Vancomycin is a popular choice because of its activity against methicillin-resistant staphylococci.

ANTIPYRETIC THERAPY

There is a tendency to reduce fever without considering the reason that the body generates a fever.

BENEFITS OF FEVER

Septic patients who are hypothermic fare worse than patients who can generate a fever, suggesting that the febrile response has a beneficial role in combating infection. Fever can inhibit viral replication and slow bacterial growth, and temperatures of 40°C can kill some bacteria like the pneumococcus.[4] In addition, fever promotes phagocytosis and lymphocyte transformation, to facilitate the immune response.[29]

ADVERSE EFFECTS OF FEVER

The physiologic effects of fever are difficult to separate from the effects of the underlying process that produces the fever. For example, an increase in heart rate during febrile infections may be caused by the septic state, and not the fever. Despite this limitation, the major concern with fever is the tachycardia, with heart rate increasing 15 beats/min for every 1°C increase in body temperature.[4] However, the syndrome of "febrile angina" has not been reported to date, so the concerns about fever in cardiac disease may be inflated.

Summary. The benefits of fever seem to outweigh the risks, so there is little reason to reduce fever unless it is producing delirium. As for patient comfort, if the fever helps reduce the stay in the ICU, a little discomfort is a small price to pay.

PERSISTENT FEVER

Fever that persists for days despite empiric antibiotics can indicate one of the following:
  1. Endocarditis
  2. Mycotic aneurysm
  3. Disseminated fungal disease

Endocarditis and mycotic aneurysm are often the result of inadequately treated bacteremia in susceptible patients. In this situation, bacteremia may be difficult to identify unless antibiotics are stopped or adsorbents are added to blood cultures to bind the circulating antibiotics. Teichoic acid antibodies in the serum can be a sign of deep-seated Staphylococcus infections.[29]

Disseminated candidiasis must always be considered in persistent fever in the ICU, particularly if the patient has received antibiotic therapy or is a chronic ICU inhabitant. Unfortunately, this diagnosis is often made postmortem. The diagnostic approach to candidal infections are presented in Chapter 45.

REFERENCES

NOSOCOMIAL FEVER

1. Felice GA, Weiler MD, Hughes RA, Gerding DN. Nosocomial febrile illnesses in patients on an internal medicine service. Arch Intern Med 1989; 149:319–324.
2. Tondberg D, Sklar D. Effect of tachypnea on the estimation of body temperature by an oral thermometer. N Engl J Med 1983; 308:945–946.
3. Mellors JW, Horwitz RI, Harvey MR et al. A simple index to identify occult bacterial infection in adults with acute unexplained fever. Arch Intern Med 1987; 147:666–671.
4. Cunha BA, Digamon-Beltran M, Gobbo PN. Implications of fever in the critical care setting. Heart Lung 1984; 13:460–465.
5. Wollschlager CM, Conrad AR, Khan FA. Common complications in critically ill patients. Disease-a-Month 1988; 34(May):221–293.

POSTOPERATIVE FEVER

6. Freischlag J, Busuttil RW. The value of postoperative fever evaluation. Surgery 1983; 94:358–363.
7. Glaciel L, Richet H. A prospective study of postoperative fever in a general surgery department. Infect Control 1985; 6:487–491.
8. Britt BA. Malignant hyperthermia. In: Orkin FK, Cooperman LH. Complications in anesthesiology. Philadelphia: J.B. Lippincott, 1983:291–307.
9. Wenzel RP, Hunting KJ, Osterman CA. Postoperative wound infection rates. Surg Gynecol Obstet 1979; 144:749–755.
10. Meyers JK, Lembeck L, O'Kane H, Baue AE. Changes in functional residual capacity of the lung after operation. Arch Surg 1975; 110:576–583.

PROCEDURES

11. Pollack VE: Adverse effects and pyrogenic reactions during hemodialysis. JAMA 1988; 260:2106–2107.
12. Periera W, Kovnat DM, Khan MA et al. Fever and pneumonia after flexible fiberoptic bronchoscopy. Am Rev Respir Dis 1975; 112:59–63.

SINUSITIS

13. Grindlinger GA, Niehoff J, Hughes L et al. Acute paranasal sinusitis related to nasotracheal intubation of head-injured patients. Crit Care Med 1987; 15:214–217.
14. Aebert H, Hunefeld G, Regel G. Paranasal sinusitis and sepsis in ICU patients with nasotracheal intubation. Intensive Care Med 1988; 15:27–30.

ABDOMINAL SOURCES

15. Orlando R, Gleason E, Drezner AD. Acute acalculous cholecystitis in the critically ill patient. Am J Surg 1983; 145:472–476.
16. Savino JA, Scalea TM, Del Guercio LRM. Factors encouraging laparotomy in acalculous cholecystitis. Crit Care Med 1985; 13:377–380.
17. Stillwell M, Caplan ES. The septic multiple-trauma patient. Crit Care Clin 1988; 4:345–373.
18. Van Thiel DH. Gastrointestinal and hepatic manifestations of chronic alcoholism. Gastroenterology 1981; 81:594–615.
19. Wood M, Anderson M eds. Neurologic infections. Philadelphia: W.B. Saunders, Co., 1988; 49–130.

NONINFECTIOUS SOURCES

20. Svensson LG, Decker G, Kinsley RB. A prospective study of hyperamylassemia and pancreatitis after cardiopulmonary bypass. Ann Thorac Surg 1984; 39:409–411.
21. Steinberg WM, Goldstein SS, Davis ND et al. Diagnostic assays in acute pancreatitis. Ann Intern Med 1985; 102:576–580.
22. Cooke M, Sande MA. Diagnosis and outcome of bowel infarction on an acute medical service. Am J Med 1983; 75:984–992.
23. Murray HW, Ellis GC, Blumenthal DS et al. Fever and pulmonary thromboembolism. Am J Med 1979; 67:232–235.
24. Mackowiak PA, LeMaistre CF. Drug Fever: A critical appraisal of conventional concepts. Ann Intern Med 1987; 106:728–733.
25. Chang YC, Gross EM. Utility of naproxen in the differential diagnosis of fever of undetermined origin in patents with cancer. Am J Med 1984; 76:597–603.
26. Lorell BH, Braunwald E. Pericardial Disease. In: Braunwald E ed, Heart Disease. A textbook of cardiovascular medicine. 2nd ed. Philadelphia: W.B. Saunders, Co., 1988; 1484–1534.

DIAGNOSIS AND THERAPY

27. Aronson MD, Bor DH. Blood cultures. Ann Intern Med 1987; 106:246–253.
28. Rubin M, Pizzo PA. Update on the management of the febrile neutropenic patient. Res Staff Physician 1989; 35:25–43.
29. Sheagren JN. Guidelines for the use of the teichoic acid antibody assay. Arch Intern Med 1984; 144:250–251.

c h a p t e r

44

NOSOCOMIAL PNEUMONIA

Pneumonia is the most fatal of the hospital-acquired (nosocomial) infections, with a mortality of 50% despite aggressive therapy and newer antibiotics.[1-5] The major issues in pneumonia are the problems associated with documenting infection and isolating the pathogen(s). This chapter will highlight these problems and will present some methods that may reduce diagnostic errors.

MICROBIOLOGY

The most common pathogen in nosocomial pneumonia is unknown because no organism is isolated in up to 50% of cases.[3] The bacteria that have been isolated, along with the prevalence of each isolate, are shown in Table 44–1. Unlike community-acquired pneumonia (where pneumococcus predominates), nosocomial pneumonia is frequently caused by gram-negative aerobic bacilli.[1-5] *Pseudomonas* species predominate

TABLE 44–1. BACTERIA ISOLATED FROM THE LOWER AIRWAYS IN ADULTS WITH NOSOCOMIAL PNEUMONIA[3,5,17]	
Organism	Total Isolates (%)
Gram-negative rods	46–75
Pseudomonas	10–30
Proteus	10–15
Haemophilus	10–17
Escherichia coli	8–23
Legionella	2–4
Anaerobic flora	3–35
Staphylococcus	26–33
Pneumococcus	6–30

in most clinical series while staphylococci emerge as the predominant gram-positive pathogens. *Legionella* is responsible for fewer than 5% of nosocomial pneumonias,[6] although epidemic outbreaks can occur when the organism gets into the hospital water supply.

The virulence of the pathogens is often given as the reason for the high mortality of nosocomial pneumonia, but there is more to the story than pathogenicity.

PATHOGENESIS

Pneumonia is produced by aspiration of mouth contents into the upper airways. **The mouth harbors up to one billion bacteria per milliliter of saliva,**[7] so aspiration of even microliters of saliva can introduce large numbers of bacteria into the upper airways. The change in spectrum of pathogens in nosocomial pneumonia is the result of a change in the resident microflora of the oropharynx.

COLONIZATION OF THE OROPHARYNX

In healthy adults, the prominent inhabitants of the oropharynx are anaerobic bacteria, with *Bacteroides melaninogenicus* being the most common isolate. In certain groups of hospitalized patients, the mouth flora changes and the predominant bacteria are aerobic gram-negative rods. This is shown in Figure 44–1. Note that the mouth flora changes only in the sicker patients in the hospital and changes little in healthy patients and hospital workers.[8] This indicates that the severity of illness plays a major role in colonization of the oropharynx while the hospital environment has little or no role in this process. This explains why debilitated outpatients from the community show the same abnormal pattern of colonization as debilitated patients in the hospital.

BACTERIAL ADHERENCE

The change in mouth flora is believed to be caused by a change in the ability of bacteria to adhere to the oral epithelium. In healthy volunteers, a layer of fibronectin (distinct from circulating fibronectin) covers the epithelium in the mouth and prevents gram-negative enteric pathogens from adhering to the underlying epithelial cells. This protective coating is lost in severe illness and the gram-negative pathogens adhere to the unprotected epithelial surface and take up residence in the mouth. This is the basis for coating the mouth with antibiotic gels to reduce the incidence of nosocomial pneumonia.[21,22]

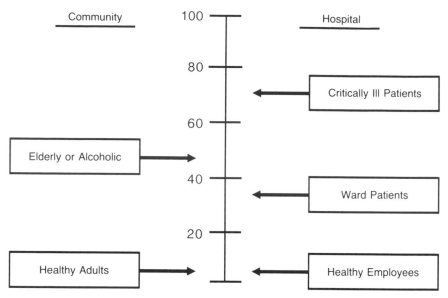

FIG. 44–1. Colonization of the oropharynx with gram-negative aerobic bacilli in different groups of adult subjects. Ordinate is the percent of all subjects in each group with positive throat cultures. From Johanson WG, Pierce AK, Sanford JP. Changing pharyngeal bacterial flora of hospitalized patients. N Engl J Med 1969; *281*:1137–1140.

GASTRIC COLONIZATION

The acid pH in the stomach is important for killing bacteria that are swallowed in the saliva (see Chapter 5). When gastric acidity is suppressed (with antacids, histamine H2 blockers, or enteral tube feedings) the bacteria in the saliva can survive in the stomach. This gastric colonization provides another reservoir for bacteria to multiply and is another source for introducing bacteria into the upper airways. This might explain why the incidence of pneumonia is higher in patients who receive gastric acid suppression therapy with antacids or histamine H2 blockers.[10] Prophylaxis for stress ulcers with sucralfate, which does not increase gastric pH in most patients, has resulted in fewer cases of nosocomial pneumonia.[9] The impact of gastric acid suppression therapy on pneumonia and disseminated sepsis is an exciting area that needs much further study.

THE CLINICAL DIAGNOSIS

The clinical diagnosis of pneumonia can be misleading. This is evident in a postmortem study showing that the clinical diagnosis of pneumonia was incorrect in 60% of cases.[10] The Centers for Disease Control has recommended the following criteria for identifying pneumonia (this applies only to adults).

CDC Definition of Pneumonia.[11] Pneumonia is present when the chest x-ray shows a new or progressive infiltrate or cavitation or a pleural effusion *and* any one of the following is present:

1. New onset purulent sputum or change in character of sputum.
2. A pathogen is isolated from blood culture, transtracheal aspirate, bronchial brushing, or biopsy. (NOTE sputum not included here).
3. A virus or viral antigen is isolated in respiratory secretions.
4. There is a diagnostic single antibody titer (IgM) or a fourfold rise in titers (IgG) from paired serum samples.
5. There is histologic evidence of pneumonia.

The most striking feature of the criteria listed here is the absence of sputum gram stain, sputum culture, and clinical signs of sepsis (fever, leukocytosis). Despite the popularity of fever and sputum analysis, neither is necessary to diagnose pneumonia.

THE CHEST X-RAY

Most clinical definitions of pneumonia require that a new infiltrate be present on the chest x-ray. This assumes a sensitivity that the routine chest radiograph is unlikely to have. The chest film may not show evidence of pulmonary edema until lung water increases by 30% (see Chapter 23), so it is very likely that chest films might not reveal small patches of inflammation. Sensitivity may be further reduced when the lungs are hyperinflated, as seen in obstructive lung disease and during mechanical ventilation.

The specificity of the chest film (the ability of infiltrates to indicate infection) is also a problem because of the multiplicity of processes that can cause pulmonary infiltrates (e.g., edema, atelectasis). This is shown in one study reporting that 40% of the pulmonary infiltrates in ICU patients did not represent infection.[13]

Specific Patterns. The pattern of infiltration can occasionally be helpful in diagnosing pulmonary infection. An example of this is shown in Figure 44–2. The chest film in this case was obtained from a patient with tricuspid valve endocarditis. The peripheral distribution of the infiltrates and the area of coalescence suggest septic emboli as the diagnosis. This is one of the few situations where the chest x-ray can be helpful in making a specific diagnosis.

Nonspecific Patterns. Most patterns of infiltration on chest x-ray are nonspecific and will not help to diagnose pneumonia. This is shown in Figure 44–3. This infiltrative pattern could represent a number of processes like hydrostatic pulmonary edema, diffuse pneumonia, or the "adult respiratory distress syndrome" (ARDS). The latter condition can coexist with pneumonia and further cloud the diagnosis (see Chapter 23). The prevalence of pneumonia in ARDS is shown by the report from one study,[12] where 60% of the patients who died with ARDS had histologic evidence of a pneumonia (usually gram-negative). Unfortunately, only 50% of the pneumonias in this study were clinically detected prior to death. Furthermore, 20% of the patients with no evidence of pneu-

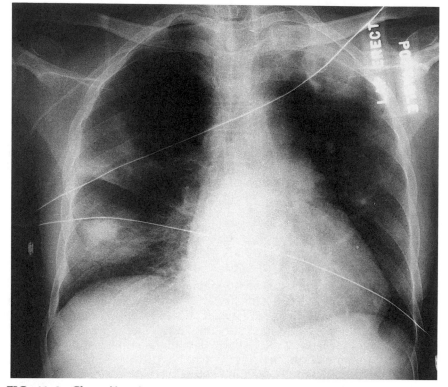

FIG. 44–2. Chest film showing peripheral infiltrates and circular areas of lung necrosis. Presumptive diagnosis: septic pulmonary emboli.

monia on postmortem exam were incorrectly diagnosed as having pneumonia while alive. Overall, 30% of the pneumonias were misdiagnosed in patients with ARDS in this study.[12]

The chest x-ray cannot be regarded as either sensitive or specific for infection. For this reason, analysis of respiratory secretions and other body fluids is used to make the diagnosis of pneumonia and to isolate the responsible pathogen.

RESPIRATORY SECRETIONS

The purulent sputum that is often associated with bacterial pneumonia can be absent in elderly patients.[3] Conversely, purulent sputum can be present without pneumonia. Infection in the upper airways can be the source of purulent sputum while the distal airspaces are clear of infection. This can occur commonly in patients with longstanding tracheal intubation. This emphasizes the importance of determining the source of respiratory secretions before interpreting the culture results.

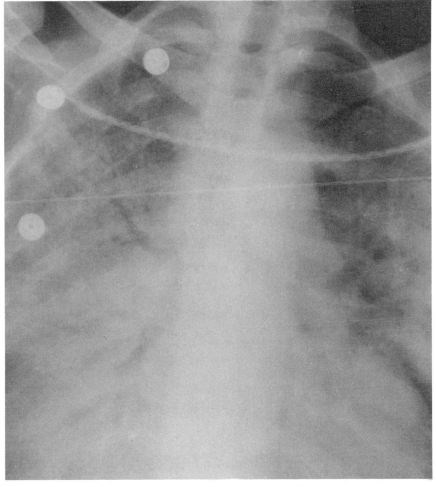

FIG. 44–3. Portable chest x-ray showing extensive infiltrates in both lungs. See text for explanation.

Microscopic Examination

The microscopic examination of secretions can be valuable for identifying infection and for locating the site of the infection (upper airways versus distal lung regions). The sputum components that are useful in this regard are listed in Table 44–2.

Leukocytes. Leukocytes are used to document inflammation or infection but not to localize the site of infection. More than 25 leukocytes per low-power field ($\times 100$) is taken as evidence for infection but is not used as evidence for pneumonia. To mark the location of an infection, the epithelial cells of the oral cavity are used as markers of the upper airways while alveolar macrophages and elastin fibers are used to mark the distal airspaces and lung parenchyma, respectively.

TABLE 44–2. SPUTUM MORPHOLOGY	
Component	**Interpretation**
Squamous Epithelial Cells >10 per LPF*	Oral contaminant
Neutrophils >25 per LPF	Inflammation in upper or lower airways
Alveolar macrophages	Lower airways specimen
Elastin fibers	Necrotizing pneumonia
*Indicates low magnification (×100)	

Squamous Epithelial Cells. The epithelial cells lining the oral cavity are large, flattened cells with abundant cytoplasm and a small nucleus. These cells are shown in Figure 44–4 and are the largest cells in the microscopic field (×400).

More than ten squamous epithelial cells per low-power field (×100) indicates that the specimen is contaminated with mouth secretions.[14]

The Alveolar Macrophage. Alveolar macrophages inhabit only distal airspaces and the presence of even one macrophage in a specimen is evidence that at least part of the specimen is from the lower regions of the lungs. The microscopic appearance of alveolar macrophages is shown in Figure 44–4. The macrophages are the oval-shaped cells with the granular cytoplasm and eccentric nucleus. The neutrophils in the figure

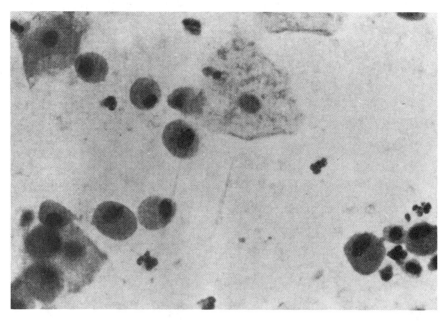

FIG. 44–4. Microscopic appearance (×400) of bronchial brushings from a ventilator-dependent patient. The large, flattened cells are squamous epithelial cells, the oval cells are alveolar macrophages, and the smallest cells are neutrophils.

are about the size of the macrophage nucleus. The largest cells in the figure are squamous epithelial cells from the oral cavity.

Elastin Fibers. Elastin fibers originate from the pulmonary parenchyma and the presence of these fibers is sometimes used as evidence for a necrotizing pneumonia.[15] These fibers are filamentous structures that can be visualized by placing a drop of 40% potassium hydroxide over a sputum sample and covering the specimen with a cover slip. Using low power magnification ($\times 100$), the elastin fibers are seen as clumps of interlacing filaments, like a ball of twine that is unravelled. When these are present, it is reasonable to assume that the specimen is from the parenchyma of the lung and that there is an ongoing destructive process in the lungs.

Screening Sputum Cultures. One of the cardinal sins in any ICU is the practice of sending tracheal aspirates to the microbiology laboratory for culture without first determining the site of origin of the specimen. The secretions from patients with artificial airways is often colonized with organisms like *Pseudomonas aeruginosa*, and a positive sputum culture does not indicate infection or pneumonia.

> Unscreened tracheal aspirates will yield spurious culture results in about half the cases of pneumonia.[13]

This means that the chances of identifying the responsible pathogen with unscreened sputum is the same as predicting heads or tails in a coin toss. The source of respiratory secretions must first be determined by microscopic analysis before the specimen is cultured.

Bronchoscopy

Routine bronchoscopy is of no value for collecting secretions for culture because the bronchoscope picks up contaminants as it passes through the upper airways. To eliminate this problem, a specialized brush has been developed that is situated in a catheter that is plugged at the distal end. The protective housing allows the catheter to be advanced through a bronchoscope without coming into contact with the upper airways.[16–18] This type of brush is available in most hospitals, and should be part of every flexible bronchoscopy performed to obtain lower airway secretions.

The specimen obtained from a protected brush is cultured quantitatively, like urine cultures. A culture yielding 10^3 organisms/ml or greater indicates a pneumonia and identifies the pathogen.[17,18] Fewer organisms may be recovered when the patient is receiving antibiotics.[17] A gram's stain of the brush specimen (separate brush specimens must be used for the culture and the gram's stain) can provide more immediate information because 10^3 organisms/ml is needed to visualize bacteria on a gram's stain.

Percutaneous Aspiration

The most reliable method for obtaining material for culture is the percutaneous lung puncture technique. A small needle (25 gauge) is

TABLE 44–3. INCIDENCE OF PARAPNEUMONIC EFFUSIONS AND
POSITIVE PLEURAL FLUID CULTURES IN BACTERIAL PNEUMONIA

Pathogen	Effusion (%)	Culture Positive (%)
Pneumococcus	50	<5
Staphylococcus aureus	40	20
Pseudomonas	50	>90
Haemophilus influenza	50	<20
Anaerobes	35	>90

From Light RW, Meyer RD, Sahn SA, et al. Parapneumonic effusions and empyema. Clin Chest Med 1985; 6:55–62.

advanced through the skin and directed to the area of consolidation. This can be done at the bedside without fluoroscopic guidance if there is evidence for consolidation by lung sounds. This technique is a lung aspirate and not a lung biopsy. It is safe in most patients but is not recommended for ventilator-dependent patients because of the high incidence of tension pneumothoraces.

PARAPNEUMONIC EFFUSIONS

Parapneumonic effusions are present in up to 50% of bacterial pneumonias, and 10% of the effusions will not resolve without chest tube drainage.[19] Table 44–3 shows the incidence of parapneumonic effusions with the pneumonias that are common in the ICU. The decision to evaluate a parapneumonic effusion is often based on the ease with which the fluid can be obtained and the response of the patient to initial antibiotic therapy. Post-thoracotomy effusions are much more likely to be infected than routine parapneumonic effusions and these warrant a more aggressive approach.

Pleural Fluid Analysis

Only 20 to 30 ml of pleural fluid is necessary for analysis. If the pleural effusion is loculated (doesn't layer on decubitus views), a bedside ultrasound is valuable for marking the location and depth of the fluid. The following studies on the fluid samples are useful: 1) Gram's stain and culture; 2) Glucose; 3) pH. There is little need to determine if the fluid is a transudate or exudate or to perform a cell count, because these tests may not separate infected from sterile fluid. The criteria for tube drainage of parapneumonic effusions are listed in Table 44–4. The only absolute indication for a chest tube is a thick, loculated, grossly purulent effusion. A positive gram's stain is also reason for some to place a tube if the effusion has not been drained during the thoracentesis, or if the effusion is post-thoracotomy (because the mortality from empyema is highest following thoracotomy).

TABLE 44–4. MANAGEMENT OF PARAPNEUMONIC EFFUSIONS	
Pleural Fluid	**Decision**
Glucose <40 mg/dl pH <7.0 Positive Gram's Stain	Tube Thoracostomy
pH = 7.0–7.2	Repeat in 12–24 hours
Glucose >40 mg/dl pH >7.20	No Rx Needed
From Light RW, et al. Parapneumonia effusions and empyema. Clin Chest Med 1985; 6:55–62.	

EMPIRIC ANTIBIOTIC THERAPY

Early antibiotic therapy is usually guided by gram stains of lower tract secretions and the clinical setting. Some popular regimens based on the results of the sputum gram stain are shown in Table 44–5. The antibiotic doses are presented in Chapter 47.

GRAM-NEGATIVE INFECTIONS

The concern here is to cover for *Pseudomonas* species and combination therapy is recommended using an aminoglycoside and an anti-

TABLE 44–5. EMPIRIC ANTIBIOTIC THERAPY		
Gram's Stain	**Antibiotic(s)**	**Comment**
GM(−) Rods:		
Single Morphology	Aminoglycoside plus ceftazidime	Good double coverage for *Pseudomonas*
Multiple Morphology	Aminoglycoside plus imipenem	Imipenem adds anaerobe coverage
GM(+) Cocci	Vancomycin	Vancomycin covers all GM(+)s, including methicillin-resistant *Staphylococcus* and anaerobes
Mixed Flora	Imipenem Vancomycin	Good for anaerobes, GM(+)s and GM(−)s, except *Pseudomonas*
No Organisms		
Immune Compromised	Aminoglycoside plus ceftazidime	Rx must cover *Pseudomonas* when immune compromised
Otherwise	No Rx	

pseudomonal penicillin or ceftazidime. If some of the gram-negative rods in the pleural fluid could be anaerobes, imipenem can be given in combination with an aminoglycoside. Although combination antimicrobial therapy is often advocated for nosocomial pneumonia because of the high mortality rate, there is no evidence that combination therapy is any better for serious gram negative pneumonias in non-neutropenic patients than single agent therapy.

GRAM-POSITIVE INFECTIONS

The concern here is *Staphylococcus aureus*, particularly methicillin-resistant organisms. Vancomycin is probably the single best agent for gram-positive cocci, including methicillin-resistant staphylococci.

ANAEROBIC INFECTIONS

Most anaerobic pneumonias are polymicrobial, with *Bacteroides fragilis* present in 15% of cultures. Penicillin remains a good drug for anaerobic pneumonias, even when *B. fragilis* is part of a polymicrobial pneumonia. However, there is a tendency to use other agents for hospitalized patients. The effective anaerobic agents are clindamycin (300 mg IV every 6 hours), metronidazole (250 to 500 mg IV every 6 hours), chloramphenicol (250 to 500 mg IV every 6 hours), and imipenem (1 gm IV every 6 hours).

THE FUTURE: PREVENTION?

The trend in recent years has been to eradicate the oral flora with locally applied antibiotics in an attempt to reduce the incidence of nosocomial pneumonia. Nonabsorbable antibiotics (usually polymyxin and an aminoglycoside) are prepared in a solution or paste and applied directly to the oral mucosa.[20,21] The results from this practice are very encouraging, with all studies showing significant decreases in the incidence of nosocomial pneumonia. Further studies are needed in this area before any firm conclusions can be drawn.

PNEUMONIA AND AIDS

Pneumonia is a hallmark of the autoimmune deficiency syndrome (AIDS) and is usually the cause of death in this illness. Several pathogens can invade the lungs in this patient population and most of them are opportunistic pathogens. *Pneumocystis carinii* is responsible for over 50% of the lung infections in AIDS patients.[22] Other pathogens include viruses (e.g., cytomegalovirus and herpes virus), fungi (cryptococcus predominating), atypical mycobacteria (avium-intracellulare), and pyogenic bacteria (streptococcus, staphylococcus, legionella, and gram-negative enteric pathogens). The fact that AIDS patients can have infections caused by routine bacterial pathogens is not mentioned enough.

CLINICAL PRESENTATION

The early presentation in *Pneumocystis* pneumonia (PCP) is marked by dyspnea, tachypnea, and an increase in the A-a PO_2 gradient. The chest film at the outset varies from being clear to showing diffuse alveolar infiltrates.[22] The lung exam in PCP is often unrewarding early in the illness despite a high A-a PO_2 gradient. If the chest film is unrevealing, a Gallium scan can detect the presence of inflammation but this is non-specific and will not identify the organism. Hilar adenopathy and pleural effusions are more common with Kaposi's Sarcoma than with lung infections.

DIAGNOSIS

The diagnostic approach is aimed at identifying *Pneumocystis carinii* in either sputum (induced with 3 to 5% saline inhalation) or in bronchial lavage specimens. The yield from sputum can be as high as 70% but this requires cytopathologists who are experienced in detecting the organism. Bronchoalveolar lavage with 100 ml saline is the standard method for retrieving the organism from the lower airways.

THERAPY

The therapy for PCP includes trimethoprim-sulfamethoxazole (Bactrim or Septra) and pentamidine isethionate. Both drugs are considered equally effective and both can be highly toxic agents as well.[23] Neither agent is successful in eradicating the organism from the airways with short courses of therapy.

Trimethoprim-Sulfamethoxazole (TMP-SMX). This agent is generally considered to be the initial drug of choice if there is no history of allergies to sulfa. (See Chapter 47 for more information on this drug.)

> Dose: Trimethoprim (20 mg/kg) and
> Sulfamethoxazle (100 mg/kg)
> Route: PO or IV
> Interval: Every 6 to 8 hours

Toxic reactions to TMP-SMX include rash, vomiting, leukopenia, thrombocytopenia, and nephritis. As shown in Table 47–7 (Chapter 47), the incidence of toxic reactions is much higher in the AIDS patient population. Toxicity may be less if the doses of the drugs are reduced to trimethoprim 15 mg/kg and sulfamethoxazole 75 mg/kg.[23]

Pentamidine Isethionate. This agent is usually reserved for patients who cannot tolerate TMP-SMX or who do not respond to TMP-SMX.

Dose: 4 mg/kg (dilute in 100 ml 5% dextrose in water)
Route: IV (Infuse over 60 minutes)
Interval: Every 24 hours

Toxic reactions to this agent are more severe than with TMP-SMX and include hypoglycemia, hyperglycemia and insulin-dependent diabetes, leukopenia, thrombocytopenia, and orthostatic hypotension.[23] All reactions except the diabetes are reversible when the drug is stopped.

Steroids. There is some enthusiasm over the use of high dose steroids in patients with refractory *Pneumocystic* pneumonia. In one study, 10 patients with rapidly progressive pneumonia on conventional therapy were given intravenous methylprednisolone (40 mg every 6 hours) and all but one of the patients recovered from the illness.[24] We are giving steroids to refractory patients at our hospital with variable results. At the present time, the value of steroid therapy in *Pneumocystis* pneumonia is undetermined.

REFERENCES

REVIEWS

1. Craven DE, Driks MR. Nosocomial pneumonia in the intubated patient. Semin Respir Med 1987; 2:20–33.
2. Hessen MT, Kaye D. Nosocomial pneumonia. Crit Care Clin 1988; 4:245–257.
3. Verghese A, Berk SL. Bacterial pneumonia in the elderly. Medicine 1983; 62:271–285.

MICROBIOLOGY

4. Ruiz-Santana S, Jiminez AG, Esteban A, et al. ICU pneumonias: A multi-institutional study. Crit Care Med 1987; 15:930–932.
5. Bartlett JG, O'Keefe P, Tally FP. Bacteriology of hospital-acquired pneumonia. Arch Intern Med 1986; 146:868–874.
6. Meyer RD. *Legionella* infections: A review of five years of research. Rev Infect Dis 1983; 5:258–278.

PATHOGENESIS

7. Higuchi JH, Johanson WG. Colonization and bronchopulmonary infection. Clin Chest Med 1983; 3:133–142.
8. Johanson WG, Pierce AK, Sanford JP. Changing pharyngeal bacterial flora of hospitalized patients. N Engl J Med 1969; 281:1137–1140.
9. Driks MR, Craven DE, Celli BR, et al. Nosocomial pneumonia in intubated patients given sucralfate as compared with antacids or histamine type-2 blockers. N Engl J Med 1987; 317:1376–1382.

CLINICAL DIAGNOSIS

10. Bryant LR, Mobin-Uddin K, Dillon ML, et al. Misdiagnosis of pneumonia in patients needing mechanical respiration. Arch Surg 1973; 106:286–288.
11. Garner JS, Jarvis WR, Emori TG, et al. CDC definitions for nosocomial infections, 1988. Am J Infect Control 1988; 16:128–140.
12. Andrews CP, Coalson JJ, Smith JD, Johanson WG, Jr. Diagnosis of nosocomial bacterial pneumonia in acute diffuse lung injury. Chest 1981; 80:254–258.
13. Berger R, Arango L. Etiologic diagnosis of bacterial nosocomial pneumonia in seriously ill patients. Crit Care Med 1985; 13:833–836.
14. Murray PR, Washington JA. Microscopic and bacteriologic analysis of expectorated sputum. Mayo Clin Proc 1975; 50:339–344.
15. Salata RA, Lederman MM, Shlaes DM. Diagnosis of nosocomial pneumonia in intubated intensive care unit patients. Am Rev Respir Dis 1987; 135:426–432.

BRONCHOSCOPY

16. Chastre J, Viau F, Brun P, et al. Prospective evaluation of the protected specimen brush for the diagnosis of pulmonary infections in ventilated patients. Am Rev Respir Dis 1984; 130:924–929.
17. Fagon J-Y, Chastre J, Hance AJ, et al. Detection of nosocomial lung infection in ventilated patients. Am Rev Respir Dis 1988; 138:110–116.
18. Richard C, Pezzang M, Bouhaja B, et al. Comparison of non-protected lower respiratory tract secretions and protected specimen brush samples in the diagnosis of pneumonia. Intensive Care Med 1988; 14:30–33.

PARAPNEUMONIC EFFUSIONS

19. Light RW, Meyer RD, Sahn SA, et al. Parapneumonic effusions and empyema. Clin Chest Med 1985; 6:55–62.

PREVENTIVE THERAPY

20. van Uffelen R, Rommes JH, van Saene HKF. Preventing lower airway colonization and infection in mechanically ventilated patients. Crit Care Med 1987; 15:99–102.
21. Stoutenbeek CP, van Saene HKF, Miranda DR, et al. The effect of oropharyngeal decontamination using topical nonabsorbable antibiotics on the incidence of nosocomial respiratory tract infections in multiple trauma patients. J Trauma 1987; 27:357–364.

AIDS

22. Rankin JA, Collman R, Daniele RP. Acquired immune deficiency syndrome and the lung. Chest 1988; 94:155–164.

23. Masur H, Kovacs JA. Treatment and prophylaxis of *Pneumocystis carinii* pneumonia. In: Sande MA, Volberding PA eds. The medical management of AIDS. Philadelphia: W.B. Saunders, 1988; 181–192.

24. MacFadden DK, Edelson JD, Hyland RH. Corticosteroids as adjunctive therapy in treatment of pneumocystis carinii pneumonia in patients with acquired immunodeficiency syndrome. Lancet 1987; 2:1477–1479.

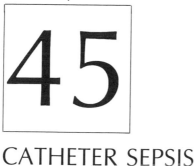

chapter

45

CATHETER SEPSIS

Vascular catheters are responsible for 10 to 15% of all hospital-acquired infections.[1] The incidence of disseminated infection from vascular catheters varies widely in different reports but averages about 7 to 8% for central venous and arterial catheters.[1-3] This chapter will present some of the practical aspects of the bedside approach to suspected sepsis from central venous catheters and arterial catheters. The following definitions will provide a framework for the discussion that follows.

> **Catheter-Related Sepsis**—When the same organism is isolated from the tip of the catheter and the blood, and there is dense growth on the catheter. Indicates that the catheter is the source of the sepsis.
>
> **Colonization**—When the organism shows sparse growth on the catheter. The blood culture can grow the same organisms or can show no growth. This indicates that the catheter is not responsible for the septic state.

A more detailed definition of dense and sparse growth is presented later in the chapter.

PATHOGENESIS

The mechanisms responsible for catheter-related sepsis are illustrated in Figure 45–1. Three pathways are described (see the enclosed numbers in the diagram).

1. Microorganisms can gain entry to the bloodstream through breaks in the infusion system (e.g., stopcocks).

2. Skin flora can migrate along the tract created by the catheter and can settle in the fibrin sheath that covers the intravascular portion of the catheter. This fibrin meshwork is avascular and provides a protective

603

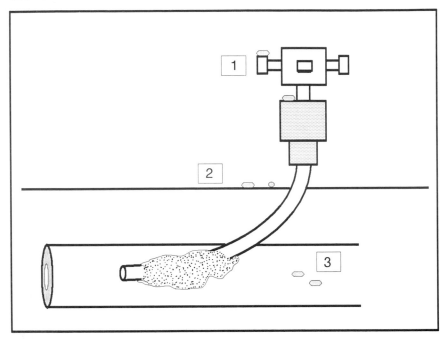

FIG. 45–1. Routes of catheter-related sepsis. See text for explanation.

environment for microbes to proliferate. Silicone catheters (e.g., Hickman and Broviac) are less thrombogenic than polyurethane catheters and show less tendency to form fibrin sheaths.

3. Organisms already in the bloodstream can settle in the fibrin sheath and proliferate. In this situation, the catheter becomes a secondary source of septicemia.

The first two routes are considered to be the primary pathways for microorganisms to gain entry to the bloodstream. The third route has received less attention than it deserves.

HOW CAN BACTERIA MIGRATE?

The notion that the skin is a primary source of organisms for catheter-associated septicemia rests on the assumption that skin microbes can move long distances along the catheter tract until they reach the fibrin sheath on the catheter tip. However, bacteria cannot move visible distances on inert surfaces like the skin. Staphylococci (the most common microbes in catheter sepsis) are non-motile organisms with no means of locomotion and cannot migrate at all without some assistance. These microbes are only one micron in diameter but they are supposed to "crawl" a distance of 12 inches (the length of a triple lumen catheter) or 300,000 times their length if they are to reach the tip of a multilumen catheter. This is analogous to a six-foot human crawling a distance of

300 miles (the distance between Boston and Philadelphia). These distances are not feasible without some form of assistance.

Microbes on the skin surface could reach the bloodstream if they were pushed along during the percutaneous insertion of the catheter. This seems unlikely because the sepsis from central venous catheters does not appear soon after the catheter is inserted but almost always takes at least 3 or 4 days to appear.[1-3]

THE ROLE OF THE BOWEL

The intravascular portion of a catheter could become seeded by microorganisms that are already in the bloodstream that entered the bloodstream from other sites, much like the situation with prosthetic valve endocarditis. The gastrointestinal tract is one of the more likely sources for introducing bacteria into the bloodstream and this risk is particularly prominent in seriously ill patients. Two factors predispose these patients to septicemia from the bowel. First, the resident flora of the stomach and small bowel increase markedly when gastric acid is suppressed with histamine H2 blockers or antacids (see Chapter 5). This allows the upper GI tract to become colonized with bacteria that are swallowed in the saliva. Second, the mucosal barrier that separates the bowel flora from the bloodstream is often atrophic or disrupted in seriously ill patients and this allows the bowel flora to "translocate" into the systemic circulation.

A recent case at our hospital points to the role of the upper GI tract in catheter tip infections. A patient in the postoperative period following an esophagogastrectomy developed fever and the workup revealed *Enterobacter cloaceae* in the blood cultures (four sets) and on the tip of a subclavian catheter (more than 100 colonies). In addition, the same organism was isolated from gastric secretions but could not be recovered from the skin around the catheter insertion site (on two occasions). The gastric pH in this patient was 5.0 at the time of the septicemia and this would explain the presence of the pathogen in the stomach (see Chapter 5). The diagnosis in this case would have been catheter-related septicemia if the cultures of the gastric aspirate were not obtained. The more likely diagnosis is bowel sepsis with secondary seeding of the catheter tip, much like an infection of any prosthetic device. We are presently culturing gastric aspirates in all cases of suspected catheter sepsis to more fully determine the role of the bowel flora in presumed catheter-related infections.

MICROBIOLOGY

The pathogens isolated from the blood in 13 prospective studies of catheter-related septicemia are shown in Table 45–1.[2] About 50% of the infections are caused by staphylococci, and the remainder are caused by *Candida* sp. and a variety of enteric pathogens.

TABLE 45–1. COMMON ORGANISMS INVOLVED IN CATHETER-RELATED SEPTICEMIA	
Organism	Total Isolates (%)
Staphylococcus epidermidis	27
Staphylococcus aureus	26
Candida sp.	17
Enterobacter	7
Serratia	5
Enterococcus	5
Klebsiella	4
Pseudomonas sp.	3
Proteus	2
Others	6

From Hampton AA, Sheretz RJ. Vascular-access infections in hospitalized patients. Surg Clin North Am 1988; 68:57–71.

STAPHYLOCOCCI

Staphylococci are common skin inhabitants but can also be found on mucous membranes (toxic shock syndrome) and in the bowel of patients receiving broad-spectrum antibiotic therapy.

Staphylococci are classified as coagulase-positive *(Staphylococcus aureus)* or coagulase-negative. The coagulase-negative strains that can be pathogenic in man are *Staphylococcus saprophyticus* (urinary tract infections) and *Staphylococcus epidermidis* (vascular catheter and bladder catheter infections).[3] They are not virulent in normal subjects but become pathogens as the severity of illness increases. Certain strains of *Staphylococcus epidermidis* produce a sticky substance called "slime" that allows the organism to attach to prosthetic materials easily and this may explain why this organism is so prevalent in infections involving prosthetic materials. This should also explain the prevalence of this microbe in cultures of vascular catheter tips.

Antibiotic Susceptibility. The coagulase-negative staphylococci can be resistant to antibiotics that eradicate the coagulase-positive strains.

As many as 80% of *Staphylococcus epidermidis* isolates are resistant to methicillin and the cephalosporins and many are also resistant to aminoglycosides.[3] The antibiotic of choice for the methicillin-resistant strains is vancomycin.

Combination therapy with vancomycin and gentamicin can be synergistic for *Staphylococcus epidermidis* and this combination is recommended for endocarditis or any other serious infections caused by these pathogens.

THE CLINICAL APPROACH

Catheter-related infection should be considered when any of the following conditions is associated with fever or other evidence for sepsis.
1. When there is no other obvious source of sepsis (e.g., pneumonia or urinary tract infection) and the catheter has been in place for at least 72 hours.
2. When there is erythema around the catheter insertion site.
3. When pus can be expressed from the catheter insertion site.

The third condition is considered proof of catheter-related sepsis.[2] Erythema around the insertion site does not correlate with the presence of bacteria in the bloodstream.

BLOOD CULTURES

The guidelines for blood cultures are presented in Chapter 43 (see Tables 43–6 and 43–7). The blood should not be withdrawn through the suspected catheter because of the risk for false-positive cultures.[3] Two sets of blood cultures (one set is one venipuncture) are adequate unless endocarditis is suspected.[6] When endocarditis is a possible diagnosis, at least three sets of blood cultures will be necessary. The volume of blood withdrawn will influence the yield from blood cultures; at least 10 ml should be taken from each venipuncture site.[6]

CATHETER REMOVAL

When catheter-related sepsis is suspected, the catheter(s) should be removed pending culture results. Silicone catheters (e.g., Hickman and Broviac) do not always require removal because infection on these catheters can be eradicated by antibiotic therapy alone.[7] This may be due to the reduced propensity for fibrin sheath formation on these catheters.

When removing a catheter, the skin around the insertion site should be cleaned with an alcohol swab and gloves should be worn. After the original catheter is withdrawn (usually over a guidewire), the distal 2 or 3 inches is cut with sterile scissors and the severed end of the catheter is immediately placed in a sterile culturette tube and taken to the microbiology lab. **Do not place the catheter tip in blood culture bottles.** The severed end of the catheter will be plated directly on blood agar plates in the microbiology lab and the number of colonies of microbes that appears will be documented. This is called a "semiquantitative" culture.[11]

GUIDEWIRE EXCHANGE

As many as 90% of the catheters removed for suspected catheter sepsis are subsequently found to be sterile.[8] This means that the routine practice of using new venipunctures for inserting replacement catheters in the

TABLE 45–2. INTERPRETATION OF SEMIQUANTITATIVE CULTURES		
Blood Culture	**Colony Count***	**Interpretation**
Positive	>15	Catheter is source of septicemia
	<15	Catheter seeded from the blood-stream
Negative	>15	Catheter infected locally Cannot rule out intermittent septicemia
	<15	Catheter is colonized

*Colonies per catheter. From Maki et al. A semiquantitative method for identifying intravenous catheter related infection. N Engl J Med 1977; 296:1305–1309.

subclavian and internal jugular veins would involve unnecessary risks in most patients. To obviate these risks, a metal guidewire is used to exchange catheters (if a replacement catheter is necessary). There has been some concern that this practice would transfer microorganisms from the infected catheter to the replacement catheter and thereby promote the persistence of the infection. However,

> Guidewire exchange has not been associated with contamination of replacement catheters,[1,2,8,9,10] and this practice is now recommended as safe unless the patient has a burn or there is purulent material at the catheter insertion site.

Replacement catheters that have been exchanged over a guidewire do not have to be removed if the original catheter is found to be infected unless there are persistent signs of sepsis after the catheter exchange.[9]

CATHETER CULTURES

Broth cultures are unreliable for distinguishing colonization of catheter tips from true infection with spread to the bloodstream.

> As many as 50% of catheters that show growth in broth culture will not be associated with septicemia.[2]

The preferred method for culturing catheter tips at the present time is a semiquantitative culture technique where the catheter is rolled over the surface of a sheep blood agar plate and the number of colonies that form are counted.[11] This "semiquantitative" culture method is interpreted according to the rules listed in Table 45–2.[11]

Guidelines for Interpretation

When the blood cultures are positive:
1. More than 15 colonies of the same organism on the catheter tip suggests that the catheter was the source of the septicemia.
2. Less than 15 colonies on the catheter tip suggests that the septi-

cemia originated elsewhere and the catheter tip was seeded by the organisms in the bloodstream.

When the blood cultures show no growth:
1. More than 15 colonies on the catheter tip suggests possible catheter-related septicemia that was missed (intermittent bacteremia).
2. Less than 15 colonies on the catheter tip indicates that the catheter is colonized and is not the cause of the fever.

Negative blood cultures should not be interpreted too rigidly when the catheter tip shows dense growth of microbes because the catheter may have seeded the bloodstream but the septicemia was missed because it was intermittent. In fact, less than 50% of catheter tips with a dense growth (> 15 colonies) are associated with positive blood cultures.[11] Blood cultures can also be misleading in catheter-related infections involving *Candida* species because this organism does not grow readily in blood cultures.[12]

GRAM'S STAIN

More immediate information is provided by staining the catheter after it is removed. This is done by making a longitudinal slit in the catheter segment (to stain both inner and outer surfaces of the catheter) and immersing the segment in gram's stain solutions using sterile forceps. An example of the yield from this method is shown in the photomicrograph in Figure 45–2. Note the rod-like bacteria, which were identified as *Klebsiella* by culture.[14]

There are several advantages to staining catheters after they are removed. First, you can identify catheter-related sepsis immediately. Second, the morphology of the organisms can help to select the appropriate antibiotic pending identification by culture. This particularly applies to *Candida*, which can be identified as large gram-positive forms that are round or oval in shape. Finally, the surface of the catheter that is involved may provide some information on the source of the problem. That is, organisms on the inner surface of the catheter may indicate a break in the infusion system while organisms attached to the outer surface of the catheter might indicate a skin source or bacteremia from a distant site.

The gram's stain is an appealing method for generating immediate information but it has been largely ignored since its first description in 1985.[14] One explanation for the lack of popularity of the gram's stain is the time involved in performing the stains and inspecting the specimen under the microscope. Routine staining of all catheters that are replaced would be time consuming and this practice may not be justified in all patients. Nevertheless, the potential value of the gram's stain should not be ignored.

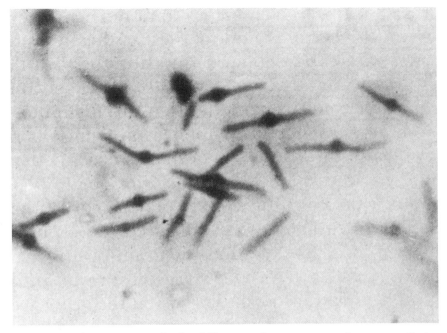

FIG. 45–2. Photomicrograph of rod-like organisms on a central venous catheter. Oil immersion field. From Cooper GL, Hopkins CC. Rapid diagnosis of intravascular catheter-associated infection by direct gram staining of catheter segments. N Engl J Med 1985; *312*:1142–1147.

AVOIDING CATHETER REMOVAL

As many as three-fourths of catheters that are removed for suspected catheter sepsis will be sterile,[1,2,11,15] which means there is an inordinate number of unnecessary catheter removal procedures. An innovative method of culturing catheters without removing them has been reported recently.[15] A narrow brush is passed through a catheter in place so that the brush collects material from the inner surface of the catheter. The brush is rolled over the surface of an agar plate, and the number of colonies that grow on the plate is documented. This is identical to the semiquantitative culture techniques used for catheters. A culture that yields over 10 colonies is considered to be positive.[15]

The major problem with this method is the possibility of leaving an infected catheter in place for 2 to 3 days while waiting for the organism to grow in culture. Catheter removal alone can be associated with improvement in the clinical signs of sepsis, even when the catheter is sterile,[16] so that catheter removal is itself a form of therapy. Keeping an infected device in the bloodstream could lead to progressive sepsis, even with the institution of antibiotics. Therefore, catheter removal is still necessary for patients who appear septic at the time of the culture. The value of *in situ* catheter culture techniques will require further study before it can be recommended.

TABLE 45–3.	APPROACHES TO SUSPECTED CATHETER SEPSIS	
Clinical Setting	Catheter Change	Empiric Antibiotics
Fever Only	Guidewire	No Antibiotics
Purulent Drainage	Remove and Use New Site	Vancomycin
Prosthetic Device in Place	Guidewire	Vancomycin plus Gentamicin
Neutropenia	Guidewire	Vancomycin plus Ceftazidime and an Aminoglycoside
Persistent Fever on Antibiotics	Remove and Use New Site	Consider Amphotericin B

ANTIMICROBIAL THERAPY

The decision to institute immediate antibiotic therapy before cultures are available is determined by the clinical situation. Some general guidelines are shown in Table 45–3. Removal of the offending catheter is often effective without the use of antibiotics.[1,2,16] However, life-threatening endocarditis can occur as a result of catheter-associated bacteremia.[13] Therefore, immediate antibiotic therapy is recommended for every patient with a prosthetic device in place, regardless of the clinical appearance of the patient. Immunosuppressed patients should also be given aggressive antibiotic therapy before the culture results are available. **Vancomycin** is the drug of choice for serious infections with coagulase-negative and methicillin-resistant strains of staphylococci. Remember that the coagulase-negative strains are usually resistant to cephalosporins as well. In neutropenic patients or those with prosthetic devices, combined therapy with vancomycin and an aminoglycoside is recommended.

The duration of antibiotic therapy needed in documented cases of catheter sepsis is also not clear. In routine cases, 4 to 5 days of therapy is probably sufficient.[2] More prolonged therapy is indicated in patients with prosthetic devices or neutropenia.

PERSISTENT SEPSIS

The persistence of positive blood cultures or clinical signs of sepsis after antibiotic therapy is underway suggests suppurative thrombophlebitis or disseminated Candidiasis, respectively.

Septic Thrombophlebitis. This endovascular infection can occur in peripheral vessels, or in the large central veins. The diagnosis is suggested by persistently positive blood cultures after catheter removal and antibiotic therapy.[17,18] In peripheral vessels, there is often evidence of local inflammation, including purulent drainage from the catheter insertion site.[17] In large central veins, evidence for obstruction is usually present (by venography or physical exam).

TABLE 45–4.   COMMON PRACTICES TO REDUCE THE RISK OF
CATHETER-ASSOCIATED INFECTION

Practice	Risk of Infection
Masks and Gowns	Not Studied
Topical Antibiotics	↓
Transparent Dressing	↑
In-Line Filters	Not Studied
Protective Sleeves	↔
Routine Changes over Guidewire	↔ ↑

Therapy for peripheral vessels is surgical excision of the involved vessel.[17] This is not feasible in the large central veins. In this situation, therapy includes catheter removal, antibiotics, and anticoagulation with heparin. The therapy can be effective in 50% of cases in central vein thrombophlebitis.[18]

Disseminated Fungal Infection. The diagnosis of disseminated *Candida* infection is often missed, because blood cultures are not positive in over 50% of cases.[19] When fever and other signs of sepsis do not abate after removing all catheters and initiating antibiotic therapy, disseminated Candidemia should be suspected. An eye exam for Candida endophthalmitis is recommended. The true incidence of endophthalmitis in disseminated Candidiasis is unknown, but it is believed to be low. However, a positive eye exam secures the diagnosis.

In neutropenic patients with persistent fever after 7 days of antibiotics, empiric therapy with amphotericin B is recommended.[20] In other patient groups, the decision to begin empiric amphotericin depends on the clinical appearance; i.e., therapy is usually considered in patients with evidence for severe sepsis or septic shock.

COMMON PRACTICES

There are several practices that have been adopted to reduce the incidence of catheter-related infection. Some are effective, while others are either not effective, not studied, or are deleterious. The more common practices are shown in Table 45–4, along with their efficacy.

MASK AND GOWN

The value of mask and gown has never been studied, but the consensus is that they make little difference in limiting the incidence of catheter sepsis.[2]

SKIN PREPARATION

Vigorous scrubbing of the skin around the insertion site is the best way to remove surface organisms. A povidone-iodine solution is used for the scrub (1 minute should be adequate), and the solution should stand on the skin for another 30 seconds before inserting the catheter. Application of a polymyxin-neomycin-bacitracin ointment around the insertion site may reduce infection.[2]

ROUTINE CATHETER CHANGES

The risk of infection can increase 1 to 2% per day after the first 72 hours,[2] so catheters should always be removed when they are no longer needed. What is probably more important than the duration of catheterization is the number of manipulations or "breaks" in the catheter-tubing system because of drug infusion or blood transfusion.

The association between duration of catheterization and infection led to the practice of replacing catheters over a guidewire every 3 to 4 days. However, this practice not only does not reduce infection,[2] it may actually increase infection rates.[21] The increase in infection rates is not surprising, because the movement of catheters up and down the tract could drag organisms into the bloodstream. At present, routine guidewire changes are recommended only for burn victims.

PROTECTIVE SLEEVES

Sterile sleeves are available for pulmonary artery catheters to allow catheter manipulation while maintaining a sterile environment for the exterior portion of the catheter. These protective sleeves are awkward to work with, and do not reduce the incidence of catheter sepsis.[22]

IN-LINE FILTERS

Filters placed in the path of infusion can trap bacteria and other debris, but there is no evidence that they reduce the rate of catheter-associated septicemia.[2] These filters are not popular because they limit the rate of infusion.

REFERENCES

REVIEWS

1. Weinbaum DL. Nosocomial bacteremia. Clin Crit Care Med 1986; 12:39–58.
2. Hampton AA, Sheretz RJ. Vascular-access infections in hospitalized patients. Surg Clin North Am 1988; 68:57–71.

COAGULASE-NEGATIVE STAPHYLOCOCCI

3. Lowy FD, Hammer SM. *Staphylococcus epidermidis* infections. Ann Intern Med 1983; *99*:834–839.
4. Sheagren JN. Significance of blood culture isolates of *Staphylococcus epidermidis*. [Editorial] Arch Intern Med 1987; *147*:635.
5. Williams JW, Wenzel RP. Coping with methicillin-resistant *S. aureus* infections. J Crit Illness 1987; *2*:65–68.

THE CLINICAL APPROACH

6. Aronson MD, Bor DH. Blood cultures. Ann Intern Med 1987; *106*:246–253.
7. Benezra D, Kiehn TE, Gold JWM, et al. Prospective study of infections in indwelling central venous catheters using quantitative blood cultures. Am J Med 1988; *85*:495–498.
8. Pettigrew RA, Lang SDR, Haydock DA, et al. Catheter-related sepsis in patients on intravenous nutrition: A prospective study of quantitative catheter cultures and guide-wire changes for suspected sepsis. Br J Surg 1985; *72*:52–55.
9. Bozzetti F, Terno G, Bonfanti G, et al. Prevention and treatment of central venous catheter sepsis by exchange via a guidewire. Ann Surg 1983; *198*:48–52.
10. Sitzmann JV, Townsend TR, Siler MC, et al. Septic and technical complications of central venous catheterization. Ann Surg 1985; *201*:766–770.
11. Maki DG, Weise CE, Sarafin HW. A semiquantitative culture method for identifying intravenous-catheter related infection. N Engl J Med *296*:1305–1309, 1977.
12. Goldstein E, Hoeprich PD. Problems in the diagnosis and treatment of systemic candidiasis. Pediatr Infect Dis J 1982; *1*:11–18.
13. Power J, Wing EJ, Talamo TS, et al. Fatal bacterial endocarditis as a complication of permanent indwelling catheters. Am J Med 1986; *81*:166–168.
14. Cooper GL, Hopkins CC. Rapid diagnosis of intravascular catheter-associated infection by direct gram staining of catheter segments. N Engl J Med 1985; *312*:1142–1147.
15. Markus S, Buday S. Culturing indwelling central venous catheters *in situ*. Infect Surg 1989; *8*:156–162.
16. Bozetti F, Terno G, Camerini E, et al. Pathogenesis and predictability of central venous catheter sepsis. Surgery 1982; *91*:383–389.
17. Garrison RN, Richardson JD, Fry DE. Catheter-associated septic thrombophlebitis. South Med J 1982; *75*:917–919.
18. Verghese A, Widrich WC, Arbeit RD. Central venous septic thrombophlebitis—the role of medical therapy. Medicine 1985; *64*:394–400.
19. Henderson DK, Edwards JE, Montgomerie JZ. Hematogenous *Candida* endophthalmitis in patients receiving parenteral hyperalimentation fluids. J Infect Dis 1981; *143*:655–661.
20. Rubin M, Pizzo PA. Update on the management of the febrile neutropenic patient. Resident & Staff Physician 1989; *35*:25–43.

COMMON PRACTICES

21. Hilton E, Haslett TM, Borestein MT, et al. Central catheter infections: Single- versus triple-lumen catheters. Influence of guide wires on infection rates when used for replacement of catheters. Am J Med 1988; *84*:667–672.
22. Heard SO. Do protective sleeves maintain sterility of pulmonary artery catheters? J Crit Illness 1987; *2*:16–17.

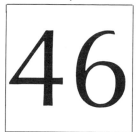

c h a p t e r

46

URINARY TRACT INFECTIONS

Urinary tract infections (UTI) account for 40% of nosocomial infections.[1,2] The major predisposing factor in nosocomial UTI is the presence of urethral drainage catheters. These devices are commonplace in ICU patients and the incidence of bacteriuria from these catheters can be as high as 10% per day.[4] This means that UTI is a constant concern in ICUs.

Like the other nosocomial infections, the diagnosis of UTI can pose problems, particularly in patients with chronic indwelling catheters. This chapter contains some practical suggestions for the diagnosis of UTI in catheterized patients. This approach is aimed at the patient with an indwelling urethral catheter. The list of references at the end of the chapter contains more information on UTI in other groups of patients.[1-4]

PATHOGENESIS

The prevailing theory for the association between urethral catheters and bladder infections involves retrograde migration of skin microbes up the urethra along the tract created by the catheter.[5] This is similar to the mechanism proposed for vascular catheter-associated septicemia presented in Chapter 45. The problem with the bacterial migration theory for either type of catheter is the assumption that bacteria can travel long distances on inert surfaces. This problem was described in Chapter 45 for vascular catheters and the same problem applies to bladder catheters.

TRAVELING MICROBES

The notion that pathogens migrate along the tract created by the urethral catheter is taken from studies that show a good correlation between the organisms isolated at the urethral orifice and those isolated in the bladder.[1-5] The problem with this theory is the distance involved in the migration path from skin to bladder. Bacteria either have no means of locomotion or they are unable to move visible distances along inert surfaces. To reach the bladder in a catheterized male, a skin organism one micron in length must travel a distance of 20 cm (the average length of the male urethra) or 200,000 times its length. This is analogous to a 6-foot tall human walking or crawling a distance of 240 miles (20 miles greater than the distance between Boston and New York). This is far from a reasonable expectation unless the bacteria are somehow aided in their journey.

Migrating Upstream

The flow of urine poses another problem for the retrograde migration theory because the microbes that finish the long journey up the urethra will be quickly washed downstream by the flow of urine as soon as they reach the bladder.[5] The flushing action of urine should protect the bladder from retrograde invasion by skin pathogens. This protection explains why the direct injection of bacteria into the bladder does not produce urinary tract infections in healthy subjects.[6]

BACTERIAL ADHERENCE

A more likely factor in the pathogenesis of urinary tract infections is the ability of pathogenic bacteria to adhere to the bladder epithelium. The photomicrograph in Figure 46-1 shows a bladder epithelial cell covered with rod-shaped bacteria.[5] These are *Lactobacillus* organisms that inhabit the lower urinary tract in healthy subjects. These commensal organisms bind to the surface epithelium of the bladder and prevent more pathogenic organisms from attaching to the bladder wall.[7] The factors that predispose patients to urosepsis (including bladder catheters) are associated with reduced adherence of commensal organisms to the bladder epithelium[4] and this allows pathogenic bacteria to establish residence in the bladder. The mechanism for bacterial adherence in the bladder is unknown at present.

MICROBIOLOGY

The pathogens isolated in more than 13,000 patients with nosocomial UTI are listed in Table 46-1.[8] Most of the isolates are gram-negative enteric pathogens with *Escherichia coli* representing one-third of all isolates. The second most common isolate is *Enterococcus*, which is becoming a prominent pathogen in the elderly. *Candida* can also be a common urinary pathogen and this organism will be discussed separately at the end of the chapter.

Coagulase-negative staphylococci were introduced in the last chapter as common isolates in sepsis from vascular catheters. These organisms

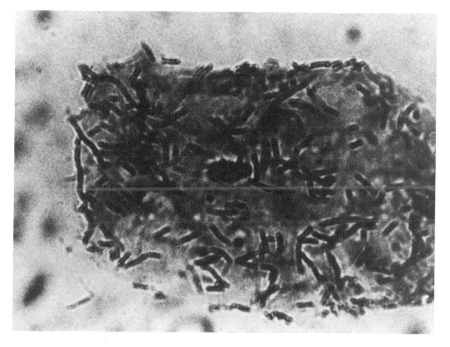

FIG. 46–1. Photomicrograph of *Lactobacillus* organisms adhering to a bladder epithelial cell. From Sobel JD. Pathogenesis of urinary tract infections: Host defenses. Infect Dis Clin North Am 1987; 1:751–772.

can also be common urinary pathogens. *Staphylococcus saprophyticus* is prevalent in young women and *Staphylococcus epidermidis* is common in patients with indwelling bladder catheters. Coagulase-positive *Staphylococcus aureus* is more invasive than the coagulase-negative strains and the presence of this pathogen in urine can signal a disseminated staphylococcal infection. Lactobacilli, Corynebacterium, and alpha-streptococci are considered to be contaminants unless they are recovered from a suprapubic aspirate in a patient who does not have a urethral catheter.

Most urinary tract infections are caused by one organism, but patients with chronic indwelling bladder catheters can have polymicrobial infection with as many as 4 or 5 organisms. A polymicrobial growth from a patient who is not chronically instrumented suggests contamination.

THE CLINICAL DIAGNOSIS

The immediate concern in any case of suspected UTI is to differentiate infection from colonization. This can be difficult in catheterized patients because urine often contains bacteria and inflammatory cells when bladder catheters have been in place for several weeks. This is why routine surveillance cultures of the urine are not recommended in asymptomatic patients.[13]

TABLE 46–1.	PATHOGENS ISOLATED FROM 13,165 URINARY TRACT INFECTIONS IN HOSPITALIZED ADULTS
Organism	Total Isolates (%)
Escherichia coli	31.0
Enterococcus	15.0
Pseudomonas	12.5
Klebsiella	7.6
Proteus	7.3
Candida sp.	5.0
Coagulase-negative *Staphylococcus*	4.4
Staphylococcus aureus	1.6

From Jarvis WR, White JM, Munn VP, et al. Nosocomial Infections Surveillance, 1983. MMWR 1985; 33:14SS.

CLINICAL PRESENTATION

Fever or some other sign of sepsis usually initiates the search for UTI. The clinical presentation is of little help in uncovering the urinary tract as a source of sepsis. Flank pain and other signs of upper tract involvement have proven neither sensitive nor specific.[2]

URINE CULTURES

Quantitative urine cultures have limited value in identifying infection in patients with indwelling bladder catheters. The definition of significant bacteriuria using 100,000 colony forming units (CFU) per ml must be viewed with caution in catheterized patients. First, infection is possible with less than 100,000 colonies on a single culture specimen.[9] Second, more than 100,000 colonies may not indicate infection in chronically instrumented patients.[10] The growth in a single urine specimen may not be as important as the growth in serial specimens. Bacteria can multiply rapidly in patients who have indwelling catheters,[9] and a urine culture that grows 100 CFU/ml one day can grow 100,000 CFU/ml in another 2 or 3 days.[9] In other words, the growth in a single urine culture may not indicate infection but a repeat culture in 2 or 3 days will uncover the infection.[9]

Urine cultures will have little role in the early decisions regarding diagnosis and antibiotic therapy. The leukocyte count in the urine can provide more immediate information for these decisions.

PYURIA

The leukocytes in an unspun urine specimen can be measured with a hemocytometer counting grid (used to count cells in cerebrospinal fluid). The number of leukocytes per cubic millimeter is used to separate infection from colonization.

A leukocyte count above 10 cells/mm³ indicates infection and fewer than 10 cells/mm³ indicates colonization.[11]

The leukocyte count can be a valuable guide for deciding about early empiric antibiotic therapy while you wait for the results of the urine culture. The interpretation of urine leukocyte counts is not applicable to leukopenic patients.

THE URINE SEDIMENT

Microscopic examination of a centrifuged urine sediment has limited value but the following statements may be useful.[12]
1. More than 5 organisms per oil-immersion field is evidence that the urine will grow 100,000 CFU/ml.
2. White blood cell casts indicate upper tract infection with renal involvement.
3. The absence of bacteria (or < 5 per oil-immersion field) does not rule out infection.
4. The density of leukocytes in a spun sediment is not reliable for separating infection from colonization.

OBTAINING URINE SPECIMENS

Catheters in place for 30 days or longer should be replaced before obtaining urine specimens to prevent contamination from bacterial colonization in the lumen of the catheters.[13] Urine samples should always be obtained through the proximal portion of the catheter, or through the sample port in the catheter system. Do not break the system and do not obtain the specimen from the urine collection bag.

TREATMENT STRATEGIES

EMPIRIC ANTIBIOTICS

Early therapy with antibiotics is indicated in the following clinical settings:
1. Hemodynamic instability.
2. Signs of upper tract infection (white cell casts in the urine)
3. Neutropenia
4. Prosthetic or damaged valve
5. Poorly controlled diabetes
6. Deteriorating renal function

SELECTION OF ANTIBIOTICS

The antibiotic selection can be guided by the urine gram stain. The following antibiotic regimens are recommended:

Gram-Negative Bacilli. Single-agent therapy is appropriate unless the patient is immunocompromised. The antibiotics most effective for single-agent therapy are the aminoglycosides. In neutropenic patients, combination therapy with an aminoglycoside plus an antipseudomonal penicillin or cetazidime is recommended.

Gram-Positive Cocci. Vancomycin is the obvious choice when gram-positive cocci are prevalent on the urine gram's stain. This drug will cover both enterococci and staphylococci (coagulase positive and negative). Combination therapy with vancomycin and gentamicin is effective for enterococcal endocarditis. Ampicillin is no longer recommended for empiric therapy of enterococcal infections because of emerging resistance to the drug.

CANDIDURIA

The presence of *Candida* in the urine can signal one of the following conditions: (1) colonization, (2) bladder infection, (3) fungus ball with risk of obstruction, (4) ascending infection with pyelonephritis, or (5) disseminated candidiasis with renal involvement. Most cases of candiduria represent simple colonization because the organism grows readily in the urine following antibiotic therapy or during prolonged urethral catheterization. The problem is to identify the occasional patient with candiduria who has disseminated candidiasis.

DISSEMINATED CANDIDIASIS

The diagnosis of disseminated candidiasis is often difficult because blood cultures do not grow the organism in over 50% of cases of disseminated disease.[15] In the absence of growth from blood cultures, the diagnosis can be secured by finding the characteristic retinal lesions or by identifying the organism in skin lesions.

The presence of high-grade lesions in the retina (fluffy white exudates protruding from the surface of the retina into the vitreous) is considered pathognomonic for disseminated disease.[15,16] Endophthalmitis is present in as many of 40% of patients with disseminated candidiasis[16] but these lesions are uncommon in neutropenic patients.[15]

Other clinical findings that suggest disseminated candidiasis include:
1. A sudden deterioration in renal function.
2. The growth of the organism from three or more sites. In neutropenic patients with unexplained fever or sepsis, growth of *Candida* from two sites is considered enough evidence to consider empiric amphotericin therapy.
3. When Candiduria (100,000 CFU/ml) occurs without the presence of indwelling bladder catheter.

AMPHOTERICIN BLADDER IRRIGATION

Local irrigation of the bladder with amphotericin is becoming commonplace despite the fact that the organism rarely disseminates from the lower urinary tract. The asymptomatic patient with an indwelling bladder catheter who is colonized with *Candida* does not require amphotericin bladder irrigation unless the organisms are numerous and the patient is neutropenic. The irrigation itself can have diagnostic value because persistence of the organism after 4 or 5 days of irrigation is taken as evidence for disseminated candidiasis or upper tract involvement.

The method for amphotericin bladder irrigation is as follows: Mix 50 mg amphotericin in 1 L of sterile water (saline precipitates the drug) and infuse at a rate of 40 ml/h using a three-way bladder catheter.[15] The response is usually prompt and the irrigation can be stopped after 3 or 4 days. Systemic absorption of the drug is negligible.

REFERENCES

GENERAL WORKS

1. Cunin CM. Detection, prevention and management of urinary tract infections. 4th ed. Philadelphia: Lea & Febiger, 1987.

REVIEWS

2. Wong ES. New aspects of urinary tract infections. Clin Crit Care Med 1987; *12*:25–38.
3. Roberts JA. Urinary tract infections. Am J Kidney Dis 1984; *4*;103–115.
4. Warren JW. Catheter-associated urinary tract infections. Infect Dis Clin North Am 1987; *1*:823–854.

PATHOGENESIS

5. Sobel JD. Pathogenesis of urinary tract infections: host defenses. Infect Dis Clin North Am 1987; *1*:751–772.
6. Howard RJ. Host defense against infection—Part 1. Curr Probl Surg 1980; *27*:267–316.
7. Daifuku R, Stamm WE. Bacterial adherence to bladder uroepithelial cells in catheter-associated urinary tract infection. N Engl J Med 1986; *314*:1208–1213.

MICROBIOLOGY

8. Jarvis WR, White JM, Munn VP, et al. Nosocomial infections surveillance, 1983. MMWR 1985; *33*:14SS.

CLINICAL DIAGNOSIS

9. Stark RP, Maki DG. Bacteriuria in the catheterized patient. What quantitative level of bacteriuria is relevant? N Engl J Med 1984; 311:560–564.
10. Platt R. Quantitative definition of bacteriuria. Am J Med 1983; 75:44–52.
11. Stamm WE. Measurement of pyuria and its relation to bacteriuria. Am J Med 1983; 75:53–58.
12. Jenkins RD, Fenn JP, Matsen JM. Review of urine microscopy for bacteriuria. JAMA 1986; 255:3397–3403.
13. Martinez OV, Civetta JM, Anderson K, et al. Bacteriuria in the catheterized surgical intensive care unit patient. Crit Care Med 1986; 14:188–191.
14. Grahn D, Norman DC, White ML, et al. Validity of urinary catheter specimen for diagnosis of urinary tract infection in the elderly. Arch Intern Med 1985; 145:1858–1860.

CANDIDURIA

15. Sobel JD. *Candida* infections in the intensive care unit. Crit Care Clin 1988; 4:325–344.
16. Parke D, Jones D, Gentry L. Endogenous endophthalmitis among patients with candidemia. Ophthalmology 1982; 89:789–792.

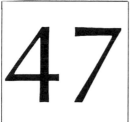

chapter

47

ANTIMICROBIAL FACTS

One simple strategy for mastering the army of antimicrobials is to limit the number of antibiotics that are used. The chart in Table 47-1 matches pathogens and antibiotics and shows the spectrum of antimicrobial agents and pathogens that you may encounter in the ICU.

The antibiotics in this table can be trimmed down to the following list:
1. Aminoglycosides
2. Amphotericin
3. Aztreonam
4. Cephalosporins
5. Clindamycin
6. Imipenem
7. Trimethoprim-Sulfamethoxazole
8. Vancomycin

This list should cover most infections that appear in any intensive care unit. Each of these antibiotics will be presented separately in the following pages. Remember that antibiotics are used in the ICU as often as any other class of critical care drugs (including hemodynamic drugs).

AMINOGLYCOSIDES

PROFILE

These agents are active against the gram-negative aerobic bacilli, enterococci, and methicillin-resistant staphylococci. They are considered to be the drugs of choice for serious gram-negative infections, particularly those caused by *Pseudomonas aeruginosa*. However, their superiority over other less toxic agents remains to be proven, at least in the non-neutropenic patient population.[6] In neutropenic patients, there is some

TABLE 47–1. ANTIMICROBIAL SELECTIONS		
Pathogen	Drug of Choice	Alternative
Gram-Positive Cocci:		
Pneumococcus or Streptococci—Groups A, B, C, G	Penicillin	Cephalosporin,* Vancomycin, Erythromycin
Enterococcus:		
Urinary Tract Infection	Ampicillin or Amoxicillin	Norfloxacillin, Ciprofloxacin
Endocarditis or Other Serious Infection	Penicillin plus Gentamicin	Vancomycin plus Gentamicin
Staph aureus or *Staph epidermidis*		
Methicillin-Sensitive	Semisynthetic Penicillin	Cephalosporin,* Vancomycin
Methicillin-Resistant	Vancomycin	Trimethoprim-Sulfamethoxazole
	← ? Add Rifampin →	
Endocarditis	← ? Add Gentamicin →	
Anaerobes		
Peptococcus *Peptostreptococcus*	Penicillin	Clindamycin, Vancomycin
Bacteroides melaninogenicus	Penicillin	Clindamycin, Metronidazole
Bacteroides fragilis	Clindamycin or Metronidazole	Imipenem, Cefoxitin
Clostridium perfringens	Penicillin	Clindamycin
Clostridium tetani	Penicillin	Tetracycline
Clostridium difficile	Vancomycin	Metronidazole
Aerobic Gram-Negative Bacilli		
Acinetobacter	Imipenem	Ticarcillin, Aminoglycoside
Escherichia coli	Ampicillin or Trimethaprim-Sulfamethoxazole	Aztreonam, Imipenem
Klebsiella *Enterobacter* *Serratia* *Proteus,* (indole positive)	Cefotaxime or Ceftriaxone	Aztreonam, Aminoglycoside
Hemophilus influenza		
Serious Infections	Cefotaxime or Ceftriaxone	Cefuroxime
Others	Ampicillin or Amoxicillin	Trimethoprim-Sulfamethoxazole, Cefotaxime, Ceftriaxone
Legionella pneumophilia	Erythromycin	Rifampin, Trimethoprim-Sulfamethoxazole
Pseudomonas aeruginosa	Ticarcillin or Ceftazidime Plus an Aminoglycoside	Aztreonam or Imipenem Plus an Aminoglycoside

*First generation cephalosporins can be used unless there is a history of a major allergic reaction (e.g., anaphylaxis) to penicillin. In the ICU, use vancomycin if there is any history of penicillin allergy (why take the risk?)
From The Med Lett 1988 (Mar); 30:33–40.

evidence that less toxic agents are as effective as aminoglycosides.[7] However, the mortality from gram-negative septicemia is high in these patients and this has created a hesitancy in eliminating the drugs traditionally considered to be the best against gram-negative infections.

DOSING

The recommended doses for adults is shown in Table 47–2. The **lean body weight** is the recommended weight to be used in the dose calculations unless the patient is morbidly obese. In obese patients, the recommended weight is the ideal body weight plus half the difference between the ideal weight and the patient's actual weight.[5] Because serum levels can vary considerably in individual patients, routine monitoring of serum levels is recommended.

These drugs are eliminated by the kidneys, therefore, dose adjustments are needed when renal function is impaired. There are two methods for adjusting the dosage.

1. Adjusting dose interval:

$$\text{Serum creatinine} \times 8 = \text{dose interval (in hours)}$$

2. Adjusting the dose:

$$\text{Dose (mg)} = \frac{\text{WT (kg)} \times \text{Standard dose (mg)}}{\text{Serum creatinine (mg\%)}}$$

The first method is called the "rule of eights" and is the traditional method of dose adjustment. However, the serum levels are subtherapeutic for longer periods of time when compared with the second method of dose adjustment. The clinical significance of this is unclear and there is no evidence that one method is superior to the other for improving clinical outcome.

TOXICITY

The major toxicities include damage to the renal tubules and the eighth cranial nerve.[8-10] **Nephrotoxicity** is the most common and most feared complication.

> Estimates are that one of every four courses of aminoglycoside therapy is complicated by acute renal failure.[8]

This may be misleading because sepsis itself can cause renal failure and many cases of deteriorating renal function during aminoglycoside therapy may not be the sole responsibility of the drugs. The features of the renal impairment are listed in Table 47–3.

There is no convincing evidence that one agent is more nephrotoxic than the other. The potential for toxicity seems to be most related to the

TABLE 47-2.	DOSE RECOMMENDATIONS FOR AMINOGLYCOSIDES			
	Loading	Daily*	Serum Levels†	
Agent	Dose	Dose	Peak	Trough
	(mg/kg)‡		(mcg/ml)	
Gentamicin	1.5–2.0	3–5	4–6	1–2
Tobramycin				
Amikacin	5.0–7.5	15	20–30	5–10

*Given in divided doses every 8 hours. Assumes renal function is normal
†Serum levels: Trough = just prior to the infusion
　　　　　　　Peak = 30 minutes after the infusion
‡Use lean body weight

length of time that trough serum levels exceed 2 mcg/ml for gentamicin and tobramicin or 10 mcg/ml for amikacin.[1] The rise in serum creatinine usually takes 5 to 7 days to appear but can appear sooner in the presence of high bilirubin levels, particularly if the hyperbilirubinemia is caused by an obstructed biliary tract.[10] The renal toxicity is also enhanced by hypovolemia and diuretic therapy.[5] The acute renal failure is usually non-oliguric and resolves with time. However, the time may be months.[5,6]

There are some early signs of renal toxicity that appear before the increase in serum creatinine. These are listed in Table 47-3. Unfortunately, these findings are prevalent in the ICU patient population as a whole and the utility of these tests is limited by lack of specificity.[5]

The **ototoxicity** from aminoglycosides is dose-related and may not be reversible.[5] The actual incidence is difficult to determine because the hearing loss is mostly in the high frequency range and requires audiometry to detect.[1]

> The hearing loss from aminoglycosides is not in the conversational range and it will not be detected without formal audiometry.

The serum levels are the best guide for determining the risk for ototox-

TABLE 47-3.	AMINOGLYCOSIDE TOXICITY		
Toxic Effect	Features	Early Detection	Aggravating Factors
Acute tubular necrosis	Nonoliguric Takes 5–7 days to appear Often resolves	Cylinduria Proteinuria Concentrating defect	Hypotension Hypovolemia Toxic dyes Biliary obstruction Renal compromise
Hearing loss	Conversational range not often affected Irreversible	Audiometry	Furosemide Other Ototoxins

icity, although the correlation between the two can vary. Furosemide may enhance the ototoxicity of these drugs.[5]

RATING

Aminoglycosides are rated as dangerous and expensive (added cost of monitoring drug levels and the cost of renal failure). These agents should be reserved for situations where serious *Pseudomonas* infections are suspected or for neutropenic patients. Industry has recognized that aminoglycosides are likely to vanish in all but select situations, and all efforts to develop new aminoglycosides have stopped.

If aminoglycoside therapy is deemed necessary, it is important to maintain intravascular volume and to limit diuretic administration, particularly the use of furosemide or other agents that may have a toxicity of their own. When using aminoglycosides in empiric regimens, the agents should be stopped in 2 to 3 days if cultures are negative or if the organism is sensitive to other antimicrobial agents. Unnecessary delays in stopping these drugs will add to the already staggering number of patients who are victims of aminoglycoside toxicity.

AMPHOTERICIN

PROFILE

This agent is reserved for serious fungal infections, either suspected or documented. It is the best agent available for mycotic infections at present, but the mortality in these infections is high despite therapy with this drug.

DOSING

The recommended dose schedules for amphotericin are shown in Table 47–4. Therapy always begins with a test dose of 1 mg given over 30 minutes because of the fever and vascular irritation associated with drug infusion (see next section). The drug is given once a day. In patients with normal renal function, a 1-hour infusion is usually safe. Otherwise, the drug is infused over 4 to 6 hours. In life-threatening infections the final daily dose is reached in 3 days, while it may take a week or so in less severe infections. The final daily dose is selected according to the severity of illness.

TOXICITY

The toxicity of this drug is high enough to limit its use in empiric antimicrobial regimens. The major toxicities are infusion-related or related to renal toxicity.

TABLE 47–4. RECOMMENDATIONS FOR AMPHOTERICIN				
Preparation:	Dilute dose in 250–500 ml D5W DO NOT USE SALINE		
Additives:	Hydrocortisone (25–50 mg) Heparin (5–50 mg)		
Infusion Time:	4–6 hours		

Seriously Ill Patients		Mild Infections	
Dose (mg/kg)	**Day**	**Dose (mg)**	**Day**
Test Dose*	1	Test Dose*	1
0.25	1	5	1
0.50	2	10	2
0.75	3	15	3
1.00	4		
Final daily dose = 0.75 – 1.0 mg/kg		Increase 5 mg per day to total daily dose of 0.4 – 0.6 mg/kg	

If serum creatinine >3 mg/dl: 1. D/C for 1 to 2 days
　　　　　　　　　　　　　2. Restart at ½ the previous daily dose, and
　　　　　　　　　　　　　　 increase as above

*Test Dose = Add 1 mg to 20 ml D5W and infuse over 30 minutes

Infusion-related toxicity includes fever, chills, vomiting, and local phlebitis. Fever is universal and can reach 40°C or higher.[11] As indicated in Table 47–4, both hydrocortisone (25 mg) and heparin (5 to 50 mg) are added to reduce the risk for fever and local phlebitis, respectively. The former agent has proven effectiveness, while the latter does not. Nothing has proven effective for reducing the vomiting that occurs in 20% of patients. Symptoms usually abate within 4 hours after stopping the drug infusion. Repeated use of the drug does not necessarily reduce the incidence of infusion-related toxicity.

Nephrotoxicity occurs in virtually every patient with hypovolemia. The distal tubules are the usual site of damage, producing a renal tubular acidosis with excessive loss of magnesium and potassium in the urine.[11] The renal magnesium and potassium wasting eventually leads to hypomagnesemia and hypokalemia unless losses are replaced.

AZTREONAM

PROFILE

This agent is effective against gram-negative aerobic bacilli, including *Pseudomonas aeruginosa*.[12] This spectrum is similar to the aminoglycosides and the drug is proving equivalent to the aminoglycosides in the treatment of gram-negative infections.[6,13]

TABLE 47-5. CEPHALOSPORINS		
Agent (Generation)	Dose	Uses in the ICU
Cephalothin (1) Cephazolin (1)	1–2 gm q 4–6 h 1–2 gm q 8 h	Used mostly for surgical prophylaxis but is also useful in *Staphylococcus* infections (not methicillin resistant)
Cefoxitin (2)	1–2 gm q 6 h	Mixed aerobic-anaerobic infection such as decubiti, perforated viscus, and aspiration pneumonia
Cefamandole (2)	1–2 gm q 6 h	Effective against *Haemophilus influenzae*
Ceftriaxone (3)	2 gm q 24 h	Once a day dosing may be an advantage, but not for serious infections
Ceftazidime (3)	1–2 gm q 8–12 h	Effective against *Pseudomonas aeruginosa* Has been used as single agent therapy with success Not always effective against *Staphylococcus aureus*

DOSING

The usual adult dose is 1 to 2 gm intravenously every 6 to 8 hours. In renal failure, the dosing is altered to a loading dose of 1 to 2 gm followed by half the loading dose given every 6 to 8 hours.

TOXICITY

At present, there is little toxicity reported. An occasional case of interstitial nephritis has appeared, but the incidence is rare.

RATING

Aztreonam is promising as an alternative to aminoglycosides, particularly in patients with renal insufficiency.[13] We are using this agent whenever possible to replace aminoglycosides in our ICUs, with no apparent deleterious results.

CEPHALOSPORINS

PROFILE

There is a virtual army of cephalosporins and they are classified into "generations" according to their time of appearance. Because the overlap between drugs is substantial, only a few drugs from each generation are presented here. These are shown in Table 47–5.

The first generation cephalosporins are primarily used for *streptococcus* and *staphylococcus* infections acquired in the community. They are not effective against methicillin resistant *Staphylococcus aureus* or *Staphylococcus epidermidis*.

The second generation agents show activity against gram-negative aerobes. Cephamandole is effective against *Haemophilus influenzae*, and cefoxitin is effective in mixed aerobic-anaerobic infections in the lung and abdomen.

The third generation cephalosporins have the most activity against gram-negative enteric organisms but lose some of their effectiveness against gram-positive cocci. They also penetrate the central nervous system more than their predecessors and can achieve significant levels when the meninges are inflamed. Ceftazidime is effective against *Pseudomonas aeruginosa* and may help replace aminoglycosides for serious pseudomonas infections.

DOSING

The usual dose in adults is 1 to 2 grams intravenously every 4 to 6 hours. Ceftriaxone is long-acting and can be administered once a day in many cases. In meningitis or infections in the ICU population, it is given every 12 hours. In renal failure, the dose of most cephalosporins is reduced to 25 to 50% of the original dose.

TOXICITY

There is no major form of toxicity. The issue of cross-allergenicity with penicillins is of little concern unless there is a history of anaphylaxis with penicillin. However, the variety of microbials available at present make it easy to find a suitable alternative to cephalosporins in penicillin-allergic patients and it is wise to withhold cephalosporins for any patient with a history of penicillin allergy.

Many patients treated with cephalosporins will develop a positive direct Coomb's test, but hemolysis is rare.[14] Other toxicities are agent-specific and will not be covered here (see reference 1 for a comprehensive presentation of all the available cephalosporins).

RATING

Ceftazidime is the lone bright star because of its value in pseudomonas infections. In fact, it has proven effective as monotherapy in neutropenic patients with gram-negative sepsis.[7] This has important implications, however, more experience with the drug is needed before any conclusions are reached about the utility of this agent in pseudomonas infections in immuno-compromised patients.

CLINDAMYCIN

PROFILE

The major use for clindamycin is for anaerobic infections, particularly those caused by *Bacteriodes fragilis*, which is the major anaerobe in the intestinal tract. Clindamycin is also active against aerobic gram-positive cocci, including *Staphylococcus aureus*, but is rarely used for infections caused by these organisms. The major uses for clindamycin are in anaerobic lung infections or as part of a multidrug regimen for empiric therapy of suspected bowel sepsis.

DOSING

The usual adult dose is 30 to 40 mg/kg per day, given in four divided doses. Dose adjustments are recommended when renal failure and hepatic failure coexist.

TOXICITY

Clindamycin made headlines in the 1970s because of its association with pseudomembranous enterocolitis, but this complication is associated with several antibiotics and is not confined to clindamycin (see Chapter 6). Diarrhea has been reported in up to 20% of patients receiving clindamycin and occurs with parenteral as well as oral administration of the drug. This subsides when the drug is stopped. Continuing the agent after diarrhea appears is dangerous and can result in life-threatening colitis.[15]

RATING

A good agent for anaerobes, but has a limited spectrum. Except for one report,[16] there is no evidence that it is superior to penicillin for anaerobic lung infections. In abdominal sepsis, it will probably be replaced by imipenem because of the wider spectrum available with imipenem.

IMIPENEM

PROFILE

The ideal antibiotic would be effective against all important pathogens while having no toxicity. Imipenem comes closer to this ideal than any other antimicrobial agent to date. The spectrum of imipenem is easier to remember by noting the pathogens that it does not cover, as shown in Table 47–6. Of the gram-positive cocci, it is not adequate for methi-

TABLE 47–6. WHAT IMIPENEM DOESN'T COVER		
Aerobes		Anaerobes
Gram-Positive Cocci	**Gram-Negative Rods**	
Methicillin-resistant *Staphylococcus aureus*	*Pseudomonas cepaciae* *Pseudomonas maltophilia*	Covers all
Some strains of *Staphylococcus epidermidis*		

cillin-resistant staphylococci or for some strains of coagulase-negative staphylococci. It is not bactericidal for enterococcus, although the significance of this is not clear. It is as good against anaerobes as any agent presently available. It also covers all the gram-negative enteric organisms, except for some uncommon species of pseudomonas. Some resistance from *Pseudomonas aeruginosa* has appeared during therapy with imipenem,[17] so monotherapy with imipenem is presently not recommended for this pathogen.

DOSING

The commercially available preparation has equal amounts of imipenem and cilastatin (Primaxin). The cilastatin is added to inhibit the renal breakdown of imipenem and to prolong its actions. The usual adult dose is 500 mg IV q 6 h. The anti-pseudomonal dose is 1 gm IV q 6 h. The drug cannot be given orally. In renal shutdown, the dose is cut by 50% and the interval is increased to 12 h.[1]

TOXICITY

No appreciable toxicity has been reported. Generalized seizures occur in 1% of patients who are predisposed to seizures.[17]

RATING

Potentially a dream agent if it proves effective against *pseudomonas* as a single agent. Can be used for abdominal sepsis, urosepsis, and nosocomial pneumonia, which is quite a mouthful. Will not be valuable for line sepsis because of the variable coverage for coagulase-negative and methicillin-resistant strains of staphylococci.

TABLE 47–7. TOXICITY OF TRIMETHOPRIM-SULFAMETHOXAZOLE IN RELATION TO AIDS

| | Patient Groups | |
Toxic Reaction	No AIDS[1]	AIDS[2]
Fever, Rash	3.4%	24%
Neutropenia	<0.1%	17%
Thrombocytopenia	<0.1%	9%

[1]From Jick H. Adverse reactions to trimethoprim-sulfamethoxazole in hospitalized patients. Rev Infect Dis 1982; 4:426–428.
[2]From Engelberg LA, et al. Clinical features of *Pneumocystis* pneumonia in the acquired immune deficiency syndrome. Am Rev Respir Dis 1984; 130:689–694.

TRIMETHOPRIM-SULFAMETHOXAZOLE (TMP-SMX)

PROFILE

This antibiotic has a wide spectrum of activity against gram-positive and gram-negative organisms, but its principal use in the ICU is to treat *Pneumocystis carinii* pneumonia in AIDS and other immune-compromised patients. It is presently considered the drug of choice for this infection in the AIDS population.

DOSING

The intravenous preparation contains 16 mg trimethoprim (TMP) and 80 mg sulfamethoxazole (SMX) per ml. The recommended daily dose for PCP is trimethoprim 20 mg/kg per day, divided into 4 doses. Serum levels of TMP-SMX are available and are drawn 90 minutes after the dose is given. These levels are used to monitor therapy in renal failure and to maximize the dose in patients who do not respond to initial therapy.

TOXICITY

Serious toxicity from TMP-SMX is rare in patients without AIDS,[18] but occurs in over 50% of patients with AIDS.[19] The reason for the enhanced toxicity in AIDS is unknown. The most common toxic reactions are listed in Table 47–7. Most reactions appear in the second week of therapy. The increase in creatinine is considered a major reaction but may not indicate diminished glomerular filtration rate because the drug interferes with the secretion of creatinine by the renal tubules.[19]

Approximately half the patients who develop toxicity will require cessation of drug therapy because of the severity of the reaction.[19] Unfortunately, pentamidine is the alternative drug for *Pneumocystis* pneumonia and this agent can be as toxic as TMP-SMX.

RATING

AIDS is a terminal illness, with the terminal event being *Pneumocystis* pneumonia in over half the cases. Therefore, it is difficult to shout praises about TMP-SMX for the therapy of this disorder. There is some suggestion that high-dose steroid therapy can improve outcome in selected AIDS patients with *Pneumocystis* pneumonia, but this requires further study.

VANCOMYCIN

PROFILE

This agent is active against all gram-positive cocci, including methicillin-resistant *Staphylococcus aureus* (MRSA), *Staphylococcus epidermidis*, *enterococcus*, diphtheroids, and *Clostridium difficile.*[21,22] It is widely used in many ICUs because of the prevalence of catheter-associated sepsis and the increasing frequency of MRSA infections in the ICU.

DOSING

Usual adult IV dose = 500 mg q 6 h

Anephric dose = 2 gm IV once a week

Infusion period = 1 hour

Enterocolitis dose = 125–500 mg po QID

The drug is not absorbed after oral ingestion. The intravenous infusion must be slow to minimize the risk for histamine release (see below). Serum levels are monitored to minimize the risk for ototoxicity. The therapeutic serum level is 18 to 26 mg/L.

TOXICITY

This agent produces little toxicity in the usual doses. The following adverse reactions are possible.
1. Local phlebitis in 10 to 15% of cases.
2. Red Man's Syndrome, produced by rapid infusion and histamine release. The features include flushing of the face and neck, pruritis, and hypotension. Fever is not common.
3. Acute chest pains that appear during the infusion and are not caused by coronary insufficiency.
4. Ototoxicity occurs when serum levels exceed 60 mg/L for several days.

5. Nephrotoxicity is uncommon but an interstitial nephritis has been reported.
6. Neutropenia is rare but can occur.

RATING

A valuable drug because of the prevalence of *staphylococcus* infections and pseudomembranous colitis in the ICU. The emergence of methicillin-resistant staphylococcus in recent years increases the value of vancomycin even more. It is usually a safe drug and it is becoming inexpensive as well. Despite being the drug of choice for *Clostridium difficile* colitis, there is a 25% relapse rate.

REFERENCES

GENERAL

1. Conte JE, Jr, Barriere SL. Antibiotics and infectious diseases. 6th ed. Philadelphia: Lea & Febiger, 1988.
2. The choice of antimicrobial drugs. The Med Let 1988; 30(Mar):33–40.
3. Neu HC ed. Update on antibiotics I. Med Clin North Am 1987; 71(Nov).
4. Neu HC ed. Update on antibiotics II. Med Clin North Am 1988; 72(May).

AMINOGLYCOSIDES

5. Pancoast SJ. Aminoglycoside antibiotics in clinical use. Med Clin North Am 1988; 72:581–612.
6. Whelton A. Treatment of gram-negative infections in patients with renal impairment: New alternatives to aminoglycosides. J Clin Pharmacol 1988; 28:866–878.
7. Rubin M, Pizzo PA. Update on the management of the febrile neutropenic patient. Resident & Staff Physician 1989; 35:25–44.
8. Sillix DH, McDonald FD. Acute renal failure. Crit Care Clin 1987; 3:909–925.
9. Kaloyanides GJ, Pastoriza-Munoz E. Aminoglycoside nephrotoxicity. Kidney Int 1980; 18:571–582.
10. Desai TK, Tsang TK. Aminoglycoside nephrotoxicity in obstructive jaundice. Am J Med 1988; 85:47 50.

AMPHOTERICIN

11. Bodey GP. Topical and systemic antifungal agents. Med Clin North Am 1988; 72:637–660.

AZTREONAM

12. Aztreonam. The Med Let 1987; 29(May):45–46.
13. Schentag JJ, Vari AJ, Winslade NE, et al. Treatment with aztreonam or tobramycin in

critical care patients with nosocomial gram-negative pneumonia. Am J Med 1985; 78(Suppl 2A):34–41.

CEPHALOSPORINS

14. Goldberg D. The cephalosporins. Med Clin North Am 1987; 71:1113–1134.

CLINDAMYCIN

15. Tedesco FJ. Pseudomembranous colitis: Pathogenesis and therapy. Med Clin North Am 1982; 66:655–665.
16. Levison ME, Mangura CT, Lorber B et al. Clindamycin compared with penicillin for the treatment of anaerobic lung abscess. Ann Intern Med 1983; 98:466–471.

IMIPENEM

17. Lipman P, Neu H. Imipenem: A new carbepenem antibiotic. Med Clin North Am 1988; 72:567–580.

TRIMETHOPRIM-SULFAMETHOXAZOLE

18. Cockerill FR, Edson RS. Trimethoprim-sulfamethoxazole. Mayo Clin Proc 1987; 62:921–929.
19. Foltzer MA, Reese RE. Trimethoprim-sulfamethoxazole and other sulfonamides. Med Clin North Am 1987; 71:1177–1194.
20. Mazur H, Kovacs JA. Treatment and prophylaxis of Pneumocystis carinii pneumonia. In: Sande MA, Volberding PA eds. The medical management of AIDS. Philadelphia: W.B. Saunders, 1988:181–192.

VANCOMYCIN

21. Levine JF. Vancomycin: A review. Med Clin North Am 1987; 71:1135–1146.
22. Southorn PA, Plevak DJ, Wright AJ, Wilson WR. Adverse effects of vancomycin administered in the perioperative period. Mayo Clin Proc 1986; 61:721–724.

appendices

1. REFERENCE TABLES

DESIRABLE WEIGHTS FOR ADULTS*			
MALES			
Height				
Feet	Inches	Small Frame	Medium Frame	Large Frame
5	2	128–134	131–141	138–150
5	3	130–136	133–143	140–153
5	4	132–138	135–145	142–156
5	5	134–140	137–148	144–160
5	6	136–142	139–151	146–164
5	7	138–145	142–154	149–168
5	8	140–148	145–157	152–172
5	9	142–151	148–160	155–176
5	10	144–154	151–163	158–180
5	11	146–157	154–166	161–184
6	0	149–160	157–170	164–188
6	1	152–164	160–174	168–192
6	2	155–168	164–178	172–197
6	3	158–172	167–182	172–202
6	4	162–176	171–187	181–207
FEMALES			
4	10	102–111	109–121	112–131
4	11	103–113	111–123	120–134
5	0	104–115	113–126	122–137
5	1	106–118	115–129	125–140
5	2	108–121	118–132	128–143
5	3	111–124	121–135	131–147
5	4	114–127	124–138	134–151
5	5	117–130	127–141	137–155
5	6	120–133	130–144	140–159
5	7	123–136	133–147	143–163
5	8	126–139	136–150	146–167
5	9	129–142	139–153	149–170
5	10	132–145	142–156	152–173
5	11	135–148	145–159	155–176
6	0	138–151	148–162	158–179

*Unclothed weights associated with the longest life expectancies. From the statistics bureau of the Metropolitan Life Insurance Company, 1983.

BASAL METABOLIC RATES		
Body Weight (kg)	kcal/24 hours	
	Male	Female
40	1340	1241
50	1485	1399
52	1505	1429
54	1555	1458
56	1580	1487
58	1600	1516
60	1630	1544
62	1660	1572
64	1690	1599
66	1725	1626
68	1765	1653
70	1785	1679
72	1815	1705
74	1845	1731
76	1870	1756
78	1900	1781
80	—	1805

From Talbot FB. Am J Dis Child 1938; 5:455–459.

TRACE ELEMENT ASSAYS		
Trace Element	Assay	Normal Range
Zinc	Plasma Zinc	12–18 mcg/100 ml
Copper	Serum Copper	15–20 mcg/100 ml
Iron	Serum Ferritin	15–200 ng/ml*
	Serum Iron	40–160 mcg/dl*
Selenium	Plasma Selenium	6–15 mcg/100 ml
	RBC Glutathione Peroxidase	30.8 ± 4.7 U/g Hb*
Chromium	Serum Chromium	0.04–0.35 mcg/L
Manganese	Serum Manganese	40–180 ng/100 ml
Molybdenum	Urine Molybdenum	20 mcg/day

*From Tietz NW. Clinical guide to laboratory tests. Philadelphia: W.B. Saunders, 1983. Otherwise, from Shenken A. Trace elements in critical illness. Intensive and Crit Care Dig, 1988; 7:20–23.

VITAMIN ASSAYS		
Vitamin	**Assay**	**Normal Range**
A	Serum Retinol	25–65 mcg/dl
C	Serum Ascorbate	0.5–1.5 mg/dl
E	Serum Tocopherol	0.5–1.5 mg/dl
D	Plasma 25–OH D3	18–37 ng/ml
	Plasma 25–OH D2	0.8–7.0 ng/dl
Thiamine	RBC Transketolase	0.9–1.27 A.C.
Riboflavin	RBC Glutathione Reductase	0.9–1.9 A.C.
Pyridoxine	Urine Pyridoxine	20–120 mcg/day
B_{12}	Serum B_{12}	200–900 pg/ml
Folate	Serum Folate	7–15 ng/ml
Biotin	Urine Biotin	6–50 mcg/day
Niacin	Urine Niacin	0.3–1.5 mg/day
Pantothenate	Urine Pantothenate	0.4–14.3 mcg/day

From Dempsey DT, et al. JPEN 1987; *11*:229–237.
A.C. = activity coefficient

ROOM AIR ARTERIAL BLOOD GASES AT SEA LEVEL			
Age (years)	**Pao_2 (mm Hg)**	**$Paco_2$ (mm Hg)**	**$(A-a)Po_2$ (mm Hg)**
20	84–95	33–47	4–17
30	81–92	34–47	7–21
40	78–90	34–47	10–24
50	75–87	34–47	14–27
60	72–84	34–47	17–31
70	70–81	34–47	21–34
80	67–79	34–47	25–38

From the Intermountain Thoracic Society Manual of Uniform Laboratory Procedures, Salt Lake City, 1984, pp. 44–45.

SERUM LEVELS OF COMMON DRUGS

Drug	Serum Level	
	Therapeutic Range	Toxic Range
Acetaminophen	10–30 mcg/ml	>200 4 h post-ingestion
N-Acetyl Procainamide	5–30 mcg/ml	>40
Amikacin	Peak: 25–35 mcg/ml	>35
	Trough: 1–4	>10
Amitryptyline	120–250 ng/ml	>500
Amobarbital	1–5 mcg/ml	>10
Chlordiazepoxide	700–1000 ng/ml	>5000
Chlorpromazine	50–300 ng/ml	>750
Desipramine	75–160 ng/ml	>1000
Diazepam	100–1000 ng/ml	>5000
Disopyramide	3–7 mcg/ml	>7
Doxepin	30–150 ng/ml	>500
Gentamicin	Peak: 5–10 mcg/ml	>10
	Trough: 1–2 mcg/ml	>2
Glutethimide	2–6 mcg/ml	>6
Imipramine	125–250 ng/ml	>500
Lidocaine	1.5–6 mcg/ml	>6
Lithium	0.6–1.2 mEq/L	>2
Methadone	100–400 ng/ml	>2000
Pentobarbital	1–5 mcg/ml	>10
	20–50 (coma)	
Phenobarbital	15–40 mcg/ml	>40 (nystagmus)
		>65 (coma)
Phenytoin	10–20 mcg/ml	>20 (nystagmus)
		>40 (mental status)
Procainamide	4–10 mcg/ml	>10
Quinidine	2–5 mcg/ml	>6
Secobarbital	1–2 mcg/ml	>5
Theophylline	10–20 mcg/ml	>20
Tobramycin	Peak: 8–10	>10
	Trough: 1–2	<2
Vancomycin		>80 mg/ml

2. PHARMACOTHERAPY

PARENTERAL DRUG INTERACTIONS		
	Serum Level	
Intravenous Drug	**Increased By**	**Decreased By**
Aminophylline	Cimetidine Erythromycin Phenytoin Propranolol	Phenobarbital Phenytoin Rifampin

Beta Blockers
  Metoprolol
  Propranolol
	Cimetidine
	Cimetidine
	Furosemide
		Rifampin

Catecholamines	Alkaline urine
	  (e.g. diamox)
		Urine acidifying agents
		  (e.g. vitamin C)

Cimetidine		Phenobarbital Rifampin
Diazepam	Propranolol	Phenytoin
Digoxin	Amiodarone Diazepam Erythromycin Quinidine Spironolactone Verapamil	Rifampin
Lidocaine	Cimetidine Beta Blockers	
Pancuronium	Clindamycin Verapamil	Theophylline
Phenytoin	Cimetidine Sulfonamides	Phenobarbital Diazepam Rifampin
Procainamide	Cimetidine Ranitidine	

1. Rudd C, Wikman J, Lumb PD. Drug interactions in critical care. In: Lumb PD, Bryan-Brown CW eds. Complications in critical care medicine. Chicago: Year Book Medical Publishers, 1988.
2. Vasko MR, Brater DC. Drug interactions. In: Chernow B ed. The pharmacologic approach to the critically ill patient. 2nd ed. Baltimore: Williams & Wilkins, 1988.
3. Dasta JF. Drug interactions in the ICU. Perspect Crit Care 1989; 2:61–85.

| INCOMPATIBILITIES FOR COMMON ICU DRUGS* ||
Drug	Incompatible With
Aminophylline	Meperidine, Morphine, Vancomycin
Amphotericin	Saline or Ringer's lactate solutions
Amrinone	Dextrose solutions, Furosemide
Dobutamine or Dopamine	Bicarbonate and other alkaline fluids
Epinephrine	Dextrose solutions, Bicarbonate
Heparin	Hydrocortisone, Hydroxysine, Meperidine, Penicillin, Vancomycin
Labetalol	Bicarbonate and other alkaline fluids
Levophed	Saline or Ringer's solutions
Morphine	Aminophylline, Bicarbonate, Heparin, Meperidine, Methicillin
Vancomycin	Aminophylline, Chloramphenicol, Dexamethasone, Heparin, Penicillin, Phenytoin, Prochlorperazine
Verapamil	Albumin, Amphotericin, Hydralazine Bicarbonate, Trimethoprim-Sulfa

*From Compendium of drug therapy. New York: McGraw-Hill, 1989.

| INTRAVENOUS FLUID INCOMPATIBILITIES |||
Category	Ringer's Lactate*	
Incompatible	Amphotericin	Cephamandole
	Ampicillin	Doxycycline
	Bicarbonate	Metaraminol
Possibly Incompatible	Amikacin	Solu-Medrol
	Arfonad	Nitroglycerin
	Azlocillin	Nitroprusside
	Bretylium	Penicillin
	Clindamycin	Procainamide
	Decadron	Propranolol
	Epinephrine	Trimethoprim
	Levophed	Vancomycin
	Mannitol	Urokinase
	Saline†	**Dextrose†**
Incompatible	Amphotericin	Epinephrine
	Levophed	Calcium Chloride
Possibly Incompatible	Aminophylline	Aminophylline

*From Griffith CA. The family of Ringer's solutions. NITA, 1986; 9:480–483.
†From Compendium of drug therapy. New York: McGraw-Hill, 1989.

PERORAL ABSORPTION AND IV ADSORPTION	
Condition	**Drugs Involved**
Absorption diminished by antacids	Ampicillin Phenytoin Benzodiazepines Propranolol Cimetidine Ranitidine Digoxin Salicylates Isoniazid Sulfonamides Penicillin Tetracyclines Phenothiazines
Drug adsorbs on polyvinyl chloride tubing	Diazepam Insulin Nitroglycerin

DOBUTAMINE

Preparation
    Concentration: 1000 mcg per ml
            Mix: 250 mg in 250 ml saline

Administration
    Usual Dose: 5 to 15 mcg/kg/min

**Infusion Rate
(gtts/min)**

Dose (mcg/kg/min) \ Weight (kg)	40	50	60	70	80	90	100
5	12	15	18	21	24	27	30
10	24	30	36	42	48	54	60
15	36	45	54	63	72	81	90
20	48	60	72	84	96	108	120
40	96	120	144	168	192	216	240

DOPAMINE						
Preparation:	1 amp (200 mg) in 250 ml diluent					
Concentration:	800 mcg/ml					

		Weight (kg)			
		40	60	80	100
Dose (mcg/kg/min)	**Desired Effect**	**Infusion Rate (gtts/min)**			
1	Renal Vasodilatation	3	5	6	8
3	↓	9	14	18	23
5	Increase Cardiac Output	15	20	27	38
7.5	↓	23	32	42	57
10	Vasoconstriction	30	45	60	75
20	↓	60	90	120	150

LIDOCAINE AND PROCAINAMIDE		

Preparation
  Concentrations: 4 mg/ml   or   8 mg/ml
         Mix: 2 g in 500 ml saline   4 g in 500 ml saline
                1 g in 250 ml saline   2 g in 250 ml saline

Administration
  Usual Dose: 1 to 4 mg/min

	Infusion Rates	
Dose (mg/min)	**(4 mg/ml) (cc/hr)**	**(8 mg/ml) (cc/hr)**
1	15	8
2	30	15
3	45	23
4	60	30

NITROGLYCERIN	
Preparation	
Concentration:	400 mcg/ml
Mix:	200 mg in 500 ml saline or
	100 mg in 250 ml saline
Administration	
Venodilator Dose:	1 to 50 mcg/min
Usual Dose:	1 to 400 mcg/min

Dose (mcg/min)	Infusion Rate (microdrops/min)
5	1
10	2
25	4
50	8
75	11
100	15
150	23
200	30
250	38
300	45
350	53
400	60

NITROPRUSSIDE	
Preparation	
Concentration:	200 mcg/ml
Mix:	100 mg in 500 ml saline or
	50 mg in 250 ml saline or
	30 mg in 150 mg saline
Administration	
Usual Dose:	0.5 to 2.0 mcg/kg/min for heart failure
	2.0 to 5.0 mcg/kg/min for hypertension

Infusion Rate (microdrops/min)

Weight (kg) Dose (mcg/kg/min)	40	50	60	70	80	90	100
0.5	6	8	9	11	12	14	15
1.0	12	15	18	20	24	27	30
1.5	18	23	27	32	36	41	45
2.0	24	30	36	42	48	54	60
2.5	30	38	45	53	60	68	75
3.0	36	45	54	63	72	81	90
3.5	42	53	63	74	84	95	105
4.0	48	60	72	84	96	108	120
4.5	54	68	81	95	108	122	135
5.0	60	75	90	105	120	135	150

NOREPINEPHRINE

Preparation
  Concentrations: 16 mcg/ml   8 mcg/ml
         Mix: 8 mg in 500 ml saline   4 mg in 500 ml saline
               4 mg in 250 ml saline   2 mg in 250 ml saline

Administration
    Beta Dose: 1 to 10 mcg/min
   Alpha Dose: >10 mcg/min

Dose mcg/min	Infusion Rates	
	(@ 16 mcg/ml) cc/hr	(@ 8 mcg/ml) cc/hr
2	8	15
4	15	30
6	23	45
8	30	60
10	38	75
12	45	90
14	53	105
16	60	120
18	68	135
20	75	150

THROMBOLYTIC THERAPY PROTOCOL

Indications

A. Chest pain plus characteristic ECG changes
B. Less than 6 hours from suspected onset
C. No contraindications

Contraindications

Absolute Contraindications

1. Pericarditis
2. Dissecting aneurysm
3. Active bleeding
4. Brain mass
5. History of CVA
6. Severe hypertension

Relative Contraindications

1. Recent Surgery
2. Recent Trauma
3. Diastolic BP >110 mmHg

Dose Recommendations

1. Streptokinase: 1.5×10^6 U by IV infusion over 1 hr
   or
2. Tissue plasminogen activator (TPA):*
                6 mg IV bolus, then
                54 mg IV over 1 hr, then
                40 mg IV over 40 min

3. Follow with one aspirin tablet (325 mg)

*Preferred if the patient has received streptokinase within 6 months

ORAL THERAPY FOR HYPERTENSIVE EMERGENCIES			
Agent	Dose	Onset of Action	Comment
Clonidine	0.2 mg initial dose Then 0.1 mg/hr to 0.8 mg	30 min	Works well Watch for sedation
Nifedipine	10–20 mg initially Repeat in 30 min PRN	5–10 min	Faster than clonidine, but can cause tachycardia in 15% of cases
Captopril	6.25 mg if acute heart failure, or hypona-tremia. Otherwise start at 25 mg PO TID	15 min	Fast onset. Watch for hypo-tension in acute heart fail-ure or any other high renin state
Minoxidil	5–10 mg initially Then 5–10 mg q 6 hr until desired effect	1–2 hrs	Slow onset

ACUTE MANAGEMENT OF GENERALIZED SEIZURES
1. If there is a history of insulin-dependent diabetes, cirrhosis, or alcoholism:
IV Bolus: 50 ml 50% dextrose plus 100 mg thiamine
2. For acute control of generalized seizures:
Diazepam: 10 mg IV @ 2 mg/minute Repeat in 3 minutes if necessary **Or** **Lorazepam:**   0.05 to 0.2 mg/kg IV bolus
3. To prevent recurrences:
Phenytoin: 18 mg/kg IV infusion DO NOT exceed a rate of 50 mg/minute to minimize the risk of hypotension. Total dose can increase to 25 mg/kg if seizures persist
Phenobarbital: IV infusion @ 100 mg/minute Total dose of 20 mg/kg
Diazepam: IV infusion @ 8 mg/hour (mix 100 mg diazepam in 500 ml saline and infuse at 40 ml/hour)
4. If seizures are refractory to the above: **CALL A NEUROLOGIST**

3. RESUSCITATION

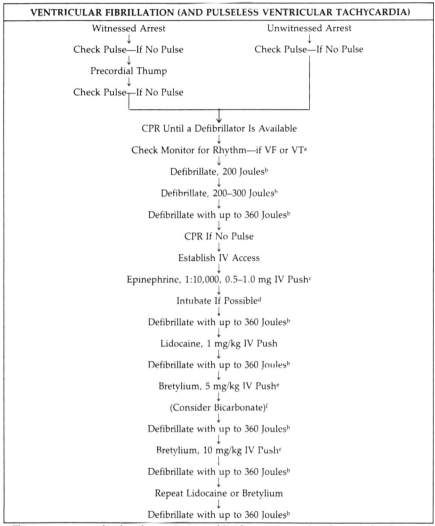

VENTRICULAR FIBRILLATION (AND PULSELESS VENTRICULAR TACHYCARDIA)

Witnessed Arrest ↓ Check Pulse—If No Pulse ↓ Precordial Thump ↓ Check Pulse—If No Pulse

Unwitnessed Arrest ↓ Check Pulse—If No Pulse

CPR Until a Defibrillator Is Available
↓
Check Monitor for Rhythm—if VF or VT[a]
↓
Defibrillate, 200 Joules[b]
↓
Defibrillate, 200–300 Joules[b]
↓
Defibrillate with up to 360 Joules[b]
↓
CPR If No Pulse
↓
Establish IV Access
↓
Epinephrine, 1:10,000, 0.5–1.0 mg IV Push[c]
↓
Intubate If Possible[d]
↓
Defibrillate with up to 360 Joules[b]
↓
Lidocaine, 1 mg/kg IV Push
↓
Defibrillate with up to 360 Joules[b]
↓
Bretylium, 5 mg/kg IV Push[e]
↓
(Consider Bicarbonate)[f]
↓
Defibrillate with up to 360 Joules[b]
↓
Bretylium, 10 mg/kg IV Push[e]
↓
Defibrillate with up to 360 Joules[b]
↓
Repeat Lidocaine or Bretylium
↓
Defibrillate with up to 360 Joules[b]

This sequence was developed to assist in teaching how to treat a broad range of patients with ventricular fibrillation (VF) or pulseless ventricular tachycardia (VT). Some patients may require care not specified herein. This algorithm should not be construed as prohibiting such flexibility. Flow of algorithm presumes that VF is continuing. CPR indicates cardiopulmonary resuscitation.

[a]Pulseless VT should be treated identically to VF.

[b]Check pulse and rhythm after each shock. If VF recurs after transiently converting (rather than persists without ever converting), use whatever energy level has previously been successful for defibrillation.

[c]Epinephrine should be repeated every five minutes.

[d]Intubation is preferable. If it can be accomplished simultaneously with other techniques, then the earlier the better. However, defibrillation and epinephrine are more important initially if the patient can be ventilated without intubation.

[e]Some may prefer repeated doses of lidocaine, which may be given in 0.5-mg/kg boluses every eight minutes to a total dose of 3 mg/kg.

[f]Value of sodium bicarbonate is questionable during cardiac arrest, and it is not recommended for routine cardiac arrest sequence. Consideration of its use in a dose of 1 mEq/kg is appropriate at this point. Half of original dose may be repeated every ten minutes if it is used.

(From 1985 National Conference on Cardiopulmonary Resuscitation (CPR) and Emergency Cardiac Care (ECC). JAMA 1986; 255:2905–2992.)

SUSTAINED VENTRICULAR TACHYCARDIA (VT)

No Pulse   **Pulse Present**
↓
Treat as VF

           Stable[a]   **Unstable**[b]
           ↓   ↓
           O_2 O_2
           ↓   ↓
  IV Access   IV Access
           ↓   ↓
Lidocaine, 1 mg/kg   (Consider Sedation)[c]
           ↓   ↓
Lidocaine, 0.5 mg/kg Every 8 min   Cardiovert 50 Joules[d,e]
Until VT Resolves, or   ↓
up to 3 mg/kg   Cardiovert 100 Joules[d]
           ↓   ↓
Procainamide, 20 mg/min   Cardiovert 200 Joules[d]
Until VT Resolves,   ↓
or up to 1,000 mg   Cardiovert With up to
           ↓   360 Joules[d]
Cardiovert as in   ↓
Unstable Patients[c]   If Recurrent, Add Lidocaine
              and Cardiovert Again Starting
              at Energy Level
              Previously Successful; Then
              Procainamide or Bretylium[f]

This sequence was developed to assist in teaching how to treat a broad range of patients with sustained VT. Some patients may require care not specified herein. This algorithm should not be construed as prohibiting such flexibility. Flow of algorithm presumes that VT is continuing. VF indicates ventricular fibrillation.

[a]If patient becomes unstable (see footnote b for definition) at any time, move to "Unstable" arm of algorithm.

[b]Unstable indicates symptoms (e.g., chest pain or dyspnea), hypotension (systolic blood pressure <90 mm Hg), congestive heart failure, ischemia, or infarction.

[c]Sedation should be considered for all patients, including those defined in footnote b as unstable, except those who are hemodynamically unstable (e.g., hypotensive, in pulmonary edema, or unconscious).

[d]If hypotension, pulmonary edema, or unconsciousness is present, unsynchronized cardioversion should be done to avoid delay associated with synchronization.

[e]In the absence of hypotension, pulmonary edema, or unconsciousness, a precordial thump may be employed prior to cardioversion.

[f]Once VT has resolved, begin intravenous (IV) infusion of antiarrhythmic agent that has aided resolution of VT. If hypotension, pulmonary edema, or unconsciousness is present, use lidocaine if cardioversion alone is unsuccessful, followed by bretylium. In all other patients, recommended order of therapy is lidocaine, procainamide, and then bretylium.

(From 1985 National Conference on Cardiopulmonary Resuscitation (CPR) and Emergency Cardiac Care (ECC). JAMA 1986; 255:2905–2992.)

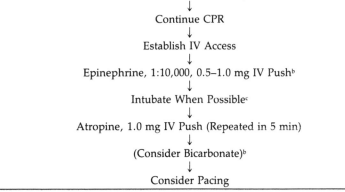

ASYSTOLE (CARDIAC STANDSTILL)
If Rhythm is Unclear and Possibly Ventricular Fibrillation, Defibrillate as for VF. If Asystole is Present[a] ↓ Continue CPR ↓ Establish IV Access ↓ Epinephrine, 1:10,000, 0.5–1.0 mg IV Push[b] ↓ Intubate When Possible[c] ↓ Atropine, 1.0 mg IV Push (Repeated in 5 min) ↓ (Consider Bicarbonate)[b] ↓ Consider Pacing

This sequence was developed to assist in teaching how to treat a broad range of patients with asystole. Some patients may require care not specified herein. This algorithm should not be construed to prohibit such flexibility. Flow of algorithm presumes asystole is continuing. VF indicates ventricular fibrillation; IV, intravenous.

[a]Asystole should be confirmed in two leads.

[b]Epinephrine should be repeated every five minutes.

[c]Intubation is preferable; if it can be accomplished simultaneously with other techniques, then the earlier the better. However, cardiopulmonary resuscitation (CPR) and use of epinephrine are more important initially if patient can be ventilated without intubation. (Endotracheal epinephrine may be used.)

[d]Value of sodium bicarbonate is questionable during cardiac arrest, and it is not recommended for the routine cardiac arrest sequence. Consideration of its use in a dose of 1 mEq/kg is appropriate at this point. Half of original dose may be repeated every ten minutes if it is used.

(From 1985 National Conference on Cardiopulmonary Resuscitation (CPR) and Emergency Cardiac Care (ECC). JAMA 1986; 255:2905–2992.)

ELECTROMECHANICAL DISSOCIATION

Continue CPR
↓
Establish IV Access
↓
Epinephrine, 1:10,000, 0.5–1.0 mg IV Push[a]
↓
Intubate When Possible[b]
↓
(Consider Bicarbonate)[c]
↓
Consider Hypovolemia,
Cardiac Tamponade,
Tension Pneumothorax,
Hypoxemia,
Acidosis,
Pulmonary Embolism

This sequence was developed to assist in teaching how to treat a broad range of patients with electromechanical dissociation. Some patients may require care not specified herein. This algorithm should not be construed to prohibit such flexibility. Flow of algorithm presumes that electromechanical dissociation is continuing. CPR indicates cardiopulmonary resuscitation; IV, intravenous.

[a]Epinephrine should be repeated every five minutes.

[b]Intubation is preferable. If it can be accomplished simultaneously with other techniques, then the earlier the better. However, epinephrine is more important initially if the patient can be ventilated without intubation.

[c]Value of sodium bicarbonate is questionable during cardiac arrest, and it is not recommended for routine cardiac arrest sequence. Consideration of its use in a dose of 1 mEq/kg is appropriate at this point. Half of original dose may be repeated every ten minutes if it is used.

(From 1985 National Conference on Cardiopulmonary Resuscitation (CPR) and Emergency Cardiac Care (ECC). JAMA 1986; 255:2905–2992.)

PAROXYSMAL SUPRAVENTRICULAR TACHYCARDIA (PSVT)

Unstable	**Stable**
↓	↓
Synchronous Cardioversion 75–100 Joules	Vagal Maneuvers
↓	↓
Synchronous Cardioversion 200 Joules	Verapamil, 5 mg IV
↓	↓
Synchronous Cardioversion 360 Joules	Verapamil, 10 mg IV
↓	(in 15–20 min)
Correct Underlying Abnormalities	↓
↓	Cardioversion, Digoxin,
Pharmacological Therapy + Cardioversion	β-Blockers, Pacing as Indicated
	(See Text)

If conversion occurs but PSVT recurs, repeated electrical cardioversion is *not* indicated. Sedation should be used as time permits.

This sequence was developed to assist in teaching how to treat a broad range of patients with sustained PSVT. Some patients may require care not specified herein. This algorithm should not be construed as prohibiting such flexibility. Flow of algorithm presumes PSVT is continuing.

(From 1985 National Conference on Cardiopulmonary Resuscitation (CPR) and Emergency Cardiac Care (ECC). JAMA 1986; 255:2905–2992.)

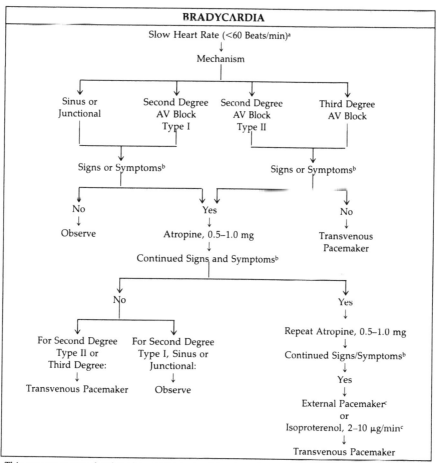

BRADYCARDIA

Slow Heart Rate (<60 Beats/min)[a]

↓

Mechanism

- Sinus or Junctional
- Second Degree AV Block Type I
- Second Degree AV Block Type II
- Third Degree AV Block

Signs or Symptoms[b]

No → Observe

Yes → Atropine, 0.5–1.0 mg

Signs or Symptoms[b]

No → Transvenous Pacemaker

Continued Signs and Symptoms[b]

No:
- For Second Degree Type II or Third Degree: ↓ Transvenous Pacemaker
- For Second Degree Type I, Sinus or Junctional: ↓ Observe

Yes:
- Repeat Atropine, 0.5–1.0 mg
- Continued Signs/Symptoms[b]
- Yes
- External Pacemaker[c] or Isoproterenol, 2–10 μg/min[c]
- Transvenous Pacemaker

This sequence was developed to assist in teaching how to treat a broad range of patients with bradycardia. Some patients may require care not specified herein. This algorithm should not be construed to prohibit such flexibility. AV indicates atrioventricular.

[a] A solitary chest thump or cough may stimulate cardiac electrical activity and result in improved cardiac output and may be used at this point.

[b] Hypotension (blood pressure <90 mm Hg), premature ventricular contractions, altered mental status or symptoms (e.g., chest pain or dyspnea), ischemia, or infarction.

[c] Temporizing therapy.

(From 1985 National Conference on Cardiopulmonary Resuscitation (CPR) and Emergency Cardiac Care (ECC). JAMA 1986; 255:2905–2992.)

ACUTE MANAGEMENT OF VENTRICULAR ECTOPY

Assess for Need for
Acute Suppressive Therapy
↓

→ Rule Out Treatable Cause
→ Consider Serum Potassium
→ Consider Digitalis Level
→ Consider Bradycardia
→ Consider Drugs

Lidocaine, 1 mg/kg
↓
If Not Suppressed,
Repeat Lidocaine, 0.5 mg/kg Every 2–5 min,
Until No Ectopy, or up to 3 mg/kg Given
↓
If Not Suppressed,
Procainamide 20 mg/min
Until No Ectopy, or up to 1,000 mg Given
↓
If Not Suppressed,
and Not Contraindicated,
Bretylium, 5–10 mg/kg Over 8–10 min
↓
If Not Suppressed,
Consider Overdrive Pacing

Once Ectopy Resolved, Maintain as Follows:
  After Lidocaine, 1 mg/kg . . . Lidocaine Drip, 2 mg/min
  After Lidocaine, 1–2 mg/kg . . . Lidocaine Drip, 3 mg/min
  After Lidocaine, 2–3 mg/kg . . . Lidocaine Drip, 4 mg/min
  After Procainamide . . . Procainamide Drip, 1–4 mg/min (Check Blood Level)
  After Bretylium . . . Bretylium Drip, 2 mg/min

This sequence was developed to assist in teaching how to treat a broad range of patients with ventricular ectopy. Some patients may require therapy not specified herein. This algorithm should not be construed as prohibiting such flexibility.
(From 1985 National Conference on Cardiopulmonary Resuscitation (CPR) and Emergency Cardiac Care (ECC). JAMA 1986; 255:2905–2992.)

DRUGS THAT CAN BE ADMINISTERED ENDOTRACHEALLY*		
Drug	**Initial Adult Dose**	**Volume**
Epinephrine (1:10,000)	1 mg	10 ml
Atropine	0.5–1 mg	5–10 ml
Lidocaine	100 mg	10 ml
Naloxone	0.4–4 mg	1–10 ml

*Instill the drug directly into the upper airway.
Do not nebulize. Follow with a series of lung inflations from an Ambu bag

BLOOD VOLUME ESTIMATES	
Males	**Females**
70 ml/kg (Lean body weight)	60 ml/kg (Lean body weight)
60 ml/kg (Obese)	50 ml/kg (Obese)
2.74 L/M$^{2\#}$	2.37 L/M$^{2\#}$
0.367 H + 0.322 W + 0.604*	0.356 H + 0.33 W + 0.183*

H = Height in cm; W = Weight in kg
#From Shoemaker W, et al. Clinical trial of survivors' cardiorespiratory patterns as therapeutic goals in critically ill postoperative patients. Crit Care Med 1982; 10:398–403.
*From Buffaloe GW, Heineken FG. Plasma volume nomograms for use in therapeutic plasma exchange. Transfusion 1983; 23:355–357.

CRYSTALLOID FLUIDS				
	Plasma*	**0.9% Saline**	**Ringer's Lactate**	**Normosol**
Na$^+$ (mEq/l)	141	154	130	140
CL$^-$ (mEq/l)	103	154	109	98
K$^+$ (mEq/l)	4–5	—	4	5
Ca/Mg (mEq/l)	5/2	—	3/0	0/3
Buffer	HCO$_3^-$ (26)	—	Lactate (28)	Acetate (27) Gluconate (23)
pH	7.4	5.7	6.7	7.4
Osmolality (mOsm/kg)	289	308	273	295

*Plasma values from Brenner BM, Rector FC, Jr. eds. The Kidney. 2nd ed. Philadelphia: W.B. Saunders 1981: 95.

COLLOID FLUIDS				
	25% Albumin	**5% Albumin**	**6% Hetstarch**	**Dextran—40**
COP (mm Hg)	70	20	30	40
Unit Size	50 ml	250 ml	500 ml	250 ml
Potency*	4:1	1.3:1	1.3:1	2:1
Bleeding	—	0.001	0.010	0.010

*Potency expressed as increased in vascular volume (mls) per milliliter of infused colloid

COMMON HYPERTONIC SOLUTIONS			
Solution	**Osmolality (mOsm/Kg H$_2$O)**	**Container Size (ml)**	**Contents Per Container (mOsm)**
3% NaCl	1026	500	513
Seawater	1000	Large	?
25% Mannitol	1374	50	69
7.5% NaHCO$_3$	1786	50	90
50% Dextrose	2525	50, 500	126, 1263

BLOOD PRODUCTS			
Blood Product	**Volume**	**Contents**	**Comments**
Whole Blood	510 ml	450 ml blood 60 ml CPD	No viable platelets after 24 hours. K$^+$ accumulates after a few days
Packed RBCs	300 ml	200 ml cells 100 ml plasma	Hct usually 60 to 70, and must be diluted with saline
Plasma	240 ml	All clotting factors	Used for clotting factors. Not used as plasma expander
Platelet Concentrate	50 ml	50 × 10^{10} platelets	Outdated after 72 hours
Cryoprecipitate	20 ml	200 mg Fibrinogen 100 mcg Factor VIII 150 mcg VWF	Rich in fibronectin Expensive and has little use in the ICU

4. SCORING SYSTEMS

GLASCOW COMA SCALE			
Eye Opening			
Spontaneous	4 points		
To Speech	3		
To Pain	2		Patient's
None	1		Score
Best Motor Response			
Obeys Commands	6 points		
Localizes	5		
Withdraws	4		
Abnormal Flexion	3		
Extends	2		Patient's
None	1		Score
Best Verbal Response			
Oriented	5 points		
Confused Conversation	4		
Inappropriate Words	3		
Incomprehensible Sounds	2		Patient's
None	1		Score
Total Glascow Coma Score			
Best Score: 15			
Worst Score: 3			

PITTSBURGH BRAIN STEM SCORE*			
Designed to complement the Glasgow Coma Scale for the evaluation of nontraumatic injury. Includes an evaluation of brainstem reflexes. This score is added to the Glasgow score, as shown below. At present, there is only limited clinical experience with the combined scale.			
Gag or cough reflex	Present = 2		
	Absent = 1		
Lash reflex (either side)	Present = 2		
	Absent = 1		
Corneal reflex (either side)	Present = 2		
	Absent = 1		
Doll's Eye or cold caloric reflex	Present = 2		
	Absent = 1		
Right pupillary light reflex	Present = 2		
	Absent = 1		
Left pupillary light reflex	Present = 2		
	Absent = 1		
	PBSS		(Best = 15) (Worst = 6)
	Add GCS		(Best = 15) (Worst = 3)
	Combined Score		(Best = 30) (Worst = 9)
*Reproduced with permission from Safar P, Bircher NG. Cardiopulmonary cerebral resuscitation. 3rd ed. Philadelphia: WB Saunders Co., 1988:262.			

CHECKLIST FOR THE DIAGNOSIS OF BRAIN DEATH*

Brain death has occurred if the following criteria are met on two consecutive occasions, at least two hours apart.

1. Does not localize in response to noxious stimuli[1] ☐

2. Body temperature above 34°C ☐

3. Serum levels of the following are negligible or
      subtherapeutic:
   a. Ethanol
   b. CNS depressant drugs ☐

4. The following movements are absent.
   a. Decorticate posturing
   b. Decerebrate posturing
   c. Shivering
   d. Spontaneous movements ☐

5. The following reflexes are absent bilaterally:[2]
   a. Pupillary light reflex
   b. Corneal reflex
   c. Oculovestibular reflex
   d. Oculocephalic reflex (Doll's eyes) ☐

6. EEG is isoelectric at maximal gain[3] ☐

7. Apnea test confirmatory[4]
   a. PaO_2 at end of test _____
   b. $PaCO_2$ at end of test _____ ☐

[1]Painful stimuli should be localized to cranial nerve areas because of the risk for spinal cord reflexes with peripheral stimuli. The favored test is supraorbital pressure.

[2]Pupillary light reflexes can be absent after eye injury, neuromuscular blocking agents, atropine, mydriatics, scopolamine, and opiates.

[3]Isoelectric EEG does not exclude brainstem activity, and is not to be used in isolation to make the diagnosis of brain death.

[4]The apnea test is confirmatory if there is no evidence of spontaneous ventilatory efforts for at least 3 minutes and the $PaCO_2$ is above 60 mmHg at the end of the test. If there is a history of chronic CO_2 retention, the PaO_2 should be below 55 mmHg at the end of the test

*Modified from the University of Pittsburgh criteria for brain death, with permission of B.C. Decker, Inc., Philadelphia.

APACHE II

Acute Physiology And Chronic Health Evaluation

The APACHE II scoring system is used to rank the severity of illness in individual patients in a medical or surgical ICU. This scoring system does NOT apply to burn patients or to postoperative coronary artery bypass graft (CABG) patients.

The graph below is from a multicenter study of 5,815 ICU patients.* Only postoperative patients are included in this graph, but the medical patients showed a similar pattern.

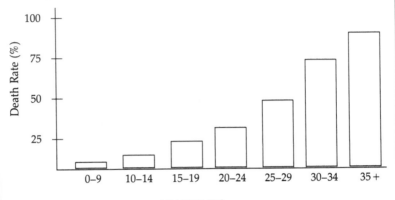

APACHE II Score

*Redrawn with permission from Knaus WA et al. APACHE II: A severity of disease classification system. Crit Care Med 1985; *13*:818–829.

The APACHE II score is generated in 3 parts.
1. **Acute Physiology Score.** This consists of 12 measurements obtained within the first 24 hours of admission to the ICU. The most abnormal measurement for each variable is selected and the total APS score is the sum of the scores from the individual measurements. The only nonobjective measure in this section is the Glasgow Coma Score (GCS). The scoring method for the GCS is included in this section of the Appendix.
2. **Age Adjustment.** A point total of zero to 6 points is alloted for the age of the patient.
3. **Chronic Health Adjustment.** Up to 5 additional points are allotted for chronic illnesses involving the major organ systems.
The final APACHE II score is the sum of the above 3 scores. The following is a list of the criteria used to generate scores in each section of the APACHE II scoring system.

APACHE II SCORING SYSTEM									
Variable	+4	+3	+2	+1	0	+1	+2	+3	+4
Temperature	≥41	39–40.9		38.5–38.9	36–38.4	34–35.9	32–33.9	30–31.9	≤29.9
Mean Arterial BP	≥160	130–159	110–129		70–109		50–69		≤49
Heart Rate	≥180	140–179	110–139		70–109		55–69	40–54	≤39
Respiratory Rate	≥50	35–49		25–34	12–24	10–11	6–9		≤5
[1]A-aPO$_2$ / [2]PaO$_2$	≥500	350–499	200–349		<200 / >70	61–70		55–60	<55
Arterial pH / [3]Serum Hco$_3^-$	≥7.7 / ≥52	7.6–7.69 / 41–51.9		7.5–7.59 / 32–40.9	7.33–7.49 / 23–31.9		7.25–7.32 / 18–21.9	7.15–7.24 / 15–17.9	<7.15 / <15
Serum Na$^+$	≥180	160–179	155–159	150–154	130–149		120–129	111–119	≤110
Serum K$^+$	≥7	6–6.9		5.5–5.9	3.5–5.4	3–3.4	2.5–2.9		<2.5
Serum Creatinine	≥3.5	2–3.4	1.5–1.9		0.6–1.4		<0.6		
Hematocrit	≥60		50–59.9	46–49.9	30–45.9		20–29.9		<20
WBC Count	≥40		20–39.9	15–19.9	3–14.9		1–2.9		<1
[4]Glascow Coma Score (GCS)									
Acute Physiology Score (APS)									

[1]If Fio$_2$ >50%
[2]If Fio$_2$ <50%
[3]Use only if no ABGs
[4]Score = 15 − Actual GCS

Age Adjustments

Age (Yrs)	Points
<44	0
45–54	2
55–64	3
65–74	5
>75	6

Chronic Health Adjustment

Points can be added if the patient has a history of the following,

1. Biopsy proven cirrhosis
2. New York Heart Association Class IV
3. Severe COPD (e.g., hypercapnia, home O_2, pulmonary hypertension)
4. Chronic dialysis
5. Immune compromised

If any of above are present, ADD: 2 points for elective surgery or for nonsurgical patients. 5 points for emergency surgery.

Apache II Score

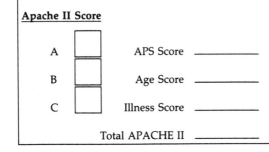

A   ☐   APS Score _____

B   ☐   Age Score _____

C   ☐   Illness Score _____

         Total APACHE II _____

5. INFECTION CONTROL

ISOLATION PRECAUTIONS[1,2]						
Illnesses	Private Room	Masks	Gowns	Gloves	Infected Material	Comments
Strict Isolation						
Chickenpox Diphtheria Smallpox	Yes Keep Door Shut	Yes	Yes	Yes	Secretions Draining Lesions	Used when several illnesses are possible, prior to Dx.
Respiratory Isolation						
Epiglottitis Meningococci Measles Mumps	Yes Door can be Open	Yes	If Soiling Likely	Yes	Respiratory Secretions	Patient wears mask when out of room.
Tuberculosis Isolation						
Pulmonary or Laryngeal TB	Yes Keep Door Shut	Yes	If Soiling Likely	If Soiling Likely	Respiratory Secretions	Patient wears mask when out of room.
Enteric Precautions						
C. difficile Hepatitis A Shigella	No	No	Yes	Yes	Feces	Institute during workup of any acute diarrhea
Contact Isolation						
Wound infection, Staph or Strep pneumonia	Yes	Only for close contact	If Soiling Likely	Yes	Wound, Any body secretion	Used for infections with highly resistant pathogens
Blood and Body Fluids Precautions						
AIDS Hepatitis B	No	No	If Soiling Likely	Yes	Blood Body Fluids	Avoid needle stick injuries. Do not cap needles.

[1]Garner J3, Simmons BP. CDC guidelines for isolation precautions in hospitals. Hospital Infections Program, Atlanta, Centers for Disease Control, 1983.
[2]Castle M, Ajemian E. Hospital Infection Control, 2nd ed., New York, John Wiley & Sons, Inc., 1987.

BODY FLUIDS AND HIV TRANSMISSION	
Transmission Documented	
Yes	No
Blood	Amniotic Fluid
Breast Milk	Cerebrospinal Fluid
Semen	Nasal Discharge
Vaginal Secretions	Saliva
	Sputum
	Sweat
	Tears
	Urine

*From Recommendations for prevention of HIV transmission in health care settings. MMWR, 1987; 36(suppl):1S–18S.

RECOMMENDED PERSONAL PROTECTION AGAINST HIV INFECTION FOR HEALTH CARE WORKERS*				
Task	**Gloves**	**Gown**	**Mask**	**Glasses**
Control Spurting Blood	Yes	Yes	Yes	Yes
Control Minimal Bleeding	Yes	No	No	No
Venipuncture	Yes	No	No	No
Starting an IV	Yes	No	No	No
Intubation or Tracheal Suction	Yes	No	No, unless there is splashing	
Measuring Blood Pressure and Temperature	No	No	No	No
Giving an Injection	No	No	No	No

*From MMWR. Atlanta: Centers for Disease Control, 1989, (Jun)38:1–37.

OUTCOME OF AIDS IN THE ICU: 1989*			
Diagnosis	**Total Number of Patients**	**Number of Patients Discharged from ICU**	**Number of Patients Alive at 3 Months**
Respiratory Failure	36	12 (33%)	6 (17%)
Hemodynamic Instability	6	4 (67%)	4 (67%)
CNS Dysfunction	4	2 (50%)	1 (25%)
Other	4	2 (50%)	2 (50%)

*From Rogers PL, et al. Crit Care Med 1989; 17:113–117.

CURRENT BIBLIOGRAPHY ON HIV INFECTION

TEXTS
1. Sande MA, Volberding PA eds. The medical management of AIDS. Philadelphia: WB Saunders, 1988.

DEFINITIONS
1. Centers for Disease Control. Classification system for human T-lymphotrophic virus type III/lymphadenopathy-associated virus infection. MMWR 1986; 35:344–360.
2. Centers for Disease Control. Revision of the CDC surveillance case definition for acquired immunodeficiency syndrome. MMWR 1987; 36:1S–18S.

INFECTION CONTROL
1. Centers for Disease Control. Guidelines for prevention of transmission of human immunodeficiency virus and hepatitis B virus to health-care and public safety workers. MMWR 1989; 38:1–37.
2. Centers for Disease Control. Update: Universal precautions for prevention of transmission of human immunodeficiency virus, hepatitis B virus, and other bloodborne pathogens in health-care settings. MMWR 1988; 37:377–387.

EPIDEMIOLOGY
1. Update: Acquired immunodeficiency syndrome—United States, 1981–1988. JAMA 1989; 261:2609–2617.

CLINICAL SYNDROMES
1. Rankin JA, Collman R, Daniele RP. Acquired immune deficiency and the lung. Chest 1988; 94:155–164.
2. Dalakas M, Wichman A, Sever J. AIDS and the nervous system. JAMA 1989; 261:2396–2399.
3. Cello JP. Gastrointestinal manifestations of HIV infection. In: Sande MA, Volberding PA eds. The medical management of AIDS. Philadelphia: WB Saunders Co. 1988:141–152.
4. Root RK. Adrenocortical function in the acquired immunodeficiency syndrome (AIDS). West J Med 1988; 148:70–73.
5. Hickey MS, Weaver KE. Nutritional therapy for the malnourished ARC or AIDS patient: Current therapeutic concepts and basic therapy outline. Contemp Surg 1988; 33(suppl):1A–32A.

CLINICAL OUTCOME
1. Rogers PL, Lane HC, Henderson DK, et al. Admission of AIDS patients to a medical intensive care unit: Causes and outcome. Crit Care Med 1989; 17:113–117.

6. HEMODYNAMIC PROFILE

COMPONENTS AND EQUATIONS

CARDIAC INDEX (CI) is the cardiac output (Q) measured by the thermodilution and divided by the body surface area (BSA).

$$CI = \frac{Q}{BSA}$$ (L/min·M²)

STROKE VOLUME INDEX (SVI) is the volume of blood ejected by the ventricles during systole. It is calculated by dividing the heart rate into the cardiac index.

$$SVI = \frac{CI}{HR} \times 1000$$ (ml/beat·M²)

STROKE WORK INDEX (SWI) is the work performed by each ventricle during one cardiac cycle. It is a function of the pressure generated in systole and the stroke volume ejected.

$$LVSWI = (MAP - PCWP) \times SVI \times 0.0136$$
$$RVSWI = (PAP - CVP) \times SVI \times 0.0136$$ (gm·M/M²)

VASCULAR RESISTANCE INDEX is a measure of the resistance to flow in the pulmonary and systemic circuits (PVRI, SVRI). Resistance is determined by dividing the pressure drop across the system by flow (CI).

$$PVRI = \frac{(PAP - PCWP)}{CI} \times 80$$

$$SVRI = \frac{(MAP - CVP)}{CI} \times 80$$ (dynes·sec/cm⁵M²)

OXYGEN DELIVERY ($\dot{D}O_2$) is the product of the cardiac output and the content of oxygen (CaO_2) in arterial blood.

$$\dot{D}O_2 = CI \times (CaO_2)$$ (ml/min M²)

OXYGEN UPTAKE ($\dot{V}O_2$) is the amount of oxygen taken up from the peripheral capillaries per minute. It is calculated as the cardiac index multiplied by the arteriovenous oxygen content difference ($CaO_2 - CvO_2$).

$$\dot{V}O_2 = CI \times (CaO_2 - CvO_2)$$ (ml/min·M²)

OXYGEN EXTRACTION RATIO (O_2ER) is the oxygen uptake divided by the oxygen delivery. It is a measure of the balance between oxygen supply and demand at the tissue level.

$$O_2ER = 1 - \frac{\dot{V}O_2}{\dot{D}O_2} \times 100$$ (%)

NORMAL HEMODYNAMIC VALUES	
Hemodynamic Parameter	**Normal Range**
Cardiac Index	2.5–3.5 L/min·m²
Stroke Volume Index	36–48 ml/beat·m²
Left Ventricular Stroke Work Index	44–56 gm·m/m²
Right Ventricular Stroke Work Index	7–10 gm·m/m²
Systemic Vascular Resistance Index	1200–2500 dynes·sec/cm⁵ m²
Pulmonary Vascular Resistance Index	80–240 dynes·sec/cm⁵ m²
Oxygen Delivery	520–720 L/min·m²
Oxygen Consumption	110–160 L/min·m²
Oxygen Extraction Ratio	22–32 %

From Marino PL, Krasner J. Hemodynamic expert. Philadelphia: WB Saunders Co., 1986.
Note: All values are referenced to body surface area.

```
10 REM        The Hemodynamic Profile
15 REM            ------------------------
20 CL = 7:COLOR CL,0
25 WIDTH 80
30 KEY OFF
35 DIM H$(10),HL(10),HH(10),L2(10),H2(10),PH$(10)
40 DIM C$(10),C(10),H(10)
45 DIM I$(13),I(20),IX$(13),IL(13),IH(13)
50 FOR I = 1 TO 9:READ H$(I), HL(I), HH(I):NEXT I
55 FOR I = 1 TO 13:READ I$(I):NEXT I
60 FOR I = 2 TO 13:READ IL(I), IH(I):NEXT I
65 DATA CI,2.4,4.0,SVI,36,48,LVSWI,44,56,RVSWI
70 DATA 7,10,SVRI,1200,2500,PVRI,80,240
75 DATA O2 DELIVERY,520,720,O2 CONSUMPTION
80 DATA 110,160,O2 EXTRACTION,22,32
85 DATA Cardiac Output,.,.,Heart Rate,Mean Arterial BP,Systolic BP
90 DATA Diastolic BP,Mean Pulm. Art. Pressure,Mean Rt. Atrial
Pressure
95 DATA Pulm. Cap. Wedge Pressure,Hemoglobin, Arterial O2
Saturation
100 DATA Mixed Venous O2 Saturation
105 DATA 30,500,40,300,30,300,30,250,40,350,0.1
110 DATA 250,0.1,200,0,50,0,50,2,20,60,100,20,90
115 L2(1) =    .5: H2(1) = 20
120 L2(2) =    10: H2(2) = 90
125 L2(3) =    10: H2(3) = 90
```

```
130 L2(4) =    2: H2(4) = 30
135 L2(5) = 400: H2(5) = 7000
140 L2(6) =   10: H2(6) = 3500
145 L2(7) =   20: H2(7) = 350
150 L2(8) =   50: H2(8) = 1000
155 L2(9) =    5: H2(9) = 70
160 CLS:LOCATE 2,20:PRINT "------ THE HEMODYNAMIC PROFILE
------"
165 LOCATE 8,7
170 PRINT"Do you want a printout of this hemodynamic profile ?
(Y/N)"
175 LOCATE 11,6:PRINT" Press <RETURN> after answering";
180 LOCATE 8,66:PRINT "          "
185 P$ = "  "
190 LOCATE 8,66: INPUT "     ", P$
195 P$ = LEFT$(P$,1):IF P$ = "Y" OR P$ = "y" OR P$ = "N" OR
P$ = "n" THEN 220 ELSE 180
200 CLS:SYSTEM
205 END
210 REM          DATA GATHERING
215 GOSUB 160
220 CLS:IF P$ = "N" OR P$ = "n" THEN 260
225 LOCATE 3,10:PRINT "Enter printout heading (3 lines)"
230 PRINT TAB(10);"Press <RETURN> after each entry"
235 PRINT:PRINT:FOR I = 1 TO 3
240 LINE INPUT PH$(I):NEXT
245 CLS
250 REM DATA FORMAT
255 PRINT
260 LOCATE 2,20:PRINT "Press <RETURN> after each entry"
265 LOCATE 5,57:PRINT "        "
270 LOCATE 5,1
275 INPUT "How many cardiac output values have you obtained?
(1-5): ",CO$
280 IF VAL(CO$) < 1 OR VAL(CO$) > 5 GOTO 265
285 N = VAL(CO$)
290 LOCATE 7,51:PRINT "        "
295 LOCATE 7,1:INPUT "Do you have an arterial catheter in place?
(Y/N): ",QP$
300 QP$ = LEFT$(QP$,1)
305 IF QP$ = "Y" OR QP$ = "y" THEN QP = 0:GOTO 320
310 IF QP$ = "N" OR QP$ = "n" THEN QP = 1:GOTO 320
315 GOTO 290
320 LOCATE 9,55:PRINT "          ":LOCATE 9,1
325 INPUT "English units (lb/in) or Metric units (kg/cm) (E/M): ",U$
```

```
330 IF U$ = "E" OR U$ = "e" THEN W$ = "Pounds":H$ =
"Inches": GOTO 345
335 IF U$ = "M" OR U$ = "m" THEN W$ = "Kilograms": H$ =
"Centimeters":GOTO 345
340 GOTO 320
345 I$(2) = "Weight (" + W$ + ")"
350 I$(3) = "Height (" + H$ + ")"
355 LOCATE 11,1
360 CLS:LOCATE 24,19
365 PRINT "          Press <RETURN> after each entry"
370 LOCATE 1,1:FOR I = 1 TO N
375 PRINT "Enter ";I$(1);" " ;I;"(0.5-20):";
380 INPUT " ",C$(I)
385 IF VAL(C$(I)) > = .5 AND VAL(C$(I)) = <20 THEN 390 ELSE 375
390 C(I) = VAL(C$(I))
395 NEXT I
400 FOR I = 2 TO 13: L=I+N+4
405 IF I = 5 AND QP = 0 THEN L = N + 9
410 IF I = 5 AND QP = 1 GOTO 445
415 IF I > 5 THEN L = L + QP - 2
420 IF I = 6 AND QP = 0 THEN I = 7:GOTO 445
425 PRINT "Enter ";I$(I);
430 INPUT ": ",IX$(I)
435 IF VAL(IX$(I)) < IL(I) OR VAL(IX$(I)) > IH(I) THEN 425
440 I(I)= VAL(IX$(I))
445 NEXT I
450 REM end data gathering
455 CLS:LOCATE 2,2
460 PRINT "You have entered the following values:"
465 PRINT
470 FOR I = 1 TO N
475 PRINT " ";I;". ";I$(1);" ";
480 PRINT I;" :";
485 PRINT TAB(35);C(I)
490 NEXT I
495 FOR I = 2 TO 13
500 P = N + I - 1
505 IF I < 5 GOTO 530
510 IF I = 5 AND QP = 0 GOTO 530
515 IF I = 5 AND QP = 1 GOTO 540
520 IF I = 6 AND QP = 0 THEN I = 8
525 P = N + I + QP - 3
530 IF P < 10 THEN PRINT " ";
535 PRINT P;". ";I$(I);" :";TAB(35);I(I)
540 NEXT I
```

```
545 GOSUB 1225
550 LOCATE 20,33:PRINT "          "
555 LOCATE 20,1:INPUT " Are these values correct? (Y/N): ",QA$
560 IF QA$ = "Y" OR QA$ = "y" THEN 925
565 IF QA$ = "N" OR QA$ = "n" THEN 570 ELSE 550
570 GOSUB 1225
575 LOCATE 20,1:PRINT "Enter the number in the left hand column
that"
580 INPUT "corresponds to the value you wish to alter and press
RETURN ",Q$
585 IF VAL(Q$) < 1 OR VAL(Q$) > P GOTO 570
590 Q = VAL(Q$)
595 IF Q > N GOTO 645
600 GOSUB 1225
605 LOCATE 20,1:PRINT "Enter ";I$(1);" ";Q;"(0.5-20) and press
RETURN :";
610 INPUT "    ",C$(Q)
615 IF VAL(C$(Q)) < .5 OR VAL(C$(Q)) > 20 THEN 600
620 C(Q) = VAL(C$(Q))
625 LOCATE 3 + Q
630 PRINT " "; Q ;". ";I$(1);" "; Q ;" :";
635 PRINT TAB(35);C(Q)
640 GOTO 545
645 I = Q - N + 1
650 IF I = 5 AND QP = 1 THEN I = 6:GOTO 675
655 IF I = 6 AND QP = 1 THEN I = 7:GOTO 675
660 IF I = 5 AND QP = 0 GOTO 675
665 IF I > 5 THEN I = I + 2 - QP
670 GOSUB 1225
675 LOCATE 20,1:PRINT "Enter ";I$(I);" and press RETURN: ";
680 PRINT TAB(52): INPUT "  ",IX$(I)
685 IF VAL(IX$(I)) < IL(I) OR VAL(IX$(I)) > IH(I) GOTO 595
690 I(I) = VAL(IX$(I))
695 LOCATE Q + 3,1
700 IF Q < 10 THEN PRINT " ";
705 PRINT Q;". ";I$(I);" :";TAB(35);I(I)
710 GOTO 545
715 LOCATE 20,1
720 PRINT "Align printer paper to top of form and press ANY
KEY          "
725 XY$ = INPUT$(1)
730 ON ERROR GOTO 1245
735 FOR I = 1 TO 3:LPRINT PH$(I):NEXT:LPRINT
740 FOR I = 1 TO N
745 LPRINT I;". ";I$(1);" ";
```

```
750 LPRINT I;" :";
755 LPRINT TAB(35);C(I)
760 NEXT I
765 IF U$ = "E" OR U$ = "e" THEN I(2) = I(2)*2.2:I(3) = I(3)/2.54
770 FOR I = 2 TO 13
775 P = N + I - 1
780 IF I < 5 GOTO 805
785 IF I = 5 AND QP = 0 GOTO 805
790 IF I = 5 AND QP = 1 GOTO 810
795 IF I = 6 AND QP = 0 THEN I = 8
800 P = N + I + QP - 3
805 LPRINT P;". ";I$(I);" :";TAB(35);I(I)
810 NEXT I
815 LPRINT
820 LPRINT
825 LPRINT"Parameter";TAB(20);"Value";TAB(35);"Normal Range"
830 LPRINT"---------";TAB(20);"-----";TAB(35);"------------"
835 LPRINT "BSA";TAB(20);INT(BSA*100)/100
840 LPRINT
845 FOR I = 1 TO 9
850 ST$ = "*"
855 LPRINT H$(I);
860 IF H(I) < HL(I) THEN LPRINT TAB(19);ST$;
865 IF H(I) > HH(I) THEN LPRINT TAB(19);ST$;
870 IF I < 5 THEN RO = .1
875 IF I > 4 THEN RO = 1
880 Y = RO*INT(H(I)/RO)
885 IF H(I) - Y > RO/2 THEN Y = Y + RO
890 H(I) = Y
895 LPRINT TAB(20);H(I);
900 TB = 39 - LEN(STR$(HL(I)))
905 LPRINT TAB(TB);HL(I);"-";HH(I)
910 LPRINT
915 NEXT I
920 RETURN
925 REM        calculations
930 CO = 0
935 FOR I = 1 TO N
940 CO = CO + C(I)
945 NEXT I
950 CO = CO/N
955 IF U$ = "E" OR U$ = "e" THEN I(2) = I(2)/2.2:I(3) = I(3)*2.54
960 BSA = .007184*I(2)^.425*I(3)^.725
965 H(1) = CO/BSA
970 H(2) = 1000*H(1)/I(4)
```

```
975  IF QP = 1 THEN I(5) = I(6)/3 + 2*I(7)/3
980  H(3) = .0136*H(2)*(I(5) - I(10))
985  H(4) = .0136*H(2)*(I(8) - I(9))
990  H(5) = 79.9*(I(5) - I(9))/H(1)
995  H(6) = 79.9*(I(8) - I(10))/H(1)
1000 H(7) = .139*I(11)*H(1)*I(12)
1005 H(8) = .139*I(11)*H(1)*(I(12) - I(13))
1010 H(9) = 100*(I(12) - I(13))/I(12)
1015 IF P$ = "Y" OR P$ = "y" THEN GOSUB 715
1020 PRINT I$;"I"
1025 PRINT
1030 CLS
1035 PRINT
1040 LOCATE 1,17:PRINT "Parameter";TAB(37);"Value";TAB(52);
"Normal Range"
1045 LOCATE 2,17:PRINT "---------";TAB(37);"-----"TAB(52);"------------"
1050 PRINT TAB(18);"BSA";TAB(37);INT(BSA*100)/100
1055 PRINT
1060 FOR I = 1 TO 9
1065 ST$ = "*"
1070 PRINT TAB(18);H$(I);
1075 IF H(I) < HL(I) THEN PRINT TAB(36);ST$;
1080 IF H(I) > HH(I) THEN PRINT TAB(36);ST$;
1085 COLOR CL,0
1090 IF I < 5 THEN RO = .1
1095 IF I > 4 THEN RO = 1
1100 Y = RO*INT(H(I)/RO)
1105 IF H(I) - Y > RO/2 THEN Y = Y + RO
1110 H(I) = Y
1115 PRINT TAB(37);H(I);
1120 TB = 57 - LEN(STR$(HL(I)))
1125 PRINT TAB(TB);HL(I);"-";HH(I)
1130 PRINT
1135 NEXT I
1140 LOCATE 24,28
1145 PRINT "Press ANY KEY to continue ";
1150 XY$ = INPUT$(1)
1155 FOR I = 1 TO 25 - N:PRINT:NEXT I
1160 CLS:LOCATE 4,2:
1165 PRINT "Which of the following do you wish to do now? ";
1170 COLOR 0,CL:PRINT"<    >":COLOR CL,0
1175 LOCATE 8,6: PRINT "1. Run another profile."
1180 LOCATE 10,6: PRINT "2. Return to DOS."
1185 LOCATE 18,6:PRINT "Press     RETURN    after entering your
choice."
```

1190 LOCATE 4,52
1195 X$ = INKEY$:IF X$ = CHR$(13) AND (X2$ = "1" OR X2$ = "2") THEN 1210
1200 IF X$ <> "1" AND X$ <> "2" THEN 1190
1205 COLOR 0,CL:PRINT X$:COLOR CL,0:X2$ = X$:GOTO 1195
1210 X$ = X2$
1215 IF X$ = "1" THEN 210
1220 IF X$ = "2" THEN 200
1225 FOR L = 1 TO 5
1230 LOCATE 18 + L,1:FOR J = 1 TO 79: PRINT "   ";:NEXT J
1235 NEXT L
1240 RETURN
1245 CLS:FOR I = 1 TO 150:LOCATE 11,1
1250 PRINT "Trouble With Printer - Aborting Printout":NEXT I
1255 GOTO 1030
1260 REM "Good Luck"

SAMPLE HEMODYNAMIC PROFILE		
Paul Marino		
4/20/91		
dobutamine @ 5 mcg/kg/min		
1 • Cardiac Output 1 :		5
2 • Weight (Pounds) :		165
3 • Height (Inches) :		72
4 • Heart Rate :		90
5 • Mean Arterial BP :		78
6 • Mean Pulm. Art. Pressure :		23
7 • Mean Rt. Atrial Pressure :		10
8 • Pulm. Cap. Wedge Pressure :		15
9 • Hemoglobin :		10
10 • Arterial O2 Saturation :		95
11 • Mixed Venous O2 Saturation :		67
Parameter	**Value**	**Normal Range**
BSA	1.96	
CI	2.5	2.4–4
SVI	* 28.3	36–48
LVSWI	* 24.2	44–56
RVSWI	* 5	7–10
SVRI	2135	1200–2500
PVRI	* 251	80–240
O2 Delivery	* 336	520–720
O2 Consumption	* 99	110–160
O2 Extraction	29	22–32

index

Page numbers in *italics* indicate figures; those folloed by *t* indicate tables.

fever from, 585-586
Myelinosis
  central pontine, 475
Myocardial energy balance
  in acute heart failure, 167, 167t
Myocardial infarction. *See* Acute
    myocardial infarction
Myoclonus
  after cardiac arrest, 196
Myonecrosis
  in renal failure, 459-460, 459t
  potassium release from, 484
Myopathy
  in selenium deficiency, 524
Myxedema coma
  in hypothyroidism, 566-567, 567t

Naloxone
  in respiratory failure, 341-342
  in septic shock, 182
Naproxen
  in tumor fever, 581
Narrow-complex tachyarrhythmia(s)
  acute management of, 265-270, 267, 268t
Nasal tube(s)
  in oxygen therapy, 322, 322t
  sinusitis from, 578, 579
Nasogastric suction
  hypokalemia from, 479, 481
Nasogastric tube(s)
  in gastric emptying evaluation, 58
National Committee on High Blood
    Pressure
  recommendations of, 89
National Heart, Lung and Blood Institute
  oxygen therapy guidelines of, 319
Necrosis
  from arterial cannulation, 97
Necrotizing enterocolitis
  from tube feeding, 68-69
Necrotizing wound infection(s)
  fever from, 574
Needle catheter jejunostomy, 536, 536
Negative pressure
  in chest tube thoracostomy, 393, 394
Negative-pressure ventilation, 355
Nephrogenic diabetes insipidus, 469
Nephrotoxic agent(s)
  aminoglycosides as, 625-627, 626t
  amphotericin as, 628
  in oliguria, 457, 458t
Neuroleptic malignant syndrome
  from haloperidol, 346
Neurologic change(s)
  after cardiac arrest, 189-200
    recovery prediction and, 196-200
  from hypertonicity, 467
  in central pontine myelinosis, 475
  in hypercalcemia, 504

in hyperglycemic nonketotic syndrome, 471
  in hypokalemia, 481
Neuromuscular excitability
  in hypocalcemia, 503
Neuromuscular weakness
  in hyperkalemia, 485
Neurosurgery
  cardiac arrest after, 190
  thromboembolism after, 76, 76t-77t
Neutropenia
  antibiotics in, 584-585, 585t
Neutrophil(s)
  in adult respiratory distress syndrome, 296, 297
  in pneumonia, 594-595, 594, 594t
  in pulmonary oxygen toxicity, 325
New CPR
  cerebral blood flow and, 194
  defined, 192-193
Nitrogen
  proteins and, 520-521, 521
Nitrogen balance
  defined, 520
Nitroglycerin
  in heart failure therapy, 163t, 166
  pharmacologic features of, 251-253, 646t
Nitroprusside
  after heart surgery, 171
  in heart failure therapy, 163t, 165, 167
  in renal failure, 458, 459t
  lactic acidosis from, 430
  pharmacologic features of, 253-255, 254, 646t
Nitroprusside test
  in ketoacidosis, 434, 435
Noncompliant ventricle
  wedge pressure in, 120
Nonhemolytic transfusion reaction(s), 226
Non-rebreathing mask(s)
  in oxygen therapy, 322t, 323, 323
Nonsteroidal anti-inflammatory agent(s)
  acute interstitial nephritis from, 451
  hyperkalemia from, 484
  nephritis from, 458
No-reflow phenomenon
  after CPR, 193
  calcium in, 504
  in shock, 136
Norepinephrine
  in treatment of shock, 135-136
  pharmacologic features of, 255-256, 647t
Normosol
  as crystalloid fluid, 207t, 208
Nosocomial diarrhea, 63-73
  antibiotic-associated, 64-67, 66t-67t
  bedside approach to, 71-73, 72
  from cimetidine, 70
  from ischemia, 71, 71t
  from magnesium, 70, 70t
  from quinidine, 71